Handbook of Nonprescription Drugs *Sixth Edition*

APhA PROJECT STAFF

Handbook of Nonprescription Drugs, ***Sixth Edition***

Richard P. Penna, Pharm.D., *Project Director*
L. Luan Corrigan, *Managing Editor*
Joan Welsh, *Project Editor*
Margaret T. Rasmussen, *Production Editor*
Samuel W. Goldstein, Ph.D., *Editorial Associate*
Janis Kelly, *Editorial Associate*
David Bohardt, *Director of Publications*

Book Design: Henry J. Bausili, *HJB Associates*
Anatomical Drawings: Walter Hilmers, Jr., *HJ Commercial Art,* with Gary Harris and Bruce Boatwright
Illustrations: Nathan Davies, *E. James White Company, Inc.*

ISBN 0-917330-27-7
Library of Congress Card Number 68-2177

AMERICAN PHARMACEUTICAL ASSOCIATION, 2215 Constitution Avenue, N.W., Washington, DC 20037
First Edition *published September 1967;* Second Edition *published January 1969;* Third Edition *published January 1971;* Fourth Edition *published March 1973;* Fifth Edition *published January 1977.*

Handbook of Nonprescription Drugs

Sixth Edition

Published by

AMERICAN PHARMACEUTICAL ASSOCIATION

2215 Constitution Avenue N.W. Washington, D.C. 20037 (202) 628-4410

THE NATIONAL PROFESSIONAL SOCIETY OF PHARMACISTS

Table of Contents

Participants

Advisory Committee

Linwood F. Tice, D.Sc., *Chairman*
Dean Emeritus, Philadelphia College of Pharmacy and Science, Philadelphia, Pennsylvania

Richard P. Penna, Pharm.D.
Associate Executive Director for Professional Affairs, Project Director, American Pharmaceutical Association, Washington, D. C.

Howard C. Ansel, Ph.D.
University of Georgia, Athens, Georgia

David Bohardt
Director of Publications, American Pharmaceutical Association, Washington, D. C.

James P. Caro, B.S.
American Society of Hospital Pharmacists, Washington, D. C.

Robert K. Chalmers, Ph.D.
Purdue University, West Lafayette, Indiana

Neil E. Esterson, B.S.
Community Pharmacist, Seaford, Delaware

George B. Griffenhagen
Associate Executive Director for Communications,
American Pharmaceutical Association, Washington, D. C.

David S. Roffman, M.S.
University of Maryland, Baltimore, Maryland

Nicholas J. Schurko, B.S.
Community Pharmacist, Woodbridge, New Jersey

Armond Welch, B.S.
Bureau of Drugs, FDA, Rockville, Maryland

Sara J. White, M.S.
University of Kansas Medical Center, Kansas City, Kansas

Authors

Glenn D. Appelt, Ph.D.
University of Colorado, Boulder, Colorado

Laurel E. Ashworth, Pharm.D.
Mercer University, Atlanta, Georgia

Kenneth J. Bender, Pharm.D.
St. Mary's Hospital, Reno, Nevada

Bobby G. Bryant, Pharm.D.
Purdue University, West Lafayette, Indiana

Nancy Burdock, B.S.
University of Mississippi, University, Mississippi

R. Keith Campbell, B.S., M.B.A.
Washington State University, Pullman, Washington

James P. Caro, B.S.
American Society of Hospital Pharmacists, Washington, D. C.

John F. Cormier, M.S.
Medical University of South Carolina, Charleston, South Carolina

Clarence E. Curry, Jr., Pharm.D.
Howard University, Washington, D. C.

Roy C. Darlington, Ph.D.
Howard University, Washington, D. C.

William R. Garnett, Pharm.D.
Virginia Commonwealth University, Richmond, Virginia

Dick R. Gourley, Pharm.D.
University of Nebraska Medical Center, Omaha, Nebraska

Lawrence J. Hak, Pharm.D.
University of North Carolina, Chapel Hill, North Carolina

Luis Hernandez, M.Sc.
Norfolk General Hospital, Norfolk, Virginia

Stephen G. Hoag, Ph.D.
North Dakota State University, Fargo, North Dakota

Benjamin Hodes, Ph.D.
Duquesne University, Pittsburgh, Pennsylvania

Raymond E. Hopponen, Ph.D.
South Dakota State University, Brookings, South Dakota

James Huff, Ph.D.
International Agency for Research on Cancer, Lyon, France

Marianne Ivey, B.S.
University of Washington, Seattle, Washington

Michael L. Kleinberg, M.S.
Ohio State University Hospitals, Columbus, Ohio

Peter P. Lamy, Ph.D.
University of Maryland, Baltimore, Maryland

Max A. Lemberger, Ph.D.
University of Florida, Gainesville, Florida

R. Leon Longe, Pharm.D.
University of Georgia, Athens, Georgia

Michael C. Makoid, Ph.D.
University of Nebraska Medical Center, Omaha, Nebraska

James W. McFadden, M.S.
Overlake Memorial Hospital, Bellevue, Washington

Michael W. McKenzie, M.S.
Purdue University, West Lafayette, Indiana

Keith O. Miller, M.S.
Medical University of South Carolina, Charleston, South Carolina

Gary M. Oderda, Pharm.D.
University of Maryland, Baltimore, Maryland

Richard M. Oksas, Pharm.D., M.P.H.
University of Maryland, Baltimore, Maryland

Frank A. Pettinato, Ph.D.
University of Montana, Missoula, Montana

Nicholas G. Popovich, Ph.D.
Purdue University, West Lafayette, Indiana

Joseph R. Robinson, Ph.D.
University of Wisconsin, Madison, Wisconsin

Farid Sadik, Ph.D.
University of South Carolina, Columbia, South Carolina

A. Jeanece Seals
Tennessee Department of Public Health, Nashville, Tennessee

Ralph F. Shangraw, Ph.D.
University of Maryland, Baltimore, Maryland

Paul Skierkowski, Ph.D.
University of Mississippi, University, Mississippi

Gary H. Smith, Pharm.D.
University of Washington, Seattle, Washington

George Torosian, Ph.D.
University of Florida, Gainesville, Florida

W. Kent Van Tyle, Ph.D.
Butler University, Indianapolis, Indiana

Charles A. Walker, Ph.D.
Florida A & M University, Tallahassee, Florida

Armond M. Welch, B.S.
Bureau of Drugs, FDA, Rockville, Maryland

Sheila West, Pharm.D.
Johns Hopkins Medical Institution, Baltimore, Maryland

Henry Wormser, Ph.D.
Wayne State University, Detroit, Michigan

Paul Zanowiak, Ph.D.
Temple University, Philadelphia, Pennsylvania

Reviewers

Kenneth Bachmann, Ph.D.
Paul Bass, Ph.D.
Robert L. Beamer, Ph.D.
Hyland A. Bickerman, M.D.
Norman F. Billups, Ph.D.
Eddie L. Boyd, Pharm.D.
George B. Browning, B.S., F.A.C.A.
W. Ray Burns, Pharm.D.
David F. Butler, M.S.
Bruce C. Carlstedt, Ph.D.
Kenneth Crahan, M.S.
D. Stephen Crawford, B.S.
Gregory R. D'Angelo, B.S.
Tom De Cillis, B.S.
Alexander F. Demetro, Pharm.D.
Robert E. Duncan, B.S.
Thomas W. Dunphy, Pharm.D.
S. Albert Edwards, Pharm.D.
Carl F. Emswiller, Jr., B.S.
Donald O. Fedder, B.S.
Stuart Feldman, Ph.D.
Earl L. Giacolini, B.S.
James Harelik, Pharm.D.
Charles I. Hicks, M.S.
George M. Hocking, Ph.D.
Linda Hogan, M.S.
James O. Inashima, Ph.D.
Raymond W. Jurgens, Jr., Ph.D.
Michael D. Kimminau
Ronald B. Kluza, Ph.D.
K. Richard Knoll, Pharm.D.
Charma A. Konnor, B.S.
Wayne A. Kradjan, Pharm.D.
Kermit E. Krantz, M.D., Litt.D.
Ruth Kroeger, Ph.D.
William S. Lackey, B.S.
Michael B. Lee, D.D.S.
Lawrence A. Lemchen, B.S.
Lawrence J. Lesko, Ph.D.
Mary M. Losey, M.S.
Irwin I. Lubowe, M.D., F.A.C.A.
Gregory A. Maggini, Pharm.D.
Shabir Z. Mosih, Ph.D.
Jeremy Matchett, Ph.D.
John W. Mauger, Ph.D.
Arthur J. McBay, Ph.D.
Richard Y. Miller, B.S., F.A.C.A.
Roger B. Miller, B.S.
William A. Miller, M.Sc., Pharm.D.
Larry D. Milne, Ph.D.
Donald W. Moore, F.A.C.A.
Timothy Moore, B.S.
Robert S. Mosser, M.D.
George Narinian, M.S.
Edward G. Nold, M.S.
Thomas W. O'Connor, Pharm.D.
James T. O'Donnell, Ph.D.
Kenneth B. Paive, Pharm.D.
Thomas F. Patton, Ph.D.
Peter M. Penna, Pharm. D.
Mark Randell Phelps, M.S.
Hugh T. Polson, B.S.
Keith W. Reichmann, Ph.D.
Arnold J. Repta, Ph.D.
Charles R. Rettig, D.P.M.
Joseph A. Romano, Pharm.D.
E. William Rosenberg, M.D.
Charles F. Ryan, Ph.D.
Roger H. Scholle, D.D.S.
Anthony J. Silvagni, Pharm.D.
Harold I. Silverman, D.Sc.
Stewart B. Siskin, Pharm.D.
Valentino J. Stella, Ph.D.
Curtis A. Taber, Ph.D.
C. Larry Thomasson, Ph.D.
Ralph W. Trottier, Jr., Ph.D.
Charles A. Walker, Ph.D.
Charles W. Weart, Pharm.D.
Matthew B. Wiener, Pharm. D.
Dennis D. Williams, Pharm.D.
Colin R. Woolf, M.D.
Thom J. Zimmerman, M.D.

Introduction

The American Pharmaceutical Association is pleased to introduce the Sixth Edition of its *Handbook of Nonprescription Drugs.* The publication of this Sixth Edition represents a continuing commitment of the Association spanning more than 12 years to provide pharmacists with reliable and practical information about drug products available to treat minor self-limiting ailments. Moreover, the changes made in the Fifth Edition and expanded in the Sixth Edition reflect the Association's desire to keep pace with the changes in pharmacy practice as pharmacists become more clinically involved in serving self-diagnosing and self-medicating patients.

ORGANIZATION

The APhA Board of Trustees appointed an advisory committee to provide general direction and guidance in designing and implementing the revision process. The advisory committee developed a procedure for processing *Handbook* chapters, determined the chapters to be included in this edition, developed content guidelines for each chapter, appointed authors and review panels, and reviewed each chapter during its various draft stages.

Each chapter also was subjected to an in-depth review by one of the 10 review panels. The panel members — pharmacists, physicians, and (when appropriate) other health professionals such as dentists and podiatrists — contributed a broad range of scientific knowledge, experience, and background so that each chapter would reflect a consensus of scientific thought.

SPECIAL FEATURES

Several new features make the Sixth Edition more informative and easier to use:

- In response to reader request, two new sections were added: an overview of the FDA OTC drug review process and a chapter on OTC products for diabetic patients.
- To make the book a handy reference tool for practicing pharmacists, the Sixth Edition contains an expanded index of drug entities by their generic names and drug products by their trade names, as well as their indications in specific disease states. Wherever possible, common names of disease states and symptoms are given along with the medical nomenclature.
- The use of margin subheadings and running heads allows the reader to determine at a glance not only which chapter is being discussed, but also specific areas within each chapter.
- Finally, since pharmacists want and need to become more clinically oriented in serving their patients' self-diagnosing and self-medicating requirements, an effort has been made to include more information to help the pharmacist make professional decisions about clinical assessment of patient symptoms.

PRODUCT TABLES

The product tables continue to be one of the most useful elements of the *Handbook.* Every effort has been made to expand the tables to include more products and more information on the quantitative amounts of active and inactive ingredients.

The information in the tables has been obtained directly from the manufacturers. However, the rate at which nonprescription drug products are reformulated is very high, especially in those drug classes that are being reviewed by FDA OTC Panels. As information regarding reformulated products reaches the *Handbook* editorial staff, tables in subsequent printings of this *Handbook* edition will reflect these new data.

The product table format follows the one established in previous editions of the *Handbook.* A concerted effort has been made to make the product tables consistent throughout, although because of the diverse nature of the product classes, consistency has not been possible in all cases. All products are listed alphabetically by trade name. Generally, column headings identify pharmacological class. Whenever a large number of products contain a particular drug entity, that drug heads the column. Rarely, where there is substantial diversity in the product contents, the column heading is simply "active ingredients." Most product tables contain an "other" column classification, which identifies active and/or inactive ingredients (no distinction is made between the two categories).

In columns specifying pharmacological class, entries are either the name of the drug entity and the quantitative amount (when supplied) or a dash. A dash indicates that the product contains no ingredients in that class.

In columns specifying drug entity, entries are identified by:

- Quantitative data, i.e., the amount of the drug entity in the product;
- NS (amount not supplied);

- A dash (product does not contain the ingredient).

A dash in the "other" column signifies that the manufacturer did not supply additional information; it should not be interpreted to mean that no other ingredients are contained in the product. For example, even though tablets contain fillers, binders, and color, dashes may appear in the "other" column for tablet preparations.

STANDARDS OF PRACTICE

The Standards of Practice for Pharmacy, published in March 1979 *(American Pharmacy;* Vol. NS19, p. 21, 1979) define clearly the responsibilities of pharmacists in serving self-diagnosing patients and detail the specific functions pharmacists should carry out in fulfilling these responsibilities.

Pharmacists apply the Standards through a five-step process:

- Identifying the problem;
- Gathering data;
- Processing data and reaching conclusions;
- Developing a plan of action;
- Monitoring and following up.

Identifying the Problem

The typical encounter between the pharmacist and a self-diagnosing patient is usually initiated when the patient presents a problem, set of symptoms, or series of questions regarding a self-diagnosed condition or proposed self-therapy.

The pharmacist's first responsibility is to identify the problem the patient is seeking to treat. Frequently, information provided by the patient is incomplete and vague. Moreover, experience has taught many pharmacists that the problems presented by the patient may be only the "tip of the iceberg."

Gathering Data

Through a series of questions the pharmacist may determine the nature of the patient's symptoms and whether they are amenable to self-treatment. Each chapter in the *Handbook* provides a number of questions to ask the patient. The reader should understand that these questions are suggestions and that specific cases may necessitate more detailed probing.

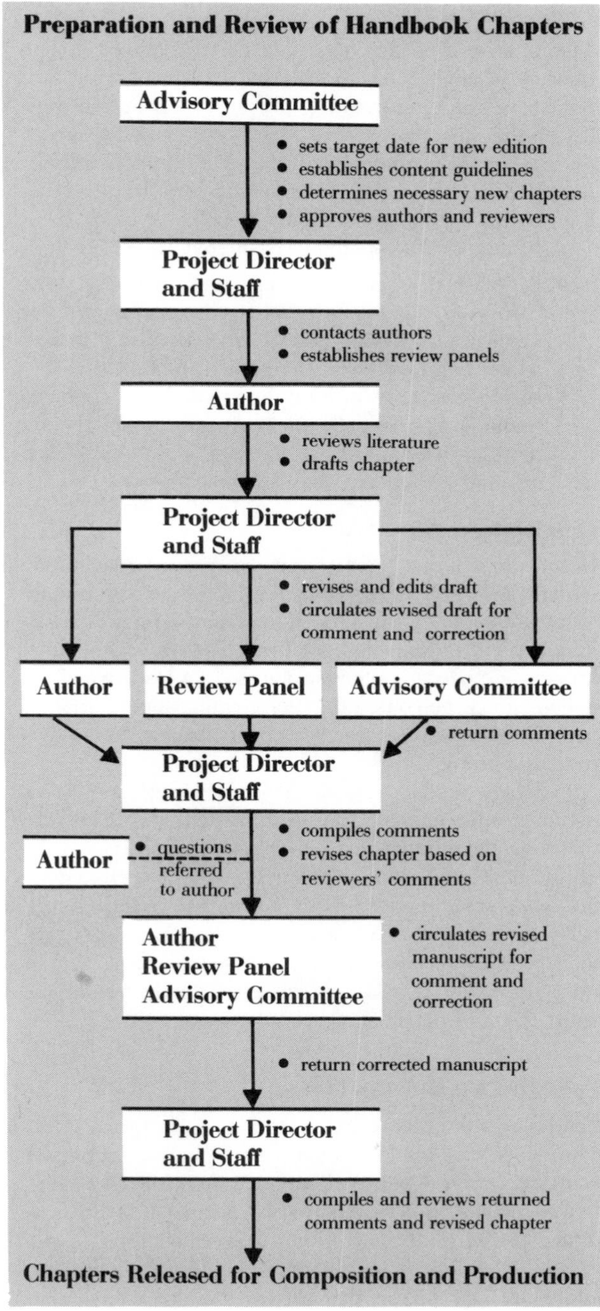

Processing the Data

The pharmacist's first and foremost judgment always must be whether to recommend self-treatment or medical referral; in the latter case the pharmacist must decide how urgent the situation is and to which practitioner or agency referral should be made. Furthermore, the patient must be made sufficiently aware of the reasons for referral so that the pharmacist's advice will be followed.

Among the factors to be considered are:

- Whether the patient is considered to be "at high risk," i.e., very young, very old, taking multiple medications, having chronic diseases, being treated by several physicians, or recently hospitalized.
- Relative severity of symptoms: high-risk patients manifesting essentially minor symptoms may require more immediate attention than low-risk patients exhibiting relatively more severe symptoms.

Developing a Plan of Action

If the pharmacist decides that the patient may safely self-medicate, the next step is to establish an appropriate "match" between the patient and a product. Product variables including dosage form, active ingredients, known side effects, potential dangers, and relative effectiveness must be considered along with patient variables such as risk status, age, sex, drug history, and other current therapy.

Whatever the decision (referral, drug therapy, or nondrug intervention), the pharmacist must make sure that the patient understands the reasons behind it and the importance of following the pharmacist's advice. If a drug product is recommended, clear and concise verbal instructions are essential. The pharmacist may use nonverbal tools such as product labeling to assure that the patient fully comprehends dosage instructions, storage conditions, warnings, and potential contraindications.

Following Up and Monitoring

Follow-up may take a number of different forms. Most commonly, it is made through direct pharmacist/patient communication—personal interview, telephone, or letter. Follow-up also can be initiated by asking the patient to return to the pharmacy within a specified time. If the patient does not seem to be responding to treatment, additional data, further data assessment, or a revised plan is necessary. Frequently, the re-evaluation results in a recommendation to refer the patient rather than attempt further treatment. The information gathered from both the initial and the follow-up evaluation should be conveyed to the referred medical practitioner.

Records are an indispensable help to the pharmacist in providing quality pharmaceutical service to self-medicating patients. Appropriately maintained records allow the pharmacist to track the steps followed in arriving at recommendations, developing a plan, and establishing the necessary monitoring procedures. Records are especially important for high-risk patients. In some cases, records may be designed for special classes of patients, e.g., diabetics. Records also provide pharmacists with a medication history to use in developing OTC recommendations and in evaluating prescribed OTC drug therapy.

Here's Your Tool

The APhA Handbook of Nonprescription Drugs is an educational and reference tool for the pharmacist. Designed to provide pharmacists with background information, suggested approaches to better patient service, and rapid, accurate retrieval of specific information, the *Handbook* is the most comprehensive publication of its kind. In our opinion, no book is better at helping pharmacists live up to their professional responsibilities and earn the trust and confidence of the self-medicating public.

Richard P. Penna, Pharm.D.
Handbook Project Director

Standards of Practice Related to Patient Care Functions

Responsibility: Reviews patient-related information for potential problems regarding drug therapy (e.g., socioeconomic factors, compliance habits, disease influences).

1. Screens existing information on patient.
   a. Reviews prior and present medical problem(s).
   b. Reviews drug usage (including OTC and prescription).
   c. Reviews patient compliance with drug regimen.
   d. Reviews drug allergies or sensitivities, i.e., date, route of administration, type of reaction.
   e. Reviews list of health care practitioners consulted.
   f. Reviews laboratory and physical examination results.
2. Collects additional information from appropriate sources if necessary.
3. Evaluates information obtained.

Responsibility: Interviews the patient or his/her representative to obtain information for entry into patient record, patient profile, or family health record.

1. Identifies patient.
2. Uses effective communication techniques in accomplishing the following:
   a. Obtains history of prior and present medical problem(s).
   b. Obtains history of drug usage (including OTC and prescription).
   c. Obtains history of patient compliance with drug regimen.
   d. Obtains history of drug allergies or sensitivities, i.e., date, route of administration, type of reaction.
   e. Obtains list of health care practitioners consulted.
   f. Verifies patient health information where possible.

Responsibility: Integrates drug-related with patient-related information in order to determine appropriate course of action (e.g., timing of dosage schedule, advising patient of possible adverse effects).

1. Determines whether patient is predisposed to side effect because of disease state(s).
2. Determines whether potential exists for significant drug interaction.
3. Determines whether patient manifests signs and/or symptoms of potential problems.
4. Assesses significance of potential problem(s) regarding drug therapy.
5. Determines alternative(s) to present regimen.

Responsibility: Confirms and further clarifies patient's understanding of medication dosage, dosage frequency, and method of administration.

1. Assesses level at which to communicate with patient.
2. Determines whether patient understands how to use medication.
3. Ascertains from patient and/or records factors affecting compliance.
4. Determines whether potential compliance problem exists.
5. Determines appropriate dosing regimen based on prescription directions, drug's characteristics, and patient's schedule, consulting with physician when necessary.
6. Explains dosing regimen to patient.

Responsibility: Advises patient of potential drug-related or health-related conditions which may develop from the use of the medication and for which the patient should seek other medical care.

1. Determines indication for drug use if possible.
2. Assesses patient's level of anxiety regarding the prescription/disease.
3. Assesses benefit versus risks of explaining side effect and/or expected response.
4. Explains possible effects of drug use to patient.
   a. Explains to patient how to recognize the signs and/or symptoms that indicate
      i. Therapeutic response.
      ii. Therapeutic failure.
      iii. Pertinent side effects.
   b. Advises patient what to do if signs and/or symptoms occur.
   c. Advises patient how to minimize side effects.
   d. Assesses whether patient understands explanation.
5. Notifies practitioner of pharmacist/patient interaction if indicated.

Responsibility: Updates the patient's history in the patient's record from information obtained by recurring patient interviews.

Responsibility: Consults with patient to properly identify symptoms in order to advise patient for self-medication.

1. Identifies patient.
2. Uses effective communication techniques in identifying major symptoms of patient.
3. Through interview, further defines symptom complex.
4. Obtains information on other medical problems, drug therapy (including OTC's), drug allergies and sensitivities.
5. Observes patient when feasible or obtains information from patient's agent.
6. Performs physical assessment (e.g., inspection of wound).
7. Makes professional judgment as to patient's condition and need for referral.
8. Recommends a product, no treatment, or other treatment or refers to appropriate health care professional.
9. Educates patient as to proper use of medications, dosage and precautions. etc.
10. Arranges for follow-up if necessary.
11. Makes appropriate entry into patient's record.

Responsibility: Refers patient to other health care providers and/or health resources where indicated.

1. Determines need for referral.
2. Recommends appropriate professional/agency for referral based on needs and severity.
3. Selects most appropriate method to facilitate meeting of patient's needs.

Responsibility: Provides information, treatment, and/or referral in emergency cases involving ingestion of toxic substances.

1. Maintains information system for dealing with emergency situation (e.g., poison control center, antidote chart, and references).
2. Obtains information to further define the ingestion situation.
3. Evaluates information and recommends treatment or referral.

Responsibility: Instructs patients in the use of medical or surgical appliances (e.g., inhalers, colostomy bags, trusses).

1. Possesses expertise in medical and surgical appliances and services offered by the pharmacy.
2. Maintains a private fitting room if applicable.
3. Instructs patient in the use and care of medical and surgical appliances.

The FDA and OTC Drugs

Although self-medication has a long history, reaching back through the centuries to various tried and true folk remedies, it is only comparatively recently that this widespread practice has received the attention it deserves. A series of legislation that began in 1906 with the Pure Food and Drug Act and culminated in 1962 — in the aftermath of the thalidomide tragedy — with the Kefauver-Harris Amendments to the Food, Drug, and Cosmetic Act included the 1951 Durham-Humphrey amendments, which divided drugs into two classes:

- Those restricted to sale by prescription only;
- Those for which directions for safe use by the public can be written, i.e., nonprescription (OTC) drugs.

This distinction was necessitated by the rapid proliferation of all drugs, particularly those amenable to use for patient self-treatment. In a relatively short time period (25 years) the dramatic expansion of the OTC market spawned a bewildering array of products claimed to cure every ailment from halitosis to hangnail. There were even some OTC products for "nondiseases," e.g., feminine cleansing products, whose only raison d'être was to impart a feeling of "freshness" to the user.

In 1972 the FDA created a program that would undertake the monumental task of evaluating the claimed safety and efficacy of active ingredients found in all nonprescription drug products, whose number is estimated at approximately 300,000. Under this program, 17 seven-member FDA OTC Panels, each consisting of at least one pharmacist, one toxicologist, physicians, and other specialists representing both consumer and industrial interests, are reviewing ingredients contained in nonprescription products to establish those agents "generally recognized as safe and effective." In addition, several prescription drugs are being investigated for possible transfer to OTC status.

In determining the logistics of the review process the FDA considered various approaches. A logical one would have been another National Academy of Sciences/National Research Council review of each marketed OTC drug product. However, the experience gained from the prescription review demonstrated that this would be a cumbersome, time-consuming, confusing procedure. Another approach would have been to bring legal action against individual products. But the vast number of products precluded this method.

FDA therefore adopted a generic approach, looking at classes of drugs instead of individual products. The estimated 300,000 marketed drug products, ranging from analgesics and laxatives to dental and vaginal/contraceptive agents, contain only about 500 significant active ingredients. Thus for example, instead of examining brand name antacid products, of which there are more than 8000, the Panels evaluated common active ingredients, such as aluminum hydroxide and magnesium carbonate.

Each drug is being classified in one of three OTC categories:

- Category I — generally recognized as safe and effective for the claimed therapeutic indication;
- Category II — not recognized as safe and effective;
- Category III — additional data needed to decide safety and/or effectiveness.

Although many of the drugs under investigation have been placed tentatively in Category III, time will determine their ultimate status.

The review process is lengthy and painstaking, involving months — even years — of sifting through many documents to determine what can be used as valid proof. The Panels base their judgments primarily on data submitted by interested parties, including industry, consumers, pharmacists, and other health professionals. Sources of information include testimonials, extensive clinical use or market success, clinical trials, both controlled and uncontrolled, and animal and human tests. The Panels also rely heavily on the published literature. Isolated case reports, random experience, testimonials, and reports lacking sufficient details to permit scientific evaluation are not considered.

In some cases, data have been generated as a result of questions raised early on regarding particular ingredients. The Panels developed specific testing criteria and parameters to be measured. This happened with the Antimicrobial Panel, which expressed safety concerns over long-term daily use of certain antimicrobial bar soaps. Appropriate studies were conducted by industry and submitted in time to be reviewed by the Panel.

After thoroughly examining all of the data, each Panel submits its findings to the FDA in the form of a report containing conclusions and recommended conditions under which OTC drugs in the particular category may be considered safe and effective and not misbranded. In addition, the report contains:

- A recommended monograph covering the drug category, to include acceptable active ingredients and their combinations, labeling indications, warnings, and adequate directions for use, prescription or OTC status, or other conditions considered necessary and appropriate (Category I);
- A statement excluding any active ingredients and their combinations, labeling claims or other statements, or conditions that have been reviewed and do not meet the standards (Category II);
- A statement of active ingredients and their combinations, labeling claims, other statements, or other conditions for which sufficient data do not exist to recommend either inclusion or exclusion from the monograph and for which further testing is therefore required (approximately 2 years) (Category III).

The Panel's report and proposed monograph are published in the *Federal Register*, and comments are invited. FDA may either agree or disagree with one or more of the Panel's recommendations. FDA's views along with changes suggested in comments (with which FDA agrees) are published again in the *Federal Register* as a tentative final monograph. An open hearing on the tentative final monograph may be scheduled if warranted. FDA then publishes a final monograph as a regulation affecting the product covered in the monograph. Category I conditions become effective 30 days after the final monograph, and Category II drugs must not be shipped 6 months after the final monograph. Any disagreement with the final monograph must be adjudicated by the courts. This final monograph may be subject to subsequent amendment.

To date, only one final product class monograph, for antacids, has been published. However, many of the Panels already have issued their reports, and their recommendations have been incorporated into pertinent chapters of this edition of the *Handbook*. Category designations have been used whenever they exist. Pharmacists interested in keeping up to date with the OTC review process should check the *Federal Register* periodically. APhA publications also report on Panel activities.

Manufacturers are not legally obligated to do any testing for any product class until the final monograph is published. Some manufacturers, in response to Panel recommendations, are conducting tests for ingredients in their marketed products (Category III ingredients represent about 30% of those reviewed thus far). In many cases, manufacturers are reformulating to use proposed Category I ingredients.

For the most part, FDA usually accepts Panel recommendations. FDA accepted the Sedative/Sleep Aid Panel's minority opinion that daytime sedatives are Category II rather than the majority opinion, which recommended Category III status. The FDA Commissioner also disagreed with the Cough/Cold Panel on several of its recommendations to switch specific prescription drugs to OTC status (e.g., diphenhydramine).

In a few cases, ingredients were found to be so unsafe that the Panels recommended immediate removal from the market. For example, the antimicrobial ingredient hexachlorophene was removed from the OTC drug market in 1972—actually while the Panel was still reviewing other antimicrobial ingredients. In 1975, tribromsalan and similar halogenated salicylanilides were removed, followed in 1977 by aerosolized zirconium products, including cosmetics.

To assure that *Handbook* authors had available to them the latest information on Panel deliberations, APhA arranged with FDA to supply minutes of Panel meetings and draft reports when allowable. Some authors were invited to meet with individual Panels. Moreover, FDA OTC Panel staff members served on a number of *Handbook* review panels.

The process of developing and publishing tentative final and final monographs is expected to require several years. After that phase, FDA will continue to review additional labeling claims, new ingredients, testing revisions, and dosage changes. Revision activities will never cease. As the years go by, more prescription drugs will be recommended for OTC use, and many new ingredients will be proposed for OTC drug marketing. In addition, FDA will begin to examine marketed products for compliance with the monographs.

Pharmacists can expect a continuing interest by FDA in nonprescription medication in terms of:

- An ongoing review of products currently on the market for safety and efficacy;
- An examination of prescription drugs for possible change to OTC status.

While each FDA OTC Panel is discharged after completing its assignment, FDA may revise the OTC monographs from time to time. Proposals for such revisions will be published in the *Federal Register* for comment. Furthermore, pharmacists may petition FDA for certain actions pertaining to the OTC monographs regardless of FDA intentions.

Thus FDA carries on its long-standing commitment to work with pharmacists to promote the rational and safe use of all drug products, especially those products sold over the counter. Because pharmacists represent a direct link to the consumer, FDA and pharmacy must maintain their partnership to assure that the public has a better understanding of the uses, hazards, and benefits of products designed for unsupervised consumer use.

Armond M. Welch, B.S., R.Ph.
Bureau of Drugs, FDA

History of OTC Drug Legislation and Regulation

Date	Event	Result
1906	Pure Food and Drug Act	Drugs must meet standards of strength and purity claimed by manufacturer; products containing opiates must so indicate on the label.
1912	Sherley Amendment	Manufacturer may not make false and fraudulent therapeutic claims about a product; difficult to enforce because burden to prove fraudulent intent is placed on government.
1938	Food, Drug, and Cosmetic Act	New drug products must be approved as safe prior to marketing.
1951	Durham-Humphrey Amendments	Drugs are divided into two classes: prescription and nonprescription (i.e., safe to use without medical supervision).
1962	Kefauver-Harris Amendments	Manufacturer must establish safety and effectiveness of all drugs marketed after 1938.
1966	NAS/NRC-FDA Drug Efficacy Study	Under contract from FDA, National Academy of Sciences/National Research Council undertakes evaluation of more than 3400 new drugs that entered market between 1938 and 1962, including 512 OTC drugs; only 15% of the OTC products are judged effective for all uses.
1972	FDA OTC Drug Products Evaluation Program	17 panels of experts commence review of active ingredients of all OTC drug products to evaluate safety and effectiveness of therapeutic claims.

Antacid Products

William R. Garnett

Chapter 1

Questions to Ask the Patient

How long has the pain been present?

When and where does the pain occur? Immediately after meals or several hours after meals?

Is the pain relieved by food? Is it aggravated by coffee or carbonated beverages?

Have you vomited blood or black "coffee ground" material?

Have you noticed blood in the stool or have the stools been black?

What medications are you currently taking? Are you taking aspirin or aspirin-containing products? Do you smoke? How much? Do you consume alcoholic beverages? Have you used antacids before? Which ones? Did they relieve the pain?

Are you on any dietary restrictions such as a low-salt diet?

Are you under a physician's care?

Every year, Americans spend millions of dollars on antacid products for relief of upper GI distress. These products may be used without a prescription both for short-term treatment of indigestion, excessive eating and drinking, or heartburn and for long-term treatment of chronic peptic ulcer disease. The pharmacist should be wary of advertising claims, evaluate on an individual patient basis the need for a medical examination before antacid therapy, and be able to select an antacid for either short-term or chronic use.

ANATOMY OF THE GI SYSTEM

The esophagus, the stomach, the duodenum, the jejunum, and the ileum comprise the upper GI tract. Short-term distress involves distention of the stomach and reflux into the esophagus, whereas chronic peptic ulcer disease involves the proteolytic action of acid and pepsin on GI mucosa and may occur at any site in the upper GI tract, usually in the stomach and duodenum (1).

Stomach

The stomach is divided anatomically and functionally. Anatomically, the stomach consists of the cardia, the fundus, the body (corpus), and the antrum. Functionally, the stomach is divided into proximal and distal areas concerned with gastric emptying.

Each anatomical area has a different type of mucosa and contributes different secretions to the gastric juice. The cardia is the smallest area of the stomach, occupying only a 0.5- to 3.0-cm strip that begins at the esophagogastric sphincter. Little is known about the function of cardiac mucosa (2).

Gastric mucosa contains surface mucous cells, mucous neck cells, argentaffin cells, parietal cells, and chief cells. It lines both the fundus and the body and is responsible for most of the components of gastric juice. The parietal cells secrete hydrochloric acid and intrinsic factor. The active proteolytic enzyme pepsin is formed from pepsinogen in the presence of hydrochloric acid. The mucosal cells of the epithelium protect the stomach from the acid–pepsin complex by releasing an alkaline mucous secretion (3). The pyloric mucosa that lines the antrum and the prepyloric canal secretes gastrin and a protective mucus.

Functionally, the proximal stomach (fundus) is responsible for the emptying of liquids, and the distal stomach (antrum) is responsible for the emptying of solids (4). A pacemaker in the greater curvature initiates peristaltic waves, and the resistance of the pyloric sphincter determines the gastric emptying rate (5).

Gastric Secretion

The three phases of gastric secretion are cephalic, gastric, and intestinal. Initiated by food, they proceed simultaneously and continue for several hours. The cephalic and gastric phases are stimulatory and synergistic. The intestinal phase is weakly stimulatory but primarily provides negative feedback (6).

Cephalic Phase

Only small amounts of gastric secretions are produced during the fasting state in the healthy individual. However, the thought, smell, taste, chewing, and swallowing of food set off a parasympathetic response via the vagus nerve called the cephalic phase (7). The vagus nerve postsynaptic transmitter, acetylcholine (the "first messenger"), then stimulates the release of hydrochloric acid, pepsinogen, and gastrin (8). The exact method of stimulation is unknown but may involve activation of a second messenger such as cyclic guanosine 3′,5′-monophosphate (9). Vagotomy or large doses of anticholinergics block this phase.

Gastric Phase

The presence of food in the stomach stimulates secretion directly and indirectly (10). The physical presence of food distends the gastric mucosa and causes a direct release of gastric secretions that requires no intermediate mechanisms. Protein also causes the release of gastrin, which is a major humoral mediator for acid and pepsinogen secretion (11). The direct and indirect processes are synergistic (2).

Food stimulates the release of gastrin by mechanical distention of the antrum, by vagal stimulation, and by a direct action on the G cells of the antrum and the duodenum (12). Gastrin release also may be stimulated by epinephrine and calcium, but this process requires amounts above physiological concentrations (13). Gastrin release is inhibited by acid, secretin, glucagon, vasoactive intestinal peptide, gastric inhibitory peptide, and calcitonin (12, 13).

mechanisms of gastric secretion

gastrins

H_2-receptors

gastric emptying rate

GI complaints

There is more than one gastrin, varying in molecular weight, site of release, and potency (14): "little" gastrin is secreted by the antrum and is the most potent; "big" gastrin, which has a longer half-life, is released from the duodenum; and "big big" gastrin is released from the jejunum (15). The gastric mucosa responds to gastrins by secreting hydrochloric acid and pepsinogen (12).

Gastrin mediates physiological functions other than acid and pepsinogen release. It may protect the stomach from the proteolytic action of acid and pepsin by stimulating gastric mucosal cell proliferation (16) and by tightening the gastric mucosal cell barrier (17). There are conflicting reports about gastrin's effect on increasing lower esophageal sphincter tone (18, 19). Because its chemical structure resembles pancreozymin and cholecystokinin, gastrin increases pancreatic secretions, bile flow, and gastric and intestinal motility (2).

The mechanism by which gastrin mediates acid and pepsin release is unknown. Gastrin may release histamine, which in turn may cause acid and pepsinogen release. Histamine receptors are divided into H_1 and H_2; H_2-receptors are responsible for acid release (20). Selective H_2-antihistamines are capable of blocking pentagastrin-mediated gastric secretion (21). This evidence suggests that gastrin acts via histamine (22). Histamine may act by releasing cyclic 3′,5′-adenosine monophosphate as a second messenger (23). The interrelationships among acetylcholine, gastrin, and histamine are unknown.

Intestinal Phase

The third phase of gastric secretion, the intestinal phase, involves both stimulation and inhibition. As long as chyme, or partly digested food, is in the intestine, there is continued gastric secretion. The mediators are "big" gastrin, cholecystokinin, and pancreozymin (6). Stimulation is weak, and the main function of the intestinal phase seems to be a negative feedback to further secretion.

Inhibition is mediated by an enterogastrone, i.e., any substance secreted from the small intestine that inhibits gastric secretion. An enterogastrone may inhibit gastric secretion by direct inhibition of either acid and pepsinogen release or gastrin or both. Cholecystokinin, pancreozymin, and glucagon inhibit gastrin release (24, 25). Secretin blocks acid secretion and inhibits glucagon release (26, 27). The stimulus for the release of enterogastrones is the presence of acid, fat, or hyperosmolar substances in the duodenum (7). Acid in the antrum diminishes gastrin release also (28).

Gastric Motility

The proximal stomach receives and stores ingested foods. By slow, sustained contractions it releases its contents into the distal stomach, where peristaltic contractions mix the contents with gastric juice before allowing them to pass through the pyloric sphincter into the duodenum. The contraction rate is regulated by a pacemaker under vagal control (7).

Gastric emptying rate depends on the resistance of the pyloric sphincter, which is controlled by many stimuli (5). Hormones (e.g., secretin, cholecystokinin, and motilin, hyperosmolar solutions, acid solutions, and fats delay gastric emptying; gastric distension increases the emptying rate (29).

The stomach is considered to be exposed to the outside environment: it receives anything capable of entering the mouth and passing down the esophagus. The stomach must react to and act on agents that are hot or cold, acid or alkaline, polar or nonpolar, liquid or solid, digestible or nondigestible. Occasionally, the protective mechanisms fail to cope with these agents, and inflammation occurs in the form of either acute or chronic upper GI distress (30).

TYPES OF GI DISORDERS

Acute Upper GI Distress

Acute upper GI distress ranges in severity from gastritis related to a single well-defined event and controlled symptomatically with antacids to acute ulcers that heal rapidly when the stressful etiology is removed to life-threatening hemorrhagic gastritis.

Gastritis

Acute gastritis is the most common GI complaint, affecting nearly 50% of the population. Patients may use terms such as "sour stomach," "acid indigestion," "heartburn," "gas," "upset stomach," or "acid stomach" for gastritis. The initiating event is usually food or alcohol overindulgence. The symptoms are usually characterized by mild epigastric discomfort, or "burning," after meals. There may be a sense of excessive stomach fullness, frequent belching or flatulence, and occasional vomiting. The most severe form involves continuous nausea and epigastric pain (31).

The syndrome is recognized mainly by patient history. Endogastroscopy is helpful in demonstrating areas of submucosal hemorrhage and superficial erosions, but there is poor correlation with histology. Radiological examination is of no use in gastritis (30).

The disease mechanism appears to be a break in the normal gastric barrier allowing hydrochloric acid to enter the mucosa, injure vessels, and cause hemorrhage, inflammation, and erosion. The process is self-limited, and symptoms can be controlled with antacids. The gastric mucosa regenerates in 2–5 days. If antacids fail to relieve the symptoms quickly, the possibility of a hiatal hernia or gallbladder disease should be considered (32).

Drug-Induced Ulceration

Alcohol, aspirin, caffeine, glucocorticosteroids, indomethacin, phenylbutazone, and tobacco smoke are often reported as being ulcerogenic. Although coffee seems to stimulate gastric secretion (33), this effect may be due to components other than caffeine. Coffee has a greater effect on stimulating gastric secretion and on lowering esophageal sphincter pressure than an equivalent amount of caffeine; decaffeinated and instant coffee and whole coffee beans seem equipotent (34). Aspirin and alcohol cause breaks in the mucosal barrier. Indomethacin causes inconsistent breaks, and the other drugs apparently are not involved (33).

Stress Ulcer

Stress ulcers are acute ulcerations that occur mainly in the stomach but also may be found in the duodenum and esophagus. They are usually shallow, small, superficial erosions but may be associated with wider ulcers if there is bleeding. Destruction and scarring seen in peptic ulcer are lacking. The real incidence is unknown, since many heal as rapidly as gastritis, but they may be the most common cause of upper GI bleeding (35). The cause is usually identifiable (36), and they have been associated with CNS lesions, trauma (Curling's ulcer), burns, sepsis, uremia, cerebrovascular accidents, and surgery.

The mechanism of stress ulcers seems to depend on an interaction among acid, changes in mucosal circulation, excretion of glycoproteins in the mucus, and mitotic rate of mucosal stomach lining. Cold, starvation, increased acidity, bile reflux, adrenalectomy, and hemorrhage favor ulceration. Vagotomy, anticholinergics, antacids, elemental diets, vitamin A, prevention of bile reflux, epinephrine, norepinephrine, serotonin antagonists, and immediate replacement of blood loss are inhibiting factors (36, 37). The major treatment is removing the precipitating event; long-term antacid therapy is rarely required.

Chronic Upper GI Distress

Antacids are used for prolonged periods in treating chronic upper GI distress, e.g., peptic ulcer disease. Peptic ulcers are chronic but may have acute exacerbations. They are most often solitary and occur at any level of the GI tract exposed to the proteolytic action of acid and pepsin. In decreasing order of incidence, they occur in the duodenum, stomach (gastric), esophagus, stoma of a gastroenterostomy, Meckel's diverticulum, and jejunum (1). However, the only significant sites of peptic ulcer disease are the duodenum and stomach. Chronic peptic ulcers differ from acute ulcers by the presence of fibrosis in the ulcer wall. They tend to be deep, burrowing through the mucosa and submucosa to the muscularis (38). While they are often considered together, duodenal and gastric ulcers have different symptoms and etiologies. However, both types may be induced by acid and pepsin stimulation (39).

Before World War I, gastric ulcers were more common, but today, duodenal ulcers predominate (40). The incidence of both types seems to have peaked and currently is on the decline (41). Males still contract the disease more often than females, but the predominance is decreasing (42). The disease is also more common in lower socioeconomic groups (41). Ulcers may recur even after surgical removal of the diseased tissue (43). Both types have a low mortality but may cause morbidity. Neither type occurs in primitive tribes or lower primates until they live in conditions of "civilization."

Gastric Ulcer

common ulcers, their origins, and symptoms

Gastric ulcers occur most often as single lesions along the lesser curvature and adjacent posterior wall of the antrum up to within 4–5 cm of the pyloric sphincter (Figure 1). They may occur occasionally in the cardia, pyloric canal, and greater curvature of the body and fundus (38). Hyperacidity is a less frequent observation in gastric ulcers than in duodenal ulcers. Gastric ulcer patients may have low or normal acid secretion. However, there are local mucosal pH differences in the stomach and duodenum, and most gastric ulcers occur in areas next to acid-secreting mucosa where the local pH is more acidic (44). Thus acid seems more important in determining where, rather than when, a gastric ulcer will occur.

role of acid and bile salts

Etiology

Several theories have been proposed for the etiology of gastric ulcer disease (45, 46), among them delayed gastric emptying distention accompanied by increased gastric secretions (47). While this hypothesis is based on experimental and clinical observations, there are reasons to question its accuracy: patients with gastric ulcers have normal gastric emptying times and low acid secretions in the presence of high gastrin levels (45).

Many gastric ulcer patients have chronic gastritis, which may damage the mucosa and make it more susceptible to peptic ulceration. However, gastritis may persist after the ulcer heals (46). Chronic gastritis may increase back diffusion of hydrogen ions that break down the gastric mucosal barrier; this process may continue even after resolution of the ulcer (17).

A theory that postulates reflux of duodenal contents, especially bile acids, due to pyloric sphincter dysfunction as a cause ties together many facts known about gastric ulcers (48). Smoking, which is associated with an increased incidence of gastric ulcer, induces duodenogastric reflux (49). Bed rest improves ulcer healing and decreases reflux (50). Hypergastrinemia occurs in gastric ulcer patients, and gastrin has been reported to inhibit the pyloric sphincter (51). Pyloric sphincter dysfunction has been shown in patients with gastric ulcer (52), whereas control and duodenal ulcer patients have normal pyloric sphincter pressure (53). A reflux of bile salts may cause gastritis in the distal portion of the stomach and a break in the mucosal barrier. The damaged mucosa next to the acid-secreting mucosa is more susceptible to ulceration. Bile salts occur more frequently and in higher

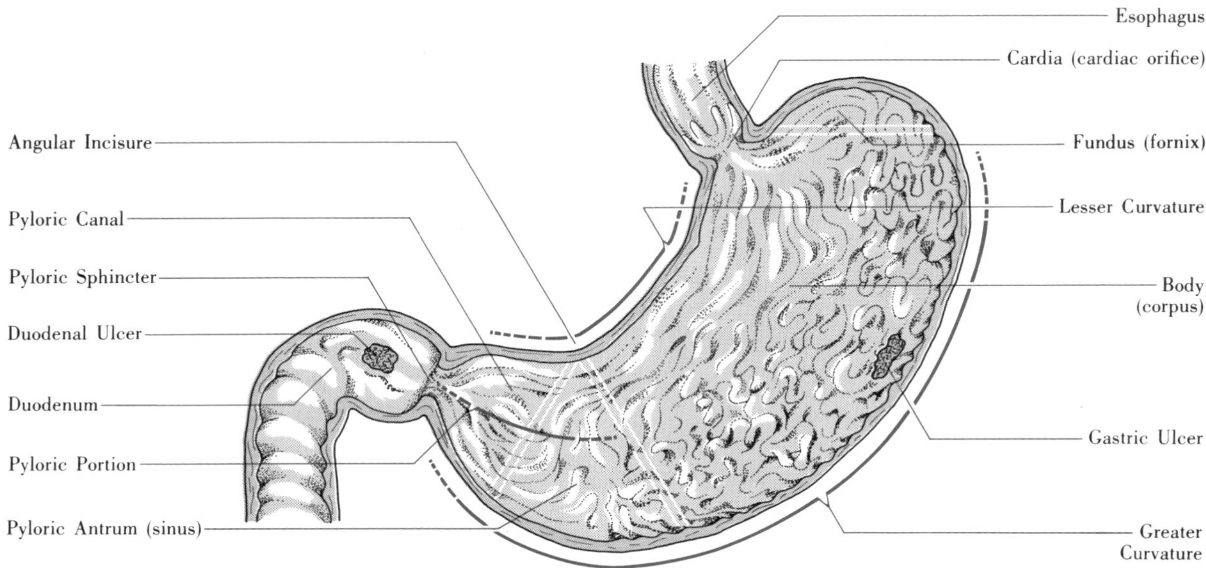

Figure 1. Sites of duodenal and gastric ulcers. Adapted from F.H. Netter, *The Ciba Collection of Medical Illustrations*, Ciba Pharmaceutical Company, New York, N.Y., 1962, p. 49, 52. Vol. 3, Part II.

reflux, pain, and GI bleeding

factors in duodenal ulcers

concentrations in gastric ulcer patients' stomachs than in normal persons or patients with duodenal ulcers (48). As attractive as this theory is, reflux has not been shown to precede either gastritis or gastric ulceration (54).

Other factors may be involved. A genetic factor is implied by the association of gastric ulcer in patients with blood group type O and nonsecretor status (55). Unknown environmental factors may cause ulcers, or the disease may be a heterogeneous group of disorders that requires the interrelation of several factors in a predisposed individual.

Symptoms

Although gastric mucosal erosion may be asymptomatic, the most common complaints are pain and GI bleeding. Gastric ulcer pain occurs within 30–60 minutes after eating and lasts 60–90 minutes. Its relationship to food intake results from distention of inflamed areas and acid release. The patient may associate the pain with eating and may stop eating, with resultant weight loss. Rhythm or chronicity associated with the pain is rare, and the pain covers a wide area of the midepigastrium. Somatic pain radiating into the back indicates penetration, perforation, or obstruction. The vomitus or stool may contain blood (the stool is black and tarry) if there is GI bleeding. Nausea, bloating, anorexia, vomiting, and weight loss also may occur.

Diagnosis

Five to ten percent of gastric ulcers are carcinomas of the stomach; therefore definitive diagnosis is needed for chronic or recurring symptoms. Bleeding, either acute or chronic, requires medical evaluation. Although a patient history is helpful, it is not as definitive for gastric as it is for duodenal ulcers. Physical examination rarely helps to locate the ulcer. Definitive gastric ulcer diagnosis is made by gastroscopy, X ray with radiopaque contrast media, gastric analysis for acid and cytogenic cells, and testing for blood (occult or frank) in the feces.

The mortality rate from gastric ulcers is low, but the morbidity is high. Gastric ulcers are less responsive to medical management than duodenal ulcers and require surgery more often.

Duodenal Ulcer

Duodenal ulcers are mucosal lesions in the anterior wall of the duodenum's proximal end just beyond the pyloric channel through which gastric contents enter the duodenum (Figure 1). Ulcers also may occur distal to the duodenal bulb or spread back into the pyloric channel or antrum. These ulcers may recur frequently or infrequently, hence the term "duodenal ulcer diathesis" (56). Duodenal ulcer is caused by excessive acid and pepsin.

Etiology

Several abnormalities may explain increased acid and pepsin delivery from the stomach to the duodenum (45, 46). There may be an increased capacity to secrete due to a large parietal cell mass (57), an increased response to agents that normally stimulate secretion (58), an increased vagal or hormonal drive to secrete (59), a defective inhibition to secretion (60), or an increased gastric emptying rate (61).

Other factors may be interrelated. Familial or genetic influence is evidenced by the frequency of occurrence of duodenal ulcer in first-degree or primary relatives of patients with duodenal ulcer, the higher concordance in monozygotic than dizygotic twins, and the greater incidence in blood type O and nonsecretors (45). Emotional and psychological factors are believed to contribute to the disease but have never been documented (42). Patients with other diseases such as arthritis, chronic pancreatitis, chronic pulmonary disease, and cirrhosis also seem to have an increased incidence of duodenal ulcers (62).

Symptoms

As in gastric ulcer, the primary symptoms are pain and GI bleeding; key differences occur in the way the patient describes the symptoms. Duodenal ulcer pain is rhythmical, periodic, and chronic. The pain usually begins 2–3 hours after meals and may continue until the next meal. It occurs when the stomach is empty and is relieved by food. The sensation is described as gnawing, burning, pressing, aching, or resembling hunger pain. The patient is often awakened at night by the pain. It is usually located in an area in the midepigastrium between the xiphoid and the umbilicus that the patient can indicate with one finger. The pain is prone to exacerbation and remission with or without therapy. Exacerbations are most common in the spring and fall and may last for days or months (56).

If there is bleeding, stool color and consistency may change. The stools become black and tarry because the blood has a chance to mix with the feces. Other GI symptoms include retrosternal burning, alteration in bowel habits, and, rarely, nausea and vomiting. The patient's appetite is good; frequently, weight gain results from the increased food intake to allay pain (62).

The major complications of duodenal ulcer are bleeding, perforation, and obstruction. The bleeding may cause anemia, iron deficiency, and hypotension. Perforation and obstruction are indications for acute surgical intervention and are manifested by acute changes in symptoms. Perforation is accompanied by a sudden, severe, generalized abdominal pain, prostration, abdominal rigidity, and pneumoperitoneum. Vomiting is the most common symptom of gastric outlet obstruction (56).

Diagnosis

A good patient history is essential in recognizing duodenal ulcer. As in gastric ulcer, physical assessment helps localize the site of pain but does little to make the diagnosis. Definitive diagnosis is made by X ray following ingestion of radiocontrast media and by duodenoscopy. Endoscopy of either the stomach or the duodenum involves passing fiberscopes down the upper GI tract (63) and is the most sensitive method of detecting ulcers (64).

ASSESSMENT

The most valuable service that the pharmacist can provide in consulting with a patient is to help the patient decide whether the ailment is amenable to self-therapy or requires medical attention. In upper GI complaints, only acute gastritis should be treated without medical intervention. Careful patient interviewing is the only method for the pharmacist to evaluate the type, severity, and duration of patient complaint.

In recommending an antacid, the pharmacist should ascertain that the complaint is acute in onset and can be related to overeating, dietary indiscretion, alcohol consumption, or tension. If the pain is acute but suggestive of perforation, the patient should be referred. If the pain is chronic or resembles peptic ulcer disease, the patient should have endoscopic evaluation (63) because symptoms of more serious diseases, such as hiatal hernia, ulcerating gastric carcinoma, duodenal neoplasm, pancreatitis, coronary artery disease, pancreatic carcinoma, and radiating pleuritic chest pain, may mimic ulcer pain (62). Patients returning frequently with complaints of acute gastritis should receive a medical examination because repeated gastritis may be associated with gastric ulcer. If relief is not obtained promptly and sustained, the pharmacist should refer the patient to a physician for evaluation.

The pharmacist should look for patient responses suggesting bleeding, vomiting, or obstruction that are life threatening and require immediate medical evaluation. Bleeding may be suspected in a patient complaining of black tarry stools or "coffee ground" vomitus. A blood loss of 50–100 ml will result in black tarry stools, whereas a blood loss of 500 ml will result in systemic symptoms of anemia. Prolonged vomiting may lead to alkalosis and dehydration. If perforation or obstruction is suspected, the patient should be referred for surgical evaluation.

duodenal ulcer complications

consulting with the patient

actions of antacids

TREATMENT

Antacids are the treatment of choice for acute gastritis and are also part of the medical management of peptic ulcer disease. Ulcer treatment is unique in that nonprescription medications are a mainstay in its medical management. A patient may find that the physician alters only the dose or dosing interval. In addition to antacids, careful dietary habits, H_2-receptor antagonists, anticholinergics, rest, and stopping smoking may prevent the need for surgery.

Antacids

Antacids have been used in the treatment of GI distress for more than 2000 years, but until the modern era of intensive antacid therapy their use was mainly empirical and subjective (65). Only recently have the actions of antacids been ecaluated closely and objectively.

Pharmacology

The primary action of antacids is to neutralize gastric acid and raise gastric pH. They do not neutralize all of the stomach acid, nor do they bring the pH to 7.0. At pH of 2.3, 90% of the acid has been neutralized, and at pH of 3.3, 99% has been neutralized (66). Raising the pH inhibits the action of pepsin. There is progressive proteolytic neutralization of pepsin, and above pH of 4.0, pepsin activity is completely inhibited (67). The main antipepsin effect of antacids is attributed to altered pH. There are conflicting reports as to pepsin's adsorbent effect (68–70).

Antacids do not coat ulcer linings (71). A possible protective effect in ulcers is the tightening of the mucosal barrier (72). Antacids increase the lower esophageal sphincter tone (73), and this action may be responsible for their effectiveness in esophageal reflux (heartburn) (74). Raising intragastric pH leads to elevated serum gastrin levels (75) and may explain the antacid effect on the gastric mucosa and lower esophageal sphincter. Of the cations in antacids, only aluminum seems to delay gastric emptying time in animals (76). In humans this effect is related to the concentration of aluminum in solution in the stomach (77). Aluminum hydroxide binds bile acids more strongly than magnesium hydroxide or aluminum phosphate (78).

All antacid products contain at least one of the four primary neutralizing ingredients: sodium bicarbonate, calcium carbonate, aluminum salts, and magnesium salts.

Sodium Bicarbonate

Sodium bicarbonate is a potent effective antacid for relief of symptoms of occasional overeating or indigestion. However, because it is completely soluble in gastric and intestinal secretions, it is contraindicated for chronic or prolonged therapy, since large doses or prolonged therapy may lead to sodium overload or systemic alkalosis (66).

important antacid ingredients

indications

recommended doses

side effects

Each gram of sodium bicarbonate contains 12 mEq of sodium. This high quantity may cause problems for individuals on low-salt diets, patients receiving diuretic therapy, or those with a tendency toward fluid overload. The suggested daily maximum intake is 200 mEq of sodium bicarbonate for patients under 60 years old and 100 mEq for those 60 and over (79).

Since the bicarbonate ion is readily absorbable, it can cause systemic alkalosis. Chronic administration with milk or calcium leads to an increase in calcium absorption and may precipitate the milk–alkali syndrome (80, 81), a possibility enhanced by a salt-losing nephropathy (82). The syndrome is characterized by hypercalcemia, renal insufficiency, and metabolic alkalosis; it improves when the antacid and calcium are discontinued (83). Symptoms include nausea, vomiting, headache, mental confusion, and anorexia (84).

Gastric distention and flatulence may occur with effervescent sodium bicarbonate. A rebound gastric hypersecretion of acid has been postulated but has not been shown in humans, even with sodium bicarbonate doses of 4–8 g (85). Some commercial forms of sodium bicarbonate contain aspirin. Ingesting such products after heavy alcohol intake may lead to hematemesis and melena (86).

Calcium Carbonate

Calcium carbonate exerts rapid, prolonged, and potent neutralization of gastric acid. It may be used safely in small doses, e.g., 0.5 g, for relief of occasional gastritis, but is not recommended for chronic use. Constipation is a limiting factor. Although there has been much enthusiasm for calcium carbonate as the antacid of choice, the recognition of its systemic side effects has prompted a re-evaluation of the agent.

Calcium carbonate reacts with hydrochloric acid to form calcium chloride, which is highly soluble and available for absorption while in the stomach. The absorption is limited because about 90% of the calcium chloride is reconverted to insoluble calcium salts, mainly calcium carbonate, in the small intestine (87). However, enough calcium may be absorbed after several days to induce hypercalcemia (88), which in turn may induce neurological symptoms, renal calculi, and decreased renal function (83, 88).

The milk–alkali syndrome is more common with sodium bicarbonate but may occur with calcium carbonate (89). When calcium is absorbed from the small intestine, bicarbonate is absorbed also. Increased bicarbonate absorption induces alkalosis, causing the hypercalcemia and alkalosis of the milk–alkali syndrome (88). This syndrome is rare, however, and when it does occur, the patient usually has a history of renal dysfunction.

Calcium carbonate may induce gastric hypersecretion (90, 91). Gastric secretory volume and acidity were found to be greater after calcium carbonate ingestion than after aluminum hydroxide or food ingestion (92).

In a study of 24 patients with chronic duodenal ulcer disease, 4–8 g of calcium carbonate induced gastric hypersecretion 3–5.5 hours after ingestion, whereas 30–60 ml of aluminum hydroxide or 4–8 g of sodium bicarbonate did not (85). This mechanism may be mediated by the calcium ion action in the GI tract.

When four equivalent neutralizing doses of calcium carbonate, sodium bicarbonate, and magnesium hydroxide were administered to 20 duodenal ulcer patients, the mean gastric output in the 60-minute period beginning 2 hours after the last dose of antacid and 30 minutes after the insertion of a nasogastric tube was twice as great with calcium carbonate as it was in the basal state or with the other antacids (93). Thus calcium carbonate itself rather than a nonspecific action of antacids may be responsible for the effects.

Observance of increased gastric secretion after calcium infusion indicates that calcium may increase serum gastrin and that hypergastrinemia may be responsible for the hypersecretion (94). A dose as small as 0.5 g of calcium carbonate (the usual dose recommended as an antacid) may increase acid secretion in male subjects with and without duodenal ulcers (95). Although several theories have been presented to explain this acid rebound, it seems most likely that the mechanism is a local effect of calcium on the gastrin-producing cells (90).

Aluminum

Aluminum is administered most often as the hydroxide but also may be given as the carbonate, phosphate, or aminoacetate. Of these, aluminum hydroxide has the greatest neutralizing capacity but still less than magnesium hydroxide, calcium carbonate, or sodium bicarbonate. Products that contain large quantities of anhydrous aluminum oxide react too slowly to be useful as antacids. Liquid preparations that lose their water content lose their neutralizing effect, and it cannot be regained by resuspending the dried powder in water (66). The drying procedure needed to convert the aluminum hydroxide gel into a powder or tablet alters the structure and results in a less reactive antacid (96).

The main side effect of aluminum antacids is constipation. Intestinal obstruction may occur in the elderly and in patients with decreased bowel motilities, dehydration, or fluid restriction (66). Impaction may be increased by agents such as sodium polystyrene sulfonate resin (Kayexalate) (97). The constipative effect may be avoided by combining aluminum with magnesium salts or by administering laxatives and stool softeners.

It was thought that aluminum was not absorbed and did not cause systemic toxicity. However, several studies reported elevated serum or bone levels of aluminum in patients receiving chronic aluminum hydroxide therapy (98–100). Systemic aluminum toxicity was postulated after elevated aluminum levels were found in brain gray matter of uremic patients who died of a neurological syndrome of unknown causes (101). These patients had taken aluminum hydroxide as a phosphate binder for 3 years or longer. Aluminum is known to be toxic to the nervous system (102), and an encephalopathy was reported in an aluminum flake powder factory worker (103). It was shown recently that aluminum is absorbed in small quantities and excreted readily in the urine (104). In patients with little or no renal function who chronically ingest aluminum salts, aluminum may accumulate and possibly be neurotoxic. The time needed for this side effect to appear is usually longer than the treatment time of either acute gastritis or peptic ulcer.

Aluminum binds with and decreases dietary phosphate absorption in the gut. This effect is useful in patients with chronic renal failure who have hyperphosphatemia, but it can cause phosphate depletion in others. Doses of 30 ml of aluminum hydroxide three times per day have adverse effects on phosphate and calcium metabolism (105). Hypophosphatemia is manifested by anorexia, malaise, and muscle weakness (66). Phosphate depletion causes release of calcium from bone with resulting osteomalacia and osteoporosis (106). Serum phosphate levels may need to be monitored bimonthly during chronic therapy with aluminum-containing antacids (107). The syndrome may occur as early as the third week of therapy and is complicated by a low-phosphate diet, diarrhea (108), or restoration of renal function after a renal transplant (109). These effects may be reversed by aluminum phosphate.

Magnesium

The magnesium salts with antacid properties are the oxide, carbonate, hydroxide, and trisilicate. (Magnesium oxide is converted to hydroxide in water.) Of these, the hydroxide, carbonate, and oxide are the most potent, falling between sodium bicarbonate or calcium carbonate and aluminum hydroxide. The major side effect of magnesium-containing antacids is osmotic diarrhea, which can have systemic effects of fluid and electrolyte depletion (87). This side effect may lead to patient noncompliance; it may be avoided by combining magnesium salts and aluminum salts.

After hydrochloric acid is neutralized by magnesium salts, magnesium chloride is formed. It is partly absorbed and is rapidly eliminated by the kidneys; but in the presence of renal disease, magnesium may accumulate, causing hypermagnesemia (87). Hypermagnesemia is manifested by hypotension, nausea, vomiting, depressed reflexes, respiratory depression, and coma (110, 111). Significant increases in magnesium levels may be seen 3–5 days after starting therapy (112). This condition may be complicated by the administration of other magnesium-containing products and may occur after renal transplant (113).

Manifestations of magnesium cardiotoxicity do not usually occur until there is severe hypermagnesemia (10–15 mEq/liter). Then depression of sinoatrial and atrioventricular conduction leads to bradyarrhythmia and asystole. However, junctional bradyarrhythmia occurred in a patient with chronic renal failure receiving 30 ml of Maalox every 2 hours (114), although the patient's blood magnesium level never rose above 4.8 mEq/liter.

An infrequent side effect of magnesium trisilicate is the development of renal stones. When this antacid is taken daily for long periods (several years), silica renal stones may develop (115–117).

Caution should be used if more than 50 mEq of magnesium is given daily to a patient with renal disease (79). Magnesium should be avoided in patients with severe renal failure.

aluminum toxicity

magnesium salts

magaldrate

other antacid ingredients

Magnesium–Aluminum Hydroxide Gels

A mixture of magnesium and aluminum hydroxide gels is a less potent acid buffer than an equal volume of magnesium hydroxide if a pH of >4.5 is desired; it is a more potent buffer if a pH of <3.5 is desired. Magaldrate is a chemical entity of aluminum and magnesium hydroxides, not a physical mixture, and has a lower neutralizing capacity than a physical mixture (118). The magnesium and aluminum ions are balanced to prevent any alteration in bowel function, but diarrhea or constipation may occur. Diarrhea seems to be more common.

Because of the presence of both salts, the mixture has the potential for any of the adverse effects of either agent. Thus it may cause hypermagnesemia in patients with chronic renal failure, hypophosphatemia, or aluminum retention.

Additional Ingredients

Many ingredients are added to antacid preparations that have no basic antacid properties but give the preparation a degree of uniqueness and added basis for advertising claims.

Simethicone

Simethicone is a gastric defoaming agent. It causes gas bubbles to be broken or coalesced into a form that can be eliminated more easily by belching or passing flatus. It has no activity as an antacid. In a randomized, double-blind, placebo-controlled trial, statistically significant improvement in symptoms with simethicone was measured by patients and physicians (119). The FDA considers simethicone safe and effective (79). It is rational to administer simethicone for acute symptoms that have components related to gas, but there is no indication for simethicone for chronic use in peptic ulcer disease.

Oxethazaine

Oxethazaine is a local anesthetic combined with antacids as a prescription antacid. It has been claimed to be more effective than an antacid alone (120). Toxicity and absorption data have not been reported.

Because the combination of oxethazaine and antacid requires a prescription, it has attracted use by physicians for patients whose insurance will not pay for nonprescription drugs. The legend precludes the pharmacist's recommending it directly to patients. It has no proven efficacy in carefully controlled trials over adequate doses of antacid for either acute gastritis or peptic ulcer.

Alginic Acid

Some antacid products contain alginic acid, sodium bicarbonate, and other antacid ingredients. In the presence of saliva in the buccal cavity, alginic acid reacts with sodium bicarbonate to form a highly viscous solution of sodium alginate. There is not enough bicarbonate, aluminum hydroxide, or magnesium trisilicate in the commercial preparations containing alginic acid to buffer gastric acid effectively. A tablet containing alginic acid is chewed, followed by a glass of water to wash the sodium alginate into the stomach, where it floats on top of the gastric contents. If there is esophageal reflux, the esophageal mucosa comes into contact with the sodium alginate rather than the acidic gastric contents (121). Effectiveness of the preparation in esophageal reflux depends on the patient's remaining in a vertical position (122–124). The patient should be instructed to sleep on pillows or to elevate the head of the bed with 15-cm blocks. The FDA considers the drug safe (79). Products containing alginic acid should be restricted to esophageal reflux and hiatal hernia and should not be used for acute gastritis or peptic ulcer disease.

sodium alginate

all antacids are not equal

dosage forms

neutralizing capacity

Bismuth

Bismuth compounds have been used for gastric distress since the 1850's but have declined in popularity in recent years since they were shown to have little antacid activity (125). There has been renewed interest in bismuth since the introduction of a new bismuth salt, tripotassium dicitratobismuthate (126). This new complex acts by chelating protein and amino acids produced by necrotic ulcer tissue to form a protective layer at the site of the ulcer crater, thus protecting the ulcer from acid pepsin digestion (127). This is a different compound and mechanism of action from the bismuth salts mixed with commercial antacids. The FDA considers bismuth compounds antacids and does not recognize them as protectants of mucosal membranes (79).

Evaluation

All antacids are not equal. The evaluation must consider the formulation, neutralizing capacity, intended use, palatability, and comparison to other agents.

Formulation

Antacids are available as chewing gums, tablets, lozenges, powders, and liquids. Insoluble antacids depend on particle size for acid neutralization. A smaller particle size increases the surface area; the greater surface area increases the wettability and ease of mixing with gastric contents. Therefore an increased surface area means an increased antacid effect. Many solid dosage forms must be masticated before they will disintegrate and react with acid in the stomach. Liquid suspensions of antacids are milled to a fine particle size and provide a greater surface area. Tablet antacids are not equal to liquid antacids on a milligram for milligram basis (87). This difference may be due to the desiccation process used in manufacturing. Tablets that do not disintegrate may lodge in the bowel and cause obstruction (128). Powders must be suspended in water before ingestion. Liquids (suspensions) generally are easier to ingest and have a greater neutralizing capacity. Tablets should be reserved for people who find liquids awkward or inconvenient.

Table 1. In Vitro Neutralizing Capacity of Various Antacids

Antacid[a]	Capacity, mEq/ml	Equivalent Volume[b], ml
Ducon[c]	7.04	11.4
Mylanta II	4.14	19.3
Titralac	3.87	20.7
Camalox	3.59	22.3
Aludrox	2.81	28.5
Maalox	2.58	31.0
Creamalin	2.57	31.1
Di-Gel	2.45	32.7
Mylanta	2.38	33.6
Silain-Gel	2.31	34.6
Marblen	2.28	35.1
WinGel	2.25	35.6
Riopan	2.21	36.2
Amphojel	1.93	41.5
A.M.T.	1.79	44.7
Kolantyl Gel	1.69	47.3
Trisogel	1.65	48.5
Malcogel[c]	1.59	50.3
Robalate	1.13	70.8
Phosphaljel	0.42	190.5

Adapted from J. S. Fordtran et al., *N. Engl. J. Med.*, *288*, 923 (1973). (Listed in decreasing order of neutralizing capacity.)
[a] For antacid components, see product table.
[b] Based on a desired 80 mEq of neutralizing capacity. To determine the amount of antacid to use for a desired neutralizing capacity, divide the milliequivalents per milliliter capacity into the desired milliequivalents of antacid. For example, the neutralizing capacity of Maalox is 2.58 mEq/ml. To achieve 156 mEq of antacid activity, 60 ml of Maalox must be given; to achieve the same antacid potency using Trisogel, 94.5 ml must be given.
[c] No longer marketed.

Potency

Several in vitro comparisons showed that all antacids are not equally potent (118, 129, 130). A 17-fold difference in acid-neutralizing capacity was found in commercial antacids following a standard test meal. The same test also correlated in vivo potency with in vitro potency. Table 1 gives these results. The FDA defines antacids in terms of minimal buffering capacity. To be called an antacid, the ingredient must contribute 25% of the total acid neutralization of the product. The product must neutralize at least 5 mEq of acid and must maintain a pH of 3.5 for 10 minutes in an in vitro test.

There has been no attempt to correlate the FDA test in terms of relative potencies or in vitro tests. The FDA test is not clinically useful. The potencies in Table 1 are the most clinically useful guidelines to antacid neutralizing capacity. Antacids that contain calcium carbonate and concentrated antacids are the most potent. However, as was previously discussed, calcium carbonate should be avoided for chronic intensive therapy. Aluminum–magnesium hydroxide gels generally offer adequate neutralizing capacity with the least toxicity potential.

Efficacy

The efficacy of antacids depends on the intended use, formulation, and dose. Any antacid with potent neutralizing capacity is effective in treating acute gastritis. However, only in the last few years have antacids been tested for efficacy in peptic ulcer disease (131, 132). These trials have shown mixed results that may be due to study design (133–137). Statistically significant improvement in healing and pain relief was reported for patients with gastric ulcers treated with calcium carbonate (133), while other studies (134–136) using small doses failed to show improvement in either healing or pain relief for gastric or duodenal ulcers. In a recent study (137) a potent liquid antacid (Mylanta II) was given in seven divided doses (1008 mEq/day) for 28 days to patients with duodenal ulcers. The treated patients showed significant improvement in ulcer healing but no difference in symptomatic relief compared with a placebo group.

Studies proclaiming no benefit have been too sweeping in their conclusions. They have summarized all antacids in all forms and in any dose when only one antacid in one form and one dose was studied. Antacids continue to be the standard of practice. However, practitioners should consider higher doses than have been traditionally used and should constantly re-evaluate efficacy.

Palatability

Patients frequently complain about the taste of antacids and refuse to take their medication. They should be questioned about palatability as a guide to compliance. The pharmacist may recommend switching to another antacid that is more palatable for a given patient. Refrigerating the antacid may help. Mylanta II has been the most accepted antacid in taste tests (138, 139).

Dosage Recommendations

Dosage recommendations depend on intended use (acute or chronic), antacid neutralizing capacity, dosage interval, and temporal relationship to meals. The dose of liquid antacids is best expressed in terms of milliequivalents (mEq) of neutralizing capacity. As has already been discussed, equal volumes are not equipotent. In acute gastritis, 40–80 mEq of liquid antacid or 2–4 g of sodium or calcium carbonate is effective. Therapy may last from one dose to several days but should never extend beyond 2 weeks without medical supervision.

Recommended regimens for antacids in peptic ulcer disease range from taking the medicine only when there is pain to taking as much antacid as can reasonably be tolerated (140). The latter protocol is favored because there are objective data to support it (137). Intensive antacid therapy for hospitalized patients who are not likely to be eating begins with 40 mEq/hour during waking hours for gastric ulcer patients and 80 mEq/hour for duodenal ulcer patients (87).

Hourly dosing is neither practical nor necessary when the patient resumes eating. Food acts as a buffer to stomach acid for about 60 minutes, and then gastric acidity increases (141, 142). Antacids taken on an empty stomach have a duration of action of only 20–40 minutes (143). However, if they are taken 1 hour after meals, their duration of action is increased to up to 3 hours (118). Thus for chronic therapy, antacids should be given 1 and 3 hours after meals and at bedtime.

Therapy should be continued for 6–8 weeks (144). The recommended dose is 80 mEq of antacid for gastric ulcer and 160 mEq of antacid for duodenal ulcer.

evaluating effectiveness
recommended regimens
duration of therapy
other drugs and diet

Other Therapy

Antacid therapy is the main treatment for acute gastritis or indigestion. The only other treatment would be avoiding the incident that precipitated the episode. Therapy other than antacids for peptic ulcer disease includes diet, anticholinergics, and H_2-antagonists (the latter two being prescription-only items).

Diet

Bland diets or ulcer diets are ineffective in treating peptic ulcers; conversely, there is no evidence that pepper or other spices cause ulceration (132). Milk increases acid production and has no antacid properties (145). Diets that alternate milk and antacids have been or should be abandoned. Bland diets are monotonous and unpalatable, resulting in poor patient compliance (146). Coffee (both caffeinated and decaffeinated), caffeine-containing beverages (e.g., cola), and alcohol are the only items that should be withheld from an ulcer patient. The patient will learn to avoid foods that cause pain (147).

Anticholinergics

Anticholinergics are prescription ingredients that have been used to prolong the duration of action of antacids. If they are used, the dose of both the antacid and the anticholinergic should be individualized; side effects from the anticholinergic may occur if it is administered in fixed combination with antacids. The FDA considers fixed dose combinations of antacids and anticholinergics unsafe (79).

Of the controlled clinical trials that have been done with anticholinergics in peptic ulcer disease, most have shown no significant benefit (132). The benefit from these drugs seldom justifies the side effects they cause. The main indications for anticholinergics in peptic ulcer disease are for persistent pain, especially nocturnal pain not responding to routine measures, for patients whose ulcers fail to heal after an adequate trial of standard therapy, and for patients with high recurrence rate (148).

Anticholinergics should be considered adjunctive therapy to antacids or H_2-antagonists.

H_2-Antagonists

The discovery of histamine H_2-receptors and the development of H_2-receptor antagonists have done much to explain gastric physiology. Cimetidine, a prescription-only drug, is the only commercially available H_2-antagonist. It has been impressive in promoting healing in duodenal ulcer and looks promising for gastric ulcer (149). The combination of cimetidine and antacid delivers a more alkaline load to the duodenum (150). Therefore cimetidine and antacids are equal therapeutically and are potentially synergistic.

Miscellaneous

Drugs under investigation for peptic ulcer treatment include carbenoxolone, dinoprostone (prostaglandin E_2), and amylopectin (140, 151). No comparison to antacids or cimetidine can be made.

cimetidine

effects of antacids on other drugs

pH alteration effects

Drug Interactions

Antacids may interfere with other drugs by altering GI absorption or renal elimination. Raising the pH with antacids may alter disintegration, dissolution, solubility, ionization, and gastric emptying time of other drugs and as a result may either increase or decrease absorption (152, 153). Enteric coats dissolve more readily, exposing acid labile drugs to digestion and exposing the upper GI tract to irritating drugs. Weakly acidic drugs have a decreased absorption because ionization is increased. Conversely, weakly basic drugs are absorbed at a faster rate. Antacids may bind or adsorb other drugs to their surface. Magnesium trisilicate and magnesium hydroxide have the greatest adsorption potential, calcium carbonate and aluminum hydroxide have an intermediate potential, and kaolin and bismuth have the least potential (154).

Antacid-induced changes in the urinary pH may alter drug elimination (155). Readily absorbed antacids such as sodium bicarbonate have the most pronounced effect. Studies in which various doses of commercial antacids were administered four times per day found that aluminum hydroxide and dihydroxyaluminum aminoacetate had no effect on urinary pH, magnesium hydroxide and calcium carbonate suspensions raised urinary pH by 0.4 and 0.5 unit, respectively, and magnesium–aluminum hydroxide gel raised urinary pH by 0.9 unit (156). A follow-up study found that the increase in urinary pH was higher on the second and subsequent days than on the first, that 15 and 30 ml of magnesium–aluminum hydroxide gel were statistically greater than 5 ml but not different from each other, and that the effect persisted 1 day after antacid treatment was stopped (157). The effect is enough to enhance the excretion of acidic drugs and inhibit the excretion of basic drugs (155).

Significant Interactions

Antacids inhibit the absorption of tetracycline antibiotics. The tetracycline molecule chelates with polyvalent ions (aluminum, calcium, and magnesium) (158). Antacids incapable of causing chelates, e.g., sodium bicarbonate, also may decrease tetracycline absorption by increasing gastric pH (159). Pharmacists should advise patients on appropriate spacing of doses of tetracyclines and antacids or calcium-containing foods such as milk (160).

Digoxin and digitoxin are adsorbed to antacids in vitro (161) and in vivo (162). Pharmacists also should advise patients on the proper spacing of doses when these drugs must be taken at the same time. Likewise, iron salts should not be given with antacids because antacids decrease iron absorption (163).

The administration of magnesium trisilicate–aluminum hydroxide antacid caused a decrease in plasma chlorpromazine levels after oral administration (164). Decreased absorption also may occur when chlorpromazine is given with magnesium–aluminum hydroxide gel (165). Antacids and chlorpromazine should not be given concurrently. Dosing at alternate times may reduce the probability of this interaction.

Antacids do not alter quinidine absorption (166). Since quinidine excretion varies inversely with urinary pH, a potentially dangerous interaction could result through alteration of urinary pH by antacids (167). Concurrent use of these drugs should be avoided or monitored closely.

In vitro, indomethacin is adsorbed by magnesium trisilicate, magnesium oxide, aluminum hydroxide, bismuth oxycarbonate, calcium carbonate, and kaolin (168). The peak concentration is delayed, and the bioavailability is reduced (169, 170). Although antacids frequently are suggested for patients taking indomethacin, the two should not be given together. Again, alternating doses may decrease the probability of this interaction.

Aspirin has been reported to be absorbed more quickly from antacid-buffered preparations, but there are no proven clinical differences (152). However, the absorption rate may increase if aspirin is given in an enteric-coated form (171–173). Renal elimination of aspirin may be increased by 30–70% by an antacid-induced increase in urinary pH (173). If aspirin and aluminum–magnesium hydroxide gel are given together and sustained levels are important, as in rheumatoid arthritis and systemic lupus erythematosus, it is advisable to monitor serum levels and to observe symptoms, checking for signs of toxicity.

Levodopa absorption is increased up to 3 times when antacids are taken concurrently (174). Alkalinization accelerates gastric emptying and delivers more levodopa to the small intestine, where it is more rapidly absorbed (175). There may be individual variation in response (176). The addition of antacids to a well-controlled parkinsonian patient may result in toxicity. If the patient is well controlled on levodopa and antacid and the antacid is removed, relapse may occur.

Potentially Significant Interactions

Isoniazid absorption is more inhibited by aluminum hydroxide than by magaldrate. The mechanism is probably due to decreased gastric emptying time. Although the clinical significance is not known, isoniazid probably should be given 1 hour before the antacid (177).

effects of antacids with other drugs

labeling requirements

advice for the patient

A potentially significant interaction between antacids and anticoagulants can be avoided by selecting the proper anticoagulant. The absorption of dicumarol was increased by 50% by 15 ml of magnesium hydroxide and 30 ml of aluminum hydroxide (178). The absorption or the effect of warfarin is not altered by antacids (178, 179). Thus only patients taking dicumarol need cautioning about antacids.

Different antacids affect naproxen differently. Sodium bicarbonate administered with naproxen resulted in earlier and higher peaks, while magnesium oxide and aluminum hydroxide delayed absorption and decreased peak plasma levels. Aluminum–magnesium hydroxide gel tended to decrease the time required to reach peak plasma levels and slightly increased the total area under the curve (180). The clinical significance of this effect is unknown. It would seem best not to administer antacids simultaneously with naproxen.

Urinary excretion of amphetamine is decreased with sodium bicarbonate (181). Because of the potential for retention and subsequent intoxication due to urinary pH alteration with all antacids, antacids and amphetamines should not be given concurrently.

Benzodiazepines react differently with antacids. When chlordiazepoxide was administered with magnesium–aluminum hydroxide gel, the absorption rate of chlordiazepoxide was slowed, but the total amount absorbed remained unchanged (182). Thus the interaction would be significant only for acute anxiety states where single doses of chlordiazepoxide are used. It would not be significant for chronic therapy. The absorption of diazepam was increased by aluminum hydroxide (183), but the clinical significance of this increase has not been determined.

The simultaneous administration of an unspecified antacid and phenytoin resulted in low phenytoin levels in three patients. When the same dose of phenytoin was given 2–3 hours before the antacid, plasma levels increased twofold to threefold (184). More complete studies are needed for confirmation.

The absorption rate of pseudoephedrine was increased in the first 4 hours in six volunteers. The antacid increased the portion of the drug that was in the nonionized and more soluble form. Total absorption was not changed, and the clinical significance is unknown (185).

Administration of a single dose of aluminum hydroxide decreased the bioavailability of a single dose of propranolol in four of five subjects (186). What effect the concomitant administration of antacids and propranolol will have on prolonged therapy has not been assessed. Likewise, the clinical significance of this interaction remains to be determined.

PRODUCT SELECTION GUIDELINES

The FDA OTC Panel on Antacid and Antiflatulent Products has defined an active ingredient in an antacid as contributing 25% of the total acid neutralization and requires that the finished product contain at least 5 mEq of acid-neutralizing capacity and maintain a pH of 3.5 for 10 minutes in an in vitro test. The label, as defined by the Panel, can list only "heartburn," "sour stomach," and "acid indigestion" as indications. The label must contain a caution if constipation or diarrhea occurs in more than 5% of the population and if there is >5 mEq of sodium, >25 mEq of potassium, >50 mEq of magnesium, or >5 g of lactose per daily dose. If the product contains >0.2 mEq (5 mg) of sodium per dosage unit, the content must be on the label. Directions for time interval between doses must be given, and a limit of 2 weeks of self-therapy is stated. A listing of the quantity of active ingredients is voluntary (79, 187).

The Panel does not make specific dosage recommendations nor give any comparative data. The label is an aid to product selection, but final selection and dosage must be based on individual evaluation and patient history. For example, antacids containing little or no sodium should be selected for individuals on a low-salt diet, e.g., patients who are pregnant or who have congestive heart failure, hypertension, edema, or renal failure. Sodium content should be compared on equipotent volumes of drug to be administered. Magnesium-containing antacids should be avoided in patients with chronic renal failure. Antacids that cause constipation or diarrhea should not be given to a patient who already has these complaints. However, a magnesium antacid may be appropriate for an elderly patient who complains of chronic constipation.

The patient's current medications should be reviewed so that a product or a dosage schedule can be selected that does not interfere with the other medication.

Although cost is not a main consideration in product selection, it should be taken into account. Cost should be computed for equipotent, not equivolume, quantities.

Specific advice to the patient should include:

- Antacids for relief of indigestion symptoms should not be taken longer than 2 weeks. If relief is not obtained, a physician should be contacted. If the antacid is being taken for peptic ulcer disease, it should be taken 1 and 3 hours after meals and at bedtime to provide a maximum duration of action.
- To prevent self-medication of an iatrogenic condition, the patient should understand that the antacid may cause diarrhea or constipation.
- Patients with restricted salt intake should be informed of the amount of sodium in the medications and advised of those products with a low sodium content. Patients with medical problems that could be influenced by potassium or magnesium should be told of the content of these ions.
- The lesser effectiveness of tablets should be made clear. If liquid antacids are unacceptable, tablets should be chewed thoroughly and followed with a full glass of water to help dissolution and dispersion in the stomach. Effervescent tablets should be dissolved in water and most of the bubbles allowed to subside before they are swallowed.
- Additional medication should be identified to enable the pharmacist to monitor for drug interactions.
- Some antacids, e.g., sodium bicarbonate and calcium carbonate, are absorbed and produce alterations in systemic and urinary pH. Others may induce nonsystemic changes.

SUMMARY

Before recommending an antacid for self-therapy, the pharmacist must ensure that the use is appropriate. If the patient's history is indicative of peptic ulcer or if there is evidence of bleeding, the patient should be referred to a physician for a medical examination.

Self-medication may be recommended if the history is indicative of acute gastritis, indigestion, heartburn, or upset stomach. Subjectively, any antacid will be effective, and therapy may be initiated with 40–80 mEq of a liquid antacid or 2–4 g of sodium bicarbonate or calcium carbonate. A product with simethicone should be recommended for the patient with gas. The pharmacist should caution against frequent use and monitor the patient for effectiveness and toxicity. If the discomfort is not relieved after 2 weeks or recurs frequently, medical help is indicated.

when self-medication is appropriate

preferred agents

Since antacids constitute part of peptic ulcer therapy, the pharmacist may be asked to recommend an antacid for the physician-supervised management of peptic ulcer disease. Aluminum–magnesium hydroxide gel is the agent of choice for initial therapy in the absence of other complications. Other agents would be more appropriate for patients with renal failure, those on low-salt diets, and those with abnormal bowel function.

All antacids are not equal. Care should be taken to select one with good buffering capacity, and equipotent volumes should be used if side effects necessitate switching to another product. Failure of antacid therapy may be due to a poor selection, a too infrequent or poorly timed administration, or an inadequate dose.

REFERENCES

(1) S. L. Robbins, "Pathologic Basis of Disease," Saunders, Philadelphia, Pa., 1974.
(2) A. C. Guyton, "Textbook of Medical Physiology," Saunders, Philadelphia, Pa., 1976.
(3) H. M. Spiro, Ed., "Peptic Ulcer," Rorer, Fort Washington, Pa., 1971.
(4) K. A. Kelley, "Surgery Annual," Appleton-Century-Crofts, New York, N.Y., 1974, p. 103.
(5) A. M. Cooperman and S. A. Cook, *Surg. Clin. North Am.*, *56*, 1277 (1976).
(6) K. J. Ivey, *Am. J. Med.*, *58*, 389 (1975).
(7) R. R. Dozois and K. A. Kelley, *Surg. Clin. North Am.*, *56*, 1267 (1975).
(8) H. T. Debas, *Am. Surg.*, *42*, 498 (1976).
(9) J. H. Eichhorn, E. W. Salzman, and W. Silen, *Nature*, *248*, 238 (1974).
(10) T. Scratcherd, *Clin. Gastroenterol.*, *2*, 259 (1973).
(11) J. E. McGuigan, *Am. J. Dig. Dis.*, *22*, 712 (1977).
(12) A. M. Ebeid and J. E. Fischer, *Surg. Clin. North Am.*, *56*, 1249 (1976).
(13) J. H. Walsh and M. I. Grossman, *N. Engl. J. Med.*, *292*, 1324 (1975).
(14) J. E. McGuigan, *Gastroenterology*, *64*, 497 (1973).
(15) D. H. Stern and J. H. Walsh, *Gastroenterology*, *64*, 363 (1973).
(16) S. Cohen and W. Lipshutz, *J. Clin. Invest.*, *50*, 449 (1971).
(17) M. L. Chapman, J. L. Werther, J. Rudick, and H. D. Janowitz, *Gastroenterology*, *63*, 962 (1972).
(18) I. W. McCall, R. F. Harvey, C. J. Owens, and B. G. Clendinren, *Br. J. Surg.*, *62*, 15 (1975).
(19) W. J. Dodds, W. J. Hogan, W. N. Miller, R. F. Barreras, R. C. Arndorfer, and J. J. Stef, *Am. J. Dig. Dis.*, *20*, 201 (1976).
(20) J. W. Black, W. A. Duncan, and C. J. Durant, *Nature*, *236*, 385 (1972).
(21) S. J. Konturek, J. Biernat, and J. Olesky, *Am. J. Dig. Dis.*, *19*, 609 (1974).
(22) J. H. Wyllie, T. Hesselbo, and J. W. Black, *Lancet*, *2*, 1117 (1972).
(23) R. R. Dozois, A. Wollin, and R. D. Rettmann, *Physiologist*, *18*, 196 (1975).
(24) A. M. Brooks and M. I. Grossman, *Gastroenterology*, *59*, 114 (1970).
(25) D. E. Wilson, B. Ginsberg, R. A. Levine, and A. Washington, *Gastroenterology*, *63*, 45 (1972).
(26) K. G. Wormsley, *Gastroenterology*, *62*, 156 (1972).
(27) J. Hansky, C. Soveny, and M. G. Korman, *Gastroenterology*, *61*, 62 (1971).
(28) M. H. Wheeler, *Gut*, *15*, 420 (1974).
(29) A. R. Cooke, *Gastroenterology*, *68*, 804 (1975).
(30) S. H. Danovitch, in "Disorders of the Gastrointestinal Tract, Disorders of the Liver, Nutritional Disorders," J. M. Dietschy, Ed., Grune and Stratton, New York, N.Y., 1976, p. 111.
(31) R. B. Hill and F. Kern, "The Gastrointestinal Tract," Williams and Wilkins, Baltimore, Md., 1977, p. 77.
(32) B. S. Wolf, *J. Am. Med. Assoc.*, *235*, 1244 (1976).
(33) A. R. Cooke, *Am. J. Dig. Dis.*, *21*, 155 (1976).
(34) *Nutrition Reviews*, *34*, 167 (1976).
(35) C. E. Lucas, C. Sugawa, J. Riddle, F. Rector, B. Rosenberg, and A. J. Walt, *Arch. Surg.*, *102*, 266 (1971).
(36) W. C. Butterfield, *Surgery Annual*, 261 (1975).
(37) P. H. Guth, *Gastroenterology*, *64*, 1187 (1973).
(38) J. E. McGuigan, in "Disorders of the Gastrointestinal Tract, Disorders of the Liver, Nutritional Disorders," J. M. Dietschy, Ed., Grune and Stratton, New York, N.Y., 1976, p. 88.
(39) M. I. Grossman, J. I. Isenberg, and J. H. Walsh, *Gastroenterology*, *69*, 1071 (1975).
(40) M. J. S. Langman, *Clin. Gastroenterol.*, *2*, 219 (1973).
(41) R. C. Brown, M. J. S. Langman, and P. M. Lambert, *Br. Med. J.*, *1*, 35 (1976).
(42) R. A. L. Sturdevant, *Am. J. Epidemiol.*, *104*, 9 (1976).
(43) B. E. Stabile and E. Passaro, *Gastroenterology*, *70*, 124 (1976).
(44) Y. Nagamachi and S. C. Skoryna, *Am. J. Surg.*, *133*, 593 (1977).
(45) M. I. Grossman, P. H. Guth, J. I. Isenberg, E. P. Passaro, Jr., B. E. Roth, R. A. L. Sturdevant, and J. H. Walsh, *Ann. Intern. Med.*, *84*, 57 (1976).
(46) A. Ippoliti and J. Walsh, *Surg. Clin. North Am.*, *56*, 1479 (1976).
(47) L. R. Dragstedt and E. R. Woodward, *Scand. J. Gastroenterol.*, *5*, Suppl. 6, 243 (1970).
(48) J. Rhodes and B. Calcraft, *Clin. Gastroenterol.*, *2*, 227 (1973).
(49) N. W. Read and P. Grech, *Br. Med. J.*, *3*, 313 (1973).
(50) F. J. Flint and P. Grech, *Gut*, *11*, 735 (1970).
(51) R. S. Fisher and G. Boden, *Gastroenterology*, *66*, 839 (1974).
(52) R. S. Fisher and S. Cohen, *N. Engl. J. Med.*, *288*, 273 (1973).
(53) J. E. Valenzuela and C. Defilippi, *Am. J. Dig. Dis.*, *21*, 229 (1976).
(54) R. A. Roverstad, *Am. J. Dig. Dis.*, *21*, 165 (1976).
(55) J. I. Rotter and D. L. Rimoin, *Gastroenterology*, *73*, 604 (1977).
(56) G. A. Hallenbeck, *Surg. Clin. North Am.*, *56*, 1235 (1976).
(57) A. J. Cox, *Arch. Pathol.*, 54, 407 (1952).
(58) J. I. Isenberg, M. I. Grossman, V. Maxwell, and J. Walsh, *J. Clin. Invest.*, *55*, 330 (1975).
(59) J. E. McGuigan and W. L. Trudeau, *N. Engl. J. Med.*, *288*, 64 (1973).
(60) J. Walsh, C. Richardson, and J. Fordtran, *J. Clin. Invest.*, *55*, 462 (1975).
(61) J. S. Fordtran and J. H. Walsh, *J. Clin. Invest.*, *52*, 645 (1973).
(62) "Harrison's Principles of Internal Medicine," 8th ed., G. W. Thorn, R. D. Adams, E. Braunwald, K. J. Isselbacher, and R. G. Petersdorf, Eds., McGraw-Hill, New York, N.Y., 1977.
(63) H. Colcher, *N. Engl. J. Med.*, *293*, 1129 (1975).
(64) M. C. Sheppard, G. R. T. Holmes, and R. Cockel, *Gut*, *18*, 524 (1977).
(65) H. M. Pollard and N. A. Augar, *Practitioner*, *201*, 139 (1968).
(66) J. F. Morrissey and R. F. Barreras, *N. Engl. J. Med.*, *290*, 550 (1974).
(67) D. W. Piper and B. H. Fenton, *Gut*, *5*, 506 (1964).
(68) J. T. Kuruvilla, *Gut*, *12*, 897 (1971).
(69) H. A. Holm, *Scand. J. Gastroenterol.*, *2*, Suppl. 42, 119 (1976).
(70) D. W. Piper and B. H. Fenton, *Am. J. Dig. Dis.*, *6*, 134 (1961).
(71) J. F. Morrissey, T. Honda, Y. Tanaka, and G. Perna, *Arch. Intern. Med.*, *119*, 510 (1967).
(72) J. E. Dill, *Gastroenterology*, *62*, 697 (1972).
(73) R. H. Higgs, R. D. Smyth, and D. O. Castell, *N. Engl. J. Med.*, *291*, 486 (1974).
(74) D. O. Castell and S. M. Levine, *Ann. Intern. Med.*, *74*, 223 (1971).
(75) G. E. Feurle, *Gastroenterology*, *68*, 1 (1975).
(76) A. Hurwitz and M. B. Sheehan, *J. Pharmacol. Exp. Ther.*, *179*, 124 (1971).
(77) A. Hurwitz, R. G. Robinson, T. S. Vats, F. C. Whittier, and W. F. Herrin, *Gastroenterology*, *71*, 268 (1976).
(78) J. E. Clain, J.-R. Malagelada, V. S. Chadwick, and A. F. Hofmann, *Gastroenterology*, *73*, 556 (1977).
(79) A. M. Schmidt, *Fed. Regist.*, *39*, 19862 (1974).
(80) C. H. Barnett, R. R. Commons, F. Albright, and J. E. Howard, *N. Engl. J. Med.*, *240*, 787 (1949).
(81) C. J. Riley, *Practitioner*, *205*, 657 (1970).
(82) A. Ansari and J. A. Vennes, *Minn. Med.*, *54*, 611 (1971).
(83) D. W. Piper, *Clin. Gastroenterol.*, *2*, 361 (1973).

(84) F. W. Green, R. A. Norton, and M. M. Kaplan, *Am. J. Hosp. Pharm.*, *32*, 425 (1975).
(85) J. S. Fordtran, *N. Engl. J. Med.*, *279*, 900 (1968).
(86) *Medical Letter*, *15*(8), 36 (1973).
(87) J. S. Fordtran, in "Gastrointestinal Disease—Pathophysiology, Diagnosis and Management," M. H. Sleisenger and J. S. Fordtran, Eds., Saunders, Philadelphia, Pa., 1973, p. 718.
(88) J. Stiel, C. A. Mitchell, F. J. Radcliff, and D. W. Piper, *Gastroenterology*, *53*, 900 (1967).
(89) D. E. McMillan and R. B. Freeman, *Medicine*, *44*, 485 (1965).
(90) R. F. Barreras, *Gastroenterology*, *64*, 1168 (1973).
(91) R. M. Case, *Digestion*, *8*, 269 (1973).
(92) H. Breuhaus, O. H. Akre, and J. B. Eyerler, *Gastroenterology*, *16*, 172 (1950).
(93) R. F. Barreras, *N. Engl. J. Med.*, *282*, 1402 (1970).
(94) D. D. Reeder, B. M. Jackson, J. Ban, B. G. Clendinnen, W. D. Davidson, and J. C. Thompson, *Ann. Surg.*, *172*, 540 (1970).
(95) J. A. Levant, J. H. Walsh, and J. I. Isenberg, *N. Engl. J. Med.*, *289*, 555 (1973).
(96) S. L. Hem, *J. Chem. Educ.*, *52*, 383 (1975).
(97) C. M. Townsend, A. R. Remmers, H. E. Sarles, and J. C. Fish, *N. Engl. J. Med.*, *288*, 1058 (1973).
(98) E. M. Clarkson, V. A. Luck, W. V. Hynson, R. R. Bailey, J. B. Eastwood, J. S. Woodhead, V. R. Clements, J. L. H. O'Riordan, and H. E. De Wardener, *Clin. Sci.*, *43*, 519 (1972).
(99) G. M. Berlyne, J. Ben-Ari, D. Pest, J. Weinberger, M. Stern, G. R. Gilmore, and R. Levine, *Lancet*, *2*, 494 (1970).
(100) V. Parsons, C. Davies, C. Goode, C. Ogg, and J. Siddiqui, *Br. Med. J.*, *4*, 273 (1971).
(101) A. C. Alfrey, G. R. LeGendre, and W. D. Kaehny, *N. Engl. J. Med.*, *294*, 184 (1976).
(102) C. A. Miller and E. M. Levine, *J. Neurochem.*, *22*, 751 (1974).
(103) A. I. McLaughlin, G. Kazantzis, E. King, D. Teare, R. J. Porter, and R. Owen, *Br. J. Ind. Med.*, *19*, 253 (1962).
(104) W. D. Kaehny, A. P. Hegg, and A. C. Alfrey, *N. Engl. J. Med.*, *296*, 1389 (1977).
(105) *Journal of the American Medical Association*, *238*, 1017 (1977).
(106) C. E. Dent and D. S. Winter, *Br. Med. J.*, *1*, 551 (1974).
(107) D. E. Abrams, R. B. Silcott, R. Terry, T. V. Berne, and B. H. Barbour, *West. J. Med.*, *120*, 157 (1974).
(108) M. Lotz, E. Zisman, and F. C. Bartter, *N. Engl. J. Med.*, *278*, 409 (1968).
(109) R. E. Chojnacki, *Ann. Intern. Med.*, *74*, 297 (1971).
(110) R. E. Randall, M. D. Cohen, C. C. Spray, and E. C. Rossmeisl, *Ann. Intern. Med.*, *61*, 73 (1964).
(111) F. J. Goodwin and F. P. Vince, *Br. J. Urol.*, *42*, 586 (1970).
(112) S. Jameson, *Scand. J. Urol. Nephrol.*, *6*, 260 (1972).
(113) A. C. Alfrey, D. S. Terman, L. Brettschneider, K. M. Simpson, and D. A. Ogden, *Ann. Intern. Med.*, *73*, 367 (1970).
(114) A. S. Berns and K. R. Kollmeyer, *Ann. Intern. Med.*, *85*, 760 (1976).
(115) J. R. Herman and A. S. Goldberg, *J. Am. Med. Assoc.*, *174*, 1206 (1960).
(116) C. Lagergren, *J. Urol.*, *87*, 994 (1962).
(117) A. M. Joekes, G. A. Rose, and J. Sutor, *Br. Med. J.*, *1*, 146 (1973).
(118) J. S. Fordtran, S. G. Morawski, and C. T. Richardson, *N. Engl. J. Med.*, *288*, 923 (1973).
(119) J. E. Bernstein and A. M. Kasich, *J. Clin. Pharmacol.*, *14*, 617 (1974).
(120) J. F. Pontes, D. J. Richards, and J. N. Sartoretto, *Curr. Ther. Res. Clin. Exp.*, *18*, 315 (1975).
(121) C. Stanciu and J. R. Bennet, *Lancet*, *1*, 109 (1974).
(122) M. Beeley and J. O. Warner, *Curr. Med. Res. Opin.*, *1*, 63 (1972).
(123) *South African Medical Journal*, *48*, 2239 (1974).
(124) G. L. Beckloff, J. H. Chapman, and P. Shiverdecker, *J. Clin. Pharmacol.*, *12*, 11 (1972).
(125) *Lancet*, *1*, 1290 (1975).
(126) *Postgraduate Medical Journal*, *51*, Suppl., 5 (1975).
(127) R. N. Brogden, R. M. Pinder, P. R. Sawyer, T. M. Speight, and G. S. Avery, *Drugs*, *12*, 401 (1976).
(128) D. Patyk, *N. Engl. J. Med.*, *283*, 134 (1970).
(129) D. W. Piper and B. H. Fenton, *Gut*, *5*, 585 (1964).
(130) E. W. Packman and A. R. Gennaro, *Am. J. Pharm.*, *145*, 162 (1973).
(131) E. Christensen, E. Juhl, and N. Tygstrup, *Gastroenterology*, *73*, 1170 (1977).
(132) J. H. Meyer (moderator), A. Schwabe, J. I. Isenberg, R. A. L. Sturdevant, M. I. Grossman, and E. Passaro, *West. J. Med.*, *126*, 273 (1977).
(133) D. Hollander and J. Harlan, *J. Am. Med. Assoc.*, *226*, 1181 (1973).
(134) M. L. Butler and H. Gersh, *Am. J. Dig. Dis.*, *20*, 803 (1975).
(135) R. A. L. Sturdevant, J. I. Isenberg, D. Secrist, and J. Ansfield, *Gastroenterology*, *72*, 1 (1977).
(136) A. Littman, R. Welch, R. C. Fruin, and A. R. Aronson, *Gastroenterology*, *73*, 6 (1977).
(137) W. L. Peterson, R. A. L. Sturdevant, H. D. Frank, C. T. Richardson, J. I. Isenberg, J. D. Elashoff, J. Q. Sones, R. A. Gross, R. W. McCallum, and J. S. Fordtran, *N. Engl. J. Med.*, *297*, 341 (1977).
(138) R. P. Schneider and A. C. Roach, *South. Med. J.*, *69*, 1312 (1976).
(139) D. Sklar, M. H. Liang, and J. Porta, *N. Engl. J. Med.*, *296*, 1007 (1977).
(140) M. J. S. Langman, *Drugs*, *14*, 105 (1977).
(141) J. S. Fordtran and J. H. Walsh, *J. Clin. Invest.*, *52*, 645 (1973).
(142) J.-R. Malagelada, G. F. Longstreth, W. H. Summerskill, and V. L. W. Go, *Gastroenterology*, *70*, 203 (1976).
(143) J. S. Fordtran and J. A. H. Collyns, *N. Engl. J. Med.*, *274*, 921 (1966).
(144) A. Littman, *Gastroenterology*, *61*, 567 (1971).
(145) A. F. Ippoliti, V. Maxwell, and J. I. Isenberg, *Ann. Intern. Med.*, *84*, 286 (1976).
(146) H. S. Caron and H. P. Roth, *Am. J. Med. Sci.*, *261*, 61 (1971).
(147) J. D. Welsh, *Gastroenterology*, *72*, 740 (1977).
(148) K. J. Ivey, *Gastroenterology*, *68*, 154 (1975).
(149) J. K. Siepler, K. D. Campagna, P. E. Donahue, and C. T. Bombeck, *Am. J. Hosp. Pharm.*, *35*, 141 (1978).
(150) J. H. B. Saunders, S. Drummond, and K. G. Wormsley, *Br. Med. J.*, *1*, 418 (1977).
(151) S. Banks and I. N. Marks, *Clin. Gastroenterol.*, *2*, 379 (1973).
(152) A. Hurwitz, *Clin. Pharmacokinet.*, *2*, 269 (1977).
(153) J. A. Romankiewicz, *Primary Care*, *3*, 537 (1976).
(154) S. Khalil and M. Moustafa, *Pharmazie*, *28*, 116 (1973).
(155) *British Medical Journal*, *2*, 405 (1975).
(156) M. Gibaldi, B. Grundhofer, and G. Levy, *Clin. Pharmacol. Ther.*, *16*, 520 (1974).
(157) M. Gibaldi, B. Grundhofer, and G. Levy, *J. Pharm. Sci.*, *64*, 2003 (1975).
(158) S. A. Khalil, N. A. Daabis, V. F. Naggar, and M. M. Motawi, *Pharmazie*, *31*, 105 (1976).
(159) W. H. Barr, J. Adir, and L. Garrettson, *Clin. Pharmacol. Ther.*, *12*, 779 (1971).
(160) *APhA Weekly*, *14*, 2 (June 21, 1975).
(161) S. A. Khalil, *J. Pharm. Pharmacol.*, *26*, 961 (1974).
(162) D. D. Brown and R. P. Juhl, *N. Engl. J. Med.*, *295*, 1034 (1976).
(163) G. Ekenved, L. Halvorsen, and L. Solvell, *Scand. J. Haematol. Suppl.*, *28*, 65 (1976).
(164) W. E. Fann, J. M. Davis, D. S. Janowsky, H. J. Sekerke, and D. M. Schmidt, *J. Clin. Pharmacol.*, *13*, 388 (1973).
(165) F. M. Forrest, I. S. Forrest, and M. T. Serra, *Biol. Psychiatry*, *2*, 53 (1970).
(166) J. A. Romankiewiez, M. Reidenberg, D. Drayer, and J. E. Franklin, *Am. Heart J.*, *96*, 518 (1978).
(167) M. B. Zinn, *Tex. Med.*, *66*, 64 (1970).
(168) V. F. Naggar, S. A. Khalil, and N. A. Daabis, *Pharmazie*, *31*, 461 (1976).
(169) H. W. Emori, H. Paulus, R. Bluestone, G. D. Champion, and C. Pearson, *Ann. Rheum. Dis.*, *35*, 333 (1976).
(170) R. L. Galeazzi, *Eur. J. Clin. Pharmacol.*, *12*, 65 (1977).
(171) B. Strickland-Hodge, T. R. Thomas, W. A. Gould, and I. Haslock, *Rheumatol. Rehabil.*, *15*, 148 (1976).
(172) S. Feldman and B. C. Carlstedt, *J. Am. Med. Assoc.*, *227*, 660 (1974).
(173) G. Levy, T. Lampman, B. L. Kamath, and L. K. Garrettson, *N. Engl. J. Med.*, *293*, 323 (1975).
(174) L. Rivera-Calimlim, C. A. Dujovne, J. P. Morgan, L. Lasagna, and J. R. Bianchine, *Eur. J. Clin. Invest.*, *1*, 313 (1971).
(175) G. B. T. Pocelinko and H. M. Solomon, *Clin. Pharmacol. Ther.*, *13*, 149 (1972).
(176) A. S. Leon and H. E. Spiegel, *J. Clin. Pharmacol.*, *12*, 263 (1972).
(177) A. Hurwitz and D. L. Scholozman, *Am. Rev. Respir. Dis.*, *109*, 41 (1974).
(178) J. J. Ambre and L. J. Fischer, *Clin. Pharmacol. Ther.*, *14*, 231 (1973).
(179) D. S. Robinson, M. B. David, and J. J. McCormack, *Clin. Pharmacol. Ther.*, *12*, 491 (1971).
(180) E. J. Segre, H. Sevelius, and J. Varady, *N. Engl. J. Med.*, *291*, 582 (1974).
(181) A. H. Beckett, M. Rowland, and P. Turner, *Lancet*, *1*, 302 (1965).
(182) D. J. Greenblatt, R. I. Shader, and J. S. Harmatz, *Clin. Pharmacol. Ther.*, *19*, 234 (1976).
(183) S. G. Nair, J. A. S. Gamble, J. W. Dundee, and P. J. Howard, *Br. J. Anaesth.*, *48*, 1175 (1976).
(184) H. L. Kutt, *Epilepsia*, *16*, 393 (1975).
(185) R. Lucarotti, J. L. Colaizzi, H. Barry, and R. L. Poust, *J. Pharm. Sci.*, *61*, 903 (1972).
(186) J. H. Dobbs, V. A. Skoutakis, S. R. Acchiardo, and B. R. Dobbs, *Curr. Ther. Res.*, *21*, 887 (1977).
(187) *FDA Consumer*, July-Aug. 1974. (DHEW Publication No. FDA-75-3003.)

Product (Manufacturer)	Dosage Form	Calcium Carbonate	Aluminum Hydroxide	Magnesium Oxide or Hydroxide	Magnesium Trisilicate	Other	Sodium Content
Albicon (Pfeiffer)	tablet suspension	560 mg/tablet	150 mg/tablet 60 mg/ml	30 mg/ml	—	magnesium carbonate (tablet)	6 mg/tablet NS[a] (suspension)
Alka-2 Chewable Antacid (Miles)	chewable tablet	500 mg	—	—	—	—	NS[a]
Alka-Seltzer Effervescent Antacid (Miles)	tablet	—	—	—	—	sodium bicarbonate, 1.008 g citric acid, 800 mg potassium bicarbonate, 300 mg	276 mg/tablet
Alkets (Upjohn)	tablet	780 mg	—	65 mg	—	magnesium carbonate, 130 mg	NS[a]
AlternaGel (Stuart)	suspension	—	120 mg/ml	—	—	—	0.4 mg/ml
Aludrox (Wyeth)	tablet suspension	—	233 mg/tablet 61.4 mg/ml	84 mg/tablet 20.6 mg/ml	—	—	1.6 mg/tablet 0.22 mg/ml
Aluminum Hydroxide Gel USP (Philips Roxane)	suspension	—	70.4 mg/ml	—	—	sorbitol peppermint sucrose	1.7 mg/ml
Alurex (Rexall)	tablet suspension	—	NS[a]	NS[a] (hydroxide)	—	—	NS[a]
Aluscop (O'Neal, Jones & Feldman)	capsule suspension	—	gel, 150 mg (suspension)	180 mg/capsule 30 mg/ml (hydroxide)	—	dihydroxyaluminum acetate, 325 mg/capsule 40 mg/ml methylparaben, 0.15% (suspension)	NS[a]
Amitone (Norcliff Thayer)	tablet	350 mg	—	—	—	mint flavor	NS[a]
Amphojel (Wyeth)	tablet suspension	—	300 or 600 mg/tablet 64 mg/ml	—	—	—	1.4 or 2.8 mg/tablet 1.4 mg/ml
A.M.T. (Wyeth)	tablet suspension	—	164 mg/tablet 61 mg/ml	—	250 mg/tablet 125 mg/ml	—	3.5 mg/tablet 1.4 mg/ml
Antacid Powder (DeWitt)	powder	—	dried gel, 15%	—	31%	sodium bicarbonate, 25% magnesium carbonate (heavy), 10%	NS[a]
Anti-Acid No. 1 (North American)	tablet	227.5 mg	—	—	—	magnesium carbonate, 130 mg bismuth subnitrate, 32.5 mg	NS[a]
Banacid (Buffington)	tablet	—	NS[a]	NS[a] (hydroxide)	NS[a]	—	NS[a]
Basaljel (Wyeth)	suspension capsule tablet	—	—	—	—	aluminum carbonate, equiv. to: 80 mg aluminum hydroxide/ml 500 mg aluminum hydroxide/capsule or tablet	0.48 mg/ml 2.8 mg/capsule 2.1 mg/tablet
Basaljel Extra Strength (Wyeth)	suspension	—	200 mg/ml	—	—	—	3.4 mg/ml
Bell-Ans (Dent)	tablet	—	—	—	—	sodium bicarbonate, 264 or 527 mg wintergreen ginger	NS[a]

Product (Manufacturer)	Dosage Form	Calcium Carbonate	Aluminum Hydroxide	Magnesium Oxide or Hydroxide	Magnesium Trisilicate	Other	Sodium Content
BiSoDol (Whitehall)	tablet powder	195 mg/ tablet	—	180 mg/tablet	—	sodium bicarbonate (powder) magnesium carbonate (powder) peppermint oil	0.036 mg/ tablet 157 mg/tsp (powder)
Camalox (Rorer)	suspension tablet	50 mg/ml 250 mg/tablet	45 mg/ml 225 mg/tablet	40 mg/ml 200 mg/tablet (hydroxide)	—	—	0.5 mg/ml 1.5 mg/tablet
Chooz (Plough)	gum tablet	NS[a]	—	—	NS[a]	—	3.15 mg/tablet
Citrocarbonate (Upjohn)	suspension powder	—	—	—	—	sodium bicarbonate, 200 mg/g (suspension) 208 mg/g (powder) sodium citrate, anhydrous, 467 mg/g (suspension) 261 mg/g (powder)	NS[a]
Creamalin (Winthrop)	tablet	—	248 mg	75 mg	—	mint flavor	41 mg
Delcid (Merrell-National)	suspension	—	120 mg/ml	133 mg/ml (hydroxide)	—	—	≦3 mg/ml
Dialume (Armour)	tablet	—	dried gel, 500 mg	—	—	—	NS[a]
Dicarbosil (Arch)	tablet	500 mg	—	—	—	peppermint oil	2.7 mg
Di-Gel (Plough)	tablet liquid	—	codried with magnesium carbonate, 282 mg/ tablet 56.2 mg/ml (liquid)	85 mg/tablet 17.4 mg/ml	—	simethicone, 25 mg/tablet 5 mg/ml	10.6 mg/tablet 1.7 mg/ml
Dimacid (Otis Clapp)	tablet	NS[a]	—	—	—	magnesium carbonate	NS[a]
Eno (Beecham Products)	powder	—	—	—	—	sodium bicarbonate, 7.6% sodium tartrate, 65.2% sodium citrate, 27.2%	156 mg/ml
Estomul-M (Riker)	tablet liquid	—	codried with magnesium carbonate, 500 mg/ tablet 183.6 mg/ml	45 mg/tablet (oxide)	—	—	NS[a]
Flacid (Amfre-Grant)	tablet	—	NS[a]	85 mg (hydroxide)	—	simethicone, 25 mg magnesium carbonate, 282 mg	NS[a]
Gelumina (Amer. Pharm.)	tablet	—	250 mg	—	500 mg	sorbitol, 18.8 mg lactose saccharin sodium	0.3 mg
Gelusil (Warner-Chilcott)	tablet suspension	—	200 mg/tablet 40 mg/ml	200 mg/tablet 40 mg/ml	—	simethicone, 25 mg/tablet 5 mg/ml mint flavor	1.7 mg/tablet 0.16 mg/ml
Gelusil II (Warner-Chilcott)	tablet suspension	—	400 mg/tablet 80 mg/ml	400 mg/tablet 80 mg/ml	—	simethicone, 30 mg/tablet 6 mg/ml orange flavor citrus flavor	2.7 mg/tablet 0.26 mg/ml

Product (Manufacturer)	Dosage Form	Calcium Carbonate	Aluminum Hydroxide	Magnesium Oxide or Hydroxide	Magnesium Trisilicate	Other	Sodium Content
Gelusil M (Warner-Chilcott)	tablet suspension	—	300 mg/tablet 60 mg/ml	200 mg/tablet 40 mg/ml	—	simethicone, 25 mg/tablet 5 mg/ml mint flavor	2.8 mg/tablet 0.26 mg/ml
Glycate (O'Neal, Jones & Feldman)	tablet	300 mg	—	—	—	glycine, 150 mg	NS[a]
Glycogel (Central Pharmacal)	tablet	325 mg	codried with magnesium carbonate, 175 mg	—	—	—	NS[a]
Gustalac (Geriatric Pharmaceutical)	tablet	300 mg	—	—	—	defatted skim milk powder, 200 mg	NS[a]
Kessadrox (McKesson)	suspension	—	67 mg/ml	11 mg/ml (hydroxide)	—	peppermint oil sorbitol	NS[a]
Kolantyl (Merrell-National)	gel tablet wafer	—	10 mg/ml 300 mg/tablet (dried gel) 180 mg/wafer (dried gel)	10 mg/ml (hydroxide) 185 mg/tablet (oxide) 170 mg/wafer (hydroxide)	—	mint flavor	<1 mg/ml ≦15 mg/tablet
Krem (Mallinckrodt)	tablet	400 mg	—	—	—	magnesium carbonate, 200 mg milk base mint or cherry flavor	NS[a]
Kudrox (Kremers-Urban)	tablet liquid	—	codried with magnesium carbonate, 400 mg/ tablet 113 mg/ml	36 mg/ml	—	sorbitol solution, 0.2 ml/ml	16 mg/tablet 3 mg/ml
Liquid Antacid (McKesson)	liquid	—	67 mg/ml	11 mg/ml (hydroxide)	—	peppermint oil sorbitol	NS[a]
Maalox (Rorer)	suspension	—	NS[a]	NS[a]	—	—	0.5 mg/ml
Maalox #1 (Rorer)	tablet	—	NS[b]	NS[b]	—	—	0.84 mg
Maalox #2 (Rorer)	tablet	—	NS[c]	NS[c]	—	—	1.80 mg
Maalox Plus (Rorer)	tablet suspension	—	dried gel, 200 mg/ tablet 45 mg/ml	200 mg/tablet (hydroxide) 40 mg/ml (hydroxide)	—	simethicone, 25 mg/tablet 5 mg/ml	1.4 mg/tablet 0.5 mg/ml
Magna Gel (North American)	suspension	—	NS[a]	NS[a] (hydroxide)	—	peppermint flavor	NS[a]
Magnatril (Lannett)	tablet suspension	—	260 mg/tablet 52 mg/ml	130 mg/tablet 26 mg/ml	454 mg/tablet 52 mg/ml	—	NS[a]
Magnesia and Alumina Oral Suspension (Philips Roxane)	suspension	—	—	0.41 g/ml	—	aluminum oxide, 24 mg/ml sorbitol saccharin sodium peppermint	1.68 mg/ml
Marblen (Fleming)	tablet suspension	NS[a]	—	—	—	magnesium carbonate peach or apricot flavor	<0.8 mg/ml
Maxamag Suspension (Vitarine)	suspension	—	gel, NS[a]	NS[a]	—	—	NS[a]

Product (Manufacturer)	Dosage Form	Calcium Carbonate	Aluminum Hydroxide	Magnesium Oxide or Hydroxide	Magnesium Trisilicate	Other	Sodium Content
Mylanta (Stuart)	tablet suspension	—	200 mg/tablet 40 mg/ml	200 mg/tablet (hydroxide) 40 mg/ml (hydroxide)	—	simethicone, 20 mg/tablet 4 mg/ml	0.043 mg/mEq of acid-neutralizing capacity 0.054 mg/mEq of acid-neutralizing capacity
Mylanta II (Stuart)	tablet suspension	—	400 mg/tablet 80 mg/ml	400 mg/tablet (hydroxide) 80 mg/ml (hydroxide)	—	simethicone, 30 mg/tablet 6 mg/ml	0.043 mg/mEq of acid-neutralizing capacity 0.054 mg/mEq of acid-neutralizing capacity
Noralac (North American)	tablet	—	codried with magnesium carbonate, 300 mg	—	100 mg	bismuth aluminate, 100 mg alginic acid, 50 mg	NS[a]
Nutrajel (Cenci)	suspension	—	60 mg/ml	—	—	—	NS[a]
Nutramag (Cenci)	suspension	—	—	NS[a] (hydroxide)	—	aluminum oxide	NS[a]
Pama (North American)	tablet	—	dried gel, 260 mg	—	260 mg	—	NS[a]
Phillips' Milk of Magnesia (Glenbrook)	suspension tablet	—	—	76–87 mg/ml 311 mg/tablet	—	—	NS[a]
Phosphaljel (Wyeth)	suspension	—	—	—	—	aluminum phosphate, 46.6 mg/ml	2.5 mg/ml
Ratio (Warren-Teed)	tablet	400 mg	—	—	—	magnesium carbonate, 50 mg	0.6–0.8 mg
Riopan (Ayerst)	tablet chewable tablet suspension	—	—	—	—	magaldrate, 400 mg/tablet 80 mg/ml	≦0.65 mg/tablet ≦0.13 mg/ml
Riopan Plus (Ayerst)	tablet suspension	—	—	—	—	magaldrate, 480 mg/tablet 80 mg/ml simethicone, 20 mg/tablet 4 mg/ml	≦0.65 mg/tablet ≦0.13 mg/ml
Robalate (Robins)	tablet	—	—	—	—	dihydroxyaluminum aminoacetate, 500 mg	<1 mg/tablet
Rolaids (Warner-Lambert)	tablet	—	—	—	—	dihydroxyaluminum sodium carbonate, 334 mg	53 mg
Silain-Gel (Robins)	suspension tablet	—	gel, 56.4 mg/ml codried with magnesium carbonate, 282 mg/tablet	57 mg/ml 85 mg/tablet	—	simethicone, 5 mg/ml 25 mg/tablet	0.96 mg/ml 7.68 mg/tablet
Soda Mint (Lilly)	tablet	—	—	—	—	sodium bicarbonate, 324 mg peppermint oil	88.7 mg/tablet
Spastosed (North American)	tablet	precipitated, 226 mg	—	—	—	magnesium carbonate, 162 mg	NS[a]

Product (Manufacturer)	Dosage Form	Calcium Carbonate	Aluminum Hydroxide	Magnesium Oxide or Hydroxide	Magnesium Trisilicate	Other	Sodium Content
Syntrogel (Block)	tablet	—	codried with magnesium carbonate, 38%	20.7% (hydroxide)	—	—	7.6 mg/tablet
Titralac (Riker)	tablet suspension	420 mg/ tablet 200 mg/ml	—	—	—	glycine, 180 mg/tablet 60 mg/ml	0.3 mg/tablet 2.2 mg/ml
Trimagel (Columbia Medical)	tablet	—	dried gel, 250 mg	—	500 mg	—	NS[a]
Trisogel (Lilly)	capsule suspension	—	100 mg/ capsule 30 mg/ml	—	300 mg/ capsule 117 mg/ml	—	3.2 mg/ml
Tums (Norcliff Thayer)	tablet	500 mg	—	—	—	peppermint oil	2.7 mg
WinGel (Winthrop)	tablet suspension	—	180 mg/tablet 36 mg/ml	160 mg/tablet 32 mg/ml	—	mint flavor	2.5 mg/tablet 0.5 mg/ml

[a] Quantity not specified.
[b] Amounts listed as 400 mg combined hydroxides of magnesium and aluminum. Individual concentrations are not listed.
[c] Amounts listed as 800 mg combined hydroxides of magnesium and aluminum. Individual concentrations are not listed.

Anthelmintic Products

Frank A. Pettinato

Chapter 2

Questions to Ask the Patient

Have you had nausea, diarrhea, or abdominal pain?

Have you been bothered by itching in the anal area?

Have you lost weight or do you become fatigued easily?

How long have the symptoms been present?

Has the problem occurred in the past? How was it treated? Was the treatment beneficial?

If the patient is not an adult, what are the age and approximate weight of the patient?

Have worms appeared in your stool?

Are other members of your family also affected?

Have you seen a physician?

Anthelmintics are used to treat worm (helminth) infections. It has been estimated that 800 million to 1.1 billion humans, or more than one-third of the world's population, harbor helminths (1). The incidence of helminth infection exceeds 90% in primitive areas where sanitation is neglected, economic conditions are poor, and preventive medicine practices are inadequate. Helminthiasis is a serious health problem, particularly in the tropics, and results in a general debilitation of large populations. Efficiency, resistance to disease, physical development in children, and productivity are reduced by these infections. In the United States and other temperate zone countries these infections are considered to be more an annoyance than a major health problem.

Helminth infections commonly encountered in the United States are trichinosis, enterobiasis (pinworm infection), ascariasis (roundworm infection), and hookworm infection. So few effective nonprescription drugs are available for helminth infections that self-medication should be discouraged. Common human helminth infections and their symptoms are listed in Table 1.

The parasitic worms that infect humans include the nematodes (roundworms), the cestodes (tapeworms), and the trematodes (flukes). Roundworms are the most frequently encountered human helminthic parasites in the United States. Tapeworm infections are rare today. Various types are included in Table 1. No nonprescription drugs are available to treat tapeworm infections.

TRICHINOSIS

Trichinosis is caused by a small nematode (*Trichinella spiralis*). Although pork is the principal source of infection, about 10% of the cases reported in this country during the last decade or so were attributed to bear meat (2). In Idaho and California, 23 people were involved in an outbreak of trichinosis from this source (3). When infected meat is eaten, the action of the gastric juices frees the larvae, which penetrate the small intestinal wall. When they develop into sexually mature adults, the males and females mate, and the female deposits larvae in the intestinal mucosa. These larvae enter the bloodstream, are carried throughout the body, and enter striated muscle fibers, where they complete their development. The areas most often affected are the muscles of the diaphragm, tongue, and eye and the deltoid pectoral and intercostal muscles. Larvae that reach other tissues such as the heart and the brain disintegrate and are absorbed.

The incidence of trichinosis in this country as determined by autopsy fell from about 15% in the years 1931–1950 to 4% in 1951–1968 (4). This decline is attributed to laws that require cooking garbage fed to hogs, storing meat at low temperatures, and developing public educational programs on the need to cook pork thoroughly.

Symptoms

Symptoms of trichinosis are extremely variable, depending on the severity of the infection. If the meat is heavily infected, the invasion into the intestinal mucosa 1–4 days after ingestion may cause nausea, vomiting, and diarrhea. In some cases, no symptoms are evident. After the seventh day the migration of the larvae may produce muscle weakness, stiffness or pain, and irregular, persistent fever of 100–105°F (37.7–40.5°C). These symptoms may be accompanied by an urticarial rash and respiratory symptoms such as cough and bronchospasm. Skeletal muscle invasion produces muscular pain, tenderness, and often severe weakness. There may be pain on chewing, swallowing, breathing, or moving the eyes or limbs. Another common symptom is edema, usually manifested as a puffiness around the eyes involving the upper eyelids. When the larvae are encysted, the only symptom may be a vague aching in the muscles.

The clinical diagnosis of trichinosis is difficult because of the asymptomatic condition of most mild infections and because of the varied and changeable nature of the symptoms. A combination of irregular fever, periorbital edema, GI disturbances, muscle soreness, hypereosinophilia, and hemorrhages in the nail beds may suggest trichinosis. The pharmacist should refer patients with these symptoms to a physician for evaluation and diagnosis. Attempting self-diagnosis is unwise, since many diseases, e.g., sinusitis, influenza, and rheumatism, mimic the symptoms of trichinosis (5).

Treatment

Treatment includes mild analgesics for relief of pain, sedatives, adequate diet, and anti-inflammatory steroids. Thiabendazole has been shown to kill the larvae in experimental animals; results in humans have been

common infestations
thiabendazole

Table 1. Human Helminth Infections

	Common Name	Source of Infestation	Symptoms
Roundworm			
Ancylostoma duodenale, Necator americanus	hookworm	spreading by contact with contaminated soil; larvae are ingested or penetrate the skin on contact	anemia caused by blood loss (0.5 ml/worm/day); indigestion, anorexia, headache, cough, vomiting, diarrhea, weakness; urticaria at the site of entry into the skin
Ascaris lumbricoides	roundworm	ingesting eggs through contact with fecally contaminated soil	mild cases may be asymptomatic; GI discomfort, pain, and diarrhea; intestinal obstruction in severe cases; occasionally, bile or pancreatic duct may be obstructed; allergic reactions
Enterobius (Oxyuris) vermicularis	pinworm seatworm threadworm	ingesting eggs by fecal contamination of hands, food, clothing, and bedding; reinfection is common; the most common worm infestation in the United States, especially in school children	indigestion, intense perianal itching, especially at night, resulting in loss of sleep; scratching may cause infection; irritability and fatigue in children
Strongyloides stercoralis	none	most frequently by larvae penetrating the skin; rarely by ingestion	similar to hookworm infestation
Trichinella spiralis	none	ingesting infected, "rare" pork; particularly prevalent in the United States	adult worms in intestinal tract cause vomiting, nausea, and diarrhea; migrating larvae cause malaise, weakness, fever, sweating, dermatitis, and cardiac and respiratory distress; can be fatal
Trichuris trichiura	whipworm	ingesting eggs through contact with fecally contaminated soil	heavy infestation causes indigestion, mild anemia, insomnia, diarrhea, and urticaria
Tapeworm			
Diphyllobothrium latum	fish tapeworm	eating raw or inadequately cooked fish	similar to beef tapeworm infestation
Hymenolepis nana	dwarf tapeworm	eating food contaminated with human feces	similar to beef tapeworm infestation
Taenia saginata	beef tapeworm	eating "rare," infected beef	no characteristic symptoms; digestive upset, diarrhea, anemia, and dizziness vary with the degree of infestation
Taenia solium	pork tapeworm	eating inadequately cooked, infected pork	similar to beef tapeworm infestation

variable. It also has been effective in reducing the fever and relieving the muscle pain, tenderness, and edema of trichinosis (6). Corticosteroids for severe symptoms in addition to thiabendazole constitute the current recommended therapy (7). There are no nonprescription drugs for the mitigation of the disease.

ENTEROBIASIS

Enterobiasis is commonly called pinworm, seatworm, or threadworm infection or oxyuriasis. The intestinal infection in humans is caused by *Enterobius vermicularis.* Unlike many helminth infections, enterobiasis is not limited to the rural and the poor but occurs in urban communities of every economic status. *E. vermicularis* is common in temperate climates and is especially prevalent among school children. The female adult is about 10 mm long, and the adult male, about 3 mm. The adult worms inhabit the first portion of the large intestine. The mature female usually does not pass her eggs into the intestinal lumen but stores them in her body until several thousand accumulate, at which time she migrates down the colon and out the anus and deposits the eggs in the perianal region. Within a few hours each egg develops into an infective larva. Ingestion of the larvae releases them in the small intestine. Within 1 month from ingestion, newly developed gravid females migrate to the anal area and discharge eggs, and the cycle continues.

The most common way of transmitting pinworm infection in children is probably direct anus-to-mouth transfer of eggs by contaminated fingers and eating food which has been touched by soiled hands. Reinfection may occur readily, because eggs are frequently found under the fingernails of infected children scratching anal areas. The eggs may be dislodged from the perianal region into the environment and may enter the mouth via hands, food, or swallowing of airborne eggs.

Symptoms

Slight infections of enterobiasis may be asymptomatic. The most important and most frequent symptom is usually an irritating itching in the perianal and perineal regions. This itching normally occurs at night when the gravid female deposits her eggs in these areas. Scratching to relieve the itching may lead to bacterial infection of the area. Nervousness, inability to concentrate, lack of appetite, and dark circles around the eyes are frequently observed in pinworm-infected children. Worms occasionally enter the female genital tract and become encapsulated within the uterus or fallopian tubes, or they may migrate into the peritoneal cavity, resulting in the formation of granulomas in these areas.

The physical symptoms are not the sole misery-inducing effects of pinworms. Parents are often dismayed to find worms near the anus of a child, and this psychological trauma or "pinworm neurosis" also must be considered one of the harmful effects of enterobiasis (8).

Perianal itching is a symptom of many other conditions mistakenly attributed to pinworm infection (9). Seborrheic dermatitis, atopic eczema, psoriasis, lichen planus, and neurodermatitis may produce severe itching when the perianal region is involved. An allergic or contact dermatitis may result from soaps or ointments used by the patient in an attempt to alleviate the initial mild symptoms. Ointments containing local anesthetics are well-known sensitizers and should be suspected as contributing to the problem. Other parasitic infestations that induce itching, such as scabies and pediculosis pubis, may involve the perianal skin in addition to the larger areas of the body. Monilial infection may be the cause of pruritis ani in patients with diabetes mellitus. Other causes include excessive vaginal discharge and urinary incontinence in women and excessive sweating during hot weather. When mineral oil is used as a cathartic, it tends to leak and may produce increased moisture and itching unless good anal hygiene is practiced. Treatment should begin with an accurate diagnosis by a medical practitioner.

Treatment

pinworm
seatworm
threadworm
oxyuriasis

Prescription-only drugs (e.g., piperazine salts, pyrvinium pamoate, pyrantel pamoate, thiabendazole, and mebendazole) may cure 80–95% of pinworm infections. Pyrantel pamoate and mebendazole are the drugs of choice because of ease of administration and patient tolerance (10).

Gentian violet is the only OTC drug available for treatment of pinworm infections. The usual adult dose is 60 mg three times per day; for children, 3 mg three times per day for each year of age up to a maximum of 90 mg per day is recommended. However, it is questionable whether this OTC drug should be recommended in view of the efficient, easily administered, and well-tolerated prescription drugs available.

The overall incidence of side effects with gentian violet is 14–28%. Used orally, gentian violet may produce nausea, vomiting, diarrhea, and mild abdominal pain. It should be used with caution in patients with cardiac, hepatic, or renal disease and intestinal disorders. Although gentian violet is a dye and can discolor tissue and clothing, staining is not a problem with the coated tablets provided they are swallowed whole, not chewed.

Simultaneous medical treatment of every family member is advised for best results. The following additional measures are recommended to prevent reinfection:

- A daily morning shower to remove eggs deposited in the perianal region during the night;
- Regular application of antipruritic ointment over the perianal region at bedtime (avoid contaminating the ointment);
- Wearing close-fitting shorts under one-piece pajamas;
- Regularly trimming an infected child's nails and brush scrubbing fingers after going to the bathroom;
- Daily use of disinfectants on the toilet seat and bathtub;
- Frequent washing of the hands, especially before meals (10).

ASCARIASIS

Ascariasis is caused by *Ascaris lumbricoides* (roundworm). The adult ascarides are 15–35 cm long and live in the small intestine, where they receive their nourishment. The female lays eggs, which are passed in the feces and develop into infective larvae in the soil. Although the mature larvae in the shell remain viable in the soil for many months, the eggs do not hatch until they are ingested by humans. Upon ingestion, the larvae are released in the small intestine. They penetrate the intestinal wall and migrate via the bloodstream to the lungs, travel up the respiratory tree to the epiglottis, where they are swallowed, and develop into male and female adults in the small intestine.

Symptoms

The larvae and adults are capable of extensive migration and therefore induce diverse symptoms involving the respiratory and GI tracts in particular (11). The most common symptoms caused by *Ascaris* infestations are vague abdominal discomfort and abdominal colic (12). Occasionally, diarrhea is present. Children characteristically have fever. The symptoms may suggest abdominal tumor or peptic ulcer disease. Migration of the worms may cause intestinal obstruction which may lead to perforation, appendicitis, and peritonitis. Light infections may be asymptomatic; heavy infestations present symptoms that may be mistaken for a variety of respiratory and GI diseases.

cycle of ascarides

available prescription drugs

hookworm cycle

Allergic reactions such as asthma, hay fever, urticaria, and conjunctivitis also may result from absorption of toxins derived from the worm. Other respiratory symptoms may include cough, wheezing, and fever.

Treatment

There are no nonprescription drugs for treating ascariasis. Cure rates of more than 90% are achieved with piperazine salts, pyrantel, and thiabendazole, which are available only by prescription.

HOOKWORM DISEASE

Hookworm infection in humans is caused by *Ancylostoma duodenale* or *Necator americanus.* The adult worms, which are about 1 cm long, attach themselves to the small intestine. Their eggs are excreted in the feces, hatch in warm, moist soil, and develop into active filariform larvae. On contact with humans the larvae rapidly penetrate the skin, enter the bloodstream, and are carried to the lungs. They then enter the alveoli, ascend the trachea to the throat, are swallowed, and pass into the small intestine, where they develop into mature adults.

Symptoms

When the larvae penetrate the exposed skin, there may be an erythematous maculopapular rash and edema with severe itching. These symptoms may persist for

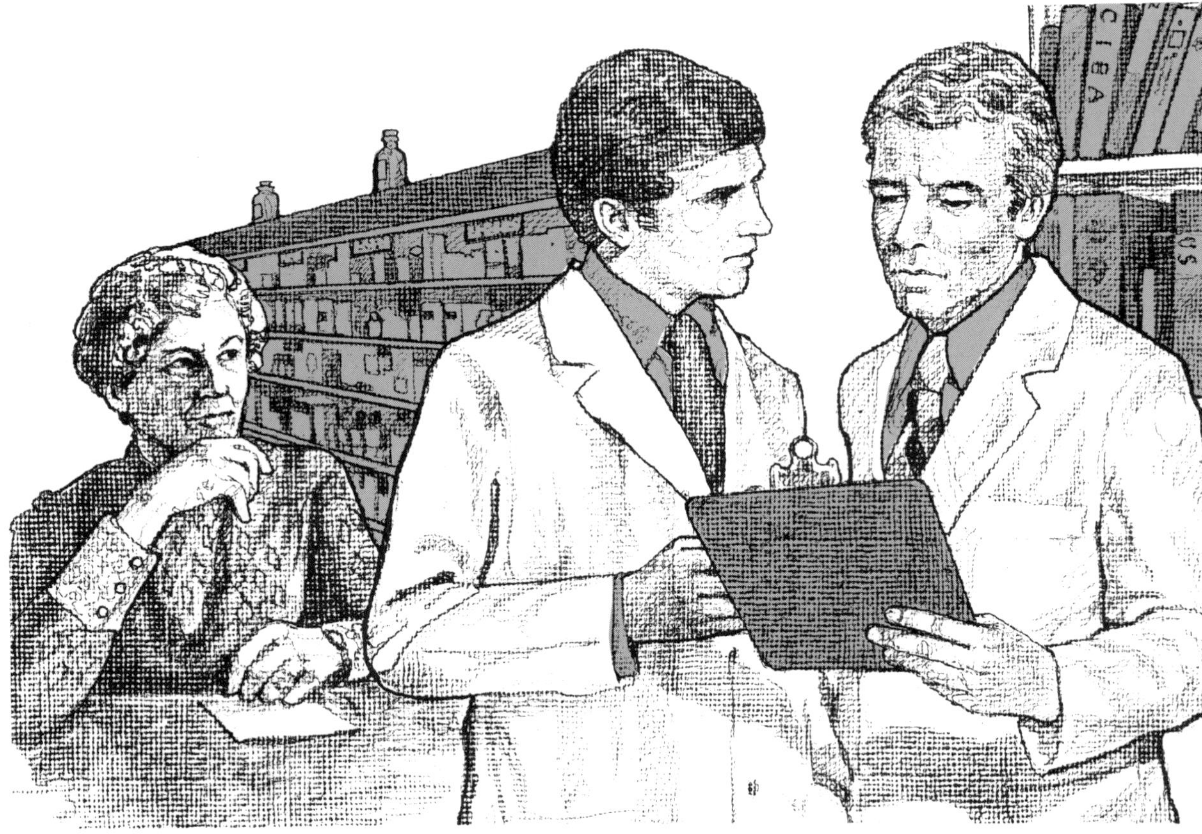

several days. The lesions occur most commonly on the feet, particularly between the toes, and have been termed "ground itch."

Heavy infestations may produce a cough and fever when the larvae migrate through the lungs. Mild intestinal infections may be asymptomatic; moderately severe infections may result in indigestion, dizziness, headache, weakness, fatigue, nausea, and vomiting. In advanced cases there is epigastric pain, abdominal tenderness, chronic fatigue, and alternating constipation and diarrhea. The epigastric pain is relieved by eating bulky food (13). As with ascariasis, these symptoms may be mistaken for those of some respiratory and GI disorders. A major clinical manifestation is iron deficiency anemia resulting from the loss of approximately 0.5 ml/worm/day of blood, which the adult extracts while it is attached to the intestinal mucosa. In areas where malaria and beriberi are common, these diseases must be differentiated from hookworm disease, or their coexistence must be established (11).

effects of hookworms

development of anemia

Treatment

tetrachloroethylene treatment

Tetrachloroethylene, a prescription drug, is effective in treating hookworm disease. It is given orally as a single dose of 0.12 ml/kg, with a maximum of 5 ml; two or more treatments at 4-day intervals are usually required to clear the infection (14). A light meal is eaten the night before treatment, no breakfast is given in the morning, and the tetrachloroethylene is given at 7–8 a.m. A relatively fat free noon meal may be eaten. (Fat aids in absorption of the drug, leading to systemic side effects.) Purgation is not necessary. The dose may need to be repeated in 4–7 days to assure complete removal of the worms. Alcohol should be avoided during treatment, since it may increase drug absorption.

Tetrachloroethylene has replaced carbon tetrachloride as an anthelmintic for the treatment of hookworm disease because it is much less toxic. In the absence of concurrent alcohol consumption it is claimed that this drug is not absorbed to any extent from the intestine (15). However, some absorption of the drug must occur, inasmuch as CNS depression has been reported frequently following its use. The depression is manifested as giddiness and inebriation. A burning sensation in the stomach, cramps, nausea, and vomiting often occur with tetrachloroethylene. Tetrachloroethylene should not be used in hookworm–*Ascaris* infections unless the *Ascaris* is treated first. The drug is irritating to the *Ascaris*, resulting in movement and possible tissue damage.

SUMMARY

The pharmacist should be familiar with the common helminth infections and their effects in order to discourage self-diagnosis and treatment. The clinical manifestations of these parasitic diseases are so general and characteristic of so many other illnesses that attempts at self-diagnosis of helminthiasis not only are difficult, but could lead to the neglect of a more serious condition. Diagnosis should be based on clinical and laboratory evidence.

Self-medication should be discouraged at every opportunity. The availability of effective, relatively safe, easy-to-take prescription drugs that can eradicate many infections in one or two doses should be reason enough to avoid self-medication. The pharmacist is the most available and capable person to encourage the patient to consult a physician for treatment.

REFERENCES

(1) "Drill's Pharmacology in Medicine," 4th ed., J. R. DiPalma, Ed., McGraw-Hill, New York, N.Y., 1971, p. 1822.

(2) "Harrison's Principles of Internal Medicine," 8th ed., G. W. Thorn, R. D. Adams, E. Braunwald, K. J. Isselbacher, and R. G. Petersdorf, Eds., McGraw-Hill, New York, N.Y., 1977, p. 1100.

(3) M. Wand and D. Lyman, *J. Am. Med. Assoc.*, *220*, 245 (1972).

(4) W. J. Zimmerman, J. H. Steele, and I. G. Kagan, *Health Serv. Rep.*, *88*, 606 (1973).

(5) S. E. Gould, "Trichinosis in Man and Animals," Charles C Thomas, Springfield, Ill., 1970, pp. 307–321.

(6) W. C. Campbell and A. C. Cuckler, *Tex. Rep. Biol. Med.*, *27*, Suppl. 2, 665 (1969).

(7) *Medical Letter*, *20*(4), 23 (1978).

(8) H. C. Wormser and H. N. Abramson, *U.S. Pharm.*, *2*(9), 46 (1977).

(9) D. L. Earnest, in "Gastrointestinal Disease," M. H. Sleisinger and J. S. Fordtran, Eds., Saunders, Philadelphia, Pa., 1973, pp. 1553–1555.

(10) "Drugs of Choice 1976–1977," W. Modell, Ed., Mosby, St. Louis, Mo., 1976, p. 362.

(11) "Harrison's Principles of Internal Medicine," 8th ed., G. W. Thorn, R. D. Adams, K. J. Isselbacher, and R. G. Petersdorf, Eds., McGraw-Hill, New York, N.Y., 1977, p. 1095.

(12) L. L. Brandborg, in "Gastrointestinal Disease," M. H. Sleisinger and J. S. Fordtran, Eds., Saunders, Philadelphia, Pa., 1973, pp. 998–999.

(13) *Ibid.*, p. 1002.

(14) "The Pharmacological Basis of Therapeutics," 5th ed., L. S. Goodman and A. Gilman, Eds., Macmillan, New York, N.Y., 1975, p. 1031.

Antidiarrheal and Other Gastrointestinal Products

R. Leon Longe

Chapter 3

Questions to Ask the Patient

Is the diarrhea associated with other symptoms such as fever, vomiting, or pain?

How long has the problem existed? Was it sudden in onset? How many times per day do you move your bowels?

Is there blood or mucus present in the stool?

Can you relate the onset of diarrhea to a specific cause such as a particular food or drug? Have you traveled recently to a foreign country?

Have you changed your diet recently?

Have other members of your family experienced similar symptoms?

Is the patient an infant or small child?

Are you currently taking or have you recently stopped taking any medications? Which ones?

Do you have diabetes or other chronic disease?

Have you tried any antidiarrheal products? Which ones? How effective were they?

Diarrhea is the abnormally frequent passage of watery stools. The frequency of bowel movements varies with the individual. Some healthy adults may have as many as three stools per day; others may defecate once in 2 or more days. The mean daily fecal weight is 100–150 g. A change from 150 to 300 g would be interpreted as diarrhea. The major factor contributing to diarrhea is excess water. Normally, about ". . . 7 liters of digestive fluid are secreted into the GI tract each day. This is made up of about 1 liter of saliva, 2 liters of gastric juice, 2 liters of pancreatic juice, about 1 liter of fluid from the liver, and 1 liter from the small bowel. In addition, another 2 liters enter the GI tract with food and drinks. Of these 9 liters all but one are reabsorbed in the small intestine. The large bowel reabsorbs about 850 milliliters of the remaining 1 liter, leaving about 150 milliliters to be excreted in the stool each day" (1). A disruption in the water absorption process that results in the accumulation of even a few hundred milliliters of water may cause diarrhea (1, 2).

Diarrhea is usually viewed and treated as a symptom of an undiagnosed and presumed minor and transient GI disorder. More than 50 conditions, including major diseases involving the kidneys, heart, liver, thyroid, and lungs, are associated with diarrhea. Diarrhea is not often the only symptom when part of a major illness (3–5).

TYPES OF DIARRHEA

If differential diagnosis and management of diarrhea are desired, a distinction must be made between acute and chronic diarrhea. Acute diarrhea is characterized by sudden onset of frequent, liquid stools accompanied by weakness, gas urgency, pain, and often fever and vomiting. Chronic diarrhea is the persistent or recurrent passage of unformed stools and is usually the result of multiple factors. The possible causes of acute and chronic diarrhea are classified below (1).

Acute
Amebic dysentery
Antibiotics
Carcinoma
Cholera
Diverticulitis
Escherichia coli toxin
Food poisoning
Giardiasis
Medication
Radiation
Regional enteritis
Salmonellosis
Shigellosis
Staphylococcal infection
Ulcerative colitis
Viral gastroenteritis

Chronic
Addison's disease
Bacterial overgrowth
Blind loops
Carcinoid syndrome
Carcinoma
Diabetic neuropathy
Dihydroxy bile acids
Diverticulitis
GI hormones
Gluten enteropathy
Hydroxy fatty acids
Hyperthyroidism
Intracranial disease
Irritable colon
Ischemic colitis
Lactase deficiency
Malabsorption syndrome
Parasitosis
Protein-losing enteropathy
Regional enteritis
Scleroderma
Stricture
Surgery
  Subtotal gastrectomy and vagotomy
  Gastroenterostomy and vagotomy
  Vagotomy and pyloroplasty
  Afferent loop syndrome from gastrojejunostomy or subtotal gastrectomy and Bilroth II anastomosis
  Ileal resection
  Short-bowel syndrome
Tuberculosis
Ulcerative colitis
Uremia
Villus tumor
Zöllinger-Ellison syndrome

The variability in the origins of diarrhea make identification of the pathophysiological mechanism difficult and may make a complete physical examination necessary, including supportive clinical laboratory tests. The causes of diarrhea can be psychogenic, neurogenic, surgical, endocrine, irritant, osmotic, dietary, allergenic, malabsorptive, and/or inflammatory.

Physiology of Digestive System

The small intestine originates at the pylorus and terminates at the cecum of the ascending colon (Figure 1). It is a convoluted tube, 6.4 meters long, made up of the duodenum, jejunum, and ileum. The small intestine is the site of digestion, absorption of nutrients, and retention of waste material; these activities depend on normal musculature, nerve tone, and digestive enzymes.

digestive system
alimentary tract
functions

The alimentary tract is basically a long, hollow tube surrounded by layers of smooth muscle—a thick, circular layer on the mucosal side of the intestine, a thinner, longitudinal one on the serosal side, and a third layer of both circular and longitudinal muscle fibers. The active contractions of the various muscles control the tone, or tension, of the intestinal wall. Normally, this tone is maintained with little expenditure of energy so that the muscles remain generally free from fatigue and capable of continued performance.

Lining the walls of the intestine is a mucous layer which protects and lubricates the walls. The mucus, composed of glycoproteins and sulfated aminopolysaccharides, is released from goblet cells interspersed among the columnar epithelial cells in the intestine. Secretion of mucus is increased by local irritation caused by foods or cathartics, and by psychic trauma, which suggests control by the autonomic nervous system. The mucus is more viscous in the upper part of the small intestine than in the colon and forms a protective physical barrier to the intestinal lining, reducing contact with irritating substances and bacteria. The alkalinity of the mucus further contributes to the protection of the intestinal lining by neutralizing acidic bacterial products.

Normal intestinal motility and peristalsis are maintained by the smooth muscles and the intrinsic nerves (Auerbach's and Meissner's plexuses). The vagus and

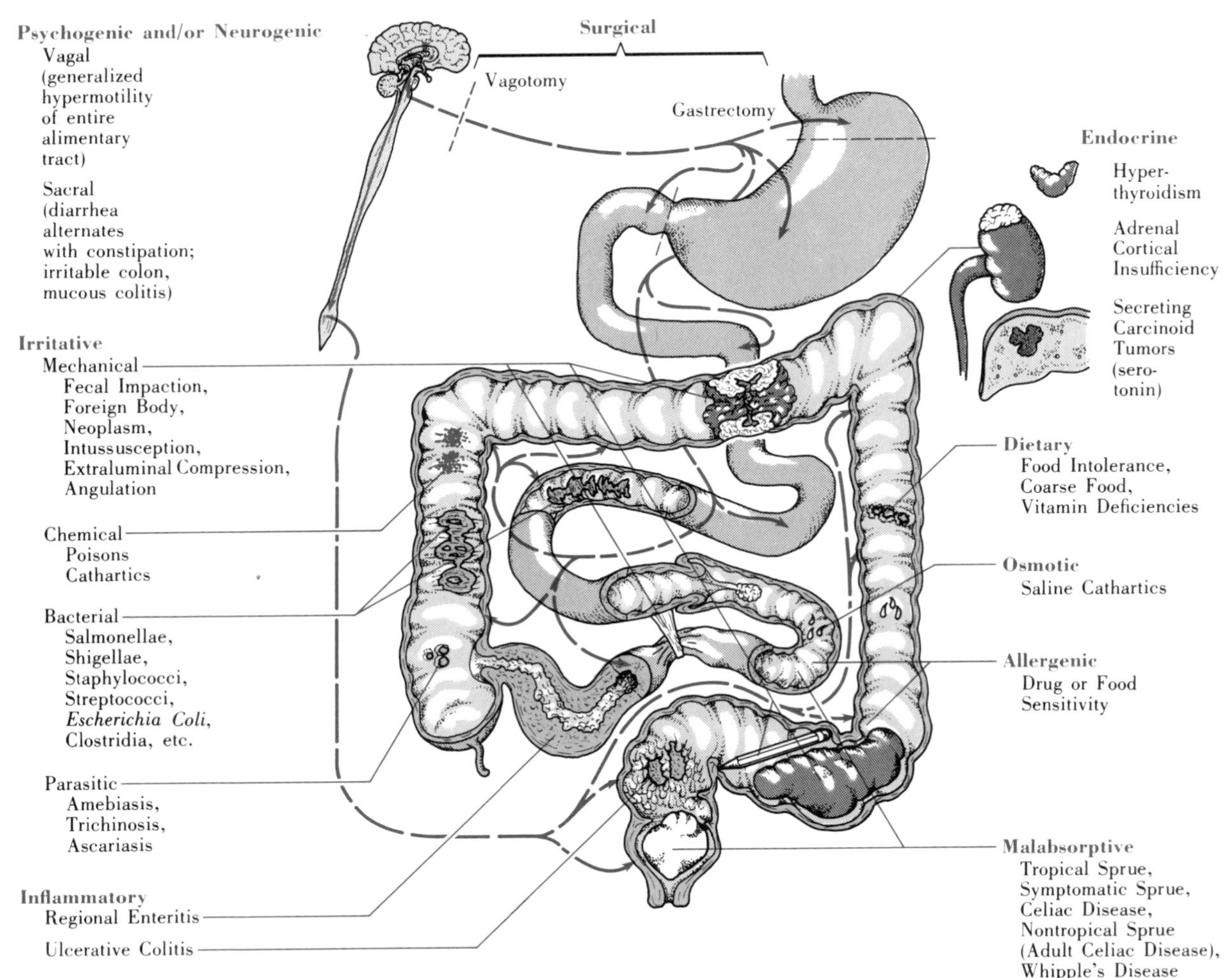

Figure 1. The lower digestive tract showing the induction of diarrhea by various causes. Adapted from F.H. Netter, *The Ciba Collection of Medical Illustrations*, Ciba Pharmaceutical Company, New York, N.Y., 1962, p. 99. Vol. 1.

parasympathetic pelvic nerves stimulate intestinal motility, whereas sympathetic innervation inhibits intestinal motility and secretion. Extrinsic autonomic innervation influences the strength and frequency of these movements and mediates reflexes by which activity in one part of the intestine influences another.

After eating, the lumen of the intestine is distended, causing the smooth muscle layers to contract. Normally, the segmental contractions of the circular muscles are accompanied by a decrease in the propulsive activity of the gut. This process retains the food in the lumen and increases the duration of its exposure to the digestive elements, enhancing digestion and absorption.

Approximately 3 liters of fluid containing electrolytes and nutrients enters the small intestine every 24 hours (4). Reabsorption reduces the quantity that reaches the large intestine to 1000 ml of an isotonic semiliquid substance (chyme).

The large intestine (about 1.5 meters long) extends from the cecum to the rectum. It is composed of the cecum, ascending colon, transverse colon, descending colon, sigmoid colon, and rectum. The colon has two primary functions: absorption and storage. The first two-thirds handles absorption, and the rest functions as storage. Chyme has an average electrolyte content of 83 mEq of sodium, 20 mEq of bicarbonate, 6 mEq of potassium, and 60 mEq of chloride (6). The proximal half (ascending and transverse parts) of the colon reduces chyme to a semisolid substance called feces, or stool. Feces is three-fourths water and one-fourth solid material, which consists of nonabsorbed food residue, bacteria, desquamated epithelial cells, unabsorbed minerals, and a small quantity of electrolytes (Table 1). The stool is stored in the descending colon until defecation.

The colon is structured like the small intestine with both circular and longitudinal muscles. The longitudinal muscles are shorter than the underlying colonic tissue and tend to draw the colon into sacs. The segmented contractions of the circular musculature further cause the division of the colon into sausagelike units which facilitate the churning of the colonic contents and the absorption of water. Thus a decrease in the occurrence or intensity of the segmental contractions and the predominance of the propulsive force of the longitudinal muscles may lead to diarrhea. In the absence of circular muscle contractions, mass colonic movements may occur during which the colon may contract to half its length and may resemble a smooth, hollow tube devoid of segmented units.

Colonic activity is increased by parasympathetic stimulation or by the administration of parasympathomimetic drugs or nicotine. Sympathetic stimulation inhibits colonic motor activity.

The normal bowel movement, or defecation, begins with the stimulation of stretch receptors in the rectum by feces. Peristaltic waves propel the feces to the anal canal where the voluntarily controlled external anal sphincter controls defecation (7).

In the colon, nonpathogenic bacterial flora produce enzymes necessary for degradation of waste products, synthesize certain vitamins, and generate ammonia. Bacteroides and anaerobic lactobacilli make up the majority of the colonic flora. Pathogenic organisms *Enterobacteriaceae* (e.g., *Escherichia coli*), hemolytic streptococci, *Clostridia*, and yeasts are also found, but only as a small proportion of the normal flora. Many factors such as diet, pH, GI disease, and drugs (e.g., antibiotics) influence the proportion of these organisms in the population. If their growth becomes uncontrolled, the increased proportion of these potential pathogens can present serious complications (8).

Table 1. Electrolyte and Water Content of Normal and Diarrheal Feces

Component	Normal[a]	Diarrheal[b]
Bicarbonate, mEq/24 hours	30	135–450
Chloride, mEq/24 hours	60	120–400
Potassium, mEq/24 hours	11.3	105–350
Sodium, mEq/24 hours	6.5	130–500
Water, ml/24 hours	111	3,000–10,000

[a] Adapted from *Documenta Geigy: Scientific Tables*, K. Diem and C. Lentner, Eds., Ciba-Geigy Limited, Basel, Switzerland, 1970, pp. 657–658.

[b] Adapted from "Manual of Medical Therapeutics," M. G. Rosenfeld, Ed., Little, Brown, Boston, Mass., 1971, p. 38.

large intestine
colon
normal bacterial flora
origins of diarrhea

Etiology of Diarrhea

Acute Diarrhea

Acute diarrhea may be of infectious, toxic, drug-induced, or dietary origin or the result of another acute or chronic illness. Of the infectious diarrhea type, most diarrhea in adults is bacterial; viral diarrhea is more frequent in pediatric patients.

Infectious Diarrhea

In the United States the bacterial pathogens most commonly responsible for acute diarrhea are *Salmonella*, *Shigella*, and enteropathic *E. coli* (9–11). Enteroviruses and adenoviruses are also suspected to cause acute diarrhea. In the majority of cases the causative agents are not identified. However, when a patient is first seen, the history often leads to identifying the source of the problem. For example, diarrhea developing in a number of patients within 12–24 hours after a common meal may be caused by a *Salmonella* infection. Fever, malaise, muscle aching, and profound epigastric or periumbilical discomfort with severe anorexia suggest an infectious, inflammatory disease of the small intestine. Severe periumbilical pain and vomiting are commonly experienced with viral gastroenteritis and are acute for 2–3 days, then gradually subside (12).

The treatment of diarrhea of infectious origin is based on combating the proliferation of the pathogen, generally with a prescribed antibiotic or other anti-infective agent and fluid support. In many instances the illness is self-limiting, and normalcy of the alimentary tract is restored, with or without treatment, in 24–48 hours.

Infantile Diarrhea

Diarrhea in infants and young children is common, and the etiology usually cannot be identified. It is often attributed to a viral infection of the intestinal tract; however, diet and systemic and local infections are other known causes of acute diarrheal episodes in children. Viral diarrhea has an abrupt onset, lasts 1–21 days, and produces a low-grade fever. The child frequently complains of upper respiratory symptoms. The disease usually is self-limiting and requires only symptomatic treatment.

Severe acute diarrhea, where water and electrolytes are lost in a short period, causes severe dehydration in children, especially infants. In the newborn, water may make up 75% of the total body weight; water loss in severe diarrhea may be 10% or more of body weight. After 8–10 bowel movements in 24 hours, a 2-month-old infant could lose enough fluid to cause circulatory collapse and renal failure. For this reason, moderate to severe diarrhea in infants should receive a physician's evaluation. The pharmacist must be cautious in recommending treatment for pediatric patients (13–17).

diarrhea in children and tourists

antibiotic-induced diarrhea

Traveler's (Turista) Diarrhea

The acute diarrhea that frequently develops among tourists visiting foreign countries with warm climates and relatively poor sanitation usually cannot be ascribed to known pathogens. However, a recent study conducted during the Fifth World Congress of Gastroenterology (18) found that enterotoxigenic *E. coli* was the most common cause of traveler's diarrhea in Mexico. It probably results from an extensive alteration in the bacterial flora of the gut caused by exposure, through food and drink, to a markedly different microbial population. Traveler's diarrhea is characterized by a sudden onset of loose stools, nausea, occasional vomiting, and abdominal cramping. Children seem particularly susceptible, and most cases develop during the first week of exposure to the new location.

In many parts of the world, iodochlorhydroxyquin has been used prophylactically to protect against traveler's diarrhea. The FDA recommended that the drug not be used for this purpose (19). Its conclusion is based on findings from Japan, Australia, and Sweden, implicating iodochlorhydroxyquin as the cause of a severe, subacute myelo-opticoneuropathy (SMON) (20). As a result, oral iodochlorhydroxyquin and diiodohydroxyquin were removed from the U.S. market (21, 22). There is no acceptable evidence that iodochlorhydroxyquin or other halogenated oxyquinolines, e.g., chiniofon, are effective in the treatment or prevention of traveler's diarrhea (23).

The FDA suggests that travelers to areas where hygiene and sanitation are poor may prevent diarrhea by eating only recently peeled or thoroughly cooked foods and by drinking only boiled or bottled water, bottled carbonated soft drinks, beer, or wine. Tap water used for brushing teeth or for ice in drinks may be a source of infection.

Drug-Induced Diarrhea

Drug-induced diarrhea is a side effect that frequently accompanies drug administration. All antibiotics produce adverse GI symptoms including diarrhea, but severity depends largely on the specific antibiotic. Antibiotics that have a broad spectrum of activity against aerobic and anaerobic organisms frequently cause diarrhea. Ampicillin, clindamycin, erythromycin, lincomycin, neomycin, and the tetracyclines are commonly prescribed broad spectrum antibiotics. Severe and persistent diarrhea has been reported by patients receiving lincomycin and clindamycin (24). Deaths have been associated with colitis induced by these drugs (25–29). Sigmoidoscopic examination reveals multiple elevated, purulent, plaquelike lesions; the surrounding mucosa may be erythematous, friable, or edematous. These antibiotic agents should be used only in serious infections when other less toxic antibiotics have not been effective. One report questioned the advisability of treating lincomycin-induced diarrhea with atropine–diphenoxylate or codeine because GI irritation was more prominent with these treatments (30).

Two processes may account for antibiotic-induced diarrhea. Diarrhea associated with the first few doses is attributed to mild irritant properties of the drug itself. Diarrhea beginning within a few days of the initial antibiotic therapy is due most likely to a disruption in the normal intestinal flora.

In general, orally administered antibiotics are not absorbed completely. The unabsorbed fraction of the dose may be irritating to the intestinal mucosa, cause alterations in intestinal motility, and induce diarrhea. Even the soluble antibiotics may cause irritation if they form strongly acid solutions, as tetracycline hydrochloride does. Some antibiotics, e.g., kanamycin and neomycin, affect intestinal absorption of nutrients, even at usual dosage levels (3).

Antibiotic-induced diarrhea also may be caused by a disruption in the normal intestinal flora or by an overgrowth of an antibiotic-resistant bacterial or fungal strain or a toxin-producing clostridium. Intestinal microorganisms that tend to proliferate during antibiotic therapy include *Staphylococcus aureus, Pseudomonas aeruginosa, Streptococcus faecalis, Candida albicans,* and species of *Salmonella* and *Proteus.* Except in cases of severe staphylococcal enterocolitis, a reduction in the dose of the drug, a change to parenteral administration, or the withdrawal of the antibiotic may relieve the problem. (Oral vancomycin and fecal enemas to restore competitive bacterial flora are indicated in staphylococcal enterocolitis.)

Other drugs, such as cathartics, which are irritating to the intestinal mucosa, may precipitate diarrhea, as may drugs that cause the retention of salts and water in the intestinal lumen. Certain antacid preparations contain magnesium to prevent the constipating effects of aluminum and calcium. Depending on the dose taken and the individual, these types of antacid preparations may induce diarrhea. Drugs that alter autonomic control of intestinal motility also may cause diarrhea. For example, it is not uncommon for the antiadrenergic, antihypertensive agents such as guanethidine, methyldopa, and reserpine to produce diarrhea. Generalized cramping and diarrhea may follow the use of a parasympathomimetic drug.

Food intolerance, caused by allergy or by the ingestion of foods that are excessively fatty or spicy or contain a high degree of roughage or a large number of seeds, also can provoke diarrhea. If diarrhea occurs in more than one person within 24 hours of ingestion of the same food, it is likely that a preformed toxin (food poison) has been ingested.

Chronic Diarrhea

Chronic diarrhea is usually the result of multiple factors and therefore can be difficult to diagnose. The pharmacist should refer patients with persistent or recurrent diarrhea to a physician. Correct causative diagnosis usually can be made only after a physician studies the patient's history carefully and performs a physical examination and appropriate laboratory tests. Chronic diarrheal illness may be caused by one of many conditions but is related generally to GI diseases.

Psychogenic factors are frequent causes of chronic diarrhea. Psychogenic diarrhea is usually characterized by small, frequent stools and abdominal pain. The stool may be watery and may follow a normal bowel movement or may appear shortly after eating. Psychogenic diarrhea is related to emotional stress which may lead to a periodic increase in parasympathetic nervous system impulses to the GI tract. It may alternate with constipation.

Some people who suffer from persistent diarrhea are aware of the cause and can manage the condition. For example, about 2.5% of adult diabetics and 22% of diabetics with evident neuropathy have chronic diarrhea. Individuals who have persistent or recurrent diarrhea and are unaware of its cause should seek prompt medical attention because conditions such as cancer of the stomach or colon or an endocrine tumor may be causing the diarrhea. One of the "seven danger signals of cancer" is a change in bowel habits. In both sexes, cancer of the colon and rectum is the most frequently reported type of cancer. The American Cancer Society estimates that almost three of every four patients might be saved by early diagnosis and proper treatment (31). A follow-up study of patients who had been suffering from "unexplained" diarrhea revealed the risk of missing a diagnosis such as neoplasm (32).

EVALUATION

The most common complaints voiced by patients with acute diarrhea are abrupt onset of frequent, watery, loose stools, abdominal cramping, fever, muscle ache, vomiting, and malaise. In chronic diarrhea the most significant finding usually is a history of previous bouts of diarrhea and complaints of anorexia, weight loss, and chronic weakness. These patients generally have histories of poor health.

In assessing the patient's complaint the pharmacist should construct the "anatomy" of a symptom by finding out:

- The patient's age;
- Mode of onset (events coincident, past episodes, acute or chronic onset, duration);
- The character and location of the symptom;
- Any factors that precipitate or aggravate the complaint;
- Any factors that relieve the symptom;
- Past treatment of the problem.

Evaluation of patient responses should enable the pharmacist to recommend an appropriate course of action.

Determining chronic diarrhea can be very difficult because it does not always involve frequent daily passage of watery stools. Three categories of chronic diarrhea can be described: frequent, small, formed stools with tenesmus (straining); large, oily, malodorous, formed stools; and frequent, voluminous, loosely formed stools. The patient may complain of weight loss, fever, anxiety/depression, nausea, vomiting, or perianal tenderness.

psychogenic factors

Alcohol abuse, ankylosing spondylitis, diverticulosis, emotional problems, gastritis, irritable bowel, and ulcerative colitis or regional enteritis are some frequently reported past medical problems. Referral to a physician is the rule and not the exception in such patients.

information needed

patients requiring physician referral

The pharmacist should obtain a history of present illness before recommending self-treatment. Four groups of patients with either acute or chronic diarrhea should as a rule be referred to a physician for a complete diagnostic evaluation:

- Children under 3;
- Patients over 60 who have a poor medical history;
- Patients with a medical history of chronic illness (e.g., asthma, peptic ulcer, or heart disease);
- Pregnant patients.

Clinical judgment must be used in evaluating these patients. For example, access to medical treatment may not be readily available, and temporary self-treatment may be needed until a medical appointment can be arranged. When a drug is implicated as a cause of diarrhea, the pharmacist should refer the patient to a physician, since the patient may need to continue taking the drug even though it is causing problems.

The medication history helps rule out drug-induced diarrhea. With this background, the pharmacist should find out about self-treatments already tried, the patient's age, symptoms, date of onset, and characteristics of stools (e.g., number, consistency, odor, and appearance). Stool character gives valuable information about diarrhea. For example, undigested food particles in the stood indicate small bowel irritation; black, tarry stool can mean GI bleeding; and red stool suggests possible lower bowel bleeding or simply the recent ingestion of red-colored food (e.g., beets) or drug products (e.g., Povan). Diarrhea originating from small bowel probably would be manifested as a marked outpouring of fluid high in potassium and bicarbonate. A pastelike or semisolid loose stool is indicative of colon-type diarrhea.

TREATMENT

Diarrhea is a symptom, and symptomatic relief must not be interpreted as being a cure for the underlying cause. Symptomatic relief generally suffices in simple functional diarrhea which is only temporary and relatively uncomplicated. More than 100 OTC products are available; however, the pharmacist should exercise caution in recommending their use in self-medication. Certain diseases that cause diarrhea might be serious or more effectively treated with agents specific for the underlying cause. The following statement is required by the FDA on all OTC antidiarrheal preparations:

> WARNING—Do not use for more than 2 days or in the presence of high fever or in infants or children under 3 years of age unless directed by a physician.

Table 2 summarizes causes of diarrhea and appropriate treatment.

Pharmacological Agents

recommended agents
paregoric
dosages
side effects

Some antidiarrheal drugs are directed against the symptoms of diarrhea, some against the cause, and some against the effect of the disease such as loss of nutrients or electrolytes. The categories of drugs generally used are opiates, adsorbents, astringents, electrolytes, nutrients, bulk laxatives, anti-infectives, digestive enzymes, intestinal flora modifiers, sedatives, tranquilizers, smooth muscle relaxants, and anticholinergic drugs. Many of the drugs used to combat diarrhea (e.g., opiates, anti-infectives, and sedatives) are prescription only.

In 1975 the FDA OTC Panel on Laxative, Antidiarrheal, Emetic, and Antiemetic Products published its report on antidiarrheal agents (33). According to the Panel, only opiates and polycarbophil were recognized as being safe and effective and thus not misbranded for OTC use. The Panel concluded that "adequate and reliable scientific evidence is not available at this time to permit final classification" of other ingredients submitted, including alumina powder, attapulgite, belladonna alkaloids, bismuth salts, calcium carbonate, calcium hydroxide, carboxymethylcellulose sodium, charcoal, kaolin, lactobacilli species, pectin, salol, and zinc phenolsulfonate. Generally, the Panel agreed that the agents are safe in recommended doses but believed that there was a lack of acceptable clinical evidence to establish their effectiveness as antidiarrheal agents.

Opiates

The opiates (opium powder, tincture of opium, and paregoric) are safe and effective in doses of 15–20 mg of opium or 1.5–2.0 mg of morphine (33). Most opiate-containing OTC antidiarrheals contain paregoric or its equivalent in the usual dose, 1 tsp (~5 ml) of paregoric containing 20 mg of powdered opium (2 mg of morphine). Several OTC products incorporate paregoric or its equivalent in a mixture with other ingredients. The pharmacist should check the labeled instructions to be certain that the preparation contains the recommended amount of paregoric per dose to achieve an antidiarrheal effect.

Because of their morphine content, paregoric-containing products exert a direct musculotropic effect to inhibit effective propulsive movements in the small intestine and colon. Thus hyperperistaltic movements decrease, and the passage of intestinal contents slows, resulting in absorption of water and electrolytes. In the usual oral antidiarrheal doses, addiction liability is low for acute diarrheal episodes because the morphine is not well absorbed orally and thus the low dose produces an effective local action in the GI tract but does not produce analgesia or euphoria. However, chronic use, as in ulcerative colitis (or acute overdose), increases the risk of physical addiction (34). Paregoric alone is a Schedule III prescription-only item, but it is a Schedule V item available for OTC purchase in combination with antidiarrheals that contain not more than 100 mg of opium (5 tsp, or about 25 ml, of paregoric per 100 ml of mixture). Opium derivatives are CNS depressants, and excessive sedation may be a problem in patients taking other CNS depressants concomitantly with the diarrhea remedy.

Antiperistaltic drugs (diphenoxylate and opiates) may worsen the effects of *Shigella* invasions. Symptoms may be prolonged in such cases (35, 36). This problem has not been reported with hydrophilic antidiarrheals (kaolin).

Polycarbophil

Polycarbophil is an absorbent which has a marked capacity to bind free fecal water. Paradoxically, it is recommended in the treatment of both diarrhea and constipation. In diarrhea, polycarbophil absorbs about 60 times its weight in water, producing formed stools; in constipation, this action prevents desiccation of fecal material and allows passage of soft stools. According to the FDA, polycarbophil is nontoxic and nonabsorbed, has no effect on digestive enzymes and nutritional status, and is metabolically inactive (33). For adults the effective oral dose is 4–6 g given in four doses (1–1.5 g/dose) per day. The dose is 0.5–1.0 g for infants under 2, 1.0–1.5 g for children between 2 and 5, and 1.5–3.0 g for children over 5 (33).

Adsorbents

The adsorbents are the most frequently used type of drug in OTC antidiarrheal preparations. Because large doses are generally used, most commercially available products are formulated as liquid flavored suspensions to improve palatability. Adsorbents generally are used in the treatment of mild functional diarrhea. The FDA Panel determined that while adsorbents are safe, there is insufficient evidence that these agents are effective in treating diarrhea (33).

Adsorption is not a specific action, and materials possessing this capability adsorb nutrients and digestive enzymes as well as toxins, bacteria, and various noxious materials when they are given orally. They also may have the effect of adsorbing drugs (e.g., lincomycin) from the GI tract. Although the systemic absorption of a drug might be expected to be poor from the GI tract during a diarrheal episode, its absorption may be further hampered by the concomitant administration of an antidiarrheal adsorbent. Thus a judgment must be made when drugs other than the antidiarrheal preparation are taken by the patient, perhaps for an unrelated condition. Depending on the medication involved, its usual rate and site of absorption, and the absolute necessity of attaining specific and consistent blood levels of the drug, an alteration of the dose

Table 2. Diarrhea and Its Treatment

Type	History	Symptoms	Usual Duration	Treatment	Prognosis
Acute					
Salmonella (infectious)	recent ingestion of contaminated food; affects all age groups	sudden onset of abdominal cramps, watery diarrhea, nausea, vomiting, fever; onset of symptoms usually within 12–24 hours after ingestion; infects perineal ileum and cecum	1–5 days	symptomatic; bed rest, fluid and electrolyte replacement; antibiotics (chloramphenicol) in life-threatening cases for 3–5 days	usually self-limiting
Shigella (infectious)	affects all age groups	sudden onset of abdominal cramps, diarrhea containing shreds of mucus and specks of blood, tenesmus (frequently), fever; infects small bowel (early) and colon (later)	4–7 days	symptomatic; bed rest, fluid, glucose, electrolyte replacement; antibiotics (ampicillin)	usually self-limiting
Escherichia coli (infectious)	affects children under 2 and the elderly in an overcrowded environment (e.g., hospital nursery or nursing home)	abdominal cramps, fever, tenesmus; infects mostly small bowel	7–21 days	fluid, glucose, electrolyte replacement	severe if not treated
Viral, infantile (infectious)	predilection for children and infants; usually occurs in summer and autumn; very contagious	abrupt onset, profuse, watery diarrhea, slight fever; frequent vomiting; upper respiratory symptoms	1–21 days	symptomatic and supportive	usually self-limiting
Traveler's	travel outside normal locus	sudden onset, nausea, abdominal cramps, tenesmus, fever, prostration	1–14 days	symptomatic and supportive	usually self-limiting
Drug-induced	broad spectrum antibiotics, autonomic drugs, laxatives, nitrofurantoin, antacids, antineoplastics, antituberculins, ferrous sulfate, colchicine	sudden onset, rectal urgency, abdominal cramps	variable	reduce dosage or discontinue drug	usually self-limiting
Chronic	history of repeated episodes, poor health history	weight loss, anorexia, mucus and/or blood in feces	weeks to years	depends on etiology	severe if not treated

From *Gastroenterology*, A. Bogoch, Ed., McGraw-Hill, New York, N.Y., 1973, pp. 33–38, 602–721; A. I. Mendeloff, in *Harrison's Principles of Internal Medicine*, 7th ed., McGraw-Hill, New York, N.Y., 1974, pp. 213–217; and S. M. Mellinkoff, *The Differential Diagnosis of Diarrhea*, McGraw-Hill, New York, N.Y., 1964, pp. 310–325.

summary of types of diarrhea and treatment

or the dosage regimen may be required. In some cases it might be better to administer the drug parenterally until the diarrheal episode is over and adsorbent drugs are discontinued.

Following the initial treatment, most antidiarrheal preparations containing adsorbents are taken after each loose bowel movement until the diarrhea is controlled. In instances in which the diarrheal episodes occur in rapid succession and for several hours, the total amount of adsorbent taken may be quite large. Because there is no systemic absorption of the adsorbent drug, the usual consequence is constipation.

The main GI adsorbents used are activated charcoal, aluminum hydroxide, attapulgite, bismuth subsalts, kaolin, magnesium trisilicate, and pectin. Adsorbents used with ion exchange resins combine their individual activities in relieving gastric distress and diarrhea. These agents are relatively inert and nontoxic except for possible interference with drugs and nutrient absorption. Kaolin, which has long been used in the Orient against diarrhea and dysentery, is a native hydrated aluminum silicate. Attapulgite is a hydrous magnesium aluminum silicate. It is activated by thermal treatment and used in a finely powdered form. Although it is seldom used as an antidiarrheal today, activated charcoal, which in a single gram has a surface area of about 100 m^2, possesses excellent adsorption properties and has been used for conditions of various origin, including cholera and infantile and nervous diarrhea (37). In a study of the treatment of acute nonspecific diarrhea, eight children, 3–11 years old, were treated for 2 days with either kaolin–pectin concentrate (Kao-Con), kaolin suspension, pectin suspension, diphenoxylate–atropine liquid (Lomotil), or placebo. The treatments did not appear to be effective in relieving the diarrhea (38).

kaolin and pectin
activated charcoal
bismuth salts
attapulgite

Pectin, a purified carbohydrate extracted from the rind of citrus fruit or from apple pomace, is widely used in the treatment of diarrhea, although its exact mechanism of action is not known. Pectin generally is found in combination with other adsorbents.

The bismuth subsalts such as the subnitrate and subsalicylates are used in antidiarrheal preparations as adsorbents, astringents, and protectives. However, subnitrate may form nitrite ion in the bowel which, upon absorption, may cause hypotension and methemoglobinemia. Bismuth subnitrate is contraindicated in infants under 2. Stools may become dark with use of a bismuth compound. According to the FDA Panel, bismuth salts are safe in amounts taken orally (0.6–2.0 g of bismuth subsalicylate every 6–8 hours), but data establishing the effectiveness of bismuth in diarrhea are deemed insufficient (33). Its effectiveness should be supported by well-controlled clinical studies.

In summary, the adsorbents—attapulgite (activated), charcoal (activated), kaolin, and pectin—are safe in the usual doses; however, there is insufficient evidence to classify these agents as effective antidiarrheals (33).

Anticholinergics

The formulations of adsorbents are frequently fortified by the addition of agents such as belladonna alkaloids (anticholinergics), making them prescription drugs. When the diarrhea is due to an increase in intestinal tone and peristalsis, belladonna alkaloids are effective "when given in doses which are equivalent to 0.6 to 1.0 milligram of atropine sulfate" (33). As a therapeutic rule, decreased intestinal motility is evidenced by a dry feeling in the mouth. However, in some available combination OTC antidiarrheal products the usual dose of belladonna alkaloids is less than the recognized effective dose. When these agents are combined with adsorbents, the possibility of inactivation by adsorption must be considered. Hence the FDA Panel recommends that "antidiarrheal products containing anticholinergics when given in doses which are equivalent to 0.6 to 1.0 milligram of atropine sulfate be available only by prescription" (33).

Anticholinergics have a narrow margin of safety, especially in young children. Their containers carry the following warning statement which should be reviewed before dispensing:

> WARNING—Not to be used by persons having glaucoma or excessive pressure within the eye, or by elderly persons (when undiagnosed glaucoma or excessive pressure within the eye occurs most frequently), or by children under 6 years of age, unless directed by a physician. Discontinue use if blurring of vision, rapid pulse, or dizziness occurs. Do not exceed recommended dosage. Not for frequent or prolonged use. If dryness of the mouth occurs, decrease dosage. If eye pain occurs, discontinue use and see your physician immediately as this may indicate undiagnosed glaucoma.

Lactobacillus Preparations

One of the most controversial forms of diarrhea treatment is the use of preparations of *Lactobacillus* organisms. The bacteriology of the intestinal tract is extremely complex, and it is difficult to explain many changes in the numbers and types of microorganisms. The flora of the GI tract plays a significant role in the maintenance of bowel function, in nutrition, and in the overall well-being of the individual. Antibiotic therapy often disrupts the balance of intestinal microorganisms, resulting in abnormal intestinal and bowel function. Seeding the bowel with viable *Lactobacillus acidophilus* and *L. bulgaricus* microorganisms has been suggested as an effective treatment for functional intestinal disturbances, including diarrhea. These microorganisms are believed to be effective in suppressing the growth of pathogenic microorganisms and in re-establishing the normal intestinal flora. However, the FDA OTC Panel states that a diet (e.g., milk or buttermilk) containing 240–400 g of lactose or dextrin is equally effective in colonizing the intestine without supplemental lactobacilli (33).

Other GI Disorders

The agents found in products recommended as GI "protectives" and antidiarrheal mixtures sometimes overlap. GI protectives are intended to soothe acutely irritated or inflamed gastric mucosa or intestinal linings resulting from the ingestion of an irritant or the contraction of an illness affecting the digestive tract. The following acute disorders may be treated with OTC protectives:

- Acute gastritis: Inflammation of the gastric mucosa is called gastritis. Acute gastritis occurs suddenly, occasionally violently, lasts for short periods, and involves the inflammation and erosion of the mucosa of the stomach.
- Acute erosive gastritis: This common disorder is caused by acute alcoholism, drugs (especially aspirin), hot spicy foods, allergenic foods in hypersensitive individuals (especially milk, eggs, and fish), bacteria or toxins in food poisoning, or an acute illness, such as a viral infection.
- Acute corrosive gastritis: This more serious disorder is caused by swallowing corrosive materials such as strong acids or alkalis, iodine, potassium permanganate, or salts of heavy metals. Such ingestion requires hospitalization and immediate emergency treatment directed toward removing or neutralizing the offending agent and providing supportive measures (39).
- Acute gastroenteritis: This condition is an acute inflammation of the lining of the stomach and intestine. It may be precipitated by excessive use of harsh cathartics, salicylates, and other irritant drugs.

The OTC products for relief of acute GI irritation and inflammation contain adsorbents, bulk formers, astringents (especially the bismuth subsalts), antacids, and GI analgesics. The commercial claims for some of the products refer to their ability to coat the stomach, reducing the irritation and inflammation. The report of the FDA OTC Panel on Antacids and Antiflatulent Products states that "the evidence currently available is inadequate to support the claim that such properties as . . . 'coating' . . . and . . . 'demulcent' . . . contribute to the relief of gastrointestinal symptoms" (40).

Patients also may be suffering from any of the following chronic GI disorders:

- Chronic gastritis: Chronic gastritis is an inflammatory reaction of the gastric mucosa. It may be associated with serious underlying diseases such as gastric carcinoma, pernicious anemia, diabetes mellitus, and thyroid disease, or it may be the result of chronic drug ingestion, e.g., aspirin.
- Colitis: Colitis is inflammation and pain of the colon. It is classified as ulcerative, amebic, bacillary, or pseudomembranous.
- Irritable colon: Irritable colon ("spastic colon" or "mucous colitis") is a motor disorder of the colon, resulting in abdominal discomfort and pain, usually with alternating episodes of diarrhea and constipation (25).

Patients with chronic conditions should be under a physician's care. Treatment is based on managing the underlying cause and avoiding the ingestion of agents that contribute to the condition. The medications prescribed may include prescription-only drugs such as antispasmodics and anti-inflammatory agents and OTC products such as bulk formers and mucilaginous products.

Many commercial products sold as "protectives" are thick, viscous suspensions which probably physically protect the mucous membranes from the irritating agents. The adsorbent drugs can bind certain offending agents. The drug substances that form bulk or thick mucilaginous fluids within the GI tract can dilute the concentration of the irritant, act as a physical barrier between it and the GI walls, and hasten the passage of the irritant toward the bowel.

PRODUCT SELECTION GUIDELINES

The information obtained during the patient interview and from the family medication record must be assessed prior to product selection. The treatment alternatives are an adsorbent such as kaolin–pectin mixture, an opiate-containing antidiarrheal product, or physician referral.

It is better to undertreat than to overtreat. No product should be recommended that the patient has tried and found unsatisfactory. A kaolin–pectin mixture should be recommended unless clear indications warrant a more potent pharmacological agent such as an anticholinergic or opiate-containing antidiarrheal product. OTC antidiarrheal products usually can manage mild to moderate acute diarrhea; severe acute diarrhea probably requires a prescription drug such as diphenoxylate, loperamide, or paregoric.

gastritis
gastroenteritis
colitis
irritable colon

The pharmacist should be contacted if control of diarrhea is not achieved in 24 hours. After this period a reassessment can be made, and another treatment chosen; i.e., the pharmacist should recommend continuing treatment for another 24 hours with the same or more potent product or advise the patient to consult a physician. If control of the symptoms is not achieved after the second 24-hour period, a physician should be consulted. Immediate physician contact is required if the patient is an infant.

The pharmacist should review the label contents as to appropriate dosage schedule based on the patient's age, the maximum number of doses per 24 hours, proper storage, and auxiliary dispensing advice (e.g., shake well before using). The patient must be questioned about special precautions on the label such as contraindications to use. Adjunctive therapy includes rest, drinking fluids, and appropriate diet. Physical and GI tract rest should be encouraged by advising bed rest and discontinuation of all solid foods.

Fluid and electrolyte losses are a primary problem, especially in infants, young children, and elderly patients. Commercial electrolyte formulas (e.g., Pedialyte and Lytren) might be helpful but must be used with caution because of possible electrolyte overload (41, 42). The diet should consist primarily of clear liquids (e.g., broth, gelatin, and fruit juices) for the first 24 hours and should progress to more solid foods as the diarrhea subsides.

SUMMARY

Diarrhea, frequent passage of unformed stools, is often treated as a simple disorder, but it can be a symptom of a more serious underlying disease. Diarrhea is either acute or chronic. Acute diarrhea is characterized by a sudden onset of loose stools in a previously healthy patient. Chronic diarrhea is characterized by persistent or recurrent episodes with anorexia, weight loss, and chronic weakness. Simple functional diarrhea usually can be treated with an OTC product.

The debilitating effect of persistent diarrhea is due largely to loss of water and electrolytes through excretion. The replacement of these vital fluids and electrolytes has become a part of diarrhea therapy, particularly in infants and children. This balance can be accomplished by the ingestion of the appropriate foods or by the use of proprietary oral electrolyte formulations which provide, in powdered form for reconstitution, a balanced formulation of important electrolytes and carbohydrates.

Complaints of GI irritation should be evaluated for their severity and nature (acute or chronic). For relatively minor acute problems, e.g., food or drink intolerance, relief may be provided by OTC protectives containing adsorbent, bulk-forming, or mucilaginous ingredients. All severely acute, uncontrolled, or chronic GI complaints should be referred promptly to a physician. The pharmacist can contribute to better patient care by being familiar with the disease processes involved in diarrhea and other GI illnesses and by appropriate selection and use of pharmacological agents.

REFERENCES

(1) E. Engler, "Dealing with Diarrhea," Science and Medical, Chicago, Ill., 1974.
(2) S. F. Phillips, *Postgrad. Med.*, *57*, 65 (1974).
(3) H. L. DuPont and R. B. Hornick, "Disease a Month," Year Book Medical, Chicago, Ill., July 1969, pp. 1–40.
(4) "The Macmillan Medical Cyclopedia," W. A. R. Thomas, Ed., Macmillan, New York, N.Y., 1955, p. 244.
(5) W. C. Matousek, "Manual of Differential Diagnosis," Year Book Medical, Chicago, Ill., 1959, p. 84.
(6) "Documenta Geigy: Scientific Tables," 7th ed., K. Diem and C. Lentner, Eds., Ciba-Geigy Limited, Basel, Switzerland, 1970, pp. 657–658.
(7) A. C. Guyton, in "Textbook of Medical Physiology," 5th ed., Saunders, Philadelphia, Pa., 1976, pp. 850–866.
(8) "Gastroenterology," A. Bogoch, Ed., McGraw-Hill, New York, N.Y., 1973, pp. 33–38, 602–721.
(9) G. F. Grady and G. T. Keusch, *N. Engl. J. Med.*, *285*, 831–841, 891 (1971).
(10) R. B. Hornick, *Adv. Intern. Med.*, *21*, 349 (1976).
(11) J. A. Shulman, *Current Prescribing*, 51 (July 1977).
(12) "Harrison's Principles of Internal Medicine," 8th ed., G. W. Thorn, R. D. Adams, E. Braunwald, K. J. Isselbacher, and R. G. Petersdorf, Eds., McGraw-Hill, New York, N.Y., 1977, pp. 210–214.
(13) S. M. Mellinkoff, "The Differential Diagnosis of Diarrhea," McGraw-Hill, New York, N.Y., 1964, pp. 310–325.
(14) "Pediatric Therapy," 5th ed., H. C. Shirkey, Ed., Mosby, St. Louis, Mo., 1975, pp. 505–509.
(15) S. Ware, *Lancet*, *1*, 252 (1977).)
(16) *Lancet*, *2*, 1126 (1976).
(17) J. O. Sherman and J. D. Lloyd-Still, *Drug Therapy* (hospital ed.), *2*, 52 (1977).
(18) M. H. Merson, G. K. Morris, D. A. Sack, J. G. Wells, J. C. Feeley, R. B. Sack, W. B. Creech, A. Z. Kapikian, and E. J. Gangarosa, *N. Engl. J. Med.*, *294*, 1299 (1976).
(19) *FDA Drug Bulletin*, 2 (May 1972).
(20) G. P. Oakley, *J. Am. Med. Assoc.*, *225*, 395 (1973).
(21) *Medical Letter on Drugs and Therapeutics*, *17*, 105 (1975).
(22) G. H. Schneller, *J. Am. Pharm. Assoc.*, *NS17*, 234 (1977).
(23) M. H. Merson and E. J. Gangarosa, *J. Am. Med. Assoc.*, *234*, 200 (1975).
(24) *FDA Drug Bulletin*, *5*, 2 (Jan.–March 1975).
(25) R. P. Hoffman, *Mich. Pharm.*, *14*, 36 (1976).
(26) A. J. Scott, G. I. Nicholson, and A. R. Kerr, *Lancet*, *2*, 1232 (1973).
(27) M. J. E. Harrod, M. S. Brown, A. G. Weinberg, W. N. Harkness, and J. L. Goldstein, *Am. J. Dig. Dis.*, *20*, 808 (1975).
(28) C. H. Ramirez-Ronda, *Ann. Intern. Med.*, *81*, 860 (1974).
(29) W. J. Ledger and O. L. Puttler, *Obstet. Gynecol.*, *45*, 609 (1975).
(30) E. Novak, J. G. Lee, C. E. Seekman, J. P. Phillips, and A. R. DiSanto, *J. Am. Med. Assoc.*, *235*, 1451 (1976).
(31) "Cancer Facts and Figures," American Cancer Society, New York, N.Y., 1975.
(32) C. F. Hawkins and R. Cockel, *Gut*, *12*, 208 (1971).
(33) *Federal Register*, *40*, 12924 (1975).
(34) "Opium Preparations," American Hospital Formulary Service, American Society of Hospital Pharmacists, Washington, D.C., Section 28:08.
(35) R. Wheeldon and H. J. Heggarty, *Arch. Dis. Child.*, *46*, 562 (1971).
(36) H. L. DuPont and R. B. Hornick, *J. Am. Med. Assoc.*, *226*, 1525 (1973).
(37) J. A. Riese and F. Damrau, *J. Am. Geriatr. Soc.*, *12*, 500 (1964).
(38) B. L. Portnoy, H. L. DuPont, D. Pruitt, J. A. Abdo, and J. T. Rodriguez, *J. Am. Med. Assoc.*, *236*, 844 (1976).
(39) "The Merck Manual of Diagnosis and Therapy," 12th ed., D. N. Holvey, Ed., Merck Sharp & Dohme, Rahway, N.J., 1972, pp. 673–731.
(40) *Federal Register*, *39*, 19874 (1974).
(41) H. F. Eichenwald and G. H. McCracken, *Med. Clin. North Am.*, *54*, 443 (1970).
(42) B. L. Nichols and H. A. Soriano, *Am. J. Clin. Nutr.*, *30*, 1457 (1977).

Product (Manufacturer)	Dosage Form	Opiates[a]	Adsorbents	Other Active Ingredients	Inactive Ingredients
Amogel (North American)	tablet	powdered opium, 1.2 mg	bismuth subgallate, 120 mg kaolin, 120 mg pectin, 15 mg	zinc phenolsulfonate, 15 mg	—
Bacid (Fisons)	capsule	—	—	carboxymethylcellulose sodium, 100 mg *Lactobacillus acidophilus* ≧500,000,000	—
Bisilad (Central)	suspension	—	kaolin, 370 mg/ml bismuth subgallate, 10 mg/ml	—	eucalyptus oil menthol methyl salicylate preservatives thymol
Corrective Mixture (Beecham Labs)	liquid	—	bismuth subsalicylate, 17 mg/ml	pepsin, 9 mg/ml phenyl salicylate, 4.4 mg/ml zinc sulfocarbolate, 2 mg/ml	alcohol, 1.5% carminatives demulcents flavoring
Corrective Mixture with Paregoric (Beecham Labs)	liquid	paregoric, 0.12 ml/ml	bismuth subsalicylate, 17 mg/ml	pepsin, 8 mg/ml phenyl salicylate, 4.4 mg/ml zinc sulfocarbolate, 2 mg/ml	alcohol, 2% carminatives demulcents flavoring
Diabismul (O'Neal, Jones & Feldman)	suspension	opium, 0.47 mg/ml	kaolin, 170 mg/ml pectin, 5.3 mg/ml	—	methylparaben propylparaben
DIA-quel (Marion Laboratories)	liquid	paregoric, 0.15 ml/ml	pectin, 4.8 mg/ml	homatropine methylbromide, 0.03 mg/ml	alcohol, 10%
Diatrol (Otis Clapp)	tablet	—	pectin	sodium bicarbonate	—
Digestalin (North American)	tablet	—	activated charcoal, 5.30 mg bismuth subgallate, 3.80 mg	pepsin, 2.00 mg berberis, 1.20 mg papain, 1.20 mg pancreatin, 0.40 mg hydrastis, 0.08 mg	—
Donnagel (Robins)	suspension	—	kaolin, 200 mg/ml pectin, 4.76 mg/ml	hyoscyamine sulfate, 0.0035 mg/ml atropine sulfate, 0.0006 mg/ml hyoscine hydrobromide, 0.0002 mg/ml	alcohol, 3.8% sodium benzoate, 2 mg/ml
Donnagel-PG (Robins)	suspension	powdered opium, 0.8 mg/ml	kaolin, 200 mg/ml pectin, 4.76 mg/ml	hyoscyamine sulfate, 0.0035 mg/ml atropine sulfate, 0.0006 mg/ml hyoscine hydrobromide, 0.0002 mg/ml	alcohol, 5% sodium benzoate, 2 mg/ml
Infantol Pink (First Texas)	liquid	opium camphorated fluid, 0.016 ml/ml	bismuth subsalicylate, 13.2 mg/ml pectin powder, 7.4 mg/ml	zinc phenolsulfonate, 3.5 mg/ml	calcium carrageenan, 3.6 mg/ml saccharin sodium, 0.27 mg/ml glycerin, 0.05 ml/ml alcohol, 0.014 ml/ml peppermint oil, 0.00016 ml/ml
Kaolin Pectin Suspension (Philips Roxane)	suspension	—	kaolin, 190 mg/ml pectin, 4.34 mg/ml	carboxymethylcellulose sodium saccharin sodium	glycerin lime mint flavor
Kaopectate (Upjohn)	suspension	—	kaolin, 190 mg/ml pectin, 4.34 mg/ml	—	—
Kaopectate Concentrate (Upjohn)	suspension	—	kaolin, 290 mg/ml pectin, 6.47 mg/ml	—	—

Product (Manufacturer)	Dosage Form	Opiates[a]	Adsorbents	Other Active Ingredients	Inactive Ingredients
Lactinex (Hynson, Westcott & Dunning)	tablet granules	—	—	*Lactobacillus acidophilus* *Lactobacillus bulgaricus*	—
Pabizol with Paregoric (Rexall)	suspension	paregoric, 0.123 mg/ml	bismuth subsalicylate, 17.2 mg/ml	aluminum magnesium silicate, 8.83 mg/ml phenyl salicylate, 3.3 mg/ml zinc phenolsulfonate, 1.7 mg/ml	alcohol, 8% carminatives
Parelixir (Purdue Frederick)	liquid	tincture of opium, 0.007 ml/ml	pectin, 4.83 mg/ml	—	alcohol, 18%
Parepectolin (Rorer)	suspension	paregoric, 0.12 ml/ml	kaolin, 180 mg/ml pectin, 5.4 mg/ml	—	alcohol, 0.69%
Pargel (Parke-Davis)	suspension	—	kaolin, 200 mg/ml pectin, 4.33 mg/ml	—	—
Pektamalt (Warren-Teed)	liquid	—	kaolin, 217 mg/ml pectin, 20 mg/ml	—	—
Pepto-Bismol (Norwich)	tablet liquid	—	bismuth subsalicylate calcium carbonate, 350 mg/tablet	—	—
Quintess (Lilly)	suspension	—	activated attapulgite, 100 mg/ml colloidal attapulgite, 30 mg/ml	—	—
Rheaban (Pfizer)	tablet suspension	—	activated attapulgite, 600 mg/tablet 140 mg/ml	—	—

[a] Schedule V drug: OTC sale forbidden in some states.

Laxative Products

Roy C. Darlington and Clarence E. Curry, Jr.

Chapter 4

Questions to Ask the Patient

For what specific reason do you wish to use a laxative?

Are you currently being treated by a physician for any illness? Have you had any abdominal surgery?

Are you experiencing symptoms such as abdominal discomfort or pain, bloating, weight loss, nausea, or vomiting?

What are the normal frequency and consistency of your bowel movement? How has it changed?

How much physical exercise do you get?

Have you attempted to alleviate constipation by dietary measures such as increasing fruit and vegetable consumption?

How long has constipation been a problem?

Are you currently taking any medicine other than laxatives?

Have you used laxatives previously to relieve constipation?

Are you allergic to any medication?

Laxative products facilitate the passage and elimination of feces from the colon and rectum (1). Because there are few recognized indications for their use, these products are misused by many people to alleviate what they consider to be constipation. Constipation is generally defined as a decrease in the frequency of fecal elimination characterized by the difficult passage of hard dry stools. It usually results from the abnormally slow movement of feces through the colon with resultant accumulation in the descending colon.

CAUSES OF CONSTIPATION

Constipation can result from the following factors:

- Neglect in responding to the defecation urge, which can weaken the defecation reflexes;
- Failure to acquire the habit of regular defecation;
- Faulty eating habits, i.e., failure to include enough bulk in diet;
- Environmental changes;
- Atony or hypertonicity of the colon;
- Hypertonicity of the ileocecal valve;
- Insensitivity of the defecation reflex initiated by fecal mass in the rectum;
- Mental stress;
- Excessive ingestion of foods that harden stools, such as processed cheese;
- Prolonged use of drugs such as aluminum hydroxide, calcium carbonate, opiates, and anticholinergic drugs (2);
- Laxative abuse;
- Surgical procedures (2).

Physiology of Lower GI Tract

The digestive and absorptive functions of the GI system involve the intestinal smooth muscle, visceral reflexes, and GI hormones (Figure 1). (See Chapter 1 for a discussion of GI tract anatomy.) Nearly all absorption (>94%) occurs in the small intestine; relatively little absorption occurs in the stomach or duodenum. Of approximately 6 liters of fluids per day ingested and supplied by secretions of the GI tract, about 1.5%, or 100 ml, is excreted with the feces (3).

Tonic contractions of the stomach churn and knead food, and large peristaltic waves start at the fundus and move food toward the duodenum. The rate at which the stomach contents are emptied into the duodenum is regulated by autonomic reflexes or a hormonal link between the duodenum and the stomach. Carbohydrates are emptied from the stomach most rapidly, proteins more slowly, and fats exhibit the slowest emptying rate. Vagotomy and fear tend to lengthen emptying time, and excitement generally shortens it. Most factors that slow the stomach emptying rate also inhibit secretion of hydrochloric acid and pepsin. When the osmotic pressure of the stomach contents is higher or lower than that of the plasma, the gastric emptying rate is slowed until isotonicity is achieved.

The mixing and passage of the contents of the small and large intestines are the result of four muscular movements: pendular, segmental, peristaltic, and vermiform. Pendular movements result from contractions of the longitudinal muscles of the intestine which pass up and down small segments of the gut at the rate of about 10 contractions per minute. Pendular movements mix, rather than propel, the contents. Segmental movements result from contractions of the circular muscles and occur at about the same rate as pendular movements. Their primary function also is mixing. Pendular and segmental movements are caused by the intrinsic contractility of smooth muscle and occur in the absence of innervation of intestinal tissue.

Peristaltic movements propel intestinal contents by

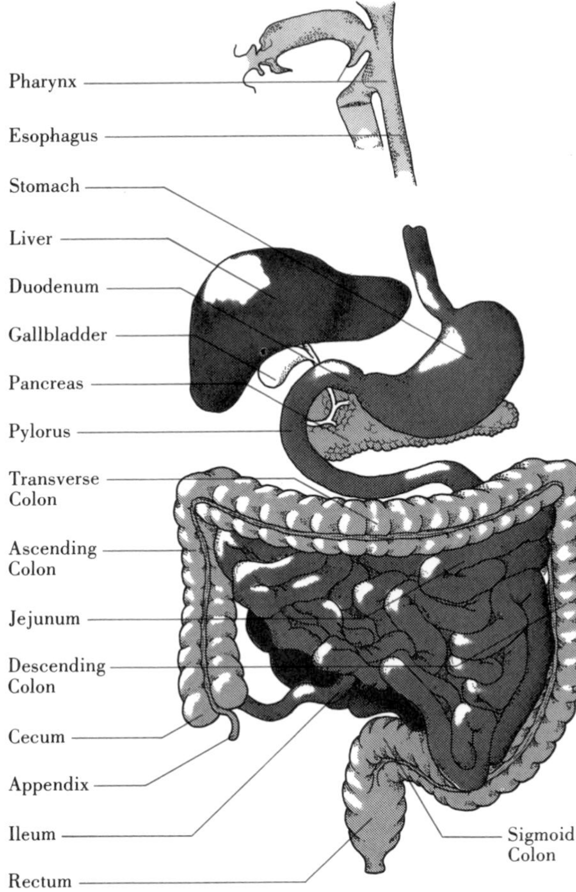

Figure 1. Anatomy of the digestive system.

peristalsis

colon

defecation

GI tract pathophysiology

circular contractions that form behind a point of stimulation and pass along the GI tract toward the rectum. The contraction rate ranges from 2 to 20 cm/sec. These contractions require an intact myenteric (Auerbach's) nerve plexus which apparently is located in the intestinal mucosa. Peristaltic waves move the intestinal contents through the small intestine in about 3.5 hours. Vermiform (wormlike) movements occur mainly in the large intestine (colon) and are caused by the contraction of several centimeters of the colonic smooth muscle at one time. In the cecum and ascending colon the contents retain a fluid consistency, and peristaltic and antiperistaltic waves occur frequently. However, the activity of the transverse, descending, and sigmoid segments of the colon is very irregular, and here through further water absorption the contents become semisolid.

Three or four times per day a strong peristaltic wave (mass movement) propels the contents about one-third (38 cm) the length of the colon. This normal reflex seems to be associated with the entrance of food into the stomach. The sigmoid colon serves as a storage place for fecal matter until defecation. Except for the fauces and anus, the entire alimentary canal normally functions involuntarily as a coordinated unit (4).

The presence of fecal material in the rectum is not sufficient in itself to initiate the defecation reflex; it must be large enough to exceed the individual threshold of the distention stimulus. The internal anal sphincter (involuntary smooth muscle) is relaxed when the rectum is distended. The nerve supply to the voluntary striated muscle of the external anal sphincter maintains it in a state of tonic contraction which, when relaxed by voluntary action, permits the reflex contraction of the distended colon to expel the feces. Defecation is a spinal reflex voluntarily inhibited by keeping the external sphincter contracted or facilitated by relaxing the sphincter and contracting the abdominal muscles. Distention of the stomach by food initiates contractions of the rectum (gastrocolic reflex) and, frequently, a desire to defecate. Children usually defecate after meals; in adults, however, habits and cultural factors may determine the time for defecation.

Pathophysiology of Lower GI Tract

Alteration in motor activities is responsible for disorders in the small intestine. Distention or irritation of the small intestine can cause nausea and vomiting; the duodenum is the most sensitive part. The motility in the small intestine is intensified when the mucosa is irritated by bacterial toxins, chemical or physical irritants, and mechanical obstruction.

Pain caused by functional disturbances of the jejunoileum is "referred" to the periumbilical region; pain in the midabdomen suggests a lesion of the small intestine. One of the most common disorders of the small intestine is the formation of gallstones in the gallbladder and bile ducts. The stones do not alter the function of the small intestine unless bile flow into the intestine is blocked, in which case, fat digestion and absorption are impaired (5). Diminished pancreatic secretion affects the digestion and absorption of fats, carbohydrates, and proteins.

The pain associated with regional ileitis is similar to that caused by appendicitis. The enterointestinal reflexes elicited from the pain cause inhibition of intestinal motility. As a result, functional obstruction often occurs in the small intestine, causing symptoms of acute intestinal obstruction.

Often, especially in older people, large masses of fecal material accumulate in a greatly dilated rectum. The loss of tonicity in the rectal musculature may be caused by ignoring or suppressing the urge to defecate. It also may be caused by the degeneration of nerve pathways concerned with defecation reflexes. Sometimes, enemas of fecal-softening laxatives may be necessary for defecation.

Painful lesions of the anal canal, such as ulcers, fissures, and thrombosed hemorrhoidal veins, impede defecation by causing a spasm of the sphincter and by promoting voluntary suppression of defecation to avoid pain.

The normal rectal mucosa is relatively insensitive to cutting or burning. However, when it is inflamed, it becomes highly sensitive to all stimuli, including those acting on the receptors mediating the stretch reflex. A constant urge to defecate in the absence of appreciable material in the rectum may occur with inflamed rectal mucosa (6).

Stress-producing situations or emotions may cause constipation, and many drugs may induce or aggravate it. These drugs include certain adrenergic agents, antacids, anticholinergics, antihistamines, diuretics, muscle relaxants, narcotics, rauwolfia preparations, and tranquilizers.

The main disorders of the colon, ulcerative colitis and excessive parasympathetic stimulation, and the chronic misuse of irritant laxative drugs may cause constipation or diarrhea. Some clinicians believe that ulcerative colitis is an infectious disease; others believe that it is caused by the digestive action of the contents of the large intestine on the mucosa. The irritation of the inflamed mucosa can initiate enough propulsive contractions to cause complete evacuation of the colon. A watery diarrhea may result.

Constipation of organic origin may be due to hypothyroidism, megacolon, stricture, or lesions (benign or malignant). Laxatives are contraindicated in such cases; proper diagnosis and medical treatment should be obtained.

EVALUATION

Signs and Symptoms of Constipation

The normal symptoms of constipation are slight anorexia and mild abdominal discomfort and distention. Constipation often results from chronic abuse or misuse of stimulant laxatives. Abdominal discomfort and inadequate response to increasing varieties and doses of laxatives are frequent complaints. Responses to questions may disclose that the patient has misconceptions concerning normal bowel movement (7). Although only limited quantitative data are available, one study indicated that the range of bowel movement frequency in humans is from three times per day to three times per week (8). Therefore constipation cannot be defined solely in terms of the number of bowel movements in any given period.

Patient Assessment

The pharmacist should try to obtain as much information about the patient as possible before making any recommendations for relief of constipation. It should be kept in mind that laxative products are both widely used and widely abused, and their use needs to be controlled. The pharmacist can apply the information gathered through the assessment process to make rational decisions based on good judgment, product knowledge, disease knowledge, and experience.

The first question that the pharmacist should ask is how the patient intends to use a laxative product. It should not be assumed that all patients purchasing a laxative are indeed constipated. The product might be needed as a result of an upcoming X ray examination of the bowel, or the purchaser may be securing it for a friend or a relative. It is important to know why the patient feels that a laxative product is necessary at the present time.

The pharmacist should find out the patient's symptoms and their duration. If symptoms have persisted for more than 2 weeks or have recurred after previous laxative use, the patient should be referred to a physician. Perhaps the patient has attempted to alleviate symptoms by dietary measures such as increasing fruit and vegetable consumption. This, too, is important information for the pharmacist.

Any patient who has an established disease affecting the GI tract presents particular concern. It is quite possible that laxative products used by these patients may affect their condition. The pharmacist should obtain accurate information regarding all diseases present. The patient should be referred to a physician when insufficient information or any doubt exists regarding disease states.

colon disorders

constipation

previous laxative use

laxative abuse

role of concurrent drug use

Although it has been suggested that the normal population experiences from three bowel movements per day to three bowel movements per week (8), individuals who fall outside this range might be classed as unusual but not always as abnormal. Thus the frequency of movements may not be the only relevant concern; the consistency of the stool and accompanying symptoms are significant as well (9).

The pharmacist should be equally concerned about the patient's current and past use of laxative products. The patient already may be using one or more products, but improper use may be preventing the desired effect. The possibility of laxative abuse also should be considered. Stimulant laxatives may be a cause of constipation in abusers due to tolerance development. An in-depth knowledge of the patient's history of laxative use provides the pharmacist with information about past patterns of drug use, effective or noneffective products, the incidence of constipation, and the use of home remedies. Depending on the pharmacist's findings, referral to a physician may be necessary.

Furthermore, all medication use by a patient is an important consideration of the pharmacist. Drugs with constipating tendencies (e.g., calcium or aluminum antacids and anticholinergic-type drugs) may counteract the effects of laxatives, whereas drugs with laxative tendencies (e.g., magnesium antacids and antiadrenergic-type drugs) may tend to intensify the effect of laxative ingredients. Pharmacists must investigate all drug use and exercise professional judgment in managing such situations.

In some cases, treatment for another ailment may relieve symptoms of constipation. In perianal disease, for example, constipation is usually the result of the patient's unwillingness to defecate due to the pain encountered. When medical and/or surgical treatment is given, the barrier to normal defecation is removed. Conditions such as hypothyroidism or depression may be responsible for a patient's complaint of constipation. Successful treatment of these disorders usually eliminates the constipation problems.

TREATMENT

Chronic constipation can often be alleviated without the use of a laxative product. The pharmacist should stress the importance of a high-fiber diet, plentiful liquid consumption, and regular exercise. However, treatment of acute constipation may require recommending a laxative.

Pharmacological Agents/Dosage Forms

Laxative drugs have been classified according to site of action, intensity of action, chemical structure, or mechanism of action. The most meaningful method is the mechanism of action, under which laxatives are classified as bulk-forming, emollient, hyperosmotic, lubricant, saline, and/or stimulant (Table 1).

Bulk-Forming Laxatives

polysaccharides
cellulose derivatives
polycarbophil
stool softeners

Because they approximate most closely the physiological mechanism in promoting evacuation, bulk-forming products are the recommended choice for simple constipation. These laxatives are natural and semisynthetic polysaccharides and cellulose derivatives that dissolve or swell in the intestinal fluid, forming emollient gels that facilitate the passage of the intestinal contents and stimulate peristalsis. They are usually effective in 12–24 hours but may require as long as 3 days. This type may be indicated for people on low-residue diets that cannot be corrected.

The hydrophilic colloid laxatives do not seem to interfere with the absorption of nutrients. They should be mixed with cold water or fruit juice just before ingestion and administered with a large amount of fluid. When they are administered properly, these agents are essentially free from systemic side effects because they are not absorbed. Esophageal obstruction has occurred in patients with strictures of the esophagus when these drugs are chewed or taken in dry form. Because of the danger of fecal impaction or intestinal obstruction, the bulk-forming laxatives should not be taken by individuals with intestinal ulcerations, stenosis, or disabling adhesions or by those who have difficulty in swallowing.

The bulk-forming drugs are derived from agar, plantago seed, kelp (alginates), and plant gums (tragacanth, chondrus, sterculia, karaya, and others). The synthetic cellulose derivatives—methylcellulose and carboxymethylcellulose sodium—are being used more frequently, and many preparations that contain these drugs also contain stimulant and/or fecal-softening laxative drugs. Polycarbophil is a synthetic cross-linked polyacrylic acid that is less frequently used.

It has been observed that making a specific choice among the different bulk products is relatively unimportant (10). More important is that each dose be taken with a full glass of water (at least 240 ml, or 8 ounces). The dose should be adjusted until the required effect has been obtained. In addition to being relatively safe, bulk-forming laxatives are suitable should long-term therapy become necessary (11).

Bulk-forming laxatives may interact and combine with other drugs, including salicylates and digitalis glycosides. They should not be taken at the same time with prescription drugs or drugs that contain a salicylate compound (12).

Emollient Laxatives

Dioctyl sodium sulfosuccinate is a surfactant which, when administered orally, increases the wetting efficiency of intestinal water and promotes the formation of oil-in-water emulsions. It facilitates admixture of aqueous and fatty substances to soften the fecal mass. Dioctyl sodium sulfosuccinate does not retard absorption of nutrients from the intestinal tract. In many cases of fecal impaction, a solution of dioctyl sodium sulfosuccinate is added to the enema fluid. Dioctyl sodium sulfosuccinate and its congeners are claimed to be nonabsorbable, nontoxic, and pharmacologically inert.

Other fecal-softening laxatives are dioctyl calcium sulfosuccinate (anionic surfactant), dioctyl potassium sulfosuccinate (anionic surfactant), and poloxamer 188 (nonionic surfactant). The latter has no irritant properties and is compatible with electrolytes. All three may be used when the sodium ion is contraindicated.

Emollient laxatives should be used only for short-term therapy (less than 1 week without physician consultation) where hard fecal masses are present: either in acute perianal disease where elimination of painful stools is desired or where the avoidance of straining at the stool is desirable.

A recognizable risk of hepatotoxicty may exist when stool softeners are used in combination with other medications (13). For example, dioctyl sodium sulfosuccinate may allow the absorption of other normally unabsorbed laxatives (14). Reports have indicated that daily use for 8 months or longer of preparations containing dioctyl sodium sulfosuccinate and oxyphenisatin acetate may produce chronic active liver disease with the attendant symptoms, including jaundice (15–18). As a result of these reports and other recommendations, laxatives containing oxyphenisatin acetate have been removed from the market (19).

Patients with hernia, severe hypertension, or cardiovascular disease should not strain to defecate; neither should those who are about to undergo or have undergone surgery for hemorrhoids or other anorectal disorders. An emollient or fecal-softening laxative is indicated in such cases.

Enemas

Enemas are used routinely to prepare patients for surgery, child delivery, and radiological examination and in certain cases of constipation. The enema fluid determines the mechanism by which evacuation is produced. Tap water, normal saline, and milk create bulk by an osmotic volume effect; vegetable oils lubricate, soften, and facilitate the passage of hardened fecal matter; and soapsuds produce defecation by their irritant action.

The popular sodium phosphate–sodium biphosphate preparations fall into the category of saline laxatives. They are usually effective evacuants in preparing patients for surgical, diagnostic, or other procedures involving the bowel and are also useful as cleansing preparations.

These agents can alter fluid and electrolyte balance significantly if they are used on a prolonged basis. Consequently, chronic use of these products in the control of simple constipation is not warranted.

A properly administered enema cleans only the distal colon, most nearly approximating a normal bowel movement (20). Proper administration requires that the diagnosis, the enema fluid, and the technique of administration be correct. Improperly administered, an enema can produce fluid and electrolyte imbalances. A misdirected or inadequately lubricated nozzle may cause abrasion of the anal canal and rectal wall or colonic perforation.

Enema fluids have caused mucosal changes or spasm of the intestinal wall. Water intoxication has resulted from the use of tap water or soapsuds enemas in the presence of megacolon (21).

To administer an enema properly, the patient should be reclining horizontally on the side; using an enema in a sitting position clears only the rectum of fecal material. The container holding the fluid should be 2.5–5 cm above the buttocks to allow free but not forcible flow of the fluid from the tube. One pint (500 ml) of properly introduced fluid usually causes adequate evacuation, if it is retained until definite lower abdominal cramping is felt. Two or three pints of nonirritating fluid usually produce a clean bowel and a nonirritated mucosa.

Hyperosmotic Agents

Glycerin suppositories are available for infants and adults and for many years were the main suppositories for lower bowel evacuation. In infants the physical manipulation usually will initiate the reflex to defecate (22), and because of this property, adverse reactions and side effects are minimal. The laxative effect of glycerin suppositories is due to the combination of glycerin's osmotic effect with the soap's irritant effect.

Lubricant Laxatives

Liquid petrolatum and certain digestible plant oils (e.g., olive oil) soften fecal contents by coating them and thus preventing colonic absorption of fecal water. There is little difference in their cathartic efficacy, although emulsions of mineral oil penetrate and soften fecal matter more effectively than nonemulsified preparations. Liquid petrolatum is useful when it is used judiciously in cases that require the maintenance of a soft stool to avoid straining, e.g., after a hemorrhoidectomy or abdominal surgery or in cases of hernia, aneurysm, hypertension, and cerebrovascular accident. However, routine use in these cases is probably not indicated. Stool softeners such as dioctyl sodium sulfosuccinate are probably better agents for these conditions.

The side effects and toxicity of mineral oil are associated with repeated and prolonged use. Significant absorption of mineral oil may occur: the oil is readily apparent in the mesenteric lymph nodes and may also be present in the intestinal mucosa, liver, and spleen, where liquid petrolatum elicits a typical foreign body reaction characterized by cells of chronic inflammation, including giant cells.

Lipid pneumonia may result from the oral ingestion and subsequent aspiration of mineral oil. The pharynx becomes coated with the oil, and droplets gain access to the trachea and the posterior part of the lower lobes of the lungs. The effect of mineral oil on the absorption of fat-soluble nutrients is controversial, but there is apparently sufficient evidence to make this property significant. The absorption of vitamins A and D may be reduced. Impaired vitamin D absorption may affect the absorption of calcium and phosphates.

Mineral oil should not be taken with meals because it may delay gastric emptying. If large doses are taken, the oil may leak through the anal sphincter. This leakage may produce anal pruritus, hemorrhoids, cryptitis, and other perianal disease and can be avoided by reducing the dose, dividing the dose, or using a stable emulsion of mineral oil. Prolonged use should be avoided. Because of the tendency of surfactants to increase the absorption of "nonabsorbable" drugs, mineral oil should not be taken with surfactant fecal softeners. Because of the greater possibility of aspiration in the very young and elderly, mineral oil is not recommended for use in these age groups.

enemas
glycerin
mineral oil

Saline Laxatives

The active constituents of saline laxatives are relatively nonabsorbable cations and anions such as magnesium and sulfate ions. The intestinal wall, acting as a semipermeable membrane to the magnesium, sulfate, tartrate, phosphate, and citrate ions, osmotically causes the retention of water in the intestinal lumen. The increased intraluminal pressure exerts a mechanical stimulus which increases intestinal motility. However, reports suggest that different mechanisms, independent of osmotic effect, also are responsible for the laxative properties of the salts. Saline laxatives have a complex series of actions, both secretory and motor, on the GI tract. For example, the action of magnesium sulfate on the GI tract is similar to that of cholecystokinin-pancreozymin (CCK-PZ). There is evidence that this hormone is released from the intestinal mucosa when saline laxatives are administered (23).

Saline laxatives are indicated for routine use only in acute evacuation of the bowel (e.g., preparation for endoscopic examination and elimination of drugs in suspected poisonings) and in ridding the gut of blood such as occurs in hepatic coma. Drugs such as these do not have a place in the long-term management of constipation.

In cases of food or drug poisoning the saline laxatives are used in purging doses. Magnesium sulfate is recommended except in cases of depressed CNS activity or renal dysfunction (2).

There are cases where the injudicious choice of a saline laxative results in serious side effects. As much as 20% of the administered magnesium ion may be absorbed from magnesium salts. If renal function is normal, the absorbed ion is excreted so rapidly that no change in the blood level of the ion can be detected. If the renal function is impaired, however, toxic concentrations of the magnesium ion accumulate in the extracellular body fluids. Magnesium exerts a depressant effect

laxatives, summary of types and properties

Table 1. Classification and Properties of Laxatives

Agent	Dosage Form	Daily Dosage Range: Adult	Daily Dosage Range: Pediatric (Age)	Site of Action	Approximate Time Required for Action
Bulk-Forming					
Methylcellulose	solid	4–6 g	1–1.5 g (>6)	small and large intestines	12–72 hours
Carboxymethyl-cellulose sodium	solid	4–6 g	1–1.5 g (>6)	small and large intestines	12–72 hours
Polycarbophil	solid	4–6 g	0.5–1.0 g (<2) 1–1.5 g (2–5) 1.5–3.0 g (6–12)	small and large intestines	12–72 hours
Plantago seeds	solid	2.5–30 g	1.25–15 g (>6)	small and large intestines	12–72 hours
Emollient					
Dioctyl calcium sulfosuccinate	solid	0.05–0.36 g	0.025 g (<2) 0.05–0.150 g (≧2)	small and large intestines	12–72 hours
Dioctyl sodium sulfosuccinate	solid	0.05–0.36 g	0.02–0.05 g (<2) 0.05–0.15 g (≧2)	small and large intestines	12–72 hours
Dioctyl potassium sulfosuccinate	solid (rectal)	0.05–0.25 g	0.1 g (children)	colon	2–15 min
Hyperosmotic: glycerin	suppository	3 g	1.15 g (<6)	colon	0.25–1 hour
Lubricant: mineral oil	liquid (oral)	15–45 ml	10–15 ml (>6)	colon	6–8 hours
Saline					
Magnesium citrate	solid	11–18 g	2.5–5.0 g (2–5)	small and large intestines	0.5–3 hours
Magnesium hydroxide	solid	2.4–4.8 g	0.4–1.2 g (2–5) 1.2–2.4 g (≧6)	small and large intestines	0.5–3 hours
Magnesium sulfate	solid	10–30 g	2.5–5.0 g (2–5) 5.0–10.0 g (≧6)	small and large intestines	0.5–3 hours
Dibasic sodium phosphate	solid (oral) solid (rectal)	1.9–3.8 g 3.8 g	¼ adult dose (5–10) ½ adult dose (≧10) ½ adult dose (>2)	small and large intestines colon (rectal)	0.5–3 hours 2–15 min

Table 1. Continued

Agent	Dosage Form	Daily Dosage Range: Adult	Daily Dosage Range: Pediatric (Age)	Site of Action	Approximate Time Required for Action
Monobasic sodium phosphate	solid (oral)	8.3–16.6 g	¼ adult dose (5–10) ½ adult dose (≧ 10)	small and large intestines	0.5–3 hours
	solid (rectal)	16.6 g	½ adult dose (>2)	colon	2–15 min
Sodium biphosphate	solid (oral)	9.6–19.2 g	¼ adult dose (5–10) ¼ adult dose (≧ 10)	small and large intestines	0.5–3 hours
	solid (rectal)	19.2 g	½ adult dose (>2)	small and large intestines	2–15 min
Stimulants					
Anthraquinones					
Aloe	solid	0.12–0.25 g	not recommended (<6) 0.04–0.08 g (6–8)	colon	8–12 hours
Cascara sagrada	fluidextract	0.5–1.5 ml	—	colon	6–8 hours
	aromatic fluidextract	2–6 ml	¼ adult dose (<2)		
	bark	0.3–1.0 g	—		
	extract	0.2–0.4 ml	½ adult dose (2–12)		
	casanthranol	0.03–0.09 ml	—		
Danthron	solid	0.075–0.15 g	not recommended (<12)	colon	8 hours
Senna	powder	0.5–2.0 g	⅛ adult dose (<2)	colon	6–10 hours
	fluidextract	2.0 ml	—		
	syrup	8.0 ml	¼ adult dose (1–6)		
	fruit extract	3.4–4.0 ml	½ adult dose (6–12)		
Sennosides A and B	solid	0.012–0.036 g	0.0015–0.018 g	colon	6–10 hours
Diphenylmethanes					
Bisacodyl	tablet	0.005–0.015 g	0.005 g (>3)	colon	6–10 hours
Phenolphthalein	solid	0.03–0.27 g	not recommended (<2) 0.015–0.020 g (2–6) 0.03–0.06 g (<6)	colon	6–8 hours
Miscellaneous: castor oil	liquid	15–60 ml	1–5 ml (<2) 5–15 ml (2–12)	small intestines	2–6 hours

laxatives, summary of types and properties

anthraquinones

emodin

on the CNS and neuromuscular activity. Cathartics that contain sodium may be toxic to individuals with edema and congestive heart disease. Since dehydration may occur from the repeated use of hypertonic solutions of saline cathartics, they should not be used by those who cannot tolerate fluid loss.

Stimulant Laxatives

A comprehensive review of stimulant laxatives has been reported, and the structure–activity relationships of the anthraquinone or emodin-containing laxatives have been investigated (22, 24–26). Stimulant laxatives increase the propulsive peristaltic activity of the intestine by local irritation of the mucosa or by a more selective action on the intramural nerve plexus of intestinal smooth muscle, thus increasing motility. Depending on the laxative, the site of action may be the small intestine, the large intestine, or both. Intensity of action is proportional to dosage, but individually effective doses vary. All stimulant laxatives produce griping, increased mucus secretion, and, in some people, excessive evacuation of fluid. Listed doses and dosage ranges are only guides to the correct individual dose. Stimulant laxatives are contraindicated with abdominal pain, nausea, or vomiting, which are symptoms of appendicitis.

Stimulant laxatives are effective but should be recommended cautiously because they may produce undesirable and sometimes dangerous side effects (11). This property becomes more important when the agents are abused. It has been said that, of all laxative products available, stimulant laxatives are the most abused (27).

stimulant laxatives
side effects
abuse potential
cascara
senna

In general, stimulant drugs are not recommended for routine use in patients with simple constipation, and they should never be used for more than 1 week of regular treatment. The dose should be within the dosage range indicated as safe and effective. These laxatives do not necessarily provide a good stimulus for the body to return to normal function. Two major hazards of stimulant laxatives are electrolyte and fluid deficiencies resulting from excessive catharsis. As with any potent laxative overdose, hypokalemia is an ever-present danger.

Stimulant laxatives, such as castor oil and bisacodyl, frequently are used before radiological examination of the GI tract and before bowel surgery. Bisacodyl also is used orally or rectally instead of an enema for emptying the colon before proctological examination.

Anthraquinones

The drugs of choice in this group are the cascara and senna compounds. Neither rhubarb, which contains an astringent (tannin), nor aloe, which is too irritating, should be recommended. The properties of each of the anthraquinone laxatives vary, depending on the anthraquinone content and the speed of liberation of the active principles from their glycosidic combinations. Crude drug formulations also may contain active constituents not found in extractive preparations or more highly purified compounds.

The precise mechanism by which peristalsis is increased is unknown. The cathartic activity of anthraquin-

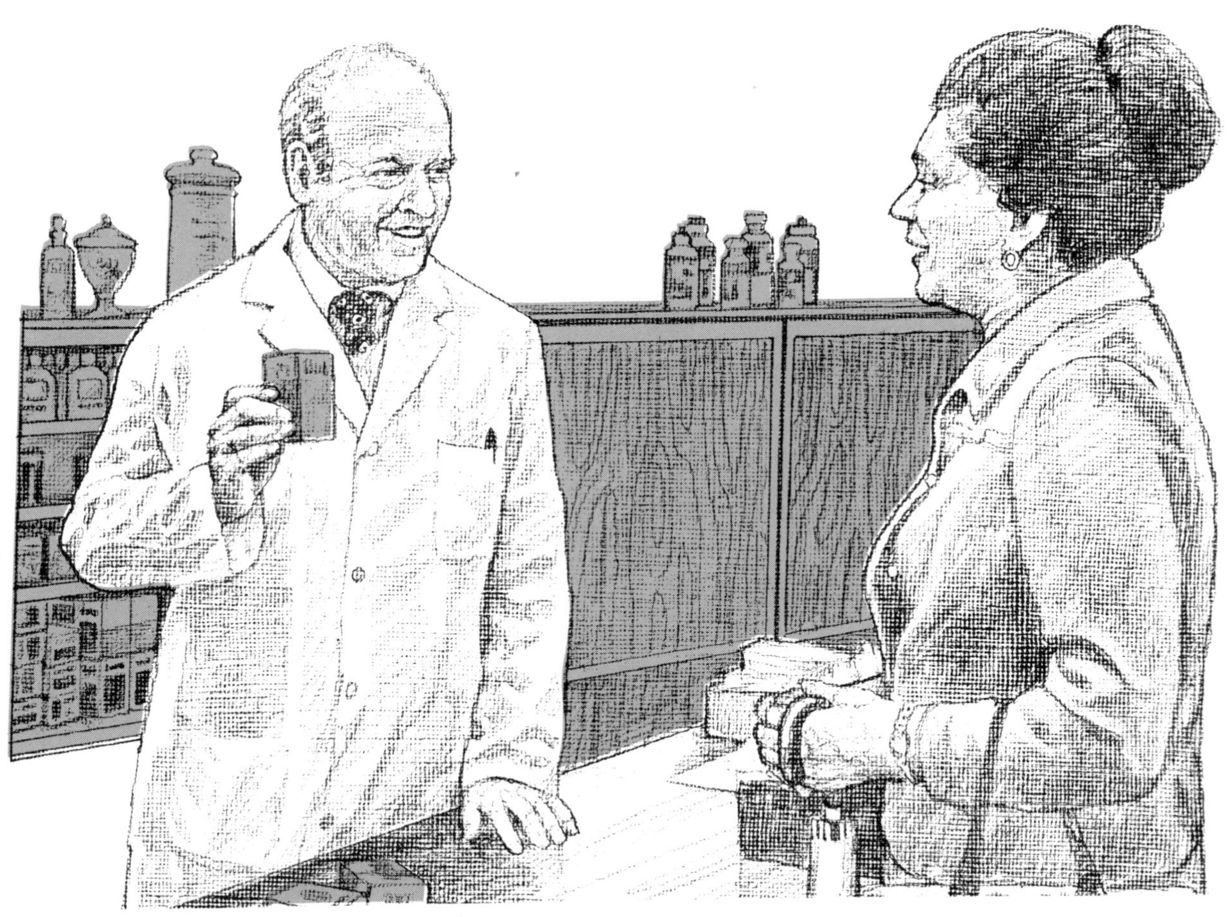

ones is limited primarily to the colon, which is reached by direct passage. Bacterial enzymes are partly responsible for the hydrolysis of the glycosides in the intestinal tract. Anthraquinones usually produce their action 8–12 hours after administration but may require up to 24 hours.

The active principles of anthraquinones are absorbed from the GI tract and subsequently appear in body secretions, including human breast milk. However, the practical significance of this finding in nursing infants is controversial. After taking a senna laxative, postpartum women reported a brown discoloration of breast milk and subsequent catharsis of their nursing infants. A follow-up study indicated that the amount of senna laxative principles in breast milk was inadequate to cause defecation (28). Another study with constipated postpartum breastfeeding women receiving a senna laxative reported that 17% of their infants experienced diarrhea (29).

Chrysophanic acid, a component of rhubarb and senna excreted in the urine, colors acidic urine yellowish-brown and alkaline urine reddish-violet. The prolonged use of anthraquinone laxatives, especially cascara sagrada, can result in a melanotic pigmentation of the colonic mucosa. The pigmentation is usually reversible 4–12 months after the drug is discontinued.

Melanosis coli is pathognomonic of prolonged use of anthraquinone laxatives. Pigment-containing macrophages appear in the mucosa, but staining reactions indicate that the pigment is not melanin but has many characteristics of lipofuscin. It may be a combination of a pigment of this type and either anthraquinone or one of its breakdown products.

The liquid preparations of cascara sagrada (fluidextracts) are more reliable than the solid dosage forms (extract and tablet). Aromatic cascara fluidextract is less active and less bitter than cascara sagrada fluidextract. Magnesium oxide, used in the preparation of the former, removes some of the bitter and irritating principles from the crude drug.

Preparations of senna are more potent that those of cascara and produce considerably more griping. Those that contain the crystalline glycosides of senna are more stable and more reliable and cause less griping than those made from the crude drug. This difference is important in making a standardized senna product the logical choice among anthracene laxatives (30).

Danthron (1,8-dihydroxyanthraquinone) is a free anthraquinone rather than a glycoside. Its action, use, properties, and limitations are similar to those of the natural anthraquinone drugs. Its site of action is the colon. It is partly absorbed from the small intestine, and a large part is metabolized by the liver; the metabolites are excreted by the kidneys, sometimes causing a harmless discoloration of the urine.

Diphenylmethane Laxatives

The most common diphenylmethane laxatives are bisacodyl and phenolphthalein.

Bisacodyl. Bisacodyl was introduced as a cathartic as a result of structure–activity studies of phenolphthalein-related compounds. Practically insoluble in water or in alkaline media, bisacodyl exerts its action in the colon on contact with the mucosal nerve plexus. Stimulation is segmented and axonal, producing contractions of the entire colon. Its action is independent of intestinal tone, and the drug is not absorbed systemically. Action on the small intestine is negligible. A soft, formed stool usually is produced 6–10 hours after oral administration and 15–60 minutes after rectal administration. Bisacodyl tablets are enteric coated to prevent irritation of the gastric lining and therefore should not be broken, chewed, or administered with alkaline materials such as antacid products.

Bisacodyl is recommended for cleaning the colon before and after surgery and prior to X ray examination. It is effective in colostomies and in reducing or eliminating the need for irrigations. No systemic or adverse effects on the liver, kidney, or hematopoietic system have been observed following its administration. Bisacodyl has not been detected in the milk of nursing women. The suppository form may produce a burning sensation in the rectum.

cascara

senna

danthron

bisacodyl

phenolphthalein

Phenolphthalein. This drug exerts its stimulating effect mainly on the colon, but the activity of the small intestine also may be increased. Its exact mechanism of action is not known; it is usually active 6–8 hours after administration.

A therapeutic dose of phenolphthalein passes through the stomach unchanged and is dissolved by the bile salts and the alkaline intestinal secretions. As much as 15% of the dose is absorbed, and the rest is excreted unchanged in the feces. Some of the absorbed drug appears in the urine, which is colored pink to red if it is sufficiently alkaline. Similarly, the drug excreted in the feces causes a red coloration if they are sufficiently alkaline (soap enemas). This effect may alarm people who are not aware of this property.

Part of the absorbed phenolphthalein is excreted back into the intestinal tract with the bile. The resulting enterohepatic cycle may prolong the action of phenolphthalein for 3–4 days. Phenolphthalein is ineffective in relieving constipation associated with obstructive jaundice. It functions as a laxative when administered intravenously and is excreted into the intestine with the bile.

Phenolphthalein is usually nontoxic. However, at least two types of allergic reactions may follow the use of phenolphthalein. In susceptible individuals a large dose may cause diarrhea, colic, cardiac and respiratory distress, or circulatory collapse. The other reaction is a polychromatic rash that ranges from pink to deep purple. The eruptions may be pinhead sized or as large as the palm of the hand. Itching and burning may be moderate or severe. If the rash is severe, it may lead to vesication and erosion, especially around the mouth and genital areas.

Osteomalacia is one untoward effect that has been attributed to excessive phenolphthalein ingestion (31). A female patient in an orthopedic clinic who had been suffering for 6 months with back and hip pain was found to have a 20-year history of ingestion of 15–20 phenolphthalein tablets per day. Discontinuance of the laxative quickly led to normal bowel habits and the resolution of the osteomalacia.

Suppositories

The bisacodyl, senna, and carbon dioxide releasing suppositories are promoted as replacements for enemas in cases where cleaning the distal colon is required. The suppositories that contain senna concentrate are advertised as effective in postsurgical and postpartum care; those that contain bisacodyl are promoted for postoperative, antepartum, and postpartum care and are adequate in the preparation for proctosigmoidoscopy. A suppository that exerts its action by the pressure of the released carbon dioxide is recommended for the same uses "or whenever the last 25 cm of the lower bowel must be emptied" (32). Although bisacodyl suppositories are prescribed and used more frequently than others, there are still strong proponents of the enema as the agent for cleaning the lower bowel.

It has been suggested that the carbon dioxide releasing suppository might serve as a beneficial replacement for some of the uses of the enema. One study reported that it was used successfully in institutionalized, spastic, and mentally retarded pediatric patients to replace enemas. It also replaced enemas in preparing these patients for intravenous pyelograms and for the installation of basal or rectal anesthetics (21).

Miscellaneous: Castor Oil

The laxative action of castor oil is due to ricinoleic acid which is produced when castor oil is hydrolyzed in the small intestine by pancreatic lipase; its mechanism of action is unknown. The assumption that defecation results from increased peristalsis due to the irritant effect of ricinoleic acid is not supported by experimental evidence.

Castor oil, a glyceride, may be absorbed from the GI tract and is probably metabolized like other fatty acids. Because the main site of action is the small intestine, its prolonged use may result in excessive loss of fluid, electrolytes, and nutrients. Castor oil generally is not recommended for the treatment of constipation.

Laxative Abuse

Regular use of most laxatives, particularly the stimulant preparations, can result in laxative abuse. The pharmacist should be aware of this possibility.

excessive use

Excessive use of laxatives can cause diarrhea and vomiting, leading to fluid and electrolyte losses, especially hypokalemia, where there is a general loss of tone of smooth and striated muscle (33). In a study of seven hospitalized female patients, 26–65 years old, the chief admitting complaints were abdominal pain and diarrhea, the number of hospital admissions ranged from 2 to 11, and the total number of days spent in the hospital ranged from 58 to 202 (33). The diagnosis of laxative abuse was difficult because the patients denied taking laxatives, and none of the colonic tissue characteristics usually associated with excessive laxative use was observed on sigmoidoscopy or radiological examination. However, additional tests revealed excessive laxative use.

Diarrhea can be a serious consequence of the overuse of laxative products, especially irritant laxatives.

anatomical changes

The prolonged misuse of laxative drugs can cause morbid anatomical changes in the colon. In a study of 12 chronic laxative users the primary anatomical changes were loss of intrinsic innervation, atrophy of smooth muscle coats, and pigmentation of the colon (34). Most users had been taking laxatives regularly for 30–40 years; two were less than 30 years old when they had their colons removed and therefore had a much shorter history. In these cases the myenteric plexus showed many swollen, but otherwise normal, neurons. This evidence suggests that the initial action of an irritant stimulation is to stimulate neurons and that prolonged and continuous stimulation causes cell death. Surgery in such cases shows that the transverse colon is often pendulous, the sigmoid section is highly dilated, and the muscle coats are thin and contain excess adipose tissue, indicating some tissue loss.

patient counseling

In counseling the patient on laxative use, the pharmacist should stress the following points:

- Laxative agents should not be used on a regular basis; more natural methods should be sought to produce regular movements.
- The use of a laxative agent in the treatment of constipation should be only a temporary measure; once regularity has returned, the laxative product should be discontinued.

high-fiber foods

A diet consisting of high-fiber foods and plenty of fluids (six to eight 8-oz. glasses of water per day) will help relieve chronic constipation. Dietary fiber is that part of whole grain, vegetables, fruits, and nuts that resists digestion in the GI tract. It is composed of carbohydrates (cellulose, hemicelluloses, polysaccharides, and pectin) and a noncarbohydrate, lignin.

Food fiber content, which is expressed in terms of crude fiber residue after treatment with dilute acid and alkali, has a significant effect on bowel habits. Because fiber holds water, stools tend to be softer, bulkier, and heavier in persons with a higher fiber intake and probably pass through the colon more rapidly.

Foods with a high fiber content take longer to chew than refined foods. Increased production of saliva and gastric juices, together with the fiber content of the food, leaves less space in the stomach to be filled with high-energy food before a sense of satiety is achieved. It is the foods that have a low energy/satiety ratio that encourage overconsumption of calories. Not only does more energy tend to be consumed with highly refined foods, but also the energy is utilized more quickly from foods in which the sugars and starches have been partially liberated from the encasing cell walls prior to ingestion. Increased consumption of highly refined foods and their subsequent rapid utilization have been implicated in the development of obesity and diabetes.

Along with a high-fiber diet, the pharmacist may encourage regular exercise provided the patient's cardiovascular system is normal and the patient is under a physician's care. Exercise in any form improves muscle tone, but that which involves abdominal muscles is the most useful in improvement of intestinal muscle tone (35). Physical activity is important in the propulsion mechanisms in the colon.

The patient should learn not to ignore the urge to defecate and should allow adequate time for elimination (30). A relaxed, unhurried atmosphere can be very important for aiding elimination. The patient should be encouraged to set a regular pattern for bathroom visits. Mornings, particularly after breakfast, seem to be a very good time. Having a specific time period set aside for elimination may help the body adjust itself to producing a regular stool.

Specific advice to patients concerning laxative products should include these reminders:

- Laxatives are not designed for long-term use; if they are not effective after 1 week, a physician should be consulted.
- Laxative products containing more than 15 mEq (345 mg) of sodium, more than 25 mEq (975 mg) of potassium, or more than 50 mEq (600 mg) of magnesium in the maximum daily dose should not be used if kidney disease or its symptoms are present.
- If a skin rash appears after the patient has taken a laxative containing phenolphthalein, the product should be discontinued.
- Saline laxatives should not be used daily and should not be administered orally to children under 6 or rectally to infants under 2.
- Mineral oil should not be given to children under 6, and castor oil should not be used to treat constipation.
- Enemas and suppositories must be administered properly to be effective.
- Laxatives should not be used in the presence of abdominal pain, nausea, vomiting, bloating, cramping, or any other related phenomena.
- Laxatives containing phenolphthalein, rhubarb, or senna may discolor urine; laxatives containing phenolphthalein may discolor feces.

PRODUCT SELECTION GUIDELINES

In considering which laxative product may be useful or best suited to a particular patient, the pharmacist should make a decision based on patient assessment. Other, more general information also can be helpful.

The overall usefulness of laxatives is determined primarily by pharmacological action, lack of side effects and adverse reactions, cost, and patient acceptability. If drug therapy for constipation is chosen, the recommendations of the FDA OTC Panel on Laxative, Antidiarrheal, Emetic, and Antiemetic Products should be noted (12). When it is necessary to use a laxative, the recommended choice is a bulk-forming product; however, the pharmacist should keep in mind the small number of situations in which its use is inappropriate. Laxatives are not recommended to treat constipation associated with intestinal pathology. They also are not a cure for functional constipation and therefore are of only secondary importance in its treatment.

The ideal laxative should be nonirritating and nontoxic, and should act only on the descending and sigmoid colon. Within a few hours it should produce a normally formed stool. Its action should then cease and permit the resumption of normal bowel activity. Unfortunately, such a laxative is not currently available.

SUMMARY

The widespread abuse of OTC laxatives is evidence of a greater need for professional consultation. As qualified professionals, pharmacists are responsible for providing this service. Their main determination, whether referral to a physician or self-therapy is indicated, requires a knowledge of the case history and current symptoms. If the case history discloses a sudden change in bowel habits that has persisted for 2 weeks, the pharmacist should refer the patient to a physician.

For most cases of simple constipation, proper diet, exercise, and adequate fluid intake will promote alleviation of the condition. Therapy with any laxative product should be limited in most cases to short-term use (1 week). If after a 1-week period of proper laxative therapy no relief has been achieved, a physician should be consulted, and the product discontinued.

advice to patient

Pharmacists who successfully perform their professional responsibilities with OTC laxatives will lessen patient demand for these products but will establish themselves as important public health consultants.

REFERENCES

(1) "New and Non-Official Drugs," Lippincott, Philadelphia, Pa., 1965, p. 615.

(2) "The Pharmacological Basis of Therapeutics," 5th ed., L. S. Goodman and A. Gilman, Eds., Macmillan, New York, N.Y., 1975, p. 976.

(3) J. R. DiPalma, "Drill's Pharmacology in Medicine," 4th ed., McGraw-Hill, New York, N.Y., 1971, p. 747.

(4) W. F. Ganong, "Review of Medical Physiology," 6th ed., Lange Medical, Los Altos, Calif., 1971, p. 357.

(5) A. C. Guyton, "Textbook of Medical Physiology," 3rd ed., Saunders, Philadelphia, Pa., 1971, p. 738.

(6) F. H. Netter, "The Ciba Collection of Medical Illustrations," Vol. 3, Part II, Ciba Pharmaceutical Company, Summit, N.J., 1962, p. 98.

(7) G. E. Sladen, *Proc. R. Soc. Med.*, *65*, 289 (1972).

(8) A. M. Connell, C. Hilton, G. Irvine, J. E. Lennard-Jones, and J. J. Misiewicz, *Br. Med. J.*, *2*, 1095 (1965).

(9) W. G. Thompson, *Can. Med. Assoc. J.*, *114*, 927 (1976).

(10) T. P. Almy, *Ann. N.Y. Acad. Sci.*, *58*, 398 (1954).

(11) K. Rutter and D. Maxwell, *Br. Med. J.*, *2*, 997 (1976).

(12) *Federal Register*, *40*, 12907 (1975).

(13) *Medical Letter on Drugs and Therapeutics*, *19*, 45 (1977).

(14) K. Naess, *J. Am. Med. Assoc.*, *212*, 1961 (1970).

(15) T. B. Reynolds, R. L. Peters, and S. Yamada, *N. Engl. J. Med.*, *285*, 813 (1971).

(16) E. Gjone, J. P. Blumhoff, S. Ritland, E. Elgjo, and G. Husby, *Scand. J. Gastroenterol.*, *7*, 395 (1972).

(17) O. Dietrichson, E. Juhl, J. O. Nielsen, J. J. Oxlund, and P. Christoffersen, *Scand. J. Gastroenterol.*, *9*, 473 (1974).

(18) R. L. Willing and R. Hecker, *Med. J. Aust.*, *1*, 1179 (1971).

(19) *Journal of the American Medical Association*, *211*, 114 (1970).

(20) "Drugs of Choice," W. Modell, Ed., Mosby, St. Louis, Mo., 1960, p. 370.

(21) H. C. Shirkey, *Nebr. State Med. J.*, *50*, 67 (1965).

(22) J. Travel, *Ann. N.Y. Acad. Sci.*, *58*, 416 (1954).

(23) R. F. Harvey and A. E. Read, *Lancet*, *2*, 185 (1973).

(24) S. J. Loewe, *J. Pharmacol. Exp. Ther.*, *94*, 288 (1948).

(25) L. Schmidt and E. Seeger, *Arzneim. Forsch.*, *b*, 22 (1965).

(26) M. H. Hubacher and S. Doernberg, *J. Pharm. Sci.*, *53*, 1067 (1964).

(27) R. G. Pietrusko, *Am. J. Hosp. Pharm.*, *34*, 291 (1977).

(28) M. W. Werthmann and S. V. Krees, *Med. Ann. D.C.*, *42*, 4 (1973).

(29) J. O. Greenhalf and H. S. Leonard, *Practitioner*, *210*, 259 (1973).

(30) K. Goulston, *Drugs*, *14*, 128 (1977).

(31) B. Frame, H. L. Guiang, H. M. Frost, and W. A. Reynolds, *Arch. Intern. Med.*, *128*, 794 (1971).

(32) "Physicians' Desk Reference," Medical Economics, Oradell, N.J., 1966.

(33) R. R. Babb, *West J. Med.*, *122*, 93 (1975).

(34) B. Smith, *Dis. Colon Rectum*, *16*, 455 (1973).

(35) *Drug Therapy*, March 1975.

Product (Manufacturer)	Dosage Form	Stimulant	Bulk	Emollient/ Lubricant	Other Laxatives	Other Ingredients
Adlerika (Last)	liquid	—	—	—	magnesium sulfate	—
Afko-Lube (Amer. Pharm.)	capsule	—	—	dioctyl sodium sulfosuccinate, 100 mg	—	—
Afko-Lube Lax (Amer. Pharm.)	capsule	casanthranol, 30 mg	—	dioctyl sodium sulfosuccinate, 100 mg	—	—
Agoral (Warner-Chilcott)	emulsion	phenolphthalein, 0.013 mg/ml	agar gel tragacanth acacia	mineral oil	—	egg albumin glycerin
Agoral Plain (Warner-Chilcott)	emulsion	—	agar gel tragacanth acacia	mineral oil	—	egg albumin glycerin
Alophen (Parke-Davis)	tablet	phenolphthalein, 60 mg	—	—	—	—
Amlax (North American)	tablet	cascara sagrada extract, 32.5 mg phenolphthalein, 32.5 mg aloin, 8 mg	—	—	bile salts, 65 mg	—
Bisacodyl (Philips Roxane)	tablet suppository	bisacodyl, 5 mg/tablet 10 mg/suppository	—	—	—	—
Black Draught (Chattem)	tablet syrup granules	senna, 180 mg/tablet 100 mg/ml (syrup) 660 mg/g (granules)	—	—	—	anise peppermint cinnamon clove nutmeg (spices only in syrup)
Caroid Laxative Tablets (Winthrop)	tablet	cascara sagrada extract, 55 mg phenolphthalein, 32.4 mg	—	—	—	—
Carter's Little Pills (Carter)	tablet	aloe, 16 mg podophyllum, 4.0 mg	—	—	—	—
Casa-Laud (Amfre-Grant)	tablet	casanthranol, 30 mg	—	dioctyl sodium sulfosuccinate, 100 mg	—	—
Cas-Evac (Parke-Davis)	liquid	cascara sagrada, 2 mg/ml	—	—	—	alcohol, 18%
Casyllium (Upjohn)	powder	cascara fluidextract, 0.5 ml/g	psyllium husk, 0.68 g/g prune powder, 0.2 g/g	—	—	—
Colace (Mead Johnson)	capsule liquid syrup	—	—	dioctyl sodium sulfosuccinate, 50 and 100 mg/ capsule, 1% (liquid), 4 mg/ml (syrup)	—	—
Coloctyl (Vitarine)	capsule	—	—	dioctyl sodium sulfosuccinate, 100 mg	—	—
Comfolax (Searle)	capsule	—	—	dioctyl sodium sulfosuccinate, 100 mg	—	—
Comfolax Plus (Searle)	capsule	casanthranol, 30 mg	—	dioctyl sodium sulfosuccinate, 100 mg	—	—

Product (Manufacturer)	Dosage Form	Stimulant	Bulk	Emollient/ Lubricant	Other Laxatives	Other Ingredients
Concentrated Milk of Magnesia (Philips Roxane)	suspension	—	—	—	magnesium hydroxide, 0.233 g/ml	glycerin sorbitol sugar, 8% lemon
Constiban (Columbia Medical)	capsule	casanthranol, 30 mg	—	dioctyl sodium sulfosuccinate, 100 mg	—	—
Correctol (Plough)	tablet	yellow phenol-phthalein, 64.8 mg	—	dioctyl sodium sulfosuccinate, 100 mg	—	—
Dialose (Stuart)	capsule	—	carboxymethyl-cellulose sodium, 400 mg	dioctyl sodium sulfosuccinate, 100 mg	—	—
Dialose Plus (Stuart)	capsule	casanthranol, 30 mg	carboxymethyl-cellulose sodium, 400 mg	dioctyl sodium sulfosuccinate, 100 mg	—	—
Dioctyl Sodium Sulfosuccinate (Philips Roxane)	capsule syrup	—	—	dioctyl sodium sulfosuccinate, 50, 100, and 250 mg/capsule, 3.33 mg/ml (syrup)	—	propylene glycol sucrose peppermint (syrup)
Dio Medicone (Medicone)	tablet	—	—	dioctyl sodium sulfosuccinate, 50 mg	—	—
Dio-Sul (North American)	capsule	—	—	dioctyl sodium sulfosuccinate, 100 mg	—	—
Diothron (North American)	capsule	casanthranol, 30 mg	—	dioctyl sodium sulfosuccinate, 100 mg	—	—
Disanthrol (Lannett)	capsule	casanthranol, 30 mg	—	dioctyl sodium sulfosuccinate, 100 mg	—	—
Disolan (Lannett)	capsule	phenolphthalein, 65 mg	—	dioctyl sodium sulfosuccinate, 100 mg	—	—
Disolan Forte (Lannett)	capsule	casanthranol, 30 mg	carboxymethyl-cellulose sodium, 400 mg	dioctyl sodium sulfosuccinate, 100 mg	—	—
Disonate (Lannett)	capsule liquid syrup	—	—	dioctyl sodium sulfosuccinate, 60, 100, and 240 mg/capsule, 10 mg/ml (liquid) 4 mg/ml (syrup)	—	—
Disoplex (Lannett)	capsule	—	carboxymethyl-cellulose sodium, 400 mg	dioctyl sodium sulfosuccinate, 100 mg	—	—
Doctate (Meyer)	capsule	—	—	dioctyl sodium sulfosuccinate, 100 and 300 mg	—	—
Doctate-P (Meyer)	capsule	danthron, 40 mg	—	dioctyl sodium sulfosuccinate, 60 mg	—	—
Dorbane (Riker)	tablet	danthron, 75 mg	—	—	—	—
Dorbantyl (Riker)	capsule	danthron, 25 mg	—	dioctyl sodium sulfosuccinate, 50 mg	—	—

Product (Manufacturer)	Dosage Form	Stimulant	Bulk	Emollient/ Lubricant	Other Laxatives	Other Ingredients
Dorbantyl Forte (Riker)	capsule	danthron, 50 mg	—	dioctyl sodium sulfosuccinate, 100 mg	—	—
Doxan (Hoechst-Roussel)	tablet	danthron, 50 mg	—	dioctyl sodium sulfosuccinate, 60 mg	—	—
Doxidan (Hoechst-Roussel)	capsule	danthron, 50 mg	—	dioctyl calcium sulfosuccinate, 60 mg	—	—
Doxinate (Hoechst-Roussel)	capsule 5% solution	—	—	dioctyl sodium sulfosuccinate, 60 and 240 mg	—	—
Dr. Caldwell's Senna Laxative (Glenbrook)	liquid	senna, 7%	—	—	—	alcohol, 4.5% peppermint oil, 0.19 mg/ml
Dual Formula Feen-A-Mint (Plough)	tablet	yellow phenolphthalein, 64.8 mg	—	dioctyl sodium sulfosuccinate, 100 mg	—	—
Dulcolax (Boehringer-Ingelheim)	tablet suppository	bisacodyl, 5 mg/tablet 10 mg/suppository	—	—	—	—
Effersyllium (Stuart)	powder	—	psyllium hydrocolloid, 3 g/tsp	—	—	—
Espotabs (Combe)	tablet	yellow phenolphthalein	—	—	—	—
Evac-Q-Kit (Warren-Teed)	liquid tablet suppository	phenolphthalein, 2 tablets (Evac-Q-Tabs), 130 mg/each	—	—	magnesium citrate (Evac-Q-Mag), 300 ml carbon dioxide releasing suppository (Evac-Q-Sert)	—
Evac-Q-Kwik (Warren-Teed)	liquid tablet suppository	phenolphthalein, 2 tablets (Evac-Q-Tabs), 130 mg/each	—	—	magnesium citrate (Evac-Q-Mag), 300 ml bisacodyl (suppository)	—
Evac-U-Gen (Walker Corp.)	tablet	yellow phenolphthalein, 97.2 mg	—	—	—	—
Ex-Lax (Ex-Lax)	chocolate tablet unflavored pill	yellow phenolphthalein, 90 mg	—	—	—	—
Feen-A-Mint (Plough)	chewing gum mint	yellow phenolphthalein, 97.2 mg	—	—	—	—
Feen-A-Mint Pills (Plough)	tablet	yellow phenolphthalein, 64.8 mg	—	dioctyl sodium sulfosuccinate, 100 mg	—	—
Fleet Bagenema (Fleet)	enema	—	—	—	liquid castile soap, 19.7 ml	—
Fleet Enema (Fleet)	enema	—	—	—	sodium biphosphate, 0.16 g/ml sodium phosphate, 0.06 g/ml	—
Fleet Enema Oil Retention (Fleet)	enema	—	—	mineral oil, 118 ml	—	—
Fleet Pediatric Enema (Fleet)	enema	—	—	—	sodium biphosphate, 0.16 g/ml sodium phosphate, 0.06 g/ml	—
Fletcher's Castoria (Glenbrook)	liquid	senna, 6.5%	—	—	—	—

Product (Manufacturer)	Dosage Form	Stimulant	Bulk	Emollient/ Lubricant	Other Laxatives	Other Ingredients
Gentlax (Blair)	tablet granules	senna concentrate, 326 mg/tablet or tsp (granules)	guar gum, 1 g/tablet or tsp (granules)	—	—	polygalacturonic acid, 100 mg/ tablet or tsp (granules)
Gentlax B (Blair)	tablet granules	senna concentrate, 108.7 mg/tablet 326.1 mg/tsp (granules)	guar gum, 333 mg/tablet 1 g/tsp (granules)	—	—	—
Gentlax S (Blair)	tablet	senna concentrate, 187 mg	—	dioctyl sodium sulfosuccinate, 50 mg	—	—
Glysennid (Dorsey)	tablet	sennosides A and B (as calcium salt), 12 mg	—	—	—	—
G-W Emulsoil (Paddock)	instant-mix liquid	—	—	—	castor oil, 30 and 60 ml	—
Haley's M-O (Winthrop)	emulsion	—	—	mineral oil, 25%	magnesium hydroxide, 75%	—
Hydrolose (Upjohn)	syrup	—	methylcellulose, 0.019 g/ml	—	—	—
Instant Mix Metamucil (Searle)	powder in single-dose packets	—	psyllium mucilloid, 3.7 g/packet	—	citric acid sodium bicarbonate (equiv. to 250 mg sodium)	—
Kasof (Stuart)	capsules	—	—	dioctyl potassium sulfosuccinate, 240 mg	—	—
Kellogg's Tasteless Castor Oil (Beecham)	liquid	—	—	—	castor oil	—
Kondremul (Fisons)	micro-emulsion	—	chondrus	heavy mineral oil, 55%	—	—
Kondremul with Cascara (Fisons)	micro-emulsion	cascara	chondrus	heavy mineral oil, 55%	—	—
Kondremul with Phenolphthalein (Fisons)	micro-emulsion	phenolphthalein	chondrus	heavy mineral oil, 55%	—	—
Konsyl (Burton Parsons)	powder	—	psyllium mucilloid, 100%	—	—	—
L. A. Formula (Burton Parsons)	powder	—	psyllium mucilloid, 50%	—	—	dextrose, 50%
Lane's Pills (Last)	tablet	casanthranol, 45 mg	—	—	—	—
Laxsil (Reed & Carnrick)	liquid	—	—	—	magnesium hydroxide, 0.08 g/ml	simethicone, 6.67 mg/ml
Magcyl (Elder)	capsule	danthron, 25 mg	—	dioctyl sodium sulfosuccinate, 100 mg	—	—
Maltsupex (Wallace)	tablet	—	malt soup extract, 750 mg	—	—	—
Metamucil (Searle)	powder	—	psyllium mucilloid, 50%	—	—	dextrose, 50%

Product (Manufacturer)	Dosage Form	Stimulant	Bulk	Emollient/ Lubricant	Other Laxatives	Other Ingredients
Milkinol (Kremers-Urban)	liquid	—	—	dioctyl sodium sulfosuccinate, 0.66 mg/ml mineral oil, 0.95 ml/ml	—	—
Milk of Magnesia USP (Philips Roxane)	suspension	—	—	—	magnesium hydroxide, 0.078 g/ml	—
Milk of Magnesia–Cascara Suspension (Philips Roxane)	suspension	cascara sagrada (equiv. to 5 ml USP fluidextract)	—	—	magnesium hydroxide, 0.078 g/ml	yellow 6
Modane (Warren-Teed)	tablet liquid	danthron, 75 mg/ tablet 7.5 mg/ml	—	—	—	—
Modane Mild (Warren-Teed)	tablet	danthron, 37.5 mg	—	—	—	—
Modane Soft (Warren-Teed)	capsule	—	—	dioctyl sodium sulfosuccinate, 120 mg	—	—
Mucilose (Winthrop)	flakes granules	—	psyllium, 100% (flakes) 50% (granules)	—	—	dextrose, 50% (granules)
Nature's Remedy Juniors (Norcliff Thayer)	tablet	aloe, 48 mg cascara sagrada, 42 mg	—	—	—	—
Nature's Remedy Regular and Candy Coated (Norcliff Thayer)	tablet	aloe, 143 mg cascara sagrada, 127 mg	—	—	—	—
Neo-Cultol (Fisons)	suspension	—	—	refined mineral oil jelly	—	chocolate flavor
Neoloid (Lederle)	emulsion	—	—	—	castor oil, 36.4% (w/w)	—
Nujol (Plough)	liquid	—	—	mineral oil	—	—
Nytilax (Pfizer)	tablet	sennosides A and B	—	—	—	—
Oxothalein (O'Neal, Jones & Feldman)	tablet	phenolphthalein, 32 mg cascara sagrada extract, 32 mg aloin, 8 mg	—	—	—	—
Peri-Colace (Mead Johnson)	capsule syrup	casanthranol, 30 mg/capsule 2 mg/ml	—	dioctyl sodium sulfosuccinate, 100 mg/capsule 4 mg/ml	—	—
Peristim Forte (Mead Johnson)	capsule	casanthranol, 90 mg	—	—	—	—
Petrogalar (Wyeth)	emulsion	phenolphthalein, 0.3%, or cascara aqueous extract, 13.2%	agar sodium alginate	mineral oil, 65%	—	acacia glycerin
Petro-Syllium No. 1 Plain (Whitehall)	liquid	—	psyllium seed	mineral oil	—	—
Petro-Syllium No. 2 with Phenolphthalein (Whitehall)	liquid	phenolphthalein, 8.126 mg/ml	psyllium seed	mineral oil	—	—
Phenolax (Upjohn)	wafer	phenolphthalein, 64.8 mg	—	—	—	sugar aromatics

Product (Manufacturer)	Dosage Form	Stimulant	Bulk	Emollient/ Lubricant	Other Laxatives	Other Ingredients
Phillip's Milk of Magnesia (Glenbrook)	suspension tablet	—	—	—	magnesium hydroxide, 0.76–0.87 g/ml 311 mg/tablet	peppermint oil, 0.038 mg/ml 1.166 mg/tablet
Phospho-Soda (Fleet)	liquid	—	—	—	sodium biphosphate, 0.48 g/ml sodium phosphate, 0.18 g/ml	artificial sweeteners flavors
Plova (Washington Ethical)	powder	—	psyllium, 100% (plain) 50% (flavored)	—	—	dextrose, 50% (cocoa flavored)
Rectalad (Wallace)	enema	—	—	dioctyl potassium sulfosuccinate, 5%	glycerin, 76% soft soap, 10%	—
Regul-Aid (Columbia Medical)	capsule syrup	—	—	dioctyl sodium sulfosuccinate, 100 mg/capsule 4 mg/ml	—	—
Regutol (Plough)	tablet	—	—	dioctyl sodium sulfosuccinate, 100 mg	—	—
Sal Hepatica (Bristol-Meyers)	granules	—	—	—	monosodium phosphate sodium bicarbonate citric acid, anhydrous sodium citrate, tribasic sodium citrate, dibasic	—
Saraka (Plough)	granules	frangula	karaya gum	—	—	—
Schoenfeld (Pfeiffer)	capsules	—	—	dioctyl sodium sulfosuccinate, 100 mg	—	—
Senokap DSS (Purdue Frederick)	capsule	senna concentrate, 163 mg	—	dioctyl sodium sulfosuccinate, 50 mg	—	—
Senokot (Purdue Frederick)	granules tablet suppository syrup	senna concentrate, 326 mg/tsp (granules) 187 mg/tablet 652 mg/suppository 43.6 mg extract/ml (syrup)	—	—	—	—
Senokot-S (Purdue Frederick)	tablet	senna concentrate, 187 mg	—	dioctyl sodium sulfosuccinate, 50 mg	—	—
Senokot with Psyllium (Purdue Frederick)	powder	senna concentrate, 65.2 mg/ml	psyllium, 0.2 g/ml	—	—	—
Serutan (J. B. Williams)	powder granules	—	psyllium, 100%	—	—	—
Siblin (Parke-Davis)	granules	—	psyllium seed husks, 50%	—	—	sugar caramel sodium chloride
Sodium Phosphate and Biphosphate Oral Solution USP (Philips Roxane)	solution	—	—	—	sodium biphosphate, 0.48 g/ml sodium phosphate, 0.18 g/ml	yellow 5 ginger/lemon saccharin

Product (Manufacturer)	Dosage Form	Stimulant	Bulk	Emollient/ Lubricant	Other Laxatives	Other Ingredients
Stimulax (Geriatric Pharmaceutical)	capsule	cascara, 30 mg	—	dioctyl sodium sulfosuccinate, 250 mg	—	—
Surfak (Hoechst-Roussel)	capsule	—	—	dioctyl calcium sulfosuccinate, 50 and 240 mg	—	—
Swiss Kriss (Modern Products)	powder tablet	senna	—	—	—	herbs flowers
Syllact (Wallace)	powder	—	psyllium seed husks, 50%	—	—	dextrose, 50%
Syllamalt (Wallace)	powder	—	malt soup extract, 50% psyllium seed husks, 50%	—	—	—
Syllamalt Effervescent (Wallace)	powder	—	malt soup extract, 25% psyllium seed husks, 25%	—	—	dextrose sodium bicarbonate citric acid
Theralax (Beecham Labs)	tablet suppository	bisacodyl, 5 mg/ tablet 10 mg/suppository	—	—	—	triglyceride base (suppository)
Tonelax (A.V.P.)	tablet	danthron, 75 mg	—	—	—	calcium pantothenate, 25 mg
Tucks Saf-Tip Oil Retention Enema (Parke-Davis)	enema	—	—	light mineral oil	—	—
Tucks Saf-Tip Phosphate Enema (Parke-Davis)	enema	—	—	—	sodium biphosphate, 0.16 g/ml sodium phosphate, 0.06 g/ml	—
Vacuetts Adult (Dorsey)	suppository	—	—	—	sodium biphosphate sodium acid pyrophosphate sodium bicarbonate	polyethylene glycols
X-Prep (Gray)	liquid powder	senna extract (liquid) senna concentrate (powder)	—	—	—	—

Emetic and Antiemetic Products

Gary M. Oderda and Sheila West

Chapter 5

Questions to Ask the Patient

Antiemetics

Will the product be used for nausea or motion sickness?

How old is the patient? Is the patient pregnant?

How long have nausea and/or vomiting been problems?

Have you noted blood in the vomitus?

Have you noted other symptoms such as abdominal pain, headache, or diarrhea?

What medications are currently being taken?

Emetics

Are you requesting the emetic for immediate emergency use or possible future use?

How old is the patient?

What has been taken?

How long ago did the ingestion occur?

How much was taken?

What symptoms is the patient showing now?

Severe nausea and the realization that one is about to vomit are two of the more unpleasant symptoms an individual may have. However disagreeable the sensation, vomiting (emesis) is an important body defense mechanism for ridding itself of a variety of toxins and poisons; vomiting may also be an irritating accompaniment to travel or pregnancy.

The OTC antiemetics are used to prevent or control the symptoms of nausea and vomiting primarily due to motion sickness, pregnancy, and mild infectious diseases. Some OTC antiemetics are promoted for the relief of such vague symptoms as "upset stomach," "indigestion," and "distention" associated with excessive food indulgence, although their value in treating these complaints is not well documented.

OTC emetic drugs are used to induce vomiting primarily in the treatment of poisoning.

Nausea and vomiting associated with radiation therapy, cancer chemotherapy, and the more serious metabolic and endocrine disorders are not appropriate diseases for self-medication and are not covered in this chapter.

THE VOMITING PROCESS

Vomiting is a complex process involving both the CNS and the GI system (Figure 1). The central involvement includes two areas of the medulla oblongata—the vomiting center and the chemoreceptor trigger zone (CTZ). The chemoreceptor trigger zone cannot produce vomiting by itself but must act through stimulation of the vomiting center. Centrally acting emetics and antiemetics work primarily by stimulating and inhibiting, respectively, the chemoreceptor trigger zone. In addition to stimuli from the chemoreceptor trigger zone, impulses from the GI tract and the labyrinth apparatus in the ear are received at the vomiting center. Stimuli are then sent to the abdominal musculature, the stomach, and the esophagus to initiate vomiting. (See Chapter 1 for the anatomy and physiology of the GI tract.)

Vomiting begins with a deep inspiration, closing of the glottis, and depression of the soft palate. A forceful contraction of the diaphragm and abdominal musculature occurs, producing an increase in intrathoracic and intra-abdominal pressure that compresses the stomach and raises esophageal pressure (1–3). The body of the stomach and the esophageal musculature relax. The positive intrathoracic and intra-abdominal pressure move food into the esophagus and mouth. Several cycles of reflux into the esophagus occur before the actual vomiting (3). Regurgitation is the casting up of stomach contents without oral expulsion. Food is expelled from the esophagus by a combination of increased intrathoracic pressure and reverse peristaltic waves (1, 2). Normally, the glottis closes off the trachea and prevents the vomitus from entering the airway. Aspiration of the vomitus may occur in some cases, e.g., in patients with significant CNS depression.

Vomiting is a symptom produced by benign processes as well as by significant, serious illnesses. It is important for the practitioner to be aware of the possibility that patients using OTC antiemetics may be self-treating the early stages of a serious illness. Nausea and vomiting may be symptomatic of digitalis toxicity, opiate use, or ingestion of other drugs and chemicals. Knowledge of the patient's drug history is important in assessing the cause of nausea and vomiting. Nausea and vomiting may also be symptoms of diverse disorders such as acute

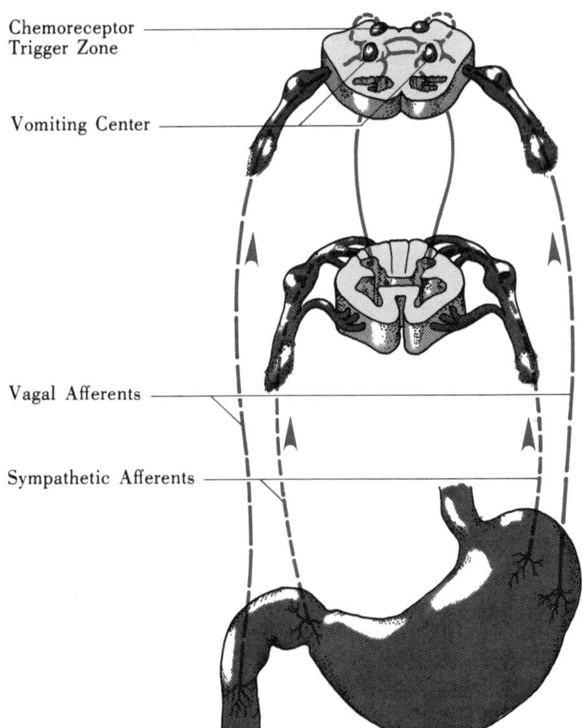

Figure 1. Mechanism of vomiting induction by emetics (apomorphine and ipecac). Adapted from A. C. Guyton, *Textbook of Medical Physiology*, 5th ed., Saunders, Philadelphia, Pa., 1976.

motion sickness
morning sickness
poisonings
referral or emetic

appendicitis, cholecystitis, migraine headache, food allergy, radiation, and cancer chemotherapy.

Overstimulation of the labyrinth apparatus produces the nausea and vomiting of motion sickness. The three semicircular canals on each side of the head in the inner ear (labyrinth) are responsible for maintaining equilibrium. Postural adjustments are made when the brain receives nervous impulses initiated by the movement of fluid in the semicircular canals. Some individuals are more tolerant than others to the effect of a particular type of motion, but no one is immune. Moreover, it appears that individuals can vary in their susceptibility to various kinds of motions, such as flying and boat riding (4). Motion sickness may be produced by unusual motion patterns in which the head is rotated in two axes simultaneously. Mechanisms other than the stimulation of the semicircular canals are also important. Erroneous interpretation of stimuli by stationary subjects who watch a film taken from a roller coaster or an airplane doing aerobatics can produce motion sickness.

The genesis of vomiting, or "morning sickness," of pregnancy is not established. Half of all pregnant women experience nausea, and about one-third of these suffer vomiting (5). Increased levels of chorionic gonadotropin have been implicated as a cause of morning sickness; levels of this hormone are maximal during the early part of pregnancy, when nausea and vomiting are most common (5, 6). Nausea and vomiting of pregnancy are difficult symptoms to treat, partly because no agent seems to be completely effective, but more important because of the concern that drug use during pregnancy should be minimal (6).

Acute transient attacks of vomiting, in association with diarrhea, are very common. Fever may be slight or absent. No precise figure is available for the incidence of this "viral gastroenteritis," although this usually harmless, self-limiting disorder may affect any age group and can occur in sizable outbreaks (5).

EMETICS

Prevalence of Poisoning

Emetics are used most commonly for the treatment of poisoning, both accidental and intentional. Poisoning is a relatively common occurrence that claims close to 3000 lives each year (7). Approximately one-half of these deaths are accidental, and about one-third occur in children under 5 (7). The number of poisoning fatalities is only a small percentage of total ingestions: during 1976, poison centers throughout the United States reported 147,277 ingestions to the National Clearinghouse for Poison Control Centers (8). Since reporting is voluntary and most large poison centers do not report, this figure does not represent all ingestions reported to poison centers. Epidemiologists estimate that only one ingestion in ten is reported to a poison center.

Emergency Treatment or OTC Emetic

Emetics remove potentially toxic agents from the stomach. It is often difficult to decide whether a patient should be referred directly to an emergency treatment facility or should be given an OTC emetic and managed at home. Taking a good history, identifying the agent, and accurately assessing the patient's condition are critical in making this decision. All ingestions where moderate to severe toxicity is expected must be referred to an emergency treatment facility. If minimal toxicity (no serious or life-threatening symptoms) is anticipated, the administration of an OTC emetic at home by a competent adult may be all that is necessary. Many ingestions reported to poison centers fall into this category. For example, a child who ingests approximately 65 mg of aspirin/0.45 kg (1 lb) of body weight can usually be managed at home. To determine whether administration of an OTC emetic is appropriate or the patient should be referred, the following information must be obtained.

Name of Product Ingested

The ingredients and the amount of each ingredient can be determined once the name of the ingested agent is known. Then the potential toxicity of each ingredient must be investigated.

Amount Ingested

This information is frequently unavailable or difficult to determine. For example, a child is found with an empty bottle of aspirin, and no one is quite sure how full the bottle was prior to ingestion. In addition, a parent will often underestimate the amount consumed or will provide unreliable information. For example, a parent reports that a child has taken two digoxin tablets. To substantiate the consumption of only two tablets, the parent may respond that the child was alone for a short period of time or that the tablets had an unpleasant taste.

It should be stressed that drugs can be both therapeutic agents and poisons, depending on the dose. Thus a 2-year-old who takes two children's aspirin tablets would obviously require no treatment; the same child who takes 15 adult aspirin tablets may be severely poisoned.

Time Since Ingestion

The amount of time since ingestion is important because an emetic will be useful only if a sufficient amount of the ingested agent remains in the stomach. Thus for quickly absorbed agents an emetic would not be recommended if several hours had elapsed after ingestion. For some agents that are slow to leave the stomach, e.g., anticholinergics and aspirin, the use of an emetic may be rational even hours after ingestion.

Symptoms

Certain symptoms (e.g., significant CNS depression) are contraindications to the use of emetics. In cases where significant symptoms such as seizures, lethargy, ataxia, or hallucinations are present, an OTC emetic at home should not be considered; the patient should be referred immediately for treatment.

Patient's Age and Weight

Much toxicity information is given on a dose per body weight basis, e.g., mg/kg. Thus knowledge of the patient's weight is needed to determine appropriate treatment. The patient's age helps to determine the appropriateness and dose of an emetic, for example.

This information should assist in answering the following questions: Is an emetic indicated? Are there any contraindications to using an emetic? Can the emetic be administered safely outside an emergency treatment facility? Poison centers are available in many communities to help pharmacists answer these questions or handle referrals. Pharmacists should be aware of how to contact their local poison center. A list of poison centers is currently printed in the *Merck Index*, the *Physician's Desk Reference*, and the *Drug Topics Red Book*.

Treatment for Poisoning

The mainstay of treatment in poisoning cases is symptomatic and supportive care. Support of vital functions, especially respiratory and cardiovascular, is critical. Treatment of specific symptoms such as seizures is also important. Many patients will detoxify themselves and survive with symptomatic and supportive care alone. Other specific treatments, including emptying the stomach and administering agents such as adsorbents, cathartics, or antidotes, do not replace the need for symptomatic and supportive care.

Stomach contents may be removed by administering an emetic or by lavage. Gastric lavage is a procedure in which a tube is placed in the stomach via the esophagus. Fluid is then instilled into the tube, allowed to mix with stomach contents, and removed by the same tube. The efficacy of ipecac treatment and lavage in removing gastric contents was compared in 20 patients, 12–20 months old, who had ingested salicylates (9). Each patient was lavaged with a small nasogastric tube and also given syrup of ipecac, and the amount of salicylate returned was measured. Approximately half the patients were lavaged first, and the others were given syrup of ipecac first. Ipecac was superior to lavage in removing salicylate, and in patients who had vomited with ipecac, little more salicylate was removed by subsequent lavage. In another study, two adult patients were first lavaged with 3 liters of normal saline through a small (20 French, or 6.7 mm) tube 10–15 minutes after ingestion and then given syrup of ipecac (10). Twenty-five tablets from one patient and 10–15 from the other were included in the vomitus following ipecac. It was also shown that under optimal conditions, dogs given sodium salicylate returned 38% of the ingested dose after lavage with a small (16 Fr., or 5.3 mm) tube and 45% after ipecac-induced emesis (11). In these studies the lavage tube used was considerably smaller than the 26–50-Fr. (8.7–16.7 mm) orogastric tubes currently recommended for acute poisoning (12). The larger lavage tubes might return significantly more stomach contents than either the smaller tubes or ipecac alone. However, there are no data to support this hypothesis, and it is felt that emesis is preferred over lavage unless a contraindication to the induction of emesis exists.

necessary information to obtain in poisoning cases

when not to use emetics

Contraindications to Emetics

An emetic is not likely to produce vomiting in patients who have significant CNS depression as evidenced by lethargy, loss of gag reflex, or unconsciousness. If vomiting is produced, the risk of aspiration of vomitus into the lungs is significant. These persons must be treated in an emergency treatment facility.

Patients who are convulsing may aspirate vomitus if given an emetic; an emetic may produce seizures in susceptible patients or worsen an existing seizure.

Patients who have ingested a caustic should not vomit. Caustic agents are strong acids and bases that produce severe burns of the mucous membranes of the mouth and esophagus. If emesis is induced, these tissues will be re-exposed to the caustic, and more damage may occur. In addition, if the esophagus is already damaged, the force of vomiting may cause esophageal perforation.

Emetics should be administered with caution in cases of undesired or excessive antiemetic drug ingestion. If an emetic is not given soon enough after an antiemetic has been ingested, a significant emetic failure rate may result. If an emetic is given in the hospital setting and vomiting does not occur, gastric lavage may become necessary to remove the antiemetic substance.

Patients who have ingested petroleum distillates traditionally have not been given emetics. It was felt that inducing vomiting would increase the likelihood of aspiration of the petroleum distillate into the lungs, leading to alveolar irritation and pneumonitis. When small amounts of petroleum distillates (less than 30 ml or 1 ml/kg) have been ingested, emptying the stomach is unnecessary, and emetics should not be considered. When large amounts of a petroleum distillate capable of producing systemic toxicity have been taken, or when a potentially dangerous chemical, e.g., a pesticide, is dissolved in a petroleum distillate base, emptying the stomach may be necessary.

A retrospective study showed that in patients who had ingested petroleum distillates a lower percentage developed aspiration pneumonitis when vomiting was induced with ipecac than with either lavage or spontaneous vomiting (13). Other research showed that aspiration pneumonitis is less likely to occur in ipecac-treated patients than in those who were lavaged (14). The pneumonitis that developed in this study was less severe in the ipecac-treated patients than in those who were lavaged (14). Therefore emetics may be used in petroleum distillate ingestions under medical supervision.

emetic of choice

doses, toxicity, interactions

Syrup of Ipecac

Syrup of ipecac is the emetic of choice for routine use. Syrup of ipecac is prepared from ipecac powder, a natural product derived from *Cephaelis ipecacuanha* or *acuminata*, and contains approximately 2.1 g of powdered ipecac/30 ml. Vomiting is probably produced by both a local irritant effect on the GI mucosa and a central medullary effect (stimulation of the chemoreceptor trigger zone) (15). The central effect is probably caused by emetine and cephaeline, two alkaloids present in ipecac.

When a patient asks to purchase syrup of ipecac, the pharmacist should determine whether it is to be used immediately to treat a poisoning ingestion or is being purchased to keep in the home in case an ingestion occurs. If the purchase is for immediate use, the pharmacist should determine whether that use is appropriate. If the purchase is for later use, the pharmacist should discuss poison prevention with the patient, distribute poison prevention materials, and provide the patient with the telephone number of a poison center. The patient must be warned that the syrup of ipecac must not be given without first consulting a pharmacist, physician, or poison center.

Ipecac Toxicity

Toxicity following the administration of ipecac is rare. After therapeutic doses, diarrhea and slight CNS depression are common. Clinical experience has shown that the ingestion of 30 ml of syrup of ipecac (the largest amount available over the counter in a single unit of purchase) is safe in children over 1. In larger doses, ipecac may produce cardiovascular toxicity including bradycardia, atrial fibrillation, and hypotension (16). Severe toxicity and death have occurred in the past when fluidextract of ipecac was given by mistake. Fluidextract of ipecac is 14 times stronger than syrup of ipecac and should no longer be found in any pharmacy (17–20).

Dosages of Ipecac

In children over 1 the recommended dose of ipecac is 15 ml (1 tbsp). Because children under 1 do not have a well-developed gag reflex, ipecac should not be administered to such patients without medical supervision. Ipecac does not work well if the stomach is nearly empty. Therefore it is recommended that at least 180–240 ml of fluid be given immediately after the ipecac to partially distend the stomach. Vomiting should occur in 15–20 minutes. If vomiting has not occurred in 20 minutes, another 15 ml of syrup of ipecac should be given.

The initial dose of ipecac for adults is 15–30 ml. No more than a total of 30 ml should be given. One study suggests that the time to vomiting is longer when milk is given with the ipecac than when other fluids are used (21). Other fluids, such as water, should be used instead of milk. The effect of other protein-containing substances that might be in the stomach when ipecac is given is not known. Syrup of ipecac is virtually 100% effective when 15 ml or more is given (22, 23). Patients who are ambulatory seem to vomit more quickly than those who are not. Stimulation of the posterior pharynx also may help to initiate vomiting.

Drug Interactions With Ipecac

The only well-documented drug interaction with syrup of ipecac involves activated charcoal. Activated charcoal is used as an adsorbent in many poisoning cases. When it is administered with ipecac, the ipecac is adsorbed by the charcoal, and emesis is prevented. In addition, the adsorptive capacity of the charcoal is reduced. If both activated charcoal and ipecac are used, the charcoal must be given after successful vomiting has been produced by the ipecac.

Other Methods of Inducing Vomiting

Vomiting may be produced in a number of ways. Syrup of ipecac is the only safe and effective OTC emetic. Home remedies other than ipecac used to induce vomiting are frequently ineffective and in some cases may be dangerous.

Mechanically induced vomiting is produced by giving the patient fluids and then stimulating the reflex with either a blunt object or a finger. Care must be taken not to injure the patient during this procedure. The percentage of persons who vomit following this procedure has been shown to be low, and the mean volume of vomitus is small compared to vomiting induced by syrup of ipecac (24).

Salt water and powdered mustard in water are unpalatable and unreliable emetics. Salt water may be quite toxic owing to sodium absorption, and in fact, fatalities have been produced in children and adults from the use of salt as an emetic (25–29). If vomiting is not produced, severe hypernatremia may result. Salt water should not be used under any circumstances, and mustard water should not be routinely recommended.

Copper and zinc sulfate have been used as emetics and act by producing direct gastric irritation leading to reflex stimulation of the vomiting center. Vomiting must occur before significant absorption of the metals takes place. In three children who vomited soon after the administration of copper sulfate as an emetic, only 54–67% of the dose was recovered in the vomitus (30).

In the same study, all six children who had been given copper sulfate as an emetic had significant increases in serum copper levels (15–105 μg/ml) as compared to one patient in the ipecac group. No evidence of copper intoxication, e.g., jaundice or oliguria, was noted. Copper sulfate administered to another patient with a three-fourths gastrectomy caused renal failure and death (31).

Although apomorphine produces rapid emesis, it is available only by prescription and must be given parenterally. Apomorphine may produce or worsen already existing CNS and respiratory depression. Naloxone has been thought to reverse these effects. In several cases, significant respiratory and/or CNS depression unresponsive to naloxone developed in patients who had been given apomorphine (32).

ANTIEMETICS

Nausea and vomiting are symptoms common to many serious and minor disorders. The pharmacist should be very cautious about patient self-medication of these symptoms and should question the patient appropriately to be satisfied that referral is not indicated.

Evaluation

The following are some of the more important considerations to determine whether an antiemetic is indicated.

Patient's Age

Vomiting in newborns can result from a number of serious abnormalities, including obstruction of the GI tract and disorders of neuromuscular control, and may quickly lead to acid–base disturbances and dehydration. Physician referral is recommended for further work-up of any vomiting in newborns. Simple causes of vomiting, such as overfeeding, feeding too quickly, or ineffective "burping" of the newborn, obviously can be resolved without drug therapy and should be excluded as causes in any evaluation (33).

One of the more common causes of vomiting in children is acute gastroenteritis. Opinions vary on whether drug therapy should be directed at the symptom, vomiting, or at the primary condition; there are no acceptable data on the effects of OTC antiemetics on vomiting with gastroenteritis in children. Some sources question the safety of treating children with antiemetics in an acute, self-limiting disorder (34, 35). It has been suggested that vomiting in gastroenteritis is a body defense that sheds the pathogen and should not be suppressed. This theory awaits confirmation.

Nondrug remedies such as Coca-Cola syrup and carbonated beverages have been used to control vomiting, apparently on an empirical basis. Vomiting may be produced by acidosis and dehydration secondary to severe diarrhea, and practitioners have noted that rehydration may control this vomiting (36).

Patient's Sex

Nausea and vomiting may be one of the earliest symptoms of pregnancy. A woman who notes nausea and vomiting in the early part of the day and who has no other symptoms except a missed menstrual cycle and perhaps weight gain should be referred for a pregnancy test and follow-up. Even if the woman is known to be pregnant, it is important to exclude "nonpregnant" causes of vomiting, such as urinary tract infections and appendicitis. Treatment of morning sickness has been characterized as "therapeutic nihilism" since the thalidomide tragedy, and most physicians are reluctant to prescribe any drug for a pregnant woman. OTC antiemetics have not been evaluated for, nor are they promoted for, use in nausea and vomiting of pregnancy. Some practitioners have suggested trying small frequent feedings to control morning sickness, although the benefits of this approach are not clear (5, 37). Nausea and vomiting also occur frequently in women during the third and fourth weeks of the menstrual cycle, possibly because of increased gonadotropin levels.

Current Drug Use

nausea and vomiting important considerations

Some drugs are known to cause nausea and vomiting as a side effect or as a toxic effect. For example, digitalis toxicity may be manifested as nausea and vomiting. One consequence of congestive heart failure is visceral congestion, which can also produce GI symptoms. Other drugs, such as tetracyclines, estrogens, and the opiate analgesics, can cause nausea and vomiting as side effects.

Vomiting Duration/Blood in Vomitus

A patient who vomits forcefully several times per day for 2–3 days or who has blood in the vomitus should be referred to a physician for diagnosis.

Other Symptoms

Patients who complain of abdominal pain, vomiting, particularly projectile vomiting, and headache should be referred to a physician. Patients with vomiting and diarrhea of gastroenteritis in whom even slight electrolyte imbalance may be critical, such as the newborn, also should be referred. Vomiting has been described as being symptomatic of a form of anorexia nervosa, when patients attempt to lose weight by repeated vomiting and chronic use of purgatives and diuretics (38). Patients with such a history should be referred for management of the underlying problem.

Ingredients in OTC Products

"There is no ailment (motion sickness), with the possible exception of the common cold and hiccoughs, for which the general populace and medical profession alike have prescribed with greater assurance and originality. The remedies have been selected on the basis of hearsay, personal experience, accident, or often apparently occult revelation. The treatments are generally uncontrolled, frequently amusing, and occasionally ingenious" (39).

The available OTC antiemetic preparations have been evaluated and are promoted only for nausea and vomiting of motion sickness (antihistamines and carbohydrates) and nausea associated with overeating or "upset stomach" (bismuth compounds). Therefore the pharmacological properties of antiemetic agents pertinent only to relieving nausea and vomiting from these causes will be reviewed in depth.

The primary agents used to prevent or control motion sickness are the parasympatholytics, antihistamines, and phenothiazines. The compounds all have CNS activity; although the precise mechanism in preventing vomiting is unknown, it is assumed to relate to increased thresholds associated with afferent input to the chemoreceptor trigger zone. Most compounds studied have varying success rates in controlling nausea and vomiting, according to the length of therapy, duration of pretreatment, duration and type of motion, and individual susceptibility to motion sickness. The ability of an agent to prevent motion sickness is not correlated with its potency as an antihistamine, anticholinergic, or phenothiazine tranquilizer (4, 39). Classic studies of the usefulness of antiemetics in motion sickness have identified scopolamine, particularly in conjunction with amphetamine, as being probably the most effective agent in preventing vomiting (40). However, these agents are available only by prescription and have produced significant side effects in therapeutic doses. Five agents have unquestionably been proven valuable in preventing motion sickness: scopolamine, promethazine, cyclizine, meclizine, and dimenhydrinate (2, 40). Only the last three are available over the counter.

recommended agents

dosages and cautions

The OTC antihistaminic preparations have all been shown to be effective antiemetics under various conditions that induce motion sickness. There is little evidence of superiority of one agent over another in all cases.

Cyclizine and Meclizine

Cyclizine and meclizine are members of the benzhydryl piperazine group of antihistamine compounds. They are reported to depress labyrinth excitability and have been shown to be safe and effective in the management of motion sickness (40–43).

Doses of meclizine for adults are 25–50 mg once per day, administered orally 1 hour before departure and repeated every 24 hours. The drug has a relatively long duration of action, and studies have suggested that it provides 24-hour protection against motion sickness (44). Meclizine is not recommended for use in children under 12.

Adult doses of cyclizine are 50 mg up to four times per day (40). For children 6–12 years old the dose is 25 mg up to three times per day. The drug should be administered 30 minutes before departure.

Drowsiness with therapeutic doses can occur, and patients should be cautioned not to drive a car or operate

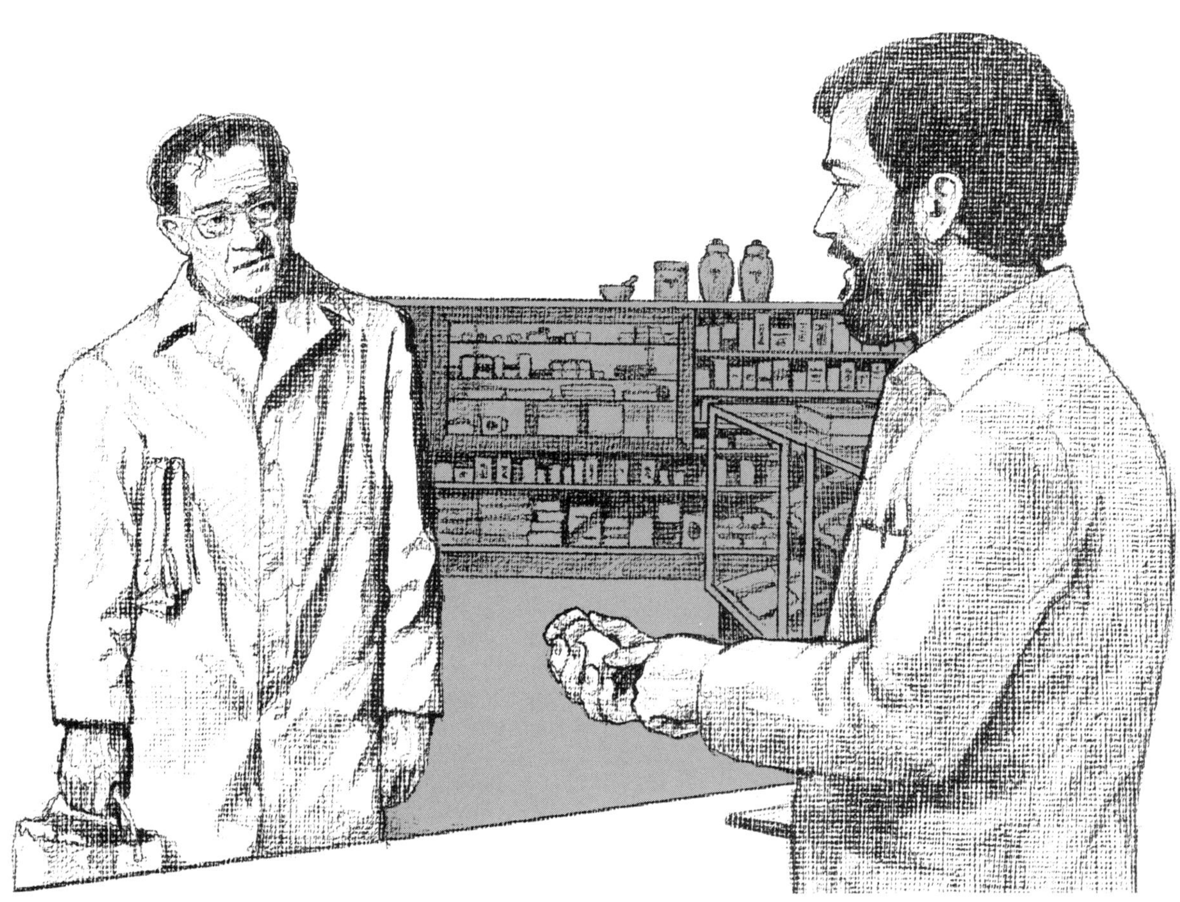

hazardous machinery while using meclizine or cyclizine. The effects are additive to those of other CNS depressants such as alcohol and tranquilizers. In large doses these agents also produce anticholinergic effects, including blurred vision and dry mouth. Patients with narrow-angle glaucoma or prostatic enlargement should be cautioned about the potential exacerbation of their symptoms.

Since 1966, the FDA has required that products containing meclizine and cyclizine carry a warning against their use by pregnant women, based on animal studies in several species that suggested that the drug may have teratogenic or embryolethal potential. Subsequent epidemiological studies of many pregnant women have not shown an increase in embryo deaths or malformations in children of women who used these drugs during early pregnancy (45, 46). The warning against the use of these drugs in pregnant women is no longer required, but pharmacists should note that these agents are not promoted for OTC use for morning sickness of pregnancy.

Dimenhydrinate

Dimenhydrinate is the 8-chlorotheophyllinate salt of the antihistamine, diphenhydramine. Both dimenhydrinate and diphenhydramine hydrochloride are effective antiemetics for motion sickness, although their precise mechanism is unknown (42, 44, 47).

Usual doses for adults are 50–100 mg, two to four times per day administered 30 minutes to 1 hour before departure (40). The dose for children 2–5 years old is 12.5–25 mg up to three times per day.

Drowsiness can occur at recommended doses, and patients should be cautioned about driving a car or operating hazardous machinery (48). In doses of 50 mg, dimenhydrinate can cause anticholinergic side effects, e.g., dry mouth (44); patients with narrow-angle glaucoma or prostatic hypertrophy should be cautioned about exacerbation of their symptoms. In one case of dimenhydrinate abuse an individual was reported to have taken between 15 and 25 tablets of dimenhydrinate (50 mg), which caused delirium, visual and auditory hallucinations, pupil dilation, and dry mouth (49). In another case report, ten 50-mg tablets were ingested, which caused cholinergic hypofunction and toxic psychosis (50). Dimenhydrinate has been implicated in one case report of allergy associated with fixed drug eruptions (51).

Oral and facial dyskinesias were reported after chronic use of antihistamines, and dystonias were reported even with acute use (52, 53). A 4-year-old manifested dystonic posture and torticollis 2 hours after taking 50 mg of diphenhydramine.

Although clinical examples are not available, it is possible that diphenhydramine salts mask the vestibular toxicity of aminoglycoside antibiotics (such as streptomycin and kanamycin) (54). A study of the control of vestibular toxic effects of streptomycin with dimenhydrinate suggests that the potential interaction warrants careful patient monitoring if both drugs are used (55).

Phosphorated Carbohydrate

Phosphorated carbohydrate solution is a mixture of levulose (fructose) and dextrose (glucose) with phosphoric acid added to adjust the pH to between 1.5 and 1.6. Studies evaluating its effectiveness in the vomiting of childhood, pregnancy, and motion sickness have been criticized as being poorly designed (56–59). The mechanism of action is suggested to be a delay in gastric emptying time because of the high osmotic pressure of the solution (60). However, there is no evidence that an increase in gastric emptying time affects nausea and vomiting, particularly if it is due to a disturbance in the semicircular canals.

The usual adult dose of the phosphorated carbohydrate is 15–30 ml (1–2 tbsp) at 15-minute intervals until vomiting ceases. Doses should be limited to five per hour. The solution should not be diluted, and the patient should not consume other liquids for 15 minutes after taking a dose. If vomiting does not cease after five doses, a physician should be contacted.

However, according to the FDA OTC Panel on Laxative, Antidiarrheal, Emetic, and Antiemetic Products, there is insufficient evidence available to establish the effectiveness of phosphorated carbohydrate, and appropriate studies should be done to document effectiveness (59).

agents for motion sickness

levulose/fructose

Large doses of levulose may cause abdominal pain and diarrhea. Levels of uric acid in urine and serum are reported to have increased in healthy volunteers when levulose (500 mg/kg) was given orally (61).

Practitioners should be aware of its high glucose content and associated problems in diabetics.

Bismuth Compounds

The OTC bismuth preparations are promoted for the relief of symptoms of nausea and upper GI distress, particularly those related to the consumption of certain foods or excess quantities of food. The proposed mechanism of action is a "coating" effect of the bismuth preparation on the gastric mucosa, although this phenomenon has been questioned (59). There is no evidence that bismuth compounds affect gastric emptying time, tone of the stomach wall, or intragastric pressure to relieve symptoms induced by overeating. Unpublished data provided by the manufacturer suggest a consumer preference for this product in treating such self-defined symptoms as "indigestion," "gas," and "full stomach" (62). However, no convincing objective data show that bismuth compounds decrease nausea and vomiting from overeating. One study of bismuth subsalicylate in dogs and humans found that bismuth subsalicylate given before or in connection with 5 ml of ipecac prevented subsequent vomiting (the effective dose of ipecac is 15 ml) (63). The bismuth subsalicylate may have bound the ipecac to prevent its absorption. The use of an ipecac model for a patient's "upset stomach" is highly questionable.

Bismuth subsalicylate may decrease subjective complaints of nausea and abdominal cramping associated with enteric infections (excluding *Shigella*) acquired in Mexico (64). In this study, 90% of subjects expressed relief after 3.5 hours of therapy, compared to 70% of placebo-treated control patients. The relationship between nausea of infectious origin and nausea associated with food consumption is not clear.

Bismuth salts appear to be poorly absorbed from the GI tract. Several studies report the absence of detectable bismuth in the urine of human subjects given high doses or treated over a long period. Detectable but unpredictable blood levels of salicylate have been reported after the ingestion of 30–45 ml of bismuth subsalicylate (equivalent to ingesting 357.5–536.3 mg of salicylic acid). Blood levels ranged from barely detectable to 6.2 mg/100 ml (65).

The manufacturer's maximum recommended dose of bismuth subnitrate provides 5.6 g for adults and 0.475 g for children (3–6 years old) within 4 hours. There is a risk of methemoglobinemia in children under 2 due to absorption of nitrates from bismuth subnitrate (65, 66). Isolated cases of eruptions like those of pityriasis rosea due to bismuth injections have been reported, but no reaction to oral use of bismuth has been noted (67). A possible relationship between toxic encephalopathy and ingestion of insoluble bismuth salts has been reported (68). A series of 45 patients treated with bismuth subnitrate (5–20 g/day) for periods ranging from 4 weeks to 30 years developed acute encephalopathies. The toxic phenomenon does not appear directly proportional to bismuth consumption and may represent an idiosyncratic reaction. Pharmacists should note that stools may darken with use of bismuth compounds.

bismuth salts
recommended doses

SUMMARY

Emetics are useful in cases of oral poisoning to remove gastric contents and to prevent further absorption of the ingested agent. Syrup of ipecac is the most effective and the safest OTC emetic for this purpose. It should be kept in all homes with young children and used if an ingestion occurs.

OTC antiemetics are useful in limited, patient-diagnosed situations, such as prevention of motion sickness. The pharmacist should ascertain the reason for purchasing an OTC antiemetic and suggest referral if necessary. Chronic unsupervised use of antiemetics, especially for an "upset stomach," should be discouraged, and the patient should be encouraged to seek additional medical help for continuous discomfort.

REFERENCES

(1) "Harrison's Principles of Internal Medicine," 7th ed., G. W. Thorn, R. D. Adams, E. Braunwald, K. J. Isselbacher, and R. G. Petersdorf, Eds., McGraw-Hill, New York, N.Y., 1974, p. 208.
(2) J. Kirsner, in "Pathologic Physiology—Mechanisms of Diseases," 5th ed., W. Sodeman and W. Sodeman, Jr., Eds., Saunders, Philadelphia, Pa., 1974, p. 711.
(3) T. R. Hendrix, in "Medical Physiology," Vol. 2, 13th ed., V. Mountcastle, Ed., Mosby, St. Louis, Mo., 1974, p. 1224.
(4) J. Brand and W. Perry, *Pharmacol. Rev.*, *18*, 895 (1966).
(5) I. Gordon et al., in "Gastroenterologic Medicine," M. Paulson, Ed., Lea and Febiger, Philadelphia, Pa., 1969, pp. 468, 1233–1234.
(6) "Williams Obstetrics," L. Hellman and J. Prichard, Eds., Meridith, New York, N.Y., 1971, pp. 343–344.
(7) J. Arena, *Mod. Treatm.*, *8*, 461 (1971).
(8) National Clearinghouse of Poison Control Centers Bulletin, U.S. Public Health Service, Washington, D.C., Feb. 1978.
(9) L. Boxer, F. P. Anderson, and D. S. Rowe, *J. Pediatr.*, *74*, 800 (1969).
(10) L. Goldstein, *J. Am. Med. Assoc.*, *208*, 2162 (1969).
(11) F. Arnold, Jr., J. B. Hodges, Jr., R. A. Barta, Jr., S. Spector, I. Sunshine, and R. Wedgewood, *Pediatrics*, *23*, 286 (1959).
(12) B. Rumack, "Poisindex," Micromedex, Denver, Colo., 1975.
(13) S. Molinas, National Clearinghouse for Poison Control Centers, U.S. Public Health Service, Washington, D.C., March-April 1966.
(14) R. C. Ng, H. Darwish, and D. A. Stewart, *Can. Med. Assoc. J.*, *111*, 537 (1974).
(15) "The Pharmacological Basis of Therapeutics," 5th ed., L. S. Goodman and A. Gilman, Eds., Macmillan, New York, N.Y., 1975, p. 1075.
(16) J. McLeod, *N. Engl. J. Med.*, *268*, 146 (1963).
(17) J. D. Speer, W. O. Robertson, and L. R. Schultz, *Lancet*, *1*, 475 (1963).
(18) T. Bates and E. Grunwaldt, *Am. J. Dis. Child.*, *103*, 169 (1962).
(19) R. Allport, *Am. J. Dis. Child.*, *98*, 786 (1959).
(20) R. Smith and D. Smith, *N. Engl. J. Med.*, *265*, 23 (1964).
(21) R. J. Varipapa and G. M. Oderda, *N. Engl. J. Med.*, *296*, 112 (1977).
(22) W. Robertson, *Am. J. Dis. Child.*, *103*, 58 (1972).
(23) W. MacLean, *J. Pediatr.*, *82*, 121 (1973).
(24) I. A. Dabbous, A. B. Bergman, and W. O. Robertson, *J. Pediatr.*, *66*, 952 (1965).
(25) J. Barer, L. L. Hill, R. M. Hill, and W. M. Martinez, *Am. J. Dis. Child.*, *125*, 889 (1973).
(26) F. DeGenaro and W. Nyhan, *J. Pediatr.*, *78*, 1048 (1971).
(27) D. Ward, *Br. Med. J.*, *2*, 432 (1963).
(28) B. Lawrence and B. Hopkins, *Med. J. Aust.*, *1*, 1301 (1969).
(29) W. Robertson, *J. Pediatr.*, *79*, 877 (1971).
(30) N. Holtzman and R. Haslam, *Pediatrics*, *42*, 189 (1968).
(31) R. S. Stein, D. Jenkins, and M. E. Korns, *J. Am. Med. Assoc.*, *235*, 801 (1976).
(32) J. Schofferman, *J. Am. Coll. Emerg. Phys.*, *5*, 22 (1976).
(33) A. Schaffer, *Surg. Clin. North Am.*, *50*, 853 (1970).
(34) O. Anderson, *Pediatrics*, *46*, 319 (1970).
(35) M. Casteels-Van Daele et al., *Arch. Dis. Child.*, *45*, 130 (1970).
(36) H. Hirschhorn and W. B. Greenough, in "Davidson's Principles and Practices of Medicine," 19th ed., A. M. Harvey, Ed., Appleton-Century-Crofts, New York, N.Y., 1976, p. 1264.
(37) *Medical Letter*, *16*, 46 (1974).
(38) P. J. Beumont, G. C. George, and D. E. Smart, *Psychol. Med.*, *6*, 617 (1976).
(39) H. I. Chinn and P. K. Smith, *Pharmacol. Rev.*, *7*, 53 (1955).
(40) C. D. Wood and A. Graybiel, *Clin. Pharmacol. Ther.*, *11*, 621 (1970).
(41) L. B. Gutner et al., *Arch. Otolaryngol.*, *59*, 503 (1954).
(42) H. I. Chinn et al. (Army/Navy/Air Force Motion Sickness Team), *J. Am. Med. Assoc.*, *160*, 755 (1956).
(43) R. Trumbull, H. I. Chinn, C. H. Maag, L. J. Milch, S. W. Handford, R. Seibert, P. Sterling, and P. K. Smith, *Clin. Pharmacol. Ther.*, *1*, 280 (1960).
(44) H. I. Chinn, S. W. Handford, P. K. Smith, T. E. Cone, Jr., R. F. Redmond, J. V. Maloney, and C. M. Smythe, *J. Pharmacol. Exp. Ther.*, *108*, 69 (1953).
(45) J. Yerushalmy and L. Milkovich, *Am. J. Obstet. Gynecol.*, *93*, 553 (1965).
(46) S. Shapiro, Data From Boston Collaborative Drug Surveillance Program, Testimony Before OTC Panel, 1974.
(47) S. W. Handford, T. E. Cone, Jr., H. I. Chinn, and P. K. Smith, *J. Pharmacol. Exp. Ther.*, *111*, 447 (1954).
(48) C. D. Wood, R. E. Kennedy, A. Graybiel, R. Trumbull, and R. J. Wherry, *J. Am. Med. Assoc.*, *198*, 1155 (1966).
(49) J. Brown and H. Sigmundson, *Can. Med. Assoc. J.*, *101*, 49 (1969).
(50) S. A. Nigro, *J. Am. Med. Assoc.*, *203*, 301 (1968).
(51) C. Stritzler and A. W. Kopf, *J. Invest. Dermatol.*, *34*, 319 (1960).
(52) R. P. Granacher, *N. Engl. J. Med.*, *296*, 516 (1977).
(53) R. Sorner, *N. Engl. J. Med.*, *296*, 633 (1977).
(54) P. Hansten, "Drug Interactions," Lea and Febiger, Philadelphia, Pa., 1973, p. 128.
(55) L. L. Titche and A. Nady, *Dis. Chest*, *20*, 324 (1951).
(56) J. E. Bradley, L. Proutt, E. R. Shipley, and R. H. Oster, *J. Pediatr.*, *38*, 41 (1951).
(57) A. B. Crunden, Jr., and W. A. Davis, *Am. J. Obstet. Gynecol.*, *65*, 311 (1953).
(58) H. A. Agerty, *Adult Child*, *1*, 66 (1969).
(59) *Federal Register*, *40*, 12935 (1975).
(60) J. B. Houston and G. Levy, *J. Pharm. Sci.*, *64*, 1504 (1975).
(61) J. Perkeentupa and K. Raivis, *Lancet*, *2*, 528 (1967).
(62) Norwich Pharmaceutical Company, unpublished data, Communication With OTC Panel on Laxative, Antidiarrheal, Emetic and Antiemetic Products, 1974.
(63) M. M. Goldenberg, L. J. Honkomp, and C. S. Davis, *J. Pharm. Sci.*, (64) H. L. DuPont, P. Sullivan, L. K. Pickering, G. Haynes, and P. B. Ackerman, *Gastroenterology*, *73*, 715 (1977).
(63) M. M. Goldenberg, L. J. Honkomp, and C. S. Davis, *J. Pharm. Sci.*, *65*, 1398 (1976).
(64) H. L. DuPont, P. Sullivan, L. K. Pickering, G. Haynes, and P. B. Ackerman, *Gastroenterology*, *73*, 715 (1977).
(65) R. E. Gosselin, H. C. Hodge, R. P. Smith, and M. N. Gleason, in "Clinical Toxicology of Commercial Products, Acute Poisoning," 4th ed., Williams and Wilkins, Baltimore, Md., 1976, pp. 251, 295.
(66) "Accumulation of Nitrate," National Academy of Sciences, Washington, D.C., 1972, pp. 46–75.
(67) W. L. Dobes and H. S. Alden, *South. Med. J.*, *42*, 572 (1949).
(68) V. Supino-Viterbo, C. Sicard, M. Risvegliato, G. Rancurel, and A. Buge, *J. Neurol. Neurosurg. Psych.*, *40*, 748 (1977).

Product (Manufacturer)	Dosage Form	Active Ingredients	Other
Bonine (Pfipharmecs)	chewable tablet	meclizine hydrochloride, 25 mg	—
Dramamine (Searle)	tablet liquid	dimenhydrinate, 50 mg/tablet 3 mg/ml	sucrose, 54% (liquid) ethanol, 5% (liquid) cherry pit flavor, 0.2% (liquid)
Eldodram (Elder)	tablet	dimenhydrinate, 50 mg	—
Emetrol (Rorer)	liquid	invert sugar, 750 mg/ml phosphoric acid, 5 mg/ml	—
Especol (Pfeiffer)	liquid	levulose (fructose) dextrose orthophosphoric acid with controlled pH	flavor
Marezine (Burroughs-Wellcome)	tablet	cyclizine hydrochloride, 50 mg	—
Ram (Scrip)	tablet	dimenhydrinate, 50 mg	—
Trav-Arex (Columbia Medical)	tablet	dimenhydrinate, 50 mg	—
Vertrol (Saron)	tablet	meclizine hydrochloride, 12.5 mg	—

Ostomy Care Products

Michael L. Kleinberg

Chapter 6

Questions to Ask the Patient

What type of ostomy do you have? Where is it located?

How long have you had the ostomy?

Do you irrigate, use a bag, or both?

What is the stoma size?

Do you have problems with the skin surrounding the stoma?

Have you noticed any change in the contents of your fecal discharge?

Are you experiencing any problems related to your ostomy such as diarrhea or gas?

Are you having any problems with odor control?

Are you taking any medication?

An ostomy is the surgical formation of an opening, or outlet, through the abdominal wall for the purpose of eliminating waste. It is usually made by passing the colon, small intestine, or ureters through the abdominal wall. The part of the intestine brought to the surface of the body is called the stoma.

The anatomy of the lower digestive tract is shown in Figure 1. The main function of the digestive system is the conversion of food into an assimilable form. Digestion begins in the mouth and then continues in the stomach and small intestine, and water absorption takes place in the large intestine. (See Chapter 1 for a complete discussion of digestion.)

Ostomy surgery necessitates the use of an appliance designed to collect the waste material normally eliminated via the bowel or bladder. Approximately 90,000 ostomies are created annually in the United States, and more than 1 million patients have established intestinal stomas (1).

The idea of cutting into the abdominal cavity and creating an artificial opening is not new. This type of surgery was first suggested in 1710 by a French physician, Alexis Littre (2). Since that time the technique of ostomy surgery has been refined greatly. The surgical creation of an ostomy is only the first step, however, in the rehabilitation of an ostomate (a person with an ostomy). Complete recovery depends on how well ostomy patients understand and adjust to their changed medical and physical circumstances.

Pharmacists involved in ostomy care must be familiar with the various types of ostomies and with the use and maintenance of the appliances for each type. They should also be prepared to provide patients with information on problems related to ostomy care such as skin care, diet, and drug therapy.

Because each ostomy patient is different, one patient may benefit from one type of appliance, while another may develop problems with it. The ostomy patient should be familiar with the techniques of applying and fitting an appliance that affords maximum benefit. Proper patient counseling on diet, fluids, and medication is necessary to prevent complications.

Pharmacy involvement in ostomy care is important. The American Pharmaceutical Association identifies ostomy care as a clinical role for the pharmacist in direct patient care. Likewise, the American Society of Hospital Pharmacists specifies experience in ostomy care in the new accreditation standards for residency training. Procurement and distribution of ostomy supplies and patient counseling are necessary services which can be provided by the pharmacist.

TYPES OF OSTOMIES

Several types of ostomies are performed regularly. They are listed below.

Colostomy

A colostomy is the creation of an artificial opening using part of the large intestine or colon. Major indications for performing a colostomy include colon or rectum obstruction, cancer of the colon or rectum, genetic malformation, diverticular disease, trauma, and loss of anal muscular control.

When certain conditions are present in the lower bowel, it may be necessary to give that part a rest. A temporary colostomy is created so that healing can take place. This healing process may take a few weeks, months, or years. Eventually, the colon and rectum will be reconnected, and bowel continuity will be restored. A permanent colostomy is formed when a significant portion of the colon is totally removed; reconstruction of the bowel is impossible. A colostomy, permanent or temporary, may be made in any part of the colon but most commonly is made in the sigmoid colon.

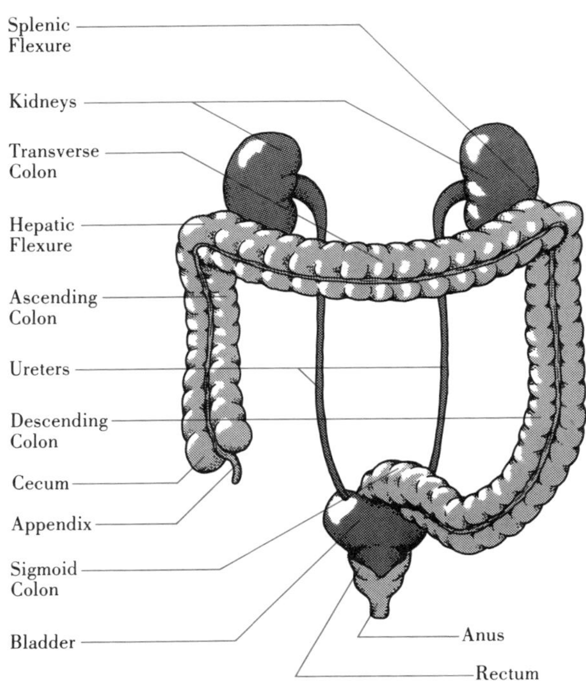

Figure 1. Anatomy of the lower digestive and urinary tracts.

colostomies
others procedures
equipment

Ascending Colostomy

This ostomy appears on the right side of the abdomen (Figure 2a). Its discharge is semisolid and requires that the patient continually wear an appliance.

Transverse Colostomy

This opening usually is created on the right side of the transverse colon (Figure 2b) in one of two ways. The first method entails lifting a loop of the transverse colon through the abdominal incision. A rod or bridge is then placed under the loop to give additional support (Figure 2c) and removed after a few days. The second method is to divide the bowel completely and have two openings (double-barrel colostomy) (Figure 2d). In this case the right ostomy discharges fecal material, and the left one discharges small amounts of mucus. The consistency of the discharge from a transverse colostomy varies, depending on the distance from the small intestine to the opening. The rest of the colon assumes the concentrating function of effluent, so that in time the stool takes on near-normal consistency. Management depends on the individual, but usually an appliance is worn continually.

Descending and Sigmoid Colostomies

These ostomies are on the left side of the abdomen (Figure 2e). They can be made as double-barrel (temporary) or single-barrel (permanent) openings. Because the fecal discharge is firm and often can be regulated by the patient, an appliance may not be needed. However, many patients prefer appliances to irrigation. There is no right or wrong method. Patient preference is the deciding factor.

Ileostomy

An ileostomy is a surgically created opening between the ileum and the abdominal wall, usually in cases of ulcerative colitis, Crohn's disease, trauma, multiple polyposis, or cancer. The entire colon is surgically removed, and the ileum is brought to the surface of the abdomen (Figure 2f). The discharge is semisolid and, because it contains pancreatic enzymes, irritating to the skin. An appliance is worn continually.

Urinary Diversions

These diversions are performed as a result of bladder loss or dysfunction usually due to cancer or genital malformation. An ileal conduit is created by implanting the ureters into a portion of the ileum and bringing the end of the ileal segment to the surface of the abdomen (Figure 2g). An appliance is worn continually. A ureterostomy involves detaching the ureters from the bladder and bringing them to the outside of the abdominal wall. This procedure is performed less frequently than the ileal conduit because patients find it more difficult to take care of themselves after surgery.

APPLIANCES AND ACCESSORIES

The appliance is an extremely important aspect of the ostomate's well-being. The ostomate has lost a normal functioning body process, and the appliance takes over that lost function and seemingly becomes a part of the body. The type of appliance depends on the type of surgery performed. The ideal appliance should be leakproof, comfortable, easily manipulated, odorproof, inconspicuous, inexpensive, and safe (3). Unfortunately, there is no one appliance that meets all these criteria. Major manufacturers of ostomy products and accessories are listed in the appendix.

Disposable (Temporary) Appliances

A disposable appliance consists simply of a plastic bag that can be attached to the skin. It is usually transparent, so that a surgeon can examine the stoma without removing the appliance. Disposable appliances save nursing time during appliance changes and are simple to apply. They generally are used immediately after surgery until the stoma has healed and inflammation has subsided. Some ostomy patients continue to use this type of appliance because of its simplicity. Disadvantages are its fragility, relative lack of adhesiveness, and cost.

Permanent (Reusable) Appliances

A permanent appliance consists of two main parts: a pouch which can be emptied and a faceplate attached to the skin. These appliances are available in one piece (with the faceplate attached to the bag) or two pieces (with a removable faceplate). Permanent appliances have the advantages of strength, better adhesiveness, and lower cost. Disadvantages include the extra care and additional

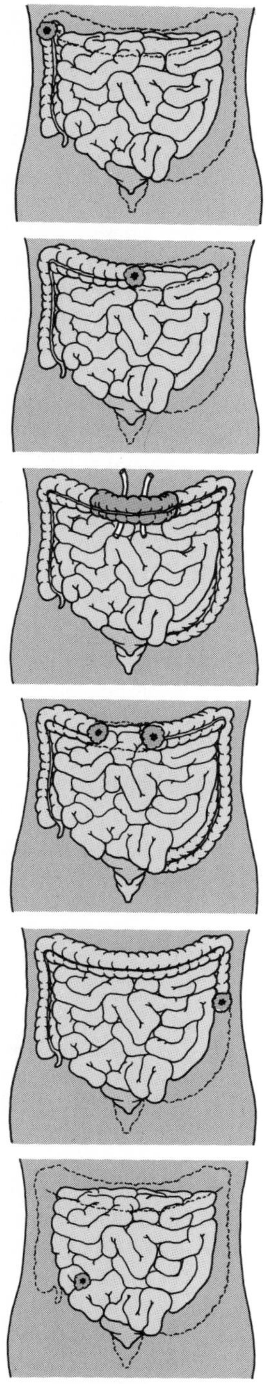

A Ascending Colostomy

B Transverse Colostomy

C Loop Ostomy

D Double-Barrel Colostomy

E Descending Colostomy

F Ileostomy

G Ileal Conduit

Figure 2. Types of ostomies. Adapted from J. R. Wuest, *J. Am. Pharm. Assoc.*, **NS15**, 626 (1975).

supplies needed. The appliance must be discarded after a few months because of its staining and retention of odor.

Accessories

Foam Pads

The foam pad is not an integral part of an appliance, but it can be very useful. Generally made of closed pore nonabsorbent foam rubber, it is cemented between the faceplate of the appliance and the skin. The pad can be used to reduce the size of the appliance orifice and to add comfort, and it may increase the number of days between appliance changes.

Belts

Special belts attached to various appliances give additional support. Belts are made for specific appliances and are not interchangeable. They provide the pressure needed for a good bond and reassure the ostomy patient that the appliance will not fall off. Belts are optional, depending on the ostomate's preference. Patients must be careful not to wear a belt too tight, since any movement by the patient may cause the faceplate to move, possibly damaging the stoma. Two fingers should fit under the belt when it is attached.

colostomies

accessory equipment

Cement

The cement that holds the appliance to the skin is usually made of latex, a hydrocarbon solvent, and a protective additive such as zinc oxide. It is waterproof and protects the skin from irritation caused by fecal material. However, the cement itself may be irritating to the skin and should not be used until a patch test is performed. The test consists of placing a small piece of material (cement) to be tested on the abdomen (not near the stoma), covering it with tape, and leaving it for 48 hours. If redness, itching, or burning occurs during this period, the test is positive, and the material should not be used. If there is no reaction, the material is safe to use. However, reactions may develop after 48 hours, and the patient should be instructed to watch for skin irritation.

Adhesive Seals

Colly-Seal, Stomahesive, and Relia-Seal are sometimes used instead of cement. Colly-Seal contains karaya, and its adhesiveness may last longer than karaya powder. Stomahesive wafers are composed of gelatin, pectin, carboxymethylcellulose sodium, and polyisobutylene. They are nonallergenic and adhere to weepy or oozing skin. Relia-Seal is a combination foam pad and adhesive. For maximum effectiveness it should be applied to dry skin.

Solvents

A solvent helps remove the cement from the appliance. It is used between the appliance and the skin, allowing easy removal of the appliance without pulling it and preventing possible skin irritation. The solvent is usually a hydrocarbon. Frequent use of solvents may defat skin, causing drying and cracking.

Karaya Gum

Karaya gum powder is made from the resin of the *Sterculia urens* tree found in India and is used for its adhesive and healing properties. Karaya becomes gelatinous in contact with moisture. Mixing aluminum hydroxide gel with the karaya instead of water increases healing. Some manufacturers produce karaya washers made of karaya mixed with glycerin and baked into a ring. The ring is moistened and stretched (molded) or cut to fit snugly around the stoma. Karaya also may be used to promote healing of irritated, weeping, or oozing areas.

Tape

A tape provides additional appliance support and waterproofs the cement–skin bond. A strip of tape is applied across the top and/or bottom of the faceplate, half on the faceplate and half on the skin.

irrigation
odor control
correct appliance fitting

Tincture of Benzoin

This product is used to make the skin more adhesive so that a better seal can be obtained, to toughen the skin, and to help prevent skin irritation. It is patted on the skin and allowed to dry, and cement is then placed over it. Some individuals may be allergic to tincture of benzoin. Tincture of benzoin compound should never be used as a substitute for tincture of benzoin because the additional ingredients (e.g., aloe) will irritate the skin.

Irrigating Sets

Some patients irrigate their colostomies to maintain bowel regularity. The irrigating set includes a reservoir for the irrigating fluid, a tube, an irrigating tip, and a collection bag.

Frequency of irrigation depends on the colostomate's normal bowel habits. Basically, colostomy irrigation is the introduction of water into the colon through the stoma by means of a catheter or conical adapter, which is safer. The water stimulates the intestinal wall, producing peristalsis, and softens the stool, allowing subsequent fecal evacuation. The patient should be very cautious in inserting the catheter because the mucosa of the colon is insensitive to pain, and perforation may occur without the patient's knowledge. The catheter should be well lubricated and inserted without pressure. Patients may continue to wear the appliance after irrigation, or they may prefer to cover the stoma with a small piece of gauze between irrigations.

Deodorizers

Odor control is either local or systemic. Some agents are placed directly in the appliance to mask the odor of the fecal discharge. Ostomates sometimes place aspirin tablets in the pouch for odor control, but this practice should be discouraged, since aspirin may irritate the stoma. Chlorophyll, charcoal tablets, and bismuth subgallate and subcarbonate are taken orally. The mechanism of action of bismuth subgallate is unknown but may involve inhibition of bacterial formation. The dose is 200 mg before each meal. Bismuth subgallate also has the advantage of decreasing peristaltic activity. However, it may have neurological side effects such as general malaise, lack of energy, and peculiar sensations in fingers and toes (4).

FITTING AND APPLICATION

Measuring the stoma to determine the proper fit of an appliance is an important part of ostomy care. An appliance whose opening is smaller than the stoma may cause stress and irritation, whereas one whose opening is larger than necessary exposes the skin around the stoma and allows excoriation and/or ulceration.

Most appliance manufacturers provide stoma gauges to assure correct faceplate fitting. The gauges usually are pieces of cardboard with premeasured and precut holes. The ostomate determines the size by selecting a precut hole and placing it over the stoma. The appliance should be 1.5–3.0 mm larger than the stoma to allow for slight swelling or motion of the stoma or for an irregularly shaped stoma and to prevent rubbing of the stoma against the faceplate edge. If a karaya appliance is used, the clearance can be much finer.

The lack of uniformity in types of ostomies and ostomy equipment makes it difficult to give standard instructions for application. Some of the procedures for applying different types of appliances and accessories are listed below (5, 6).

Disposable Adhesive Appliances

- Assemble the equipment.
- Remove the used appliance by gently peeling away the pouch from the skin. Solvent may be applied with a medicine dropper, one drop at a time, between the body and bag. Karaya may be removed with water.
- Measure the stoma (only when selecting an appliance, not routinely).
- Clean the skin around the stoma with soap and water. Be sure to remove all the soap. Pat dry.
- If a skin barrier is used, place it snugly around the stoma.
- Peel the paper backing from the adhesive. If the appliance has a karaya backing, moisten with water.
- Grasp both sides of the appliance and place the center opening over the stoma. Press gently around the stoma.
- Close the pouch by turning the bottom up twice. Secure it with a rubber band or clip supplied by the manufacturer.
- Apply tape and belt, if desired.

Permanent Appliances

- Assemble the equipment.
- If a two-piece appliance is used, attach the pouch to the faceplate by stretching the opening in the pouch over the faceplate. Secure the attaching device around the pouch.
- Old cement should be removed from the faceplate by rubbing with a cotton ball or gauze pad dipped in solvent.
- Apply two thin coats of cement to the clean faceplate. Allow each coat to dry thoroughly.

- Remove the used appliance by gently peeling away the pouch from the skin. Solvent may be applied as for a disposable appliance. Karaya may be removed with water.
- Clean the skin with soap and water. A little solvent may be used to remove excess cement. Allow to dry.
- Apply two thin coats of cement to the clean skin. Spread it slightly beyond the area to be covered by the faceplate. Allow each coat to dry thoroughly.
- If a skin barrier (e.g., karaya) is used, place it snugly around the stoma.
- Grasp both sides of the appliance and place the center opening over the stoma. Press gently around the stoma.
- Clamp the bottom of the pouch.
- Apply tape and belt, if desired.

Karaya Rings

- Cut the karaya sheet into squares and cut a hole 3 mm smaller than the stoma, or use precut karaya washers which are 3 mm smaller than the stoma.
- Moisten the karaya with water.
- Stretch the karaya around the stoma to fit snugly.
- Apply as directed.

Adhesive Seals

Instructions differ depending on whether the seal is a pad or a wafer.

Relia-Seal

- Cut a hole in the Relia-Seal about the same size as the stoma. Use one pad per application.
- Peel the white paper covering from the pad and apply the Relia-Seal over the stoma.
- Peel the blue paper covering from the pad.
- Place the appliance over the Relia-Seal.

An adhesive barrier may be needed between the Relia-Seal and the appliance for added adhesion.

Stomahesive

- Cut a hole in the wafer about the same size as the stoma. Use one wafer per application.
- Cut a hole in the double-faced adhesive disc the same size as the opening in the faceplate.
- Apply one side of the adhesive disc to the shiny surface of the Stomahesive.
- Remove the paper backing from the dull side of the Stomahesive and apply this side to the skin.
- Remove the paper backing from the adhesive disc.
- Place the appliance over the Stomahesive and the adhesive disc.

IMPORTANCE OF DIET

The diet for an ostomate should be individualized. Some patients are placed on a low-residue diet (a diet low in fruits and vegetables) for the first few weeks following surgery so as to minimize waste discharge and intestinal obstruction. After this initial period the ostomate may be allowed to eat all foods. It might be wise for the patient to try a different type of food each day, enabling selective avoidance of foods that produce unfavorable reactions. Some foods may cause cramps or diarrhea; fish, onions, and eggs may produce odor (cranberry juice, yogurt, and buttermilk may help reduce odor); and peas, beans, asparagus, cabbage, radishes, cucumbers, and carbonated beverages may produce gas. Patients with a urinary ostomy, ileostomy, or ascending colostomy must ensure an adequate amount of fluid in their diets to prevent the precipitation of crystals or kidney stones in the urine. Absence of the large bowel may not allow normal absorption of water needed to maintain urinary volume.

POTENTIAL COMPLICATIONS

Ostomates may experience both psychological and physical complications. The pharmacist should be prepared to treat either type.

Psychological Complications

Following ostomy surgery, depending on prior mental status and self-confidence, the patient may be psychologically depressed. There also may be the fear of not being able to engage in former work, participate in sports, perform sexually, or have children. The pharmacist should reassure the patient that the ability to carry out these activities or functions generally remains unchanged.

The United Ostomy Association, formed in 1962, is made up of various ostomy organizations around the country whose main purpose is to help ostomy patients by giving moral and physical support and supplying information. The United Ostomy Association sponsors a yearly meeting and publishes a quarterly journal and other literature. The address is 1111 Wilshire Boulevard, Los Angeles, California 90017. Many local organizations provide free counseling that may be helpful to patients.

procedures for application

diet considerations

complications

Physical Complications

Physical complications of ostomy are stenosis of the stoma, fistula formation, prolapse, retraction, and skin irritation. The pharmacist may deal for the most part with skin irritation.

Stenosis

Stenosis, or narrowing, of the stoma is caused by the formation of excess scar tissue. To overcome this problem, a physician may try dilation of the stoma with a lubricated finger. If this does not work, surgery may be indicated.

Fistula

The formation of an opening, or fistula, in the area projecting external to the abdomen may be caused by an injury to the stoma, a poorly fitting appliance, or poor surgical technique. The fistula allows direct drainage onto the skin, which can lead to other problems. Treatment is surgical repair.

Prolapse

Prolapse, the abnormal extension of the bowel beyond the abdominal wall, frequently results from too large an opening in the abdominal wall. The danger of prolapse is the decrease in blood supply to the bowel outside the abdominal cavity. Treatment is surgical intervention.

Retraction

Retraction is the recession of the stoma to a subnormal length caused by a stretched opening in the abdominal wall. It also may damage the skin surface. Treatment is surgical intervention.

Skin Irritation

Skin irritation usually occurs when an appliance is not used correctly (7). Irritation leads to leakage, and leakage causes more irritation. Sensitization to materials used and frequent appliance changes also may further this complication. Excessive sweating around the stoma and in the skin under the rubber appliance may increase skin irritation, since sweating will decrease the adhesion between the skin and the appliance. The ostomate should therefore delay appliance changes for a time after a hot bath or shower, when the skin normally sweats.

complications

drug use by ostomates

suppliers

To avoid skin irritation, the ostomate may purchase or make a cover for the appliance. When the skin around the stoma is irritated, the ostomate may wish to use karaya gum powder on the inflamed skin between the skin and the cement. It may be necessary to use an anti-inflammatory cream containing a steroid. Ointments should be avoided, since they are greasy and do not allow a tight bond. A method under investigation is the use of cholestyramine (8). The local application of this ointment may bind bile acids and therefore minimize skin inflammation.

USE OF DRUGS

Because part or all of the colon is removed and intestinal transit time may be altered, the ostomate may have difficulty in taking prescription or nonprescription medication.

Coated or sustained-release preparations may pass through the intestinal tract without being absorbed, and the patient may receive a subtherapeutic dose. The ostomate should look for any undissolved drug particles in the pouch. Liquid preparations or preparations crushed or chewed before swallowing are best.

The ostomate also must be careful in taking antibiotics, diuretics, and laxatives. Antibiotics may alter the normal flora of the intestinal tract, causing diarrhea or fungal infection of the skin surrounding the stoma. If diarrhea occurs, fluid and electrolyte intake should be increased. Antidiarrheal and antimotility drugs may affect ileal excreta (9). The physician may prescribe nystatin powder to treat fungal overgrowth.

Diuretics should be given with care, since additional loss of fluid may cause dehydration, especially in patients with ileostomies, whose fluid and electrolyte balance is more difficult to maintain (10). Laxatives may be used in colostomy patients but only under close supervision. Ostomates tend to become obstructed, and the laxative's particular action may cause perforation. If the colostomate is having constipation, a stool softener may be recommended. Ileostomates should never need a laxative.

SUMMARY

With proper instructions and equipment, ostomates can lead normal healthy lives. Pharmacists can help by giving patients the necessary information and treatment for ostomy supply service.

REFERENCES

(1) J. R. Benfield, E. Fowler, and P. V. Barrett, *Arch. Surg.*, *107*, 62 (1973).
(2) C. D. Cromar, *Dis. Colon Rectum*, *7*, 256 (1968).
(3) M. Sparberg, "Ileostomy Care," Charles C Thomas, Springfield, Ill., 1971, p. 18.
(4) D. Lowe, *Med. J. Aust.*, *2*, 664 (1974).
(5) L. Gross, "Ileostomy: A Guide," United Ostomy Association, Inc., Los Angeles, Calif., 1974, p. 28.
(6) N. N. Gill, J. Kerr, and R. B. Turnbull, "Instructions for the Care of the Ileostomy Stoma," Cleveland Clinic Foundation, Cleveland, Ohio.
(7) I. Scott, *Practitioner*, *199*, 657 (1967).
(8) J. T. Rodriguez, T. L. Huang, G. D. Ferry, W. J. Klish, F. J. Harberg, and B. L. Nichols, *J. Pediatr.*, *88*, 659 (1976).
(9) P. Kramer, *Dig. Dis.*, *22*, 327 (1977).
(10) N. D. Gallagher, D. D. Harrison, and A. P. Skyring, *Gut*, *3*, 219 (1962).

APPENDIX: MAJOR MANUFACTURERS

- Atlantic Surgical Co., Inc.
  1834 Landsdowne Avenue
  Merrick, Long Island, NY 11566
  (516) 868-4545

  Full line of appliances, adhesive foam pads, stoma paper guide strips, and karaya powder.

- Blanchard Ostomy Products
  2216 Chevy Oaks Circle
  Glendale, CA 91206
  (213) 242-6789

  Appliances and karaya wafers.

- Byram Surgical, Inc.
  2 Armonk Street
  Byram, CT 10573
  (203) 531-6400

  Appliances and supplies.

- Cipa
  17 Fields Court
  Brockton, MA 02401

  Temporary pouches.

- Coloplast/Bard, Inc.
  73 Central Avenue
  Murray Hill, NJ 07974
  (201) 277-8000

  Disposable pouches.

- Richard Daniels
  P.O. Box 2181
  Dublin, CA 94556

  Cellu-Rings.

- Davol, Inc.
  Box D
  Providence, RI 02901
  (401) 463-7000

  Appliances and Relia-Seal.

- The DePress Co.
  130 Central Avenue
  Holland, MI 49423
  (616) 392-3145

  Deodorant tablets.

- Duke Labs, Inc.
  P.O. Box 529
  South Norwalk, CT 06856
  (203) 838-4737

  Double-backed adhesive.

- Thomas Fazio Laboratories
  P.O. Box 35
  Assonet, MA 02702
  (617) 823-0753

  Appliances, supplies, and karaya powder.

- Ferndale Labs and Surgical, Inc.
  780 West Eight-Mile Road
  Ferndale, MI 48220
  (313) JO4-5780, LI8-0900

  Deodorant tablets.

- Graham-Field Surgical Co., Inc.
  32-56 Sixty-second Street
  Woodside, NY 11377
  (212) 728-8770

  Appliances and supplies.

- John F. Greer Co.
  5335 College Avenue, P.O. Box 2898
  Oakland, CA 94618
  (415) 652-2213

  Appliances and supplies.

- Gricks, Inc.
  Hollis, NY 11423
  (212) 465-4440

  Appliances and supplies.

- Hollister, Inc.
  211 East Chicago Avenue
  Chicago, IL 60611
  (312) 642-2001

  Disposable pouches with built-in karaya, karaya washers, karaya paste, and skin gel.

- Imex Company
  222 West 17th South
  Salt Lake City, UT 84115
  (801) 486-1057

  Disposable pouches.

- Johnson and Johnson Company
  501 George Street
  New Brunswick, NJ 08903
  (201) 524-0400

  Dermicel paper tape.

- Eli Lilly and Co.
  740 S. Alabama Street
  Indianapolis, IN 46206

  Oral deodorant (bismuth subcarbonate).

- Marlen Mfg. and Dev. Co.
  5150 Richmond Road
  Bedford, OH 44146
  (216) 292-7060

  Full line of appliances, stoma paper guide strips, and karaya powder.

- Marsan Mfg. Co., Inc.
  Packer Drive
  Wausau, WI 54401
  (715) 842-3391

  Full line.

- Mason Laboratories
  P.O. Box 194
  Willow Grove, PA 19090
  (215) 659-1815, 659-1819

  Colly-Seal and Colly-Seal appliances.

- Medicon, Inc.
  Hollbrook, MA 02343

  Karaya washers.

- The Medical Specialty Co., Inc.
  P.O. Box 3663, Dilweg Station
  Green Bay, WI 54303
  (414) 494-5082

  Appliances and supplies.

- Moran Medical Supplies
  P.O. Box 24, MIT Branch
  Cambridge, MA 02139
  (617) 862-7848

  Karaya washers.

- 3M Medical Products Division
  3M Center
  St. Paul, MN 55101
  (612) 733-1110

  Double-backed adhesive, adhesive foam pads, and micropore paper tape.

- Nu-Hope Labs., Inc.
  2900 Rowene Avenue
  Los Angeles, CA 90039
  (213) 666-5249

  Appliances and supplies.

- Osteolite Company, Inc.
  842 East 18th Avenue
  Denver, CO 80218
  (303) 266-9063

  Appliances and supplies.

- Osto Care Company
  P.O. Box 2131
  Sepulveda, CA 91343
  (213) 782-3100

  Carbo zinc stoma gaskets.

- The Parthenon Co., Inc.
  P.O. Box 11274
  Salt Lake City, UT 84111
  (801) 355-7630

Deodorant tablets and Devrom oral deodorant (bismuth subgallate).

- The Perma-Type Co., Inc.
  P.O. Box 175
  Farmington, CT 06032
  (203) 677-7388

  Appliances, supplies, and karaya powder.

- Perry Products
  3803 East Lake Street
  Minneapolis, MN 55406
  (612) 722-4783

  Nonadhesive appliances.

- Pettibone Labs., Inc.
  11 E. 44th St.
  New York, NY 10017
  (212) 661-8117

  Ostobon deodorant.

- Requa Manufacturing Co., Inc.
  4510 Bullard Avenue
  Bronx, NY 10470
  (212) FA5-8888

  Charcoal deodorant.

- Robinson Surgical Appliance Co.
  21 East Main Street
  Auburn, WA 98002
  (206) TE3-3161

  Appliances.

- H.W. Rutzen and Son
  345 West Irving Park Road
  Chicago, IL 60618

  Appliances.

- Rystan Company
  Dept. OR, 470 Mamaroneck Avenue
  White Plains, NY 10605
  (914) 761-0044

  Derifil deodorant.

- E.R. Squibb and Sons, Inc.
  Hospital Division
  Princeton, NJ 08540
  (609) 921-4000

  Kenalog spray, Mycostatin powder, and Stomahesive.

- Sween Corporation
  Rapidan, MN 56079

  Deodorant and cleansing supplies.

- Torbot Co.
  1185 Jefferson Boulevard
  Warwick, RI 02886
  (401) 739-2241

  Appliances.

- United Surgical Corp.
  11775 Starkey Road
  Largo, FL 33540
  (813) 392-1261

Full line of appliances, adhesive foam pads, stoma paper guide strips, bismuth subgallate, and skin prep.

In addition to these products, the following general items are sold: mild detergents, available at grocery stores (Dreft, Lux, Vel, Joy); small (No. 2) and large (No. 4 or 5) binder clips available at stationery stores; G.E. Silicone Seal, available at hardware stores; girdles for men (Carter's "Trimmer," Arrow's "Mandate and Highrise," Jockey's "Vitalizer"); Stretch girdles for women by Vassarette, Olga, Warner, Formfit, and Gossard; Tupperware; aluminum hydroxide gel (Maalox, Amphojel); "glucose" drinks (e.g., Gatorade, Olympade, Bulldog Punch, Sportade, Quick Kick).

Information taken from the *Ileostomy Guide*, United Ostomy Association, Los Angeles, Calif., 1974.

Cold and Allergy Products

John F. Cormier and Bobby G. Bryant

Chapter 7

Questions to Ask the Patient

How old are you?

What are the symptoms? Is there runny nose, sore throat, cough, fever, earache?

How long have the symptoms been present?

Do you have a history of allergies?

Do you have any respiratory disease such as asthma or bronchitis?

Do you have diabetes, glaucoma, heart disease, thyroid problems, or high blood pressure?

What medications are you taking?

Which products have you used? Were they effective?

Does your job require you to remain alert to prevent an accident?

Although the common cold and allergic rhinitis are etiologically different, they present similar symptoms and respond to similar management approaches. This chapter provides the pharmacist with the information necessary to identify and distinguish between these disorders, as well as other disorders that may mimic them, and to advise the patient on the proper use of cold and allergy products.

TYPES OF DISORDERS

The common cold is a mixture of symptoms affecting the upper respiratory tract (Figure 1). It is also called a "cold," acute rhinitis, infectious rhinitis, coryza, or catarrh. The symptoms, which are usually acute and self-limiting, may be caused by one of many viruses. The main anatomical sites of infection may vary, and therefore a cold may present symptoms, individually or in combination, of the nose (rhinitis), throat (pharyngitis), larynx (laryngitis), or bronchi (bronchitis). The intensity of symptoms may vary from hour to hour. The only reasonable approach is to treat individual symptoms with individual drugs (1).

Allergic rhinitis is the reaction of the nasal mucosa resulting from an antibody-mediated reaction to one or more inhaled antigens. It may be perennial because of the year-round presence of antigenic substances, or it may be seasonal to correspond with the periodic appearance of offending antigens. The most common type of allergic rhinitis is seasonal and is called hay fever or pollinosis.

Upper Respiratory Tract

The nose is a respiratory organ. As a passageway for airflow into and out of the lungs, it humidifies and warms inspired air and filters inhaled particles. Several anatomical features facilitate the performance of these functions. The nasal cavity is divided by a central septum and fingerlike projections (turbinates) that extend into the cavity, increasing the nasal surface area.

The nasal passageway surface is coated with a continuous thin layer of mucus, which is a moderately viscous, mucoproteinaceous liquid secreted continuously by the mucus glands. Under normal conditions, foreign bodies such as dust, bacteria, powder, and oil droplets are trapped in the film and carried out of the nose into the nasopharynx. The turbinates cause many eddies in the flowing air, forcing it to rebound in different directions before finally completing its passage through the nose. This rapid change in airflow enables air-suspended particles to precipitate against the nasal surfaces. High vascularity and resultant high blood flow within the nasal mucosa help warm and humidify the inspired air.

Nerve control of the nasopharyngeal vascular bed is derived from both sympathetic and parasympathetic divisions of the autonomic nervous system. Stimulation of the sympathetic fibers (or the action of adrenergic or anticholinergic drugs) causes decreased activity of the mucus glands and vasoconstriction that reduces the size of the turbinates, widening the airway. Parasympathetic stimulation (or the action of cholinergic or antiadrenergic drugs) increases mucus production and narrows the airways by vasodilation and vascular engorgement of the mucosal tissue.

The epithelium of the nasal passageways is ciliated. The constant beating of the cilia causes the mucus film to be moved continually toward the nasopharynx, carrying with it trapped particles to be expectorated or swallowed (2). Because this ciliary movement is one of the body's main defense mechanisms, care should be taken in administering agents that impair this movement. Oils, especially mineral oil, and the overuse of topically applied decongestants interfere with normal ciliary movement.

The mucus blanket is rich in lysozyme and contains

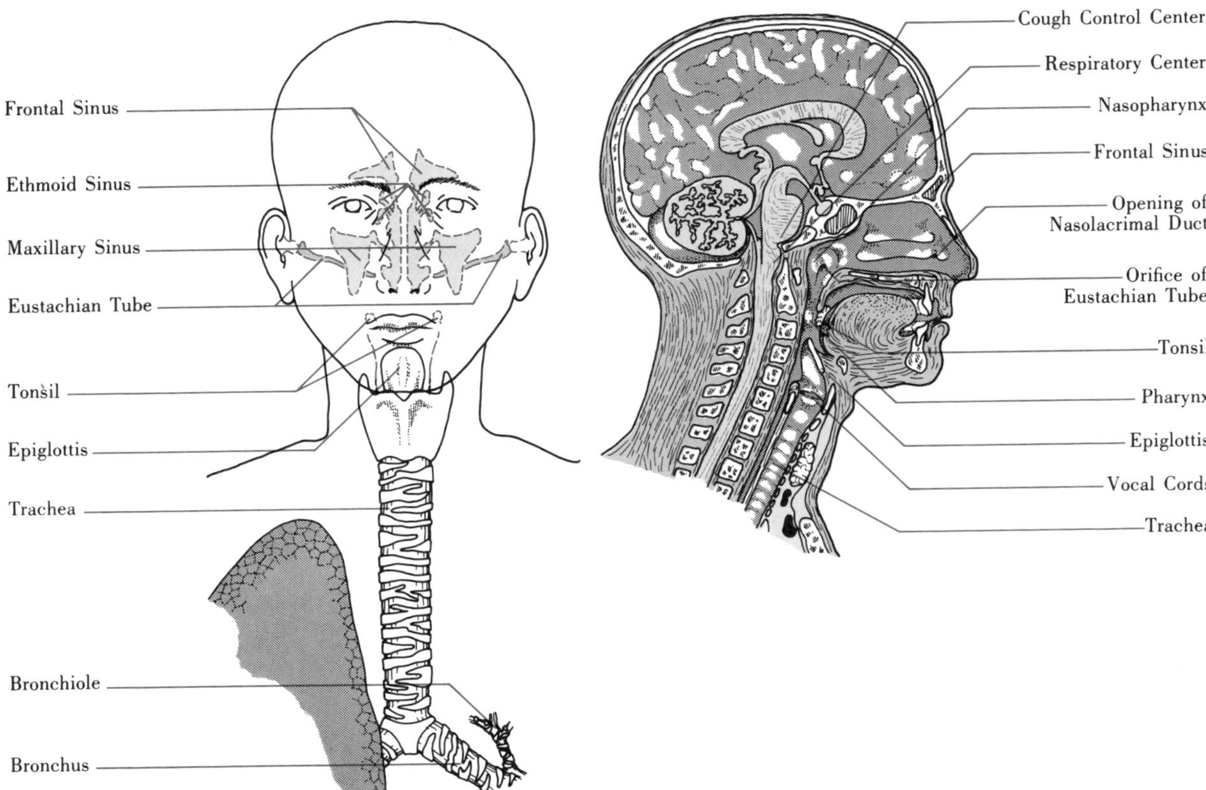

Figure 1. Anatomy of the respiratory passages.

respiratory tract physiology

interferon

cough reflex

sneeze reflex

glycoproteins and immunoglobulins (3). Lysozyme is an important defense against bacteria because it readily digests the lipid and carbohydrate cell wall of some bacteria. It is also responsible for the digestion of the cell wall of pollens and the subsequent release of antigenic substances. Mucus glycoproteins may temporarily inhibit some viruses by combining with the virus protein coat. The union of inhibitor and virus is reversible, and therefore these inhibitors probably do no more than delay host cell invasion by virus particles. Immunoglobulins of low molecular weight, mainly IgA and IgG, also are contained in the mucous secretion. Although they are present in low concentrations, they also may decrease the infectivity of certain viruses.

Viruses that attach to and invade respiratory tract host cells stimulate the infected cell to produce interferon. Interferon is active not only against the virus that caused its production, but also against other unrelated viruses. It protects neighboring, noninfected cells against subsequent viral infection (4). Research is being done on safe ways to increase interferon production but has not yet led to the development of any approved drugs.

The cough reflex is an essential body defense mechanism by which the respiratory airways leading to the lungs are kept free of foreign matter. It occurs in health as well as disease and is frequently the symptom in various pathological states. All areas of the respiratory tract, i.e., the trachea, larynx, bronchi, and terminal bronchioles, are sensitive to foreign matter or other causes of irritation such as irritant corrosive gases and infection. A cough may be caused by the stimulation of receptors (mechanoreceptors and chemoreceptors) located in the mucosa of the airways and lungs. Afferent impulses pass along nerve pathways to the cough center in the medulla, which coordinates efferent impulses to the diaphragm and to the intercostal and abdominal muscles. The cough response is an automatic sequence of events leading to the rapid expulsion of air from the lungs designed to carry with it foreign bodies that have initiated the reflex. Localized bronchoconstriction also may play an important role in stimulation of the cough reflex. Although the evidence is inconclusive at this time, this "bronchomotor theory" is believed by some to be the mechanism whereby irritation causes bronchoconstriction which triggers the cough reflex (5).

The sneeze reflex is very similar to the cough reflex, except that it is intended to clear the nasal passages instead of the lower respiratory tract. Irritation in the nasal passages initiates the sneeze reflex. The afferent impulses from the nose travel to the medulla, where the reflex is triggered. A series of reactions similar to those for the cough reflex takes place. In addition, the uvula is depressed, so that large amounts of air pass rapidly through the nose, as well as through the mouth, helping to clear the nasal passages of foreign matter (2).

The passageways of the trachea and lungs are similarly lined with a ciliated, mucus-coated epithelium that aids in removing foreign matter. As in the nasal passageways, the cilia in the trachea and lungs also beat toward the pharynx, carrying mucus and trapped particles out of the respiratory tract.

Differential Diagnosis

Conditions Mimicking the Common Cold

Other infectious diseases present initial manifestations identical to those of the common cold (6). It is important that the pharmacist be aware of these disorders because some of them have potentially serious implications for which a physician should be consulted. Using strictly palliative therapy in situations that may not be self-limiting has little effect on the underlying problem. For example, a patient's "sore throat," alone or in conjunction with other symptoms, may be caused by bacteria, by a virus, or by another irritative process. The only conclusive means by which bacterial pharyngitis may be excluded is by culture. This test is not always practical, however, nor is it always needed. Table 1 may assist the pharmacist in evaluating a sore throat complaint in adults. Sore throat in children should be evaluated by a physician as soon as possible, and symptomatic therapy should be employed only to provide relief until a physician can be seen. In this situation, if symptomatic therapy alone is recommended and the child is actually suffering from β-hemolytic streptococcal pharyngitis, the relatively rare but possible sequela of rheumatic heart disease or glomerulonephritis may develop due to inappropriate treatment, i.e., lack of antibiotic therapy.

Influenza

A viral respiratory tract infection that may mimic a cold is called influenza, or the "flu." Flu is usually distinguishable from the common cold by its epidemic occurrence and by fever, dry cough, joint and muscle ache, and more significant general malaise. Although treatment is symptomatic, it usually is more vigorous than cold treatment, and complications, especially secondary bacterial infections, are more likely to develop. This is especially true in elderly and debilitated patients, who should be referred to a physician when influenza is suspected.

flu

Measles

The incidence of measles (rubeola) has been drastically reduced by immunization; when it does occur, it is associated with a prodrome (premonitory symptoms) which includes fever, rhinitis, dry cough, and conjunctivitis. Initially, it is difficult to distinguish from the common cold. However, in about 3 days, a red rash indicative of measles develops over the face, trunk, and extremities. The appearance of Koplik's spots is pathognomonic of measles. These spots usually appear 1–2 days prior to the rash as tiny "table salt crystals" usually on the mucous membranes of the cheek. Although treatment is symptomatic (along with patient isolation), a physician should be notified because secondary bacterial infections and postmeasles encephalitis may develop. Also, local public health regulations may require reporting measles.

sore throat characteristics

rubeola

German Measles

Another viral disease in which fever, malaise, and rhinitis coincide with the eruption of a fine red rash is German measles (rubella). It is recommended that this disorder also be brought to a physician's attention because of possible complications. An important concern is the devastating effect that rubella may have on a fetus in utero. If a pregnant woman is exposed to a case of rubella (actual or suspected), she must be referred to a physician to determine her degree of immunity to the virus.

rubella

Allergy

A history of allergy and a review of symptoms help differentiate allergic rhinitis from the common cold. Hay fever may be suspected in young children who suffer from repeated coldlike symptoms.

Conditions Mimicking Allergic Rhinitis

It is also important for pharmacists to recognize common disease entities that may mimic signs or symptoms of allergic rhinitis. The main clinical entity in differential diagnosis of seasonal allergic rhinitis is infectious rhinitis. A mucopurulent discharge, the possibility of fever and other systemic symptoms, and the lack of pruritus often distinguish infectious from allergic rhinitis (Table 2). Chronic sinusitis, recurrent infectious rhinitis, abnormalities of nasal structures, and nonseasonal, nonallergic, noninfectious rhinitis of unknown etiology (vasomotor rhinitis) may be confused with perennial allergic rhinitis (7). A physician should be consulted to differentiate between these conditions.

Other conditions that may mimic the symptoms of allergic rhinitis are rhinitis medicamentosa, reserpine rhinitis, foreign bodies in the nose, and cerebrospinal rhinorrhea. Rhinitis medicamentosa is a condition resulting from the overuse of topically applied vasoconstricting agents. The pharmacist may identify this condition by questioning the patient about past use of nose drops or sprays for nasal congestion. Preparations containing re-

Table 1. Characteristics of a Sore Throat

Parameter	Bacterial	Nonbacterial
Onset	rapid	slower
Soreness	marked	seldom marked
Constitutional symptoms	marked	mild
Upper and lower respiratory symptoms	present in 50% of cases	usual
Lymph nodes	large, tender	slight enlargement, not tender

Adapted from V. Bulteau, *Med. J. Aust.*, *2*, 1053 (1966).

Table 2. Characteristics of Various Types of Rhinitis

Characteristic	Allergic Seasonal	Allergic Perennial	Infectious	Nonallergic (Vasomotor)
Etiology	IgE-mediated immunological	IgE-mediated immunological	respiratory infection	autonomic nervous system disorder
Seasonal pattern	yes	present year round	often worse in winter	worse in changing seasons
Recurrences	mild symptoms between attacks	mild symptoms between attacks	clears completely	frequently continuous
Recurrences	mild symptoms between attacks	mild symptoms between attacks	clears completely	frequently continuous
Family history of allergy	common	common	occasional	occasional
Systemic symptoms	rare	rare	common	rare
Other allergic symptoms (asthma, eczema)	common	common	occasional	occasional
Pruritus	yes	yes	no	mild or absent
Fever	no	no	occasional	no
Conjunctivitis	yes	yes	no	no
Discharge	waterlike	waterlike	mucopurulent	waterlike
Paroxysmal sneezing	yes	yes	no	yes

types of rhinitis

incidence of colds and related factors

serpine or other antiadrenergic antihypertensives may cause marked nasal congestion. Often, this side effect is transient and subsides with continued antihypertensive administration. However, if it persists and is bothersome, topical decongestant treatment may be necessary. Although a dosage reduction may help clear nasal congestion, such a reduction may sacrifice blood pressure control. Another alternative is to try a different antihypertensive agent.

In rare instances the presence of a foreign body in the nose may be mistaken for chronic allergic rhinitis. Examination by a physician is necessary. Cerebrospinal rhinorrhea may follow a head injury; it is characterized by the discharge of a clear, watery fluid from one nostril.

The Common Cold

The common cold has been rated as the most expensive single illness in the United States. In fact, more time is lost from work and school because of the common cold than because of all other diseases combined. Among approximately 60 million industrial employees in the United States the common cold accounts for nearly 1 million person-years lost from work annually. This amounts to about one-half of all absences and approximately one-fourth of the total work time lost each year in industry (7).

The patient's age is related to the incidence of the common cold and to its complications. Children 1–5 years old are most susceptible, and each child averages 6–12 respiratory illnesses per year, most of which are common colds. Some practitioners feel that infants less than 6 months old are somewhat resistant to these viruses, but this finding may be attributed to infants' relatively infrequent exposure to different environments. Individuals 25–30 years old average about six respiratory illnesses per year; older adults average two or three. Young children are more prone to complications of the common cold, such as middle ear inflammation (otitis media) and pneumonia, than older cold sufferers. However, many adults also suffer from these complications (e.g., sinusitis) (3, 8).

There is an apparent relationship between the season of the year and the common cold. It is not known what the exact relationship is, but it is usual to observe three peak seasons of common colds per year. One of these occurs in the autumn, a few weeks after schools open; another occurs in midwinter; and a third occurs in the spring. These separate epidemics are associated with different viruses, each of which may have its own seasonal epidemiology. U.S. Public Health Service studies show that during the winter quarter of the year, about 50% of the population experience a common cold; during the summer quarter, only about 20% are stricken with a cold (8).

Body chills or wet feet in themselves do not induce the common cold. However, if the virus is a recent invader, the effects of exposure probably are distinct contributory factors because such exposure is associated with a vasomotor effect that decreases the nasal mucosal temperature by several degrees. As a result of this temperature change, many people experience symptoms of nasal irritation such as sneezing and serous discharge. These changes in the nasal mucosa and a subsequent change in the character of the mucus may then facilitate viral invasion (8). Poor nutritional state, fatigue, and emotional disturbances are associated with greater susceptibility to infection as well as increased severity of infection and greater likelihood of complications (8).

Respiratory disease such as the common cold is spread directly from person to person with no intermediate source such as food, water, or animals. The only means by which spreading may be prevented is by isolating the infected individual. However, by the time a cold has been detected, the virus undoubtedly has already been transmitted to others via respiratory droplets (4).

Allergic disorders involving the nasopharynx, e.g., hay fever, also seem to play a part in facilitating infection. The probable cause for this is the inflammatory changes occurring in the mucosa as a result of the antigen–antibody reaction which may facilitate subsequent viral invasion.

The American public buys approximately $500–700 million of OTC cough, cold, and allergy preparations each year; about 50% are purchased in pharmacies. Pharmacists should take advantage of the many opportunities thus afforded to interact with and assist the self-medicating patient in proper product selection and administration.

Etiology

Viruses cause the common cold. More than 120 different viral strains that produce common cold symptoms in humans have been isolated (8). Known causative agents include the rhinoviruses (approximately 60 different serological types), adenoviruses, coxsackieviruses, echoviruses, influenza viruses, and parainfluenza viruses. Of these, the rhinoviruses comprise the largest etiological group (8), probably accounting for more than one-half of all common colds in adults. A significant number, 5–10%, of common colds are associated with more than one virus, and definite evidence of simultaneous infection with two viruses is not rare (3, 8).

Viruses differ from bacteria by their existence within the host cell, their chemical composition, their mode of replication, and their responsiveness to drug therapy (4). The process of a viral infection is divided into three stages: entry into the host cell and nucleic acid release; genome replication and viral protein synthesis; and assembly of new virus particles and their release from the cell to infect additional host cells (9). There probably are several mechanisms by which the virus penetrates the host cell, but none is well defined. Once inside the host cell, the virus is attacked by host cell enzymes and possibly other substances, releasing the viral nucleic acid. In the second stage of infection the virus uses metabolic pathways of the host cell itself to duplicate the viral genome and synthesize viral proteins. Finally, these components are assembled into new, mature virus particles and are released by the host cell. The release may be rapid and may be accompanied by lysis and death of the host cell, although cell death may not always result. The new virus particles then infect adjacent cells by the same cycle.

causes of common cold

viruses

process of viral infection

cold symptoms

When host cell injury or death occurs, the body's inflammatory defense mechanism is activated, causing pathological changes and subsequent symptoms. These clinical manifestations of infection are not evident, however, until after extensive viral replication and inflammation have occurred.

A specific immune response (serum-neutralizing antibody) is initiated against the infecting virus, conferring a clinical immunity that may be apparent for up to 2 years. Reinfection, however, is not entirely prevented and usually results in a modified illness. The specificity of the antibody and its concentration at the infection site appear to be critical in the likelihood and extent of reinfection (3). These characteristics also underscore the difficulty of developing comprehensive vaccines to prevent the common cold.

Pathophysiology and Symptoms

The symptoms associated with the common cold are a manifestation of the pathological changes (inflammation) that occur in the respiratory epithelium, secondary to viral invasion. The pathological changes that make up the inflammatory response to one or more viruses are excess blood flow in the area (hyperemia), abnormal fluid accumulation in the intercellular spaces (edema), and profuse watery discharge from the nasal mucous membrane (rhinorrhea) (8).

The severity of the cellular damage (and hence the degree of inflammation and symptoms) is related to the type and virulence of the infecting virus and the extent of the infection. Various strains of influenza virus, for example, do a great deal more damage to the respiratory epithelium than those that cause the cold. Therefore "flu" symptoms are usually more severe than cold symptoms, and the predisposition to secondary bacterial complications is greater.

Although colds commonly involve the nasal structure, other sites along the respiratory tract also may be affected. This condition is due to the predilection of certain viruses for pharyngeal, laryngeal, or bronchial cells and to the extension of the infectious process from the original invasion site (4).

Because the incubation period for these viral infections is relatively short (1–4 days), patients often report a rapid onset and progression of symptoms. Virus shedding usually begins 1–2 days prior to the onset of symptoms and is associated with epithelial sloughing and regeneration. A few days later, during the symptomatic phase, peak viral replication and host cell injury occur. With the intervention of body defenses, such as interferon, virus excretion ceases after several days, and symptoms decrease (3).

rhinorrhea—hallmark of common cold

frequency of cold symptoms

pharyngitis

laryngitis

secondary bacterial infections

The clear, watery fluid that initially flows from the irritated nasal epithelium (nasal discharge or rhinorrhea) is the hallmark of the common cold. Although it is initially clear, it is followed shortly by a much thicker and tenacious mucoid or purulent secretion, largely composed of dead epithelial cells and white blood cells. The quantity of epithelial cells shed may be so high at times as to give the appearance of purulence. It is commonly assumed that these mucopurulent secretions are the result of secondary bacterial infection. However, this is not always the case. Viruses may cause inflammatory reactions on their own, and the secretions occur even when there has been no change in the nasal bacterial flora.

Nasal congestion (swelling of the nasal turbinates) encroaches on the nasal lumen, which is also burdened with the increased secretions. Nasal discharge and congestion are the most commonly described discomforts associated with the common cold (Table 3).

The combination of nasal irritation, nasal discharge, and nasal congestion (which cause further irritation) gives rise to sneezing. Sneezing is not as discomforting as the discharge and congestion and subsides when the infection and secretions clear.

Pharyngitis also may occur during a cold. This throat symptom is usually described as a "dryness" or "soreness" rather than actual pain such as that associated with bacterial pharyngitis or acute tonsillitis. Pharyngitis is attributed to edema of the pharyngeal mucosa which activates sensory nerve fibers as the infection spreads to deeper tissue.

This irritation of the pharynx ("tickling") also may cause a nonproductive cough. The cough also may result from irritation of tracheal or bronchial mucous membranes due to the direct extension of the inflammation or from infectious material dripping from the nasopharynx (postnasal drip). At its onset the cough is usually dry and nonproductive. Later stages of the common cold are characterized by heavy bronchial congestion resulting from the cellular debris of local phagocytic activity added to the respiratory tract fluids in the bronchial and nasal passage secretions and draining into the lower respiratory tract. Ciliary activity may not be sufficient to remove these fluids, and coughing is necessary to clear the lower tract of accumulated phlegm.

Another possible manifestation of the common cold is laryngitis, which is associated with hoarseness or loss of voice. It also may be caused by the spread of infection, or it may be an irritation secondary to drainage from the nasopharynx. A hot or warm sensation ("feverishness") is another fairly common complaint. In general, little or no fever is actually present. Headache, which usually occurs in the early stages of the cold, may be caused by the infection and inflammation of the nasal passages and paranasal sinuses.

Complications

In an otherwise healthy individual the common cold is self-limiting; the course of symptoms is 5–7 days. It is not uncommon (but not inevitable) for complications to develop during or immediately following a common cold. The pharmacist should be familiar with possible complications, their causes, and how they are treated. Viral infection induces swelling and some exudation, but it causes no significant change in the bacterial flora of the nasopharynx. If the inflammatory changes are of sufficient magnitude, passages connecting the paranasal sinuses and middle ear become obstructed, and under these conditions, infection may occur from secondary bacterial growth.

The most common bacterial complications are sinusitis, otitis media, and pneumonia (6). Obstruction of the various respiratory and auditory passages resulting in stasis of infected mucus is usually the predisposing factor to bacterial infection.

Young children are especially prone to otitis media and pneumonia. Children's eustachian tubes are short, relatively horizontal, and rather narrow. This facilitates fluid accumulation in the middle ear as well as rapid blockage in response to only a slight degree of inflammation. A young child's bronchiolar passages also are smaller in diameter than those of older children and adults and become blocked easily. The smaller passages

Table 3. Frequency of Common Cold Symptoms

Symptoms	Frequency, %
Severe	
Nasal discharge	100
Nasal obstruction	99
Moderate	
Sore or dry throat	96
Malaise	81
Postnasal discharge	79
Headache	78
Cough	76
Mild	
Sneezing	97
Feverishness	49
Chilliness	43
Burning eyes and mucous membranes	28
Aching muscles	22

and the child's lack of conscious effort to "cough up" accumulated fluids in the lower tract lead to stasis of the fluids, inflammation, and secondary bacterial infection. During the first few years of life, the "cold" problem is potentially serious.

These complications usually manifest themselves by worsening of local symptoms and signs (e.g., earache, headache, or cough), development of a fever, and failure of the cold to improve in the expected time. Such manifestations in a person with a recent cold probably are caused by secondary bacterial invaders for which culture and sensitivity tests and appropriate prescribed antibiotic therapy are indicated.

Treatment

Self-medication of the common cold is intended to provide palliation of symptoms. There are no curative remedies, only drugs that bring temporary relief while the cold runs its course and the normal body defenses attempt to remove the viral invaders and repair the damage. In general, additional bed rest and prevention of chilling add to the patient's comfort. Adequate fluid intake is necessary to prevent dehydration and to decrease the viscosity of respiratory secretions. A well-balanced diet should be maintained.

Nasal Congestion and Nasal Discharge

Treating nasal congestion is valuable in that it not only relieves the discomfort but also prevents excessive nose blowing which may further irritate mucous membranes and the nostrils. Excessive nose blowing also may force infected fluids into nasal sinuses and the eustachian tubes, extending the infection and discomfort. Decongestants (sympathomimetic amines) applied as drops or spray to the nasal mucosa or administered systemically are effective vasoconstrictors that help decrease edema and swelling of the nasal mucosa. The watery nasal discharge found in the early stages of the common cold may be minimized by decongestant use.

Cough

The first step in attempting to control a cough is to provide the respiratory tract with adequate fluids either by increasing oral fluid intake or by humidifying the inspired air. If the cough is dry, nonproductive, hyperactive, and annoying, a cough suppressant is indicated; an expectorant agent, by virtue of its action, theoretically would be useful in providing a demulcent effect, but none has been proven effective (1). These two agents are frequently found together in OTC products. If the cough is productive and frequency is tolerable, ensuring adequate fluid intake may be all that is needed. An expectorant agent may be recommended as adjunctive therapy to facilitate the removal of phlegm and to prevent the frequency of the cough from causing exhaustion, although there is no proof that this effect will occur.

The "tickling" sensation in the pharynx that causes a cough may be treated initially with a demulcent, e.g., hard candy or cough drop, but if the cough becomes more intense, a cough suppressant may be recommended (1).

Dry or Sore Throat

In the absence of definite pharyngeal pain and fever associated with the sore throat complaint, bacterial pharyngitis probably can be ruled out. However, a sore throat in a child is difficult to evaluate and should not be self-medicated; the child should be seen by a physician.

Lozenges and gargles containing antiseptics and/or topical anesthetics are promoted quite heavily for treating sore throat. However, aside from a demulcent effect, the use of an antibacterial lozenge or gargle is irrational because the antibacterial ingredients are not effective against viruses.

If the throat is dry or "raspy," hard, sour candy may be used to stimulate saliva flow, which acts as a demulcent. A frequently overlooked measure in soothing an inflamed throat is the regular use of a warm, normal saline gargle (2 tsp/qt of water). If these measures do not provide adequate relief, lozenges or sprays containing a local anesthetic (e.g., phenol, hexylresorcinol, or benzocaine) may be used every 3–4 hours for temporary symptomatic relief.

Laryngitis

Acute laryngitis presents a therapeutic problem—the only direct way to reach the inflamed laryngeal tissue is by inspired air. Lozenges and gargles do nothing to relieve hoarseness; their ingredients or the saliva that they stimulate do not reach this area. Water vapor inhalation (steam or cool mist) several times a day has proven beneficial in acute laryngitis. The value of adding any medications to steam has not been proven. Inhaling irritants (smoking) should be avoided, and the voice should be rested as much as possible.

Feverishness and Headache

Vague complaints of feverishness and headache, although not necessarily occurring together, may be treated with the same remedies. Aspirin or acetaminophen, in the proper dosage, is usually effective. In conjunction with fluids and rest, aspirin or acetaminophen is very useful because of its analgesic/antipyretic properties. Fever (orally measured temperature greater than 37.2–37.6°C) is seldom associated with the common cold, and the lasting benefit of the antipyretic property of aspirin or acetaminophen is doubtful. When a true fever is present and persists for more than 24 hours in spite of treatment with OTC drugs, a physician should be consulted. In the interim, aspirin or acetaminophen will provide temporary relief of fever symptoms. If fever persists in spite of these medical measures, the patient should be sponged or bathed in cool or tepid, not cold, water. The use of diluted isopropyl alcohol (e.g., 50:50 in water) also has been recommended as adjunctive antipyretic therapy. In spite of this sponging solution's proven effectiveness, its use has been associated with two drawbacks (10). First, coma following acute alcohol poisoning has been reported in patients sponged with isopropyl alcohol, and second, it has been found that there is significantly more discomfort associated with its use than with tepid water (10, 11). Therefore the most

symptomatic relief

nasal discomforts

cough control

suppressants, expectorants, and demulcents

pharyngeal pain

fever

rational approach to fever reduction in adults and children is aspirin or acetaminophen and/or tepid water sponging (12).

Physician-directed treatment is usually unnecessary unless there is concern that the patient has something other than a cold, the symptoms are severe, or secondary complications are present or suspected. Severely debilitated patients, however, should seek advice from their physicians, as should patients with other chronic disorders (e.g., emphysema) in which a respiratory infection may pose serious problems or the usual nonprescription remedies may be contraindicated.

Allergic Rhinitis

Etiology and Pathophysiology

incidence and symptoms of allergic rhinitis

seasonal and perennial

Allergic rhinitis may begin at almost any age, although the incidence of first onset is greatest in children and young adults and decreases with age. Heredity seems to play a role. Allergic rhinitis itself is not genetically transmitted; however, the heightened predisposition to become sensitized following exposure to adequate concentrations of an allergen is transferred (7).

Pollens from plants that depend on the wind for cross-pollination and mold spores are the main agents responsible for seasonal allergic rhinitis. Ragweed pollen accounts for ~75% of seasonal rhinitis patients in the United States; grass pollens, 40%; and tree pollens, ~9%. Approximately 25% suffer from both grass and ragweed allergic rhinitis, and ~5% suffer from all three allergies (13).

The seasonal appearance of symptoms is a reflection of the pollen or spores in the air. Of the airborne mild spores, *Alternaria* and *Hormodendrum* are the most common and also may cause seasonal allergic rhinitis (14). These spores are most prevalent from mid-March to late November. Tree pollination begins in late March and extends to early June. Grasses generally pollinate from mid-May to mid-July. Ragweed pollen has a long season, extending from early August to early October or to the first killing frost. For a particular plant in a given locale the pollinating season is relatively constant from year to year. Weather conditions such as temperature and rainfall influence the amount of pollen produced but not the actual onset or termination of a specific season (7). Thus appearance of seasonal allergic rhinitis symptoms is influenced by the patient's geographic location and specific hypersensitivities.

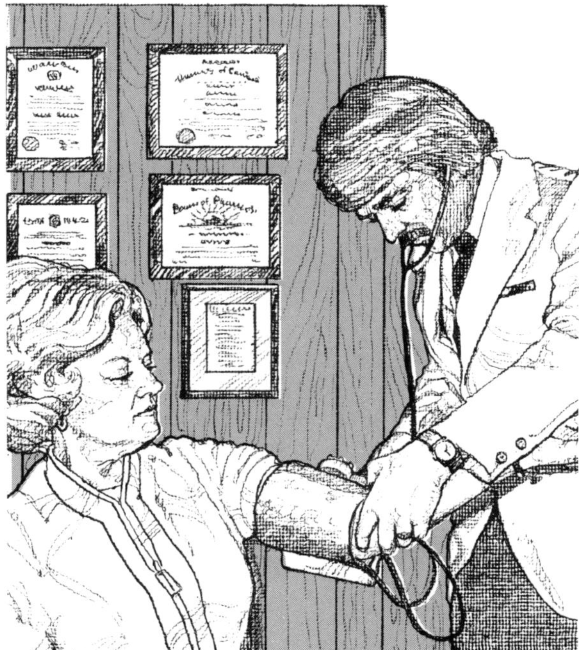

Perennial allergic rhinitis symptoms are usually caused by house dust, animal dander, and feathers. Occupational causes may include wheat flour, various grains, cotton and flax seeds, and enzymes used in detergents. The continued presence of the allergens results in patient symptoms that are persistent more or less year round.

Allergic rhinitis symptoms may be due to many different etiological allergens. These allergens, which are primarily protein in nature, may, when deposited on the nasal mucosa, initiate an inflammatory response by the body and produce symptoms characteristic of allergic rhinitis.

The pathological inflammatory process of seasonal allergic rhinitis develops within minutes after an allergen is deposited on the nasal mucous membrane of an allergy-prone individual. Pollen itself is not believed to be directly antigenic. However, the lysozyme component of nasal mucus may degrade the pollen cell wall to allow for the release of the proteinaceous contents. This released protein may be an antigen. The antigen stimulates lymphoid tissue in the respiratory tract to produce a specific type of immunoglobulin, IgE (reagin). These reaginic antibodies have a special affinity for circulating basophils and tissue mast cells. The cells pick up many IgE molecules on their surfaces and thus become sensitized. Subsequent exposure to the same antigen, by its deposition on nasal mucosa, causes an antigen–antibody reaction, which causes vasoactive chemical mediators to be released from these sensitized host cells. These mediators include histamine, slow-reacting substances of anaphylaxis, eosinophilic chemotactic factor, and possibly others.

The nasal mucosa is particularly vulnerable to this immediate type of allergic reaction because the allergen is deposited directly where it may act locally and because the mediators are very active vasodilators that are released in a highly vascularized area. The immediate effects are vasodilation, increased vascular permeability, and increased mucus secretion, all of which are responsible for the symptoms.

The longer the symptoms persist, from whatever cause, more chronic and irreversible changes such as thickening of the mucosal epithelium, connective tissue proliferation, loss of epithelial cilia, and development of polyps of the nose or sinuses may be noted.

Signs and Symptoms

The major signs and symptoms of allergic rhinitis are edema and symptoms resulting from the engorgement of the nasal mucosa—sneezing, rhinorrhea, nasal pruritus, and nasal congestion are the most common. Sudden sneezing attacks may consist of 10–20 sneezes in rapid succession.

The rhinorrhea is typically a watery, thin discharge that may be quite profuse and continuous. Purulent discharge does not occur in uncomplicated allergic rhinitis; its presence indicates a secondary infection. The nasal congestion of allergic rhinitis is due to swollen turbinates. If the nasal obstruction is severe, it may cause headaches or earaches. With continuous, severe nasal congestion, loss of smell and taste may occur. Itching of the nose also may be a prominent feature, particularly in children, and causes frequent nose rubbing.

Conjunctival eye symptoms commonly associated with allergic rhinitis include itching and lacrimation. These symptoms are caused by the trapping of pollen grains in the conjunctival sac and subsequent antigen–antibody reaction as well as possible lacrimal duct congestion caused indirectly by the nasal congestion. Patients with severe eye symptoms often complain of photophobia and sore, tired eyes. Dark circles or greater than normal discolorations beneath the eyes are called "allergic shiners." This symptom is more common in perennial rhinitis than in the seasonal variant.

A characteristic of seasonal allergic rhinitis is the periodicity of its appearance. Careful patient history indicates when the symptoms first began and the intervals at which they were exacerbated. With seasonal rhinitis the allergic reaction often begins with sneezing and progresses to rhinorrhea, then possibly to severe nasal obstruction, at which time sneezing may be absent and rhinorrhea minimal. Perennial rhinitis is more likely to begin with nasal obstruction and postnasal discharge than with sneezing and rhinorrhea (15).

The symptoms of allergic rhinitis may exhibit periodicity even within the season. Most patients tend to exhibit more intense symptoms in the morning and on windy days due to increased pollen in the air. Symptoms may diminish when it rains and pollen is cleared from the air.

It is more difficult to associate perennial rhinitis than seasonal rhinitis with the environment; the patient history may be helpful in these cases. The most common perennial allergens are house dust and household pet dander, which may be in contact with the patient during all seasons.

Generally, allergic rhinitis tends to show increasingly severe symptoms for 2–3 years until a somewhat stabilized condition is reached. With seasonal allergic rhinitis, symptoms then tend to be exacerbated annually. There is no effective means of predicting whether symptoms will increase or decrease in severity. In fact, for reasons not well understood, hypersensitivity may disappear after several years. The pharmacist may differentiate seasonal allergic rhinitis from perennial allergic rhinitis by questioning the patient concerning the appearance and disappearance of symptoms. The treatment is similar with both of these conditions.

Complications

Patients with allergic rhinitis may develop complications due to chronic nasal inflammation including recurrent otitis media with hearing loss, sinusitis, loss of epithelial celia, and nasal or sinus polyps. Complications of allergic rhinitis seem to be more prominent in children. Nasal allergy in children also leads to bony structural changes in the palate and a depression of cheek bone prominence. The resulting crowding of incisor teeth is called the "Gothic arch." Children with chronic, recurrent rhinitis may develop a hearing impairment due to the involvement of the eustachian tubes and middle ear. Often a child develops a characteristic manner of rubbing the nose with the palm of the hand to relieve itching and spread the nasal wall to produce better nasal ventilation. This persistent rubbing is called the "allergic salute."

allergic rhinitis symptoms

possible complications

progression to asthma

steps in treatment

Another possible complication of rhinitis, especially in children, is its progression to asthma or other atopical disorders. Although asthma is difficult to predict, allergic rhinitis and asthmatic attacks often may be precipitated by the same agents. If allergic rhinitis symptoms are prolonged, a slight cough and a feeling of constriction in the chest or asthmatic wheezing may follow. These are dangerous signals—a warning of possible asthma onset. Because one-third or more of all patients with allergic rhinitis may develop asthma, these signs should be the basis for directing the patient to a physician for diagnosis and treatment (15).

Perennial allergic rhinitis is associated with chronic symptoms that may lead to anatomical changes within the nasal and sinus cavities. The resulting complications include loss of epithelial celia and development of nasal polyps. Because the symptoms are chronic and complications may develop, all perennial allergic rhinitis sufferers should be under a physician's care.

Treatment

Allergic rhinitis treatment steps involve:

- Avoidance of allergens to prevent the immunological response;
- Injection of allergen extracts to alter the immunological response to the allergens (immunotherapy);
- Pharmacological treatment to minimize or counteract the consequences of the immunological response once it has occurred.

In most cases of allergic rhinitis, total avoidance of the allergen is difficult because airborne allergens are so widely distributed and, in most cases, patients are sensitive to more than one allergen. However, avoidance of certain situations (e.g., burning leaves, sleeping with bedroom windows open, and driving in the countryside when pollen counts are especially high) decreases exposure to environments or situations conducive to encountering potential allergens. The mechanical filters in most air conditioners help reduce the number of allergens if they are changed regularly (e.g., monthly), if doors and windows are kept closed, and if the air is recirculated. An electrostatic precipitator in conjunction with a central heating and air conditioning unit is even more effective in reducing house dust and other potential allergens.

When brief exposure to an allergen is unavoidable, a proper face mask effectively filters the inhaled air. Such masks are sold by industrial or scientific supply firms as well as pharmacies for protection against noxious dust. The commonly used gauze masks are ineffective. The pharmacist should explain to the patient specific measures that decrease the likelihood of exposure to the offending allergen.

immunotherapy (hyposensitization)

histamine and mechanism of action of antihistamines

commonly used antihistamines

Immunotherapy (hyposensitization) attempts to raise a person's threshold for symptoms following exposure to the allergen. Although the mechanisms of immunotherapy are not understood completely, it is believed that blocking antibodies are produced when the patient is given a continuing series of allergen injections in specified incremental doses. Successful treatment regimen enables the patient to develop increased allergen tolerance. The indications for immunotherapy, a relatively long-term treatment modality, are relative rather than absolute. For example, if a patient's symptoms are mild and last only a few weeks, the patient may be well managed by symptomatic therapy alone. For those whose reaction to the allergens is much more severe or who cannot tolerate symptomatic treatment, immunotherapy may be considered.

Immunotherapy begins with the proper identification of the offending allergen, most commonly by skin tests measuring the patient's response to test allergens introduced intracutaneously. After the offending allergen is identified, an extract is injected in small amounts at frequent intervals. Most studies indicate that in pollen allergy, 70–80% of the patients treated with immunotherapy experience beneficial results (7, 17, 18).

Immunotherapy does not cure the disease but reduces the number of symptoms, making it easier to control the allergy by symptomatic medication. Patients who experience allergic rhinitis symptoms throughout the year, whose allergic reactions tend to be severe, and who do not demonstrate a beneficial response from self-medication may be candidates for immunotherapy and should be advised by the pharmacist to seek the aid of a physician.

INGREDIENTS IN OTC PRODUCTS

The primary pharmacological agents employed in treating these disorders are the antihistamines and the α-adrenergic agonists (decongestants). Antihistamines are valuable because they prevent the effects of histamine released as a result of the antigen–antibody reaction. The α-adrenergic agonists, on the other hand, reverse the effects of histamine or viral inflammation by constricting dilated blood vessels, thereby diminishing nasal congestion.

Antihistamines

Histamine is a common biogenic amine found in every body tissue; most, however, is found in the mast cells. In these cells, histamine is localized and stored in granules and generally becomes active only when the cells are lysed. It may be released to exert its effects as a result of an antigen–antibody reaction (e.g., allergy) or physical damage (e.g., trauma or infection). Histamine has the most significant effects on the cardiovascular system, exocrine glands, and smooth muscles. Its major effects in the common cold and allergic rhinitis are the ability to cause profound vasodilation, increased capillary permeability, and edema. These effects are more pronounced in highly vascularized areas such as the nose.

Histamine is released in both the common cold and the allergy, but the actual cause of its release and the amount released differ, and therefore the magnitude of its contribution to the symptoms is different in the two disorders. In hay fever the antigen–antibody reaction leads to cellular damage of specific sensitized cells (e.g., mast cells) and consequent release of histamine that initiates the local, inflammatory response. In colds the local inflammatory response results from widespread cell injury caused by virus particle invasion. Therefore the vasodilation and resultant edema associated with a cold may be attributed not only to histamine release but also (and perhaps predominantly) to the body's inflammatory defense and the release of inflammatory mediators in addition to histamine.

Antihistamines are chemical agents that exert their effect in the body primarily by competitively blocking the actions of histamine at receptor sites (19, 20). They are therefore classified as "pharmacological antagonists" of histamine with a mechanism of action analogous to other pharmacological antagonists such as antiadrenergics and anticholinergics. They do not prevent histamine release, and because they act by competitive inhibition, if the histamine concentration at the receptor site exceeds the drug concentration, histamine effects predominate. Although antihistaminic activity is the dominant effect of these agents, antihistamines are structurally similar to other pharmacological classes of drugs (e.g., anticholinergic, local anesthetic, and ganglionic-blocking and adrenergic-blocking agents) and exert various combinations and degrees of side effects. In some cases the side effects have been used to achieve a therapeutic goal (e.g., CNS depression for insomnia and local anesthetic effects for pruritus). However, these side effects, especially drowsiness, may be bothersome and potentially dangerous.

The most commonly used nonprescription antihistamines and their usual dosages are shown in Table 4. Brompheniramine maleate (which has been recommended for OTC status but has not yet appeared on the OTC market), chlorpheniramine maleate, doxylamine succinate, methapyrilene hydrochloride, phenindamine tartrate, pheniramine maleate, and pyrilamine maleate are recognized by the FDA OTC Panel on Cold, Cough, Allergy, Bronchodilator, and Antiasthmatic Products as being safe for OTC use and effective in suppressing the symptoms of allergic rhinitis when taken in the dosage specified. Conclusive evidence is still lacking as to the safety and effectiveness of phenyltoloxamine citrate (1). (This chapter contains references to the Panel's report. The reader should be aware that the FDA Commissioner has disagreed with some of the Panel's recommendations. Proposed regulations based on the Panel's report have not been published by FDA as of this writing.)

Antihistamines are most effective in controlling allergic rhinitis (1, 21). They are rarely effective in vasomotor rhinitis.

Some regular antihistamine users may find that they do not obtain the same degree of relief after a period of weeks or months. One reason for this apparent decreased effectiveness is that some antihistamines are capable of hepatic enzyme induction, resulting in metabolism increase in the liver. The enzyme induction also has implicated antihistamines as a possible cause of diminished effectiveness of several other types of drugs. However, the clinical significance of such interactions is open to question. The various antihistamine classes differ in their capacity to induce hepatic enzymes. Therefore because only a few antihistamines have been studied in this regard, when tolerance develops, switching to a different antihistamine is a practical recommendation.

Although antihistamines have no ability to prevent or abort the common cold, they are found in almost all cold remedies. A rationale for their inclusion in these products probably stems from their anticholinergic action, which decreases the amount of mucus secretion, relieving the rhinorrhea. Moreover, studies did not exclude patients with allergic rhinitis (1). Although some people experience a "drying" effect, the anticholinergic activity of the antihistamines is actually very weak, and this action may be insignificant at the dosage levels of the various nonprescription preparations.

In general, antihistamines possess a high therapeutic index (toxic dose/therapeutic dose), and serious toxicities

effects of antihistamines

antihistamine dosages for commonly used agents

Table 4. Antihistamine Dosage

Drug (by Chemical Class)	Dosage (Maximum Daily Dose) Adults	Children 6 to <12	Children 2 to <6
Ethanolamines			
Diphenhydramine hydrochloride	25–50 mg every 4–6 hours (300 mg)	12.5–25 mg every 4–6 hours (150 mg)	6.25 mg every 4–6 hours (37.5 mg)
Doxylamine succinate	7.5–12.5 mg every 4–6 hours (75 mg)	3.75–6.25 mg every 4–6 hours (37.5 mg)	professional labeling only: 1.9–3.125 mg every 4–6 hours (18.75 mg)
Phenyltoloxamine citrate	50 mg every 4–6 hours (300 mg)	information inadequate to establish dosage	
Ethylenediamines			
Methapyrilene	50 mg every 4–6 hours (300 mg)	25 mg every 4–6 hours (150 mg)	12.5 mg every 4–6 hours (75 mg)
Pyrilamine maleate	25–50 mg every 6–8 hours (200 mg)	12.5–25 mg every 6–8 hours (100 mg)	6.25–12.5 mg every 6–8 hours (50 mg)
Thonzylamine hydrochloride	50–100 mg every 4–6 hours (600 mg)	25–50 mg every 4–6 hours (300 mg)	12.5–25 mg every 4–6 hours (150 mg)
Alkylamines			
Pheniramine maleate	12.5–25 mg every 4–6 hours (150 mg)	6.25–12 mg every 4–6 hours (75 mg)	3.125–6.25 mg every 4–6 hours (37.5 mg)
Brompheniramine maleate	4 mg every 4–6 hours (24 mg)	2 mg every 4–6 hours (12 mg)	1 mg every 4–6 hours (6 mg)
Chlorpheniramine maleate	4 mg every 4–6 hours (24 mg)	2 mg every 4–6 hours (12 mg)	1 mg every 4–6 hours (6 mg)
Miscellaneous:			
phenindamine tartrate	25 mg every 4–6 hours (150 mg)	12.5 mg every 4–6 hours (75 mg)	6.25 mg every 4–6 hours (37.5 mg)

The FDA OTC Panel on Cold, Cough, Allergy, Bronchodilator, and Antiasthmatic Products has recommended all of these ingredients as safe and effective (Category I) except phenyltoloxamine citrate, for which there is insufficient evidence (Category III).

antihistamine toxicity

contraindications to use

drowsiness

side effects

sympathomimetic amines as topical decongestants

rebound congestion

are seldom noted in adults. At recommended labeled doses, most OTC antihistamines also are safe for use in children. As with most drugs, however, accidental overdose in children may lead to profound symptoms, such as excitement, ataxia, incoordination, muscular twitching, generalized convulsion with pupillary dilation, and skin flushing. Treatment is symptomatic and usually requires supportive therapy with artificial respiration.

The major contraindication to antihistamine use—the agent's sedative properties—is relative. Degrees of drowsiness associated with antihistamines vary, depending on the agent's chemical class, but none are entirely free of this side effect. The ethanolamines (e.g., diphenhydramine hydrochloride) have a pronounced tendency to induce sedation. The alkylamines (e.g., chlorpheniramine maleate), on the other hand, possess minimal sedative properties, and the ethylenediamines (e.g., pyrilamine maleate and methapyrilene hydrochloride) are approximately intermediate in their sedative properties (21). Although most individuals acquire a tolerance to this effect, it would appear that alkylamines are in most cases the most suitable agents for daytime use (21). Should drowsiness persist, switching to another antihistamine may alleviate the problem; reducing the dosage also may be helpful unless the dosage used is less than effective as an antihistamine. If a person's job or other activities require a high degree of mental alertness, any antihistamine must be used cautiously until its effect is determined by the individual. The effects of alcohol and other CNS depressants including hypnotics, sedatives, analgesics, and antianxiety agents may be enhanced by the antihistamines. If concurrent administration is necessary, caution must be exercised because of the increased possibility of drowsiness (21, 22).

A paradoxical effect frequently seen in children is CNS stimulation rather than depression, causing insomnia, nervousness, and irritability (e.g., phenindamine). For this reason, antihistamines must be used cautiously in children with convulsive disorders (1, 18). The anticholinergic properties of an antihistamine may predominate in some individuals. Antihistamines may cause dry mouth, blurred vision, urinary retention (in older males suffering from an enlarged prostate), and constipation as a result of their anticholinergic effects; these effects, however, are usually associated with high doses. Because of the drying effect on respiratory secretions and potential airway obstruction, some practitioners believe that antihistamines should not be given to asthmatics (23). The agents may be useful, however, in special situations where the physician may elect a trial course of adjunctive antihistamine therapy in patients not adequately controlled with the usual antiasthmatic regimen (3). The cholinergic-blocking properties of the antihistamines may pose a problem for patients whose glaucoma is being controlled with an anticholinesterase. Such an effect is unpredictable, but because of the potential consequences a patient being treated for narrow-angle glaucoma probably should take antihistamines only under a physician's supervision.

The cholinergic-blocking effect of antihistamines has a quantitatively unpredictable additive effect with anticholinergic drugs. Although excessive cholinergic blockade effects are usually of minor clinical significance, effects such as urinary retention, constipation, and dry mouth may be bothersome (1).

Hypersensitivity reactions may develop with the antihistamines, but this effect is more common with topical application than with oral use (21).

Topical Decongestants

Various sympathomimetic amines have been used to provide relief from the nasal stuffiness of colds and allergic rhinitis. These drugs, which differ primarily in their duration of action, are contained in many nonprescription products promoted for hay fever and colds. Nasal decongestants stimulate the α-adrenergic receptors of the vascular smooth muscle, constricting the dilated arteriolar network within the nasal mucosa and reducing blood flow in the engorged edematous nasal area. This constriction results in shrinkage of the engorged mucous membranes, which promotes drainage, improves nasal ventilation, and relieves the feeling of stuffiness.

The ideal topical decongestant agent should have a prompt and prolonged effect. It should not produce systemic side effects, irritation to the mucosa with resultant harmful effects on the cilia of the respiratory tract, or rebound congestion. An ideal topical sympathomimetic amine has not yet been found (24).

The intranasal application of commercially available decongestants provides a prompt and dramatic decrease of nasal congestion. The shrinking of the mucous membrane not only makes breathing easier but also permits the sinus cavities to drain.

It is very important that the patient follow the label directions as to frequency and duration of use. The topical application of these drugs is often followed by a rebound phenomenon (rhinitis medicamentosa): the nasal mucous membranes become even more congested and edematous as the drug's vasoconstrictor effect subsides. This secondary congestion is believed to result from ischemia caused by the drug's intensive local vasoconstriction and local irritation of the topically applied agent itself. If the use of a topical nasal decongestant is restricted to 3–4 days or less, the rebound congestion is minimal; with chronic use and/or overuse of these agents, rebound nasal stuffiness may become quite pronounced. This rebound phenomenon represents a vicious cycle because it leads to more frequent use of the agent that causes it. To determine the possible existence of this condition, the pharmacist should question a patient concerning prior use of nasal sprays, drops, or inhalants. If, in the pharmacist's judgment, the patient is experiencing this rebound phenomenon, topical decongestant therapy should be discontinued, and systemic decongestants and/or an isotonic saline drop should be used.

The patient should be instructed on the proper administration of topical decongestants to obtain maximum relief without encountering side effects from the drug's systemic absorption. These products are available as drops or sprays. Nasal decongestant sprays are packaged in flexible plastic containers that produce a fine mist when squeezed. The patient should administer nasal sprays in the upright position, squeezing once into each nostril. The nose should be blown to remove mucus 3–5 minutes after spraying. If there is still congestion, another dose should be administered which should reach further into the nasal cavities and to the surfaces of the turbinates.

Some people may prefer to administer the decongestant solution with a nasal atomizer. Most commercial spray containers are designed to deliver the approximate dose with one squeeze; the atomizer, however, is not so calibrated. Also, using an atomizer may increase the possibility of contaminating the solution. If the patient prefers to use a nasal atomizer, instructions should be provided on the proper use of the particular atomizer, including the liquid level and proper placement within the nostril, and the hazards of misuse. The patient should be instructed to remove the solution and rinse the atomizer after use to guard against solution contamination. Naphazoline solutions should not be used in atomizers containing aluminum parts because drug degradation will result.

Nasal drops usually do not cover the entire nasal mucosa and may pass to the pharynx, where they may be swallowed. Although systemic absorption through the nasal mucosa is minimal because of the local vasoconstriction induced by the drug, if an excess amount drains through the nasal passage and is swallowed, absorption and systemic effects are then possible. The amount of medication swallowed may be minimized by proper administration. To administer nasal drops, the patient should recline on a bed with the head tilted back over the edge or should recline on the side, holding the head lower than the shoulders. The drops should be placed in the lower nostril without touching the nasal surface with the dropper. After the drops have been instilled into each nostril, the patient should breathe through the mouth and remain in the reclining position for about 5 minutes. To ensure that the medication spreads, the head may be turned from side to side while the patient is reclining. A topical decongestant in spray form is probably more convenient for adults and older children. Sprays also may afford better decongestion by reaching greater areas of the mucous membranes. Drops are the most effective means of administering a topical decongestant to children under 6 because of their smaller nostril openings.

Several agents are commonly used as topical nasal decongestants. The primary difference lies in their intensity and duration of action (see Table 5).

Ephedrine

Ephedrine is the prototype of the topical sympathomimetic decongestants. The various ephedrine salts provide rapid nasal decongestion applied topically in 0.5–1.0% concentrations. Ephedrine's peak effects are achieved 1 hour after administration. The aqueous solution of topical ephedrine as drops or sprays is the only vehicle recommended by the FDA OTC Panel, since oily solutions may lead to lipid pneumonia (1). Products containing ephedrine should be shielded from direct light, since decomposition will be hastened by such exposure. Ephedrine should be administered as two to three drops or sprays not more frequently than every 4 hours and is not recommended in children less than 6 years of age.

Phenylephrine

Phenylephrine hydrochloride is one of the most effective OTC topical nasal decongestants (25). It is commonly applied as two or three drops or sprays of a 0.25–0.5% solution every 4 hours. The use of stronger solutions except under a physician's direction is hazardous. This agent may produce a marked irritation of the nasal mucosa in some individuals, in addition to the irritation already present from the pathological condition of the allergic disorder or cold. If this reaction occurs, phenylephrine use should be stopped immediately.

Phenylephrine hydrochloride is also commercially available as an aqueous jelly. A small amount of the jelly is placed in each nostril and snuffed well back into the nasal passage. This product is not convenient and is not widely used. The effectiveness of this dosage form has not been established. Nasal decongestants in jelly form are used most commonly by otorhinolaryngologists for office examination or treatment. Theoretically, a more prolonged decongestant effect may be achieved with nasal jellies, which may have an emollient and protective action on the nasal mucosa (26), but these effects also have not been proven.

proper topical decongestant administration

nasal drops

doses and effects of topical decongestants

Naphazoline

Naphazoline hydrochloride is a more potent vasoconstrictor than phenylephrine hydrochloride. It produces CNS depression rather than stimulation when it is absorbed systemically. Because of its systemic effects this agent is not recommended for use in children under 6 years old except on the advice and supervision of a physician (1). Naphazoline hydrochloride is commonly administered as one to two drops or sprays of a 0.05% solution every 6 hours. It may be irritating to the mucosa and may sting when administered; use should be discontinued if this adverse effect persists or worsens.

Oxymetazoline and Xylometazoline

Longer-acting topical nasal decongestants, such as oxymetazoline hydrochloride and xylometazoline hydrochloride, have a decongestant effect that may last 6–12 hours, with a gradual decline thereafter (1, 27, 28). Because of their longer duration these agents are easier to use, but because they are used only twice per day, potential rebound congestion or rhinitis medicamentosa is not less likely to occur. Oxymetazoline may be administered as two to three drops or sprays in the morning and evening; xylometazoline may be administered in the same amount every 8–10 hours (1).

Levodesoxyephedrine/Propylhexedrine

These sympathomimetic amines are volatile and commonly used in inhalants. Controlled studies comparing the efficacy and safety of these aromatic amines to other nasal decongestants are lacking. The use of these volatile substances through an inhaler seems to be an efficient and convenient way of reaching the desired areas of the nasal mucosa, provided there is some nasal airflow.

One problem is the loss of the agent when the cap

Table 5. Topical Nasal Decongestant Dosage

Drug and Concentration	Dosage: Adults, Drops or Sprays	Children 6–12, Drops or Sprays	Children 2–6, Drops[a]
Ephedrine, 0.5% (various salts)	2–3 (≧4 hours)	1–2 (≧4 hours)	—
Naphazoline hydrochloride, 0.05%	1–2 (≧6 hours)	not recommended (refer to 0.025%)	—
0.25%	—	1–2 (≧6 hours)	—
Oxymetazoline hydrochloride, 0.05%	2–3 (morning and evening)	same as for adults	not recommended (refer to 0.025%)
0.025%	—	—	2–3 (morning and evening)
Phenylephrine hydrochloride, 0.5%	2–3 (≧4 hours)	not recommended (refer to 0.25%)	not recommended (refer to 0. 125%)
0.25%	same as 0.5%	2–3 (≧4 hours)	not recommended (refer to 0. 125%)
0. 125%	—	—	2–3 drops (≧4 hours)
Xylometazoline hydrochloride, 0. 1%	2–3 (8–10 hours)	not recommended (refer to 0.05%)	not recommended (refer to 0.05%)
0.05%	—	2–3 (8–10 hours)	2–3 (8–10 hours)

The FDA OTC Panel on Cold, Cough, Allergy, Bronchodilator, and Antiasthmatic Products has recommended these ingredients as safe and effective (Category I) at the dosages specified. Only drops should be used in children 2 to <6, since the spray is difficult to use in the small nostril.

[a] For children under 6 there is no recommended dosage of ephedrine, naphazoline, or oxymetazoline except under the advice and supervision of a physician.

dosages of topical decongestants

effects of oral decongestants

is not properly replaced. Also, there may not be sufficient nasal airflow to distribute the agent throughout the nasal cavity. These agents have been implicated as being irritating to the nasal mucosa and as interfering with ciliary action, as have all effective topical nasal decongestants. As with other topical amines, overuse produces side effects of local irritation and rebound congestion.

Oral Decongestants

Administering sympathomimetic amines orally distributes the drug via the systemic circulation to the vascular bed of the nasal mucosa. The oral decongestant agents have the advantage of a longer duration of action in comparison with certain topically applied decongestants. However, they cause less intense vasoconstriction than the topically applied sprays or drops. The oral agents have not been associated with rebound congestion or rhinitis medicamentosa because of their lesser degree of vasoconstriction and the lack of local drug irritation (21).

These agents, of course, do not exert their action exclusively on the vasculature of the nasal mucosa; in doses large enough to bring about nasal decongestion they also affect other vascular beds (21). Although the vasoconstriction produced by oral decongestants usually does not increase blood pressure, individuals predisposed to hypertension may experience a change in blood pressure. These decongestants may cause cardiac stimulation and the development of arrhythmias in individuals so predisposed. In a prediabetic or a brittle or juvenile diabetic, sympathomimetic administration may be a problem because these drugs increase the blood glucose level. Labeling instructions on products containing sympathomimetics should indicate that patients with hypertension, hyperthyroidism, diabetes mellitus, or ischemic heart disease should use these products only on the advice of a physician. Sympathomimetic amines should not be administered to patients receiving monoamine oxidase inhibitor (MAOI) therapy because a hypertensive crisis may result. They should be used cautiously in hypertensive patients stabilized with guanethidine (29). These warnings apply largely to the oral agents, since they are not likely to occur with topically applied drugs.

Ephedrine, phenylpropanolamine hydrochloride, phenylephrine hydrochloride, and pseudoephedrine are sympathomimetic amines commonly incorporated into cold and allergy products (see Table 6). Only phenylpropanolamine, phenylephrine, and pseudoephedrine have been shown to be effective as oral decongestants.

Ephedrine

Ephedrine is effective as a bronchodilator for asthma but has not been proven effective as a nasal decongestant. Orally, in doses of 12.5–25 mg every 4 hours for adults and children 12 or over, ephedrine is effective as a bronchodilator for use in treating symptoms of asthma. The effects usually appear within 30 minutes to 1 hour following oral administration. Ephedrine has CNS stimulatory effects.

Phenylpropanolamine

Phenylpropanolamine hydrochloride resembles ephedrine in its action but is somewhat more active as a vasoconstrictor and less active as a CNS stimulant and bronchodilator. Oral doses of 25–50 mg three times per day are recommended for the symptomatic treatment of nasal congestion. The peak effect occurs approximately 3 hours after administration.

Phenylephrine

Phenylephrine hydrochloride in doses of 10 mg every 4 hours is recommended. This drug is rapidly hydrolyzed in the GI tract, and the amount delivered to the bloodstream via the oral route is hard to predict, but effectiveness as an oral decongestant has been demonstrated (1). Phenylephrine is a common ingredient of cold preparations but is usually present at inadequate dosage levels.

Pseudoephedrine

Pseudoephedrine is another effective vasoconstrictor. It has less vasopressor action than ephedrine and causes little CNS stimulation. The peak effect of a 60-mg dose occurs approximately 4 hours after administration.

Antitussives and Expectorants

The cough associated with the common cold may be either productive or nonproductive (dry cough). The productive cough is useful and essential if it helps to remove accumulated secretions and debris (phlegm) from the lower tract. Although a patient with "chest congestion" is expected to expectorate phlegm ("productive" cough) during coughing, this does not necessarily occur. It would be inappropriate, however, to describe the cough as "nonproductive" because this description usually is related to dry, noncongested coughing. For the sake of distinction in this section as well as rationale for product selection later, a cough will be classified in one of the following categories:

- Congested/productive—cough associated with the expectoration of phlegm;
- Congested/nonproductive—cough associated with chest congestion and scant expectoration of phlegm;
- Dry/nonproductive—cough not associated with chest congestion.

By referring to these categories the pharmacist will be able to determine when and which type of antitussive agent should be used.

oral nasal decongestants, actions and dosages

cough preparations

types of cough

Excessive coughing, particularly if it is dry and nonproductive, not only is discomforting but also tends to be self-perpetuating because the rapid air expulsion further irritates the tracheal and pharyngeal mucosa. The general types of antitussive agents available for self-medication are expectorants and cough suppressants. Table 7 indicates the sites at which the cough reflex may be blocked as well as the mechanism of the agents.

Expectorants

The use of expectorants in clinical practice is a highly controversial issue revolving around doubts of therapeutic efficacy. The controversy stems from the lack of objective experimental data showing that an expectorant decreases sputum viscosity or eases expectoration more than a placebo. In fact, in spite of the widespread use of guaifenesin, one study states that "from a scientific point of view . . . , [this drug] probably has no rational use in clinical medicine as an expectorant" (30). Other literature also questions the efficacy of expectorants, stating that "the use of expectorants is based primarily on tradition and the widespread subjective clinical im-

Table 6. Oral Nasal Decongestant Dosage

	Dosage (Maximum Daily Dose)		
Drug	**Adults**	**Children 6 to <12**	**Children 2 to <6**
Phenylephrine	10 mg every 4 hours (60 mg)	5 mg every 4 hours (30 mg)	2.5 mg every 4 hours (15 mg)
Phenylpropanolamine	25 mg every 4 hours or 50 mg every 8 hours (150 mg)	12.5 mg every 4 hours or 25 mg every 8 hours (75 mg)	6.25 mg every 4 hours or 12.5 mg every 8 hours (37.5 mg)
Pseudoephedrine	60 mg every 4 hours (360 mg)	30 mg every 4 hours (180 mg)	15 mg every 4 hours (90 mg)

The FDA OTC Panel on Cold, Cough, Allergy, Bronchodilator, and Antiasthmatic Products has recommended these ingredients as safe and effective (Category I) at the dosages specified.

Table 7. Blockade of Cough Reflex

Site	Mechanism	Blocking Agents
Sensory nerves	reduction of primary irritation; inhibition of bronchoconstriction; inhibition of afferent impulses	demulcents/ expectorants; bronchodilators; local anesthetics
Cough center (medulla)	depression	opiate and nonopiate suppressants
Motor nerves	inhibition of efferent impulses	local anesthetics

Adapted from H. Salem and D. M. Aviado, *Drug Inform. J.*, *8*, 111 (Oct.–Dec. 1974).

cough reflex inhibition

water in cold therapy

commonly used expectorants, dosages, regimens, and side effects

cough suppressants

pression that they are effective" (21). The apparent difficulty in accumulating objective evidence stems from two factors: insufficient evidence as to which physicochemical property of respiratory secretions correlates best with ease of expectoration and lack of appropriate techniques and instrumentation (1). The FDA OTC Panel was unable to classify any claimed expectorant as Category I.

Fluid intake and maintaining adequate humidity of the inspired air are important to respiratory tract fluid mucus production and therefore are essential in cold therapy. These measures may be accomplished by increasing fluid intake (six to eight glasses per day) and by using a cool mist or hot steam vaporizer.

Subjective findings constitute the basis for continued expectorant use. In fact, according to the FDA OTC Panel on Cold, Cough, Allergy, Bronchodilator, and Antiasthmatic Products, "until such objective methods become available, the Panel will consider well-controlled, double-blind subjective studies in the assessment of efficacy" (1). Table 8 lists the usual dose and dosage range of the most commonly used expectorants.

There are no apparent absolute contraindications to the use of orally administered expectorants. The toxicity associated with expectorant drugs varies among agents. In general, the most common adverse effect to anticipate is gastric upset.

Ammonium Chloride

Administered in doses of 300 mg every 2–4 hours, ammonium chloride is believed to increase the amount of respiratory tract fluid by reflex stimulation (irritation) of the gastric mucosa. It may cause serious illness in a healthy person if 50 g or more is ingested. In the presence of renal, hepatic, or chronic heart disease, doses of 5 g have caused severe poisoning (31). A relative contraindication exists when ammonium chloride is used in patients with hepatic, renal, or pulmonary insufficiency; doses larger than those recommended may be predisposing to metabolic acidosis. Because ammonium chloride acidifies the urine, it may affect the excretion of other drugs (29). This effect probably is not significant because the usual daily dosage range as a systemic acidifier is 4–12 g (32), which is greatly in excess of the safe range for OTC use.

Guaifenesin

Guaifenesin also is thought to act by reflex gastric stimulation in doses of 200–400 mg every 4 hours. In spite of its mechanism of action its use is seldom associated with gastric upset and nausea. In vitro studies demonstrate guaifenesin's ability to reduce platelet agglutination, an effect associated with clotting time in vivo. The in vitro concentration to produce this effect translates into an oral dose much larger than normal, and thus the effect does not seem to be clinically significant (1, 28).

Ipecac Syrup

Administration of 0.5–1.0 ml three or four times per day of ipecac syrup (see Table 8 for concentration) is believed to increase respiratory secretion flow by gastric irritation. Little is known regarding the toxicity associated with ipecac per se. The chief alkaloids, emetine and cephaeline, however, are very toxic. There is no information on the absorption of small oral doses from the GI tract or on the cumulative effects of repeated oral administration (1). For this reason the Panel has recommended a 1-week time limit when ipecac preparations are used for self-medication. Ipecac is not recommended for use in children less than 6 years of age.

Terpin Hydrate

This volatile oil derivative, believed to act by direct stimulation of lower respiratory tract secretory glands, is recommended in doses of 200 mg every 4 hours. Because of the elixir's high alcohol content the potential for alcohol abuse should be recognized; however, misuse is associated far more frequently with terpin hydrate and codeine elixir. Terpin hydrate elixir is not recommended for use in children younger than 12 years old (1). Some GI distress, such as nausea and vomiting, has been noted in the recommended dosage.

Other ingredients (effectiveness unproven) in cold products associated with expectorant claims include:

- Beechwood creosote;
- Benzoin preparations;
- Camphor;
- Eucalyptus oil;
- Menthol;
- Peppermint oil;
- Pine tar;
- Potassium guaiacolsulfonate;
- Sodium citrate;
- Tolu;
- Turpentine oil.

Antitussives

Antitussives (cough suppressants) are indicated when there is a need to reduce the frequency of a cough, especially when it is the dry/nonproductive type (21, 33).

Table 8. Expectorant Dosage

Drug	Dosage (Maximum Daily Dose) Adults	Children 6 to <12	Children 2 to <6
Ammonium chloride	300 mg every 2–4 hours	150 mg every 2–4 hours	75 mg every 2–4 hours
Guaifenesin	200–400 mg every 4 hours (2400 mg)	100–200 mg every 4 hours (1200 mg)	50–100 mg every 4 hours (600 mg)
Ipecac syrup	0.5–1.0 ml (of syrup containing not less than 123 mg and not more than 157 mg of total ether-soluble alkaloids of ipecac/100 ml) 3 or 4 times/day	0.25–0.5 ml (of syrup containing not less then 123 mg and not more than 157 mg of total ether-soluble alkaloids of ipecac/100 ml) 3 or 4 times/day	not recommended
Terpin hydrate	200 mg every 4 hours (1200 mg)	100 mg (of terpin hydrate alone or in a nonalcoholic mixture, not the elixir for children under 12) every 4 hours (600 mg)	50 mg every 4 hours (300 mg)

The FDA OTC Panel on Cold, Cough, Allergy, Bronchodilator, and Antiasthmatic Products has concluded that the available data are insufficient to permit classification of these ingredients (Category III).

dosages of expectorants

codeine—the standard of comparison for antitussives

other cough suppressants, mechanisms and side effects

The mechanism by which the narcotic and non-narcotic agents affect a cough's intensity and frequency depends on the principal site of action: CNS depression of the cough center in the medulla or suppression of the nerve receptors within the respiratory tract (1).

Codeine

Codeine is the antitussive against which all other antitussives are compared (17). The dependence liability of codeine is much less than that of morphine, but tolerance and addiction may occur when codeine is taken in excessive amounts. The average adult antitussive dose is 15 mg (with a range of 10–20 mg). At this dosage, codeine provides effective cough relief. (See Table 9 for children's dosage.) Stringent controls have been placed on codeine-containing nonprescription products as a result of their misuse. There is no danger of psychological and physical dependence when codeine is used in recommended amounts for short periods. On a weight basis, the respiratory depressant effect of codeine is about one-fourth that of morphine. Even when the dose is increased, commensurate increase in respiratory depression does not necessarily occur. In doses commonly used in OTC cough products, in an otherwise healthy person the effects on respiration are not apparent. Codeine is thought by some investigators to have a drying effect on the respiratory mucosa; this property would be detrimental in asthma and/or emphysema because of the increased viscosity of respiratory fluids and decreased cough reflex (24).

In clinical practice the adverse effects most commonly encountered with codeine include nausea, drowsiness, and constipation, especially when recommended dosage levels are exceeded. Allergic reactions and pruritus also may occur but are not as common. In general, antitussive codeine doses are well tolerated.

Codeine may enhance the effects of oral anticoagulants, but this effect is probably not significant with short-term antitussive doses. Codeine's CNS depressant effect is additive to that of other CNS depressants, and such agents should be used cautiously when given concurrently.

The contraindications to codeine use include its use in individuals with chronic pulmonary disease, where mucosal drying and slight respiratory depression, in addition to impairing the clearing of the airway of secretions, may be additionally detrimental (1). Codeine should be avoided by patients who have experienced codeine-induced allergic manifestations (e.g., pruritus or rash). Codeine is safe and effective used as directed for cough.

Dextromethorphan

Dextromethorphan is a methylated dextro-isomer of levorphanol, but, unlike its analgesic counterpart, it has no significant analgesic properties and does not depress respiration or predispose to addiction (33). Some investigators believe that dextromethorphan and codeine are equipotent; others give a slight edge to codeine (33). Unlike codeine, increasing the dose of dextromethorphan to 30 mg does not increase its antitussive effects (33).

Adverse effects produced by dextromethorphan hydrobromide at recommended OTC dosages are mild and infrequent. Drowsiness and GI upset are the most common complaints. Accidental poisonings in children have resulted in stuporousness and disturbances in gait, with rapid recovery after emesis (33).

Dextromethorphan hydrobromide at OTC dosages (Table 9) is a safe and effective antitussive for which there are no apparent contraindications unless, of course, the patient is hypersensitive to it (1).

Diphenhydramine

Diphenhydramine hydrochloride, a potent antihistamine, is a safe and effective OTC antitussive, according to the FDA OTC Panel. However, the Commissioner has disagreed with this recommendation and as of January 1, 1979, had not issued any decision on the question of exempting diphenhydramine from prescription requirement.

Objective results of clinical studies indicate that diphenhydramine, in 25- and 50-mg doses, significantly reduced coughing in chronic cough patients (34). The recommended adult dose is 25 mg every 4 hours, not to exceed 150 mg in 24 hours (see Table 9). The safe OTC dosage for children under 6 has not been established (1).

cough suppressants, mechanisms and side effects

dosage of antitussives

The adverse effects associated with diphenhydramine hydrochloride are typical of other antihistamines. The most commonly encountered adverse effects are sedation and anticholinergic (atropinelike) effects. Because of these properties, diphenhydramine hydrochloride should not be taken by individuals in whom anticholinergics are contraindicated (those with narrow-angle glaucoma or prostatic hypertrophy) or in situations where mental alertness is required (e.g., driving a car).

Diphenhydramine should be used cautiously in individuals taking "tranquilizers," sedatives, or hypnotics, because of its additive CNS depressant effect. Likewise, ingesting alcohol will have additive depressant effects, and caution must be exercised in taking diphenhydramine hydrochloride. Diphenhydramine hydrochloride should not be given to patients receiving monoamine oxidase inhibitors and should be used cautiously in patients taking other anticholinergic drugs because of additive effects (35). It should not be used in patients with a history of asthma, because of its anticholinergic properties (1). Diphenhydramine hydrochloride, like codeine and dextromethorphan hydrobromide, is a safe and effective antitussive but has a propensity for side effects, which must be kept in mind when recommending it.

Noscapine

Noscapine is an opium alkaloid related to papaverine. Although it is used in only a few nonprescription preparations, its limited availability is not an indication of its effectiveness—it has been reported to reduce the frequency and severity of allergic cough (32, 33). Nevertheless, the FDA Panel has suggested additional testing to establish its effectiveness (1). Noscapine's antitussive effectiveness is dose related, and although some investigators believe that it is equipotent on a weight basis to codeine, safe OTC dosages range from 15 to 30 mg every 4–6 hours, not to exceed 180 mg/day (Table 9).

In therapeutic doses, noscapine shows little or no effect on the CNS or respiratory system and has neither analgesic properties nor addictive liabilities. Constipation and other GI reactions have not been encountered to a significant degree. Noscapine is apparently safe at currently available OTC dosages, but effectiveness has yet to be proven.

Other ingredients that may have antitussive properties include (1):

- Beechwood creosote;
- Camphor (topical/inhalant);
- Caramiphen edisylate (ethanedisulfonate);
- Carbetapentane citrate;
- Cod liver oil;
- Elm bark;
- Ethylmorphine hydrochloride;
- Eucalyptol/eucalyptus oil (topical/inhalant);
- Horehound (horehound fluidextract);

Table 9. Antitussive Dosage

Drug	Dosage (Maximum Daily Dose)		
	Adults	**Children 6 to <12**	**Children 2 to <6**
Codeine	10–20 mg every 4–6 hours (120 mg)	5–10 mg every 4–6 hours (60 mg)	2.5–5 mg every 4–6 hours (30 mg)
Dextromethorphan	10–20 mg every 4 hours or 30 mg every 6–8 hours (120 mg)	5–10 mg every 4 hours or 15 mg every 6–8 hours (60 mg)	2.5–5 mg every 4 hours or 7.5 mg every 6–8 hours (30 mg)
Diphenhydramine hydrochloride [a]	25 mg every 4 hours (150 mg)	12.5 mg every 4 hours (75 mg)	6.25 mg every 4 hours (37.5 mg) [b]
Noscapine hydrochloride	15–30 mg every 4–6 hours (180 mg)	7.5–15 mg every 4–6 hours (90 mg)	3.75–7.5 mg every 4–6 hours (45 mg)

The FDA OTC Panel on Cold, Cough, Allergy, Bronchodilator, and Antiasthmatic Products has recommended all of these ingredients as safe and effective (Category I) except noscapine hydrochloride, for which there is insufficient evidence (Category III).

[a] Currently (as of January 1, 1979) requires a prescription at all doses.

[b] Only on physician recommendation.

- Menthol/peppermint oil (topical/inhalant);
- Thymol (topical/inhalant);
- Turpentine oil (spirits of turpentine) (topical/inhalant).

These ingredients need to be tested for effectiveness.

Bronchodilators

Bronchoconstriction has been implicated in the cough reflex. Drugs known to inhibit bronchoconstriction may have antitussive action (1). It is on the basis of the "bronchomotor theory" that some investigators contend that a sympathomimetic bronchodilator is indicated for reducing cough resulting from the common cold or bronchitis (nonchronic). Currently, methoxyphenamine in certain OTC drug products is the only bronchodilator ingredient associated with this claim (1). This consideration requires further investigation.

Oral Antibacterials and Anesthetics

Pharyngitis, or sore throat, is a symptom of the common cold and, less commonly, of allergic rhinitis. In allergic rhinitis it may result from the drying effect of constant mouth breathing caused by nasal congestion or from swelling in the pharynx due to a pollen sensitivity reaction. Treating the nasal congestion and administering antihistamines are measures that help diminish the pharyngitis resulting from allergic response. With the common cold, pharyngitis is usually the result of the infectious process, and histamine release is not the target-offending agent. Most commonly, the symptom is soreness or dryness rather than actual pain, as in the more severe cell injury and inflammation of bacterial infections. Pharyngitis also is believed to result from continuous postnasal mucous discharge impinging on the pharynx.

Other environmental factors also may lead to pharyngitis. Overusing tobacco products and ingesting large amounts of concentrated alcohol-containing beverages or other irritating substances are factors associated with pharyngeal irritation and sore throat. More rarely, irritant gas inhalation also may be an etiological factor.

Diseases in which pharyngitis may be a symptom include not only the common cold but also streptococcal infection of the throat, scarlet fever, tonsillitis, influenza, measles, and smallpox. It is important that the etiology be uncovered so that appropriate measures may be taken. An acute sore throat with a nonbacterial infection has a much slower onset than bacterial pharyngitis. The soreness and the constitutional symptoms are milder, temperature is usually normal or only slightly elevated, and there is a dry, raspy, possibly tickling sensation in the throat when swallowing.

A sore throat may indicate a more serious disease that demands medical attention (e.g., streptococcal pharyngitis), and self-treatment may mask the symptoms. When the sore throat symptom is not related to environmental factors, to allergic rhinitis, or to a cold, a physician should be consulted. Failure to consult a physician may result in a worsening of the condition and development of complications. If the sore throat symptoms can be self-medicated, there are many products to choose from that are promoted for relief, but only those containing local anesthetics have any basis for effectiveness. Since most of these products are lozenges, sprays and mouthwashes, gargles, and throatwashes, effectiveness is limited to the mucous membranes of the oral tract which can be reached by the dosage form.

The primary purpose of a mouthwash is to cleanse and soothe. Most mouthwashes are promoted for bad breath with the suggestion that these products kill germs. The Council on Dental Therapeutics does not recognize substantial contributions to oral health from medicated mouthwashes (36). Much of the controversy surrounding the use of these products stems from the problems associated with substantiating germicidal or germistatic claims. There is no method that effectively compares the germicidal activity in the test tube with that in the oral cavity. There is also no adequate evidence that individuals benefit from a nonspecific change in the oral cavity flora; it is possible that alteration of the normal oral cavity flora actually may allow invasion by pathogenic organisms. In addition, most infectious sore throats are viral in origin, and using a lozenge or gargle promoted as an "antibacterial" does not influence the viral pharyngitis.

antibacterials and anesthetics for sore throat

dosage forms

mechanisms and effectiveness

The antimicrobial substances in most commercial mouthwashes are phenols, alcohol, quaternary ammonium compounds, volatile oils, oxygenating agents, and iodine-containing preparations. These agents are believed to be of little value in treating sore throat symptoms.

A possible benefit of oral mouthwashes and gargles is derived from the anesthetic compounds they contain. These agents temporarily desensitize the sensory nerves in the pharyngeal mucosa, affording transient relief. The danger remains, however, in masking a symptom of a condition which may be harmful. Many commercially available lozenges also are promoted to treat sore throat symptoms. They usually contain an antibacterial agent in combination with a local anesthetic. The beneficial effect of this combination is probably caused by the anesthetic agent.

There is much controversy surrounding the effectiveness of the different anesthetic ingredients in lozenges and mouthwashes promoted for sore throats. The value and effectiveness of a local anesthetic agent usually are established by testing on human skin, oral mucosa, or tongue, not by pharyngeal tests. Consequently, patient satisfaction is probably the best indicator of these products' effectiveness until they meet the FDA regulations being proposed by the FDA OTC Panel on Oral Cavity Drug Products.

Benzocaine

Benzocaine is beneficial in diminishing sore throat symptoms in concentrations of 5–20%. Concentrations of less than 5% are not considered beneficial. There are currently no OTC preparations containing an effective benzocaine concentration.

Phenol and Phenol-Containing Salts

These agents are included in several OTC lozenges. They are effective in concentrations of 0.5–1.5%.

Benzyl Alcohol

Benzyl alcohol is an effective oral anesthetic agent used in concentrations of as much as 10%.

The pharmacist should recommend a product that contains an effective dose of a local anesthetic and a minimum of extraneous compounds whose effectiveness or value is doubtful. The pharmacist also should try to follow up on patient response to recommended agents for future suggestions as to alternative OTC therapy for pharyngeal soreness.

Anticholinergics

Some nonprescription cold remedies contain atropine or a mixture of belladonna alkaloids. The rationale for their inclusion is that their drying effect provides symptomatic relief from the "runny nose" associated with the cold and allergic rhinitis.

atropine and other belladonna alkaloids

interactions and hypersensitivity

fever-reducing agents

effects, interactions, and adverse reactions of aspirin and acetaminophen

role of vitamin C

Although anticholinergics can dry excess nasal secretions, the doses commonly found in nonprescription remedies (e.g., 0.06–0.2 mg total alkaloids) have not been shown to accomplish this objective. To make up for this therapeutic shortcoming, these agents are usually found in products that also contain an antihistamine. The additive anticholinergic effect obtained from such a combination theoretically may help reduce secretions resulting from the common cold, but this claim remains to be proven for specific combinations. Such a combination exposes the patient to the antihistamine's unwanted sedative effects. It hardly seems rational to combine the therapeutic effect of one drug (in subtherapeutic amounts) with the unpredictable side effect of another in an attempt to achieve the effects obtainable with a larger (therapeutic) dose of the former.

Drug interactions involving anticholinergics are unlikely at the doses used in a cold or allergy remedy when no other ingredients are present that have anticholinergic effects. However, hypersensitivity to these relatively small amounts does occur. If a hypersensitive individual also suffers from asthma, narrow-angle glaucoma, or enlarged prostate, a physician should be contacted before a preparation containing an anticholinergic is taken.

Pending further definitive dosage data the anticholinergics available in OTC products should not be considered significant contributors to the relief of cold or allergy symptoms (1). Therefore their presence in a product should not be a criterion for product selection.

Antipyretics/Analgesics

In the common cold there is seldom an actual clinical fever. More often it is a feeling of warmth but with little or no temperature elevation. The usefulness of aspirin or acetaminophen lies in relieving the discomforts of generalized aches and pains or malaise associated with the viral infection. (See Chapter 9 for a complete discussion of internal analgesic products.)

In adults, 325–650 mg of aspirin or acetaminophen every 4–6 hours should help relieve discomfort and slight fever. In children, aspirin may be given as follows: 65 mg per year of age up to a maximum of 650 mg for a 10-year-old or older, every 4–6 hours. Some practitioners may prefer to avoid possible aspirin toxicity in small children and recommend acetaminophen. Acetaminophen doses for children are: under 1 year, 60 mg; 1–2 years, 60–120 mg; 2–6 years, 120 mg; and 6–12 years, 250 mg. They should be repeated every 4–6 hours (12, 37).

Both aspirin and acetaminophen have been reported to increase the response to oral anticoagulants, although any effect from acetaminophen is likely to be small and not clinically significant (22, 29). Although acetaminophen might be preferred when an analgesic/antipyretic is indicated for a patient also taking an oral anticoagulant, it should not be added to the regimen without first ensuring adequate follow-up of clinical and laboratory parameters by checking with the patient's physician.

Patients taking either probenecid or sulfinpyrazone to control their serum uric acid levels should avoid aspirin because of its inhibitory effect on the uricosuric action of these drugs (29). Aspirin also has been shown to diminish indomethacin effectiveness and should likewise be avoided when conditions such as rheumatoid arthritis are treated with the latter (22).

GI disturbances are common with aspirin. Pharmacists should recommend that patients with a history of peptic ulcer disease avoid aspirin and take acetaminophen instead. Patients with a history of asthma or hay fever and nasal polyps also should avoid aspirin because it has been established that some of these individuals are allergic (hypersensitive) to aspirin (21).

Adverse reactions to acetaminophen are rare in the recommended dosage. An overdose, however, may be associated with acute hepatic necrosis, which may be fatal. Although acetaminophen does not share the adverse GI, hemorrhagic, and acid–base side effects of aspirin, when it is ingested in large quantities, it may be more lethal than aspirin and considerably more difficult to treat (38). In light of this finding the American Academy of Pediatrics Committee on Drugs has made several recommendations regarding acetaminophen, one of which would require the use of "childproof" containers; for products to be taken by children the containers would hold no more than a total of 2 g of acetaminophen (38).

It is important in considering patients with the aforementioned problems to realize that many combination products incorporate both aspirin and acetaminophen in the same product.

Ascorbic Acid (Vitamin C)

The claim that ascorbic acid is effective in preventing and treating the common cold is controversial. Linus Pauling, who popularized its use for the cold, recommends 1–5 g daily as a prophylactic measure and as much as 15 g daily to treat a cold (39). Many studies have been conducted, and although some have shown trends in favor of ascorbic acid's effectiveness, they have not shown the vitamin to be unequivocally effective in any dosage in either preventing or reducing the severity or duration of colds (40).

The potential for adverse effects associated with these large doses is also a debated issue. The most frequently noted adverse effect is diarrhea. Precipitation of urate, oxalate, or cystine stones in the urinary tract has been seen, although the potential for this problem at doses of ≧1 g per day increases with higher doses. The effects on the urinary excretion of other drugs also must be investigated because of ascorbic acid's ability to acidify the urine (41).

Urine acidification increases the possibility of aminosalicylic acid crystalluria in patients receiving aminosalicylic acid in the free acid form. It also increases the excretion of drugs that are weak bases (e.g., amphetamines), reducing their effect, and increases renal tubular salicylate reabsorption, increasing serum salicylate concentrations. Ascorbic acid in doses large enough to acidify the urine (4–12 g per day) should not be given with aminosalicylic acid and should be used cautiously when salicylates are taken in large doses (e.g., 3–5 g per day). There is no apparent problem in taking this vitamin with amphetamines as long as the decreased effect of the amphetamines is anticipated (29).

Ascorbic acid has been implicated in an interaction with warfarin in which the anticoagulant's hypoprothrombinemic effect was diminished (22, 29). Only isolated incidents were reported, however, and it is felt that the interaction either was dose dependent or occurred only in certain patients. Until further clarification is provided, practitioners should be aware of this possible interaction and inquire about ascorbic acid intake in patients who respond erratically to an anticoagulant. The possibility of an exaggerated hypoprothrombinemic response also must be kept in mind when these patients stop taking the vitamin.

Diabetics taking ascorbic acid and testing the urine by the glucose oxidase "dip" test may encounter false negative results; the copper reduction method may produce false positive results (29).

ADJUNCTIVE THERAPY

Inhaling water vapor is an adjunctive therapeutic measure that provides a demulcent action on the respiratory mucosa and adds to and dilutes respiratory tract fluid, decreasing its viscosity (33). Humidifying the inspired air usually aids in relieving the cough and hoarseness associated with laryngitis. Humidification may be a prophylactic measure against upper respiratory infections when people are exposed to low relative humidities. This is usually the case during the winter months, when doors and windows are closed and the heat is on. The relative humidity may be as low as 10% in the home on a cold day; 40–50% is necessary for comfort, and 60–80% is better for persons with respiratory problems. However, at this level, condensation on windows and walls is a limiting factor. With inspiration of dry air the mucus viscosity increases, and irritation of the respiratory mucosa may develop, creating a predisposition to viral or bacterial invasion.

The oldest method of humidifying the air involves generating steam from a pot of boiling water or, more commonly, from an electric steam vaporizer. A newer method involves a cool mist vaporizer from which fine droplets of water are formed by pumping water through a fine screen. Therapeutically, the steam vaporizer does not seem to offer an advantage over the cool mist type. The cool mist type vaporizers are safe in that they do not generate heat or hot water; however, they are noisier, they humidify somewhat more slowly than the steam vaporizers, and they become quickly contaminated because the water particles absorb heat from the surrounding air, chilling the air and causing air saturation at a lower temperature. It is important to follow the manufacturer's directions for cleaning the unit to avoid bacterial overgrowth (a problem not encountered with steam vaporizers). Steam vaporizers do not incur the hazards of contamination and do not lower room temperature.

If humidification is supplemented with a volatile substance (menthol or compound benzoin tincture), a steam vaporizer must be used. It has not been established whether these volatile substances are of therapeutic value, and therefore they may have no advantage over inhaling plain water vapor. In some cases they may even cause irritation of the respiratory tract.

As an adjunctive measure, humidifying the inspired air is important. Either a steam-generated unit or a cool mist vaporizer may be used as prophylaxis and should be used at the cold's onset. It is also important to increase oral fluid intake to prevent dehydration during a cold.

effects of ascorbic acid on other drugs

nondrug measures

PRODUCT SELECTION GUIDELINES

The effectiveness of many products available for self-medication of colds may be questionable, but they are generally safe when used as directed. Allergic rhinitis treatment provides comfort until the acute symptoms subside. Past experience may influence selection. Nevertheless, the pharmacist must be prepared to distinguish between the common cold and allergic rhinitis on the basis of symptoms, recognize complications that may arise or have arisen, and recommend the proper approaches for control of the symptoms (i.e., self-medicate or consult a physician), including drugs, adjunctive measures, and duration of treatment.

Patient Considerations

When symptoms usually associated with the common cold are present, recognizing the underlying disorder is not difficult. However, recognition of the allergic rhinitis condition is often more involved. In both conditions the pharmacist should conduct a brief but careful history of the present illness. This history should provide information that is useful in distinguishing one disorder from another, identifying those disorders which should or should not be self-medicated. The following specific points should be investigated:

- Abruptness of onset;
- Symptomatology;
- Intensity;
- Duration;
- Recurrence.

Common cold onset generally is associated with a prodrome (e.g., "running nose" or dry throat); in fact, it is very common for people to predict that they are "coming down with a cold." Allergic rhinitis is much more abrupt in onset—the condition develops immediately after exposure to the allergen. It is usually initially manifested by a paroxysmal attack of repetitive sneezing.

Early in a cold's development the symptoms are not very intense. As the infection runs its course, the symptoms may get worse, subject to patient variability and depending on the infecting organism. The intensity of symptoms in allergic rhinitis is based on the amount of allergen encountered and the degree of individual hypersensitivity. Generally, the symptoms are most intense following allergen exposure and subside over time unless additional exposures are encountered.

Duration of cold symptoms is a very important detail in deciding which course of action should be taken. Typically, the common cold lasts 4–7 days. If the problem persists beyond this time with no apparent improvement or if the cold symptoms tend to be recurrent, a physician should be consulted for an evaluation. Duration of allergic rhinitis symptoms is extremely variable, partially because of individual sensitivity to the allergen. If the patient has received no relief in 10 days of self-treatment, physician follow-up evaluation and proper management are indicated.

patient and product considerations in cold therapy

The recurrent nature of seasonal allergic rhinitis is a hallmark in differentiating this condition from other nonallergic respiratory conditions. The recurrence of symptoms often follows high pollen counts or patient activities that result in increased allergen exposure. If the symptomatology is present throughout the year or if it persists after the first killing frost, the condition may be perennial allergic rhinitis. Referral to a physician is desirable with perennial allergic rhinitis because of the prolonged duration of symptoms and the potential for developing complications.

Information on medications that have already been tried will aid the pharmacist not only in assessing the patient's current status but also in selecting a product. If, in the pharmacist's judgment, the measures were appropriate and were not effective, the patient should be encouraged to see a physician. If no medication was tried or if inadequate or inappropriate measures were taken, the pharmacist should recommend a more appropriate course of therapy. When a patient seeks the pharmacist's assistance in selecting a cold or allergy remedy, the pharmacist should question the individual as to the presence of other acute or chronic illnesses. This process may identify patients for whom many preparations should be used cautiously, if at all.

Orally administered preparations containing sympathomimetics should be given only on the advice of a physician to patients with hyperthyroidism (the patient is already predisposed to tachycardia and arrhythmias), hypertension (especially moderate to severe, where additional peripheral vasoconstriction may cause significant blood pressure elevation), diabetes mellitus (especially in insulin-dependent diabetics and in cases where glycogenolysis may cause the diabetes to go out of control), and ischemic heart disease or angina (where an increase in heart rate may precipitate an acute angina attack and possibly a subsequent myocardial infarction). These concerns center primarily around the oral administration of sympathomimetic decongestants, where systemic effects are predictable. Judiciously administered decongestant drops, sprays, or inhalations provide a local intranasal action without significant concern of systemic absorption.

Theoretically, all of these effects may occur when the sympathomimetics reach the systemic circulation. In actual practice, however, the effect on a diabetic has not been a particular problem, except in an extremely unstable (brittle) diabetic. Should a diabetic patient take a liquid cough/cold preparation containing sugar? The syrup vehicle may contain as much as 85% (weight per volume) sucrose, and each gram of sucrose has about 4 cal (17 cal/tsp). If 4 tsp (about 70 cal) are taken in 1 day, the additional (nondietary) calories may be clinically significant in a brittle diabetic. Consequently, a sugar-free preparation is preferable. In a stable diabetic, however, these additional calories probably would be of little concern.

Another factor that pharmacists should take into consideration in dealing with a diabetic patient is the alcohol contained in the product. Alcohol, like sucrose, also will provide calories—more calories, in fact, than an equal weight of sucrose. Because most liquid cough remedies contain alcohol (1–25%, each gram providing about 7 cal), it is clear that a brittle diabetic taking a "usual" dose might experience some difficulty with diabetes control. Persons taking disulfiram also must be cautious of alcohol in cough syrups. The minimum amount necessary to trigger an adverse reaction has not been established.

The anticholinergic properties of antihistamines are usually not prominent in OTC preparations. However, the anticholinergic effects of atropine and other belladonna alkaloids in some allergy and cold remedies pose a potential problem. In cases of glaucoma or urinary retention secondary to prostatic hypertrophy, preparations containing anticholinergic agents and antihistamines, especially in combination, should be used only on a physician's advice.

The pharmacist should have a medication history to avoid possible drug interactions and to identify and avoid drug allergies or idiosyncrasies. In addition, a history of chronic topical nasal decongestant use may help identify rhinitis medicamentosa.

Product Considerations

In view of the number of cold and allergy products (single-entity and combinations) it is important that the pharmacist become familiar with a few preparations, especially those found safe and effective by FDA OTC Panels and those found empirically useful, and recommend these preferentially. In trying to single out a preparation the pharmacist needs to know what effect is sought, which drug entity will produce this effect, how much of the drug is necessary to produce this effect, and which nonprescription product satisfactorily meets these needs.

If only one effect is sought (e.g., nasal decongestion), a preparation with a single agent in a full therapeutic dose should be used. When more than one effect is desired, selection becomes more complex. Several single-entity products may be used, but this solution is not usually acceptable to the patient—a combination product is preferred. The pharmacist should be selective in recommending a combination because many of these preparations carry the idea of "shotgun therapy" to its extreme. One study states that "the numerous compounded remedies, including those with vitamins, bioflavonoids, quinine, alkalinizers, multiple analgesics, antihistamines, decongestants, and tranquilizers, are developed for sales profit in a large market of uninformed and uncritical people and are not for the benefit of the patient . . ." (3). Combinations recommended by FDA OTC Panels provide a reasonable basis for selection when directions for use are followed carefully.

The pharmacist should select a combination product containing the desired agents in full therapeutic doses, with as few additional ingredients as possible. This goal, however, seldom is achievable. The pharmacist must decide which effect is most important and select the combination on the basis of the agent that will produce this effect. For example, antihistamine efficacy in common cold treatment is doubtful, and this drawback is magnified by the subtherapeutic doses contained in most nonprescription remedies. An antihistamine–decongestant therefore should be selected on the basis of the decongestant, only secondary consideration being given to the antihistamine.

The opposite is probably indicated in selecting a combination product for allergic rhinitis. There is no proven evidence that incorporating other ancillary agents or other ingredients of the same pharmacological class in a subtherapeutic dose provides more relief or even as much relief as one agent in its full therapeutic dose.

Combination products containing analgesic/antipyretic agents generally should not be recommended. Their routine use carries the risk of masking a fever that may indicate a bacterial infection. Such agents should be administered separately and only when needed. Similarly, preparations that do not disclose the amounts of ingredients on the package should not be recommended. It would be difficult for a pharmacist to justify recommending a product to ameliorate a symptom when there is no indication as to how much of the active ingredients the product contains.

The use of timed-release preparations allows better patient compliance and increased patient convenience. However, some practitioners feel that these advantages may be outweighed by the fact that drug bioavailability in this dosage form may be neither uniform nor reliable (21). The pharmacist's recommendation of a timed-release preparation should be based on the presence of indicated agents in therapeutic doses and, in the pharmacist's experience, the product's success record.

There is much controversy concerning the advantages of oral nasal decongestants over the topical agents. Proponents of oral decongestants state that these agents can affect all respiratory membranes, that they are unaffected by the character of mucus, that they do not induce pathological changes in the nasal mucosa, and that they relieve nasal obstruction without the additional irritation of locally applied medication.

There is also evidence to support the value of topically applied vasoconstrictors. Although nasal sprays and drops do not represent the ideal dosage form, they do provide rapid relief. Because the relief is so dramatic, the patient tends to overuse topical agents, risking drug-induced irritation of the nasal mucosa, alteration of the mucosal ciliary movement, and possibly rhinitis medicamentosa.

Combining topical therapy with oral decongestant therapy is also a controversial procedure. However, judicious use of an oral decongestant proven safe and effective along with a fast-acting topical agent presents a definite advantage. With this combination the patient experiences rapid relief from the topically applied decongestant and possibly a greater degree of relief via the systemic circulation from the oral agent if given in an adequate dose. Depending on the topical agent being used, a longer lasting effect also is possible with this combined therapy.

product and patient considerations

Patient Consultation

advising the patient

In almost all cases of self-medication the pharmacist is the first and only knowledgeable professional contacted. If the pharmacist takes the time to identify the patient's problem and ensure proper product selection, advice regarding proper use also must be considered essential to fulfilling professional responsibility.

Patients cannot always be depended on to read and/or follow the package instructions. There is a tendency to believe in the philosophy that "if one is good, two are better." This is not always the case, however. Pharmacists should caution against increasing the dose and/or frequency of administration of any medication, especially antihistamines and topical decongestants.

Even when antihistamines are taken in recommended amounts, they may cause transient drowsiness. Patients should be advised of this effect, especially if they are taking a prescription medication that also depresses the CNS. They should be advised as to the possible effects and should determine what effect the medication has on them before engaging in activities requiring mental alertness.

Nasal solutions may become contaminated. The pharmacist should recommend that the tip of the dropper or the spray applicator be rinsed in hot water after use, that only one person use the spray or drop applicator, and that the bottle or spray be discarded when the medication is no longer needed. Contamination of the nasal dropper also may be minimized by not touching the nose or the nasal surface with the dropper itself.

Nondrug measures (humidification, increased fluid intake, and local heat) may be recommended, and although these suggestions may not seem acceptable to the patient who desires a medication, they may be quite beneficial in combination with a medication. The pharmacist's recommendation that the patient use humidification and/or increase fluid intake is in the patient's best interest. Normal saline gargles several times per day help relieve an inflamed throat, and the tepid water sponge bath with or without aspirin or acetaminophen usually causes an elevated temperature to fall dramatically.

It is important that the patient realize that a cold will go away in spite of the medication recommended, that the medication is intended only to relieve discomfort, and that relief should occur in a week or less. The concern for duration of self-medication stems not only from the potential adverse effects of some of the medications but also from the minority of cold sufferers who may develop complications, such as secondary bacterial infections. If the pharmacist does not stipulate a time limit for therapy, patients may unknowingly continue self-medicating with little effect, prolonging their discomfort and delaying the time for a physician's diagnosis and appropriate treatment.

advising the patient

A cold usually lasts 7 days. The duration of therapy depends on which day in the course of the cold the medication is begun. If symptoms persist beyond the arbitrary, yet fairly reliable, 7-day limit in spite of adequate therapy, a physician should be consulted. If after 2–3 days of therapy the symptoms do not improve or become more intense, or if a fever, a very painful sore throat, or a cough productive of a mucopurulent sputum develops, the patient also should seek a physician's diagnosis.

Product selection must be based not only on the presence of an effective agent in a therapeutic amount but also on underlying disorders that may be influenced adversely by the recommended therapy. Having chosen the product, the pharmacist must then ensure that the patient knows how to take the medication and what to expect from it with regard to symptomatic relief as well as adverse effects. The patient must be told for how long the medication should be taken. Realizing that questions may arise later, the pharmacist should encourage the patient to return or call back.

SUMMARY

By evaluating the presenting symptoms the pharmacist usually can distinguish the common cold from disorders such as the "flu" or allergic rhinitis and offer proper suggestions for treatment. The pharmacist also can offer the allergic rhinitis sufferer medications to provide symptomatic relief. By conducting a careful history and recognizing the pertinent symptoms a partial diminution of the symptoms may be achieved through advice and medication.

Recommendations for common cold and allergic rhinitis treatment should be directed at relieving the symptoms. The pharmacist's endorsement of a "shotgun" remedy is irrational, since the intensity of symptoms will vary from hour to hour. Recommending a particular product is also irresponsible if the product contains agents in less than therapeutic amounts.

Common cold treatment objectives are drying nasal secretions, opening congested nasal passages, reducing frequency of a cough, soothing a sore throat, overcoming the hoarseness of laryngitis, and relieving feverishness and headache. For allergic rhinitis the treatment is directed at blocking or competing with the effect of released histamine, relieving nasal congestion, and palliating secondary symptoms such as pharyngitis and headache. For nasal congestion, topically applied phenylephrine hydrochloride (0.25–0.5%) used every 4 hours if needed or oxymetazoline hydrochloride (0.05%) used twice per day if needed is a very effective decongestant. To augment the effects of the topical decongestant, an oral nasal decongestant also may be recommended. Pseudoephedrine, 60 mg every 4 hours, or phenylpropanolamine, as much as 50 mg three times per day, is usually effective for this purpose.

The very few oral nasal decongestants available as single-entity products should be recommended. Topically applied products should contain only the decongestant. For example, antihistamines add no beneficial effect to a topical decongestant preparation. Oral antihistamines in combination with nasal decongestants may be indicated in allergic rhinitis.

The frequency of cough resulting from colds usually may be controlled by humidification of the inspired air (vaporizers), a demulcent/expectorant to the mucosa (hard candy or cough drop), and/or a cough suppressant (codeine or dextromethorphan). Humidification should be started early in the course of a cold and continued throughout. Products that contain a cough suppressant in combination with an expectorant should not be recommended. In the case of a dry cough, the dose of the cough suppressant is the criterion by which a product is selected. Administration of 15 mg of codeine or dextromethorphan usually decreases the cough's frequency and intensity.

The dry, sore throat present in colds and to a lesser extent in allergic rhinitis may be relieved by dissolving a piece of hard candy in the mouth to stimulate saliva flow. Frequent warm normal saline gargles may relieve symptoms. Topical antibacterials for a viral infection or allergic rhinitis are unwarranted. Significant relief may be obtained from a lozenge or throat spray containing an anesthetic such as hexylresorcinol or phenol in sufficient concentration.

Laryngitis may be managed by water vapor inhalation, by voice rest, and by avoiding inhaled irritants (e.g., tobacco smoke). Dissolving lozenges in the mouth or gargling does little to reach the inflamed laryngeal tissues.

Relief from feverishness and headache may be provided by using an analgesic/antipyretic, either aspirin or acetaminophen. Products containing these agents in combination with several other ingredients are not recommended. Taking aspirin or acetaminophen regularly during the common cold or acute allergic rhinitis masks the possible development of a fever, which may indicate secondary bacterial infection. An antipyretic agent should be used to bring relief only as needed.

Antihistamines are effective in allergic rhinitis; their role in common cold treatment is at best only adjunctive by virtue of mild anticholinergic drying effects. Chlorpheniramine maleate, administered orally in doses of as much as 4 mg, is effective and only slightly sedative. There is marked individual variability to the different antihistamines. The pharmacist should be aware of this variability and should be prepared to suggest an alternative if relief is not obtained with the original agent. As with the nasal decongestants, most antihistamines are found in combination with other ingredients in commercial preparations and should not be recommended. The only rational combination for allergic rhinitis treatment is an oral antihistamine with an oral nasal decongestant. Other ingredients found in OTC products are of dubious efficacy.

The duration of therapy depends on when during a cold the patient decides to start treatment. In any case, the patient should be able to stop treatment on the sixth or seventh day of the cold. Slight symptoms, e.g., cough, may persist for another day or so and, if necessary, should be treated.

The duration of treatment of allergic rhinitis should be limited to 3 days when topical nasal decongestants are used, in order to minimize the chances of rhinitis medicamentosa. Generally, oral decongestant therapy should be limited to 10 days. The patient's need of the oral agents for longer than 10 days may indicate the development of complications, and the patient should be referred to a physician. An antihistamine product may be used prophylactically in acute allergic rhinitis. The duration of antihistamine therapy should coincide with the appearance and disappearance of the particular allergen.

Patients who have a common cold or allergic rhinitis offer the pharmacist many opportunities to be involved. Although pharmacists often cannot counsel every cold and/or hay fever sufferer, they should be available on request and voluntarily as other professional responsibilities permit.

REFERENCES

(1) *Federal Register, 41,* 38312 (1976).
(2) A. C. Guyton, "Textbook of Medical Physiology," Saunders, Philadelphia, Pa., 1976, pp. 525–527.
(3) "Cecil-Loeb Textbook of Medicine," P. B. Beeson and W. McDermott, Eds., Saunders, Philadelphia, Pa., 1975, pp. 184–187, 829.
(4) A. G. Christie, "Infectious Disease—Epidemiology and Clinical Practice," Churchill Livingstone, New York, N.Y., 1974, pp. 316–318, 359–360, 363.
(5) H. Salem and D. M. Aviado, *Drug Inform. J., 8,* 111 (1974).
(6) "Current Medical Diagnosis and Treatment," M. A. Krupp and M. J. Chatton, Eds., Lange Medical, Los Altos, Calif., 1977, p. 96.
(7) J. I. Tennenbaum, in "Allergic Diseases—Diagnosis and Management," R. Patterson, Ed., Lippincott, Philadelphia, Pa., 1972, pp. 161–195.
(8) "Medical Notes on the Common Cold," Burroughs Wellcome, Research Triangle Park, N.C., 1972.
(9) W. B. Pratt, "Fundamentals of Chemotherapy," Oxford University Press, New York, N.Y., 1972, p. 232.
(10) R. W. Steele, P. T. Tanaka, R. P. Lara, and J. W. Bass, *J. Pediatr., 77,* 824 (1970).
(11) S. W. McFadden and J. E. Haddow, *Pediatrics, 43,* 622 (1969).
(12) *Federal Register, 42,* 35346 (1977).
(13) W. B. Sherman, "Hypersensitivity Mechanisms and Management," Saunders, Philadelphia, Pa., 1968.
(14) J. M. O'Loughlin, *Drug Ther., 4,* 47 (April 1974).
(15) P. M. Seebohm, *Postgrad. Med., 53,* 52 (1973).
(16) L. Tuft, "Allergy Management in Clinical Practice," Mosby, St. Louis, Mo., 1973, pp. 185–238.
(17) A. W. Frankland, *Int. Arch. Allergy Appl. Immunol., 6,* 45 (1955).
(18) L. H. Criep, *J. Am. Med. Assoc., 166,* 572 (1965).
(19) "Basic Pharmacology in Medicine," J. R. DiPalma, Ed., McGraw-Hill, New York, N.Y., 1976, pp. 280–290.
(20) "International Encyclopedia of Pharmacology and Therapeutics," Vol. 1, Section 74, M. Schachter, Ed., Pergamon, New York, N.Y., 1973, p. 127.
(21) "AMA Drug Evaluations," 3rd ed., Publishing Sciences Group, Littleton, Mass., 1977, pp. 644, 647, 655, 662, 673, 681.
(22) "Evaluations of Drug Interactions," 2nd ed., APhA, Washington, D.C., 1976.
(23) "Manual of Medical Therapeutics," 22nd ed., Little, Brown, Boston, Mass., 1977, p. 157.
(24) "Drill's Pharmacology in Medicine," J. R. DiPalma, Ed., McGraw-Hill, New York, N.Y., 1971, p. 655.
(25) D. M. Aviado, "Sympathomimetic Drugs," Charles C Thomas, Springfield, Ill., 1970, pp. 282, 288, 382.
(26) E. W. Martin, "Techniques of Medication," Lippincott, Philadelphia, Pa., 1969, p. 91.
(27) J. T. Connell, *Ann. Allergy, 27,* 541 (1969).
(28) G. Aschan and B. Drettner, *Eye Ear Nose Throat Mon., 43,* 66 (1964).
(29) P. D. Hansten, "Drug Interactions," Lea and Febiger, Philadelphia, Pa., 1975.
(30) S. R. Hirsch, *Drug Ther., 5,* 179 (April 1975).
(31) C. J. Polson and R. N. Tattersall, "Clinical Toxicology," Lippincott, Philadelphia, Pa., 1969, p. 92.
(32) "The United States Dispensatory," 27th ed., A. Osol and R. Pratt, Eds., Lippincott, Philadelphia, Pa., 1973, p. 794.
(33) "Drugs of Choice, 1978–1979," W. Modell, Ed., Mosby, St. Louis, Mo., 1978, pp. 461–475.
(34) Parke, Davis and Company, product information, 1976.
(35) Parke, Davis and Company, package literature.
(36) "Accepted Dental Therapeutics," 36th ed., American Dental Association, Chicago, Ill., 1975.
(37) H. C. Shirkey, "Pediatric Drug Handbook," Saunders, Philadelphia, Pa., 1977.
(38) Committee on Drugs, American Academy of Pediatrics, *Pediatrics, 61,* 108 (1978).
(39) L. Pauling, "Vitamin C and the Common Cold," Freeman, San Francisco, Calif., 1970.
(40) *Medical Letter on Drugs and Therapeutics, 16,* 85 (1974).
(41) *Medical Letter on Drugs and Therapeutics, 12,* 105 (1970).

Product[a] (Manufacturer)	Cough Suppressant	Expectorant	Sympathomimetic	Antihistamine	Other
Actol Expectorant (Beecham Labs)	noscapine, 6 mg/ml	guaifenesin, 40 mg/ml	—	—	alcohol, 12.5% fruit flavoring
Acutuss Expectorant With Codeine (Philips Roxane)	codeine phosphate[b], 2 mg/ml	guaifenesin, 20 mg/ml	phenylephrine hydrochloride, 1 mg/ml	—	sucrose corn syrup alcohol, 5%
Alamine (North American)	—	—	phenylephrine hydrochloride, 1 mg/ml	chlorpheniramine maleate, 0.2 mg/ml	menthol, 0.2 mg/ml alcohol, 5% green mint flavor
Alamine-C (North American)	codeine phosphate[b], 1 mg/ml	—	phenylephrine hydrochloride, 2 mg/ml	chlorpheniramine maleate, 0.4 mg/ml	menthol, 0.2 mg/ml alcohol, 5% grape flavor
Alamine Expectorant (North American)	codeine phosphate[b], 1 mg/ml	guaifenesin, 20 mg/ml	phenylephrine hydrochloride, 2 mg/ml	chlorpheniramine maleate, 0.4 mg/ml	menthol, 0.2 mg/ml alcohol, 5% grape flavor
Alo-Tuss Tablets (North American)	dextromethorphan hydrobromide, 10 mg	—	phenylephrine hydrochloride, 5 mg	chlorpheniramine maleate, 2 mg	—
Amonidrin Tablets (O'Neal, Jones & Feldman)	—	ammonium chloride, 200 mg guaifenesin, 100 mg	—	—	—
Atussin D.M. Expectorant (Amfre-Grant)	dextromethorphan hydrobromide, 3 mg/ml	guaifenesin, 20 mg/ml	phenylephrine hydrochloride, 1 mg/ml phenylpropanolamine hydrochloride, 1 mg/ml	chlorpheniramine maleate, 0.4 mg/ml	sucrose
Atussin Expectorant[c] (Amfre-Grant)	—	guaifenesin, 20 mg/ml	phenylpropanolamine hydrochloride, 1 mg/ml phenylephrine hydrochloride, 1 mg/ml	chlorpheniramine maleate, 0.4 mg/ml	—
Baby Cough Syrup (DeWitt)	—	ammonium chloride, 2.6 mg/ml	—	—	glycerin, 68.6 mg/ml licorice extract, 2.4 mg/ml
Bayer Cough Syrup for Children (Glenbrook)	dextromethorphan hydrobromide, 1.5 mg/ml	—	phenylpropanolamine hydrochloride, 1.8 mg/ml	—	alcohol, 5%
Benylin DM (Parke-Davis)	dextromethorphan hydrobromide, 2 mg/ml	—	—	—	alcohol, 5% ammonium chloride sodium citrate
Breacol (Glenbrook)	dextromethorphan hydrobromide, 2 mg/ml	—	phenylpropanolamine hydrochloride, 7.5 mg/ml	chlorpheniramine maleate, 0.8 mg/ml	alcohol, 10%
Broncho-Tussin[c] (First Texas)	codeine phosphate[b], 2.17 mg/ml	terpin hydrate, 8.7 mg/ml	—	—	alcohol, 40%
C3 Capsules (Menley & James)	dextromethorphan hydrobromide, 30 mg	—	phenylpropanolamine hydrochloride, 50 mg	chlorpheniramine maleate, 4 mg	—
Cerose[c] (Ives)	codeine phosphate[b], 2 mg/ml	potassium guaiacolsulfonate, 17.2 mg/ml ipecac fluidextract, 0.034 mg/ml	phenylephrine hydrochloride, 1 mg/ml	phenindamine tartrate, 2 mg/ml	sodium citrate, 39 mg/ml citric acid, 13 mg/ml glycerin, 8 min/ml alcohol, 2.5%

Product [a] (Manufacturer)	Cough Suppressant	Expectorant	Sympathomimetic	Antihistamine	Other
Cerose DM [c] (Ives)	dextromethorphan hydrobromide, 2 mg/ml	potassium guaiacolsulfonate, 17.2 mg/ml ipecac fluidextract, 0.034 mg/ml	phenylephrine hydrochloride, 1 mg/ml	phenindamine tartrate, 1 mg/ml	sodium citrate, 39 mg/ml citric acid, 13 mg/ml alcohol, 2.5%
Cetro-Cirose [c] (Ives)	codeine phosphate [b], 1 mg/ml	potassium guaicolsulfonate, 17.2 mg/ml ipecac fluidextract, 0.034 mg/ml	—	—	sodium citrate, 39 mg/ml citric acid, 13 mg/ml alcohol, 1.5%
Cheracol (Upjohn)	codeine phosphate [b], 2 mg/ml	guaifenesin, 20 mg/ml	—	—	alcohol, 3%
Cheracol D (Upjohn)	dextromethorphan hydrobromide, 2 mg/ml	guaifenesin, 20 mg/ml	—	—	alcohol, 3%
Children's Hold 4 Hour Cough Suppressant (Beecham)	dextromethorphan	—	phenylpropanol-amine	—	—
Chlor-Trimeton Expectorant (Schering)	—	ammonium chloride, 20 mg/ml guaifenesin, 10 mg/ml	phenylephrine hydrochloride, 2 mg/ml	chlorpheniramine maleate, 0.4 mg/ml	sodium citrate, 10 mg/ml alcohol, 1%
Chlor-Trimeton Expectorant with Codeine (Schering)	codeine phosphate [b], 2 mg/ml	ammonium chloride, 20 mg/ml guaifenesin, 10 mg/ml	phenylephrine hydrochloride, 2 mg/ml	chlorpheniramine maleate, 0.4 mg/ml	sodium citrate, 10 mg/ml alcohol, 5.25%
Codimal DM [c] (Central)	dextromethorphan hydrobromide, 2 mg/ml	potassium guaiacolsulfonate, 16.66 mg/ml	phenylephrine hydrochloride, 1 mg/ml	pyrilamine maleate, 1.66 mg/ml	sodium citrate, 43.2 mg/ml citric acid, 10 mg/ml alcohol, 4%
Codimal Expectorant (Central)	—	potassium guaiacolsulfonate, 20 mg/ml	phenylpropanola-mine hydro-chloride, 5 mg/ml	—	sodium citrate, 43.2 mg/ml citric acid, 10 mg/ml
Codimal PH (Central)	codeine phosphate [b], 2 mg/ml	potassium guaiacolsulfonate, 16.66 mg/ml	phenylephrine hydrochloride, 1 mg/ml	pyrilamine maleate, 1.66 mg/ml	sodium citrate, 43.2 mg/ml citric acid, 10 mg/ml
Colrex [c] (Rowell)	dextromethorphan hydrobromide, 2 mg/ml	—	phenylephrine hydrochloride, 1 mg/ml	chlorpheniramine maleate, 0.2 mg/ml	cherry flavor alcohol, 4.5%
Colrex Expectorant [c] (Rowell)	—	guaifenesin, 20 mg/ml	—	—	alcohol, 4.7%
Conar [c] (Beecham Labs)	noscapine, 3 mg/ml	—	phenylephrine hydrochloride, 2 mg/ml	—	mint flavor
Conar Expectorant (Beecham Labs)	noscapine, 3 mg/ml	guaifenesin, 20 mg/ml	phenylephrine hydrochloride, 2 mg/ml	—	orange flavor
Conex (O'Neal, Jones & Feldman)	—	guaifenesin, 5 mg/ml	phenylpropanola-mine hydro-chloride, 2.5 mg/ml	chlorpheniramine maleate, 0.2 mg/ml	methylparaben, 0.13% propylparaben, 0.03%
Conex with Codeine (O'Neal, Jones & Feldman)	codeine phosphate [b], 1 mg/ml	guaifenesin, 5 mg/ml	phenylpropanola-mine hydro-chloride, 2.5 mg/ml	chlorpheniramine maleate, 0.2 mg/ml	methylparaben, 0.13% propylparaben, 0.03%
Consotuss (Merrell-National)	dextromethorphan hydrobromide, 3 mg/ml	—	—	doxylamine succinate, 0.75 mg/ml	alcohol, 10%

Product[a] (Manufacturer)	Cough Suppressant	Expectorant	Sympathomimetic	Antihistamine	Other
Coricidin (Schering)	—	ammonium chloride, 20 mg/ml guaifenesin, 10 mg/ml	phenylpropanolamine hydrochloride, 2.5 mg/ml	chlorpheniramine maleate, 0.4 mg/ml	—
Coryban-D[c] (Pfipharmecs)	dextromethorphan hydrobromide, 1.5 mg/ml	guaifenesin, 10 mg/ml	phenylephrine hydrochloride, 1 mg/ml	—	alcohol, 7.5% acetaminophen, 24 mg/ml
Cosanyl DM Improved Formula (Health Care Industries)	dextromethorphan hydrobromide, 3 mg/ml	—	*d*-pseudoephedrine hydrochloride, 6 mg/ml	—	alcohol, 6% peach flavor
Cotussis (Merrell-National)	codeine phosphate[b], 2 mg/ml	terpin hydrate, 4 mg/ml	—	—	alcohol, 20%
Creomulsion (Creomulsion Co.)	—	creosote ipecac	—	—	white pine menthol cascara wild cherry alcohol
Creo-Terpin (Roberts)	—	creosote, 4.3 mg/ml terpin hydrate, 4.3 mg/ml	—	—	sodium glycerophosphate, 8.76 mg/ml alcohol, 25%
Dimacol Liquid and Capsules (Robins)	dextromethorphan hydrobromide, 3 mg/ml 15 mg/capsule	guaifenesin, 20 mg/ml 100 mg/capsule	pseudoephedrine hydrochloride, 6 mg/ml 30 mg/capsule	—	alcohol, 4.75% (liquid)
DM-4 Children's Cough Control (DeWitt)	dextromethorphan hydrobromide, 0.8 mg/ml	ammonium chloride, 8 mg/ml potassium guaiacolsulfonate, 7.6 mg/ml	—	—	glycerin, 15 mg/ml alcohol, 1.5%
DM-8 (DeWitt)	dextromethorphan hydrobromide, 1.6 mg/ml	ammonium chloride, 16 mg/ml potassium guaiacolsulfonate, 15 mg/ml	—	—	alcohol, 3%
Dondril Anticough Tablets (Whitehall)	dextromethorphan hydrobromide, 10 mg	guaifenesin, 50 mg	phenylephrine hydrochloride, 5 mg	chlorpheniramine maleate, 1 mg	—
Dorcol Pediatric (Dorsey)	dextromethorphan hydrobromide, 1.5 mg/ml	guaifenesin, 7.5 mg/ml	phenylpropanolamine hydrochloride, 1.75 mg/ml	—	alcohol, 5%
Dr. Drake's (Roberts)	—	ipecac fluidextract	—	—	castor oil
Dristan (Whitehall)	dextromethorphan hydrobromide, 1.5 mg/ml	—	phenylephrine hydrochloride, 1 mg/ml	chlorpheniramine maleate, 0.2 mg/ml	—
Efricon (Lannett)	codeine phosphate[b], 2.19 mg/ml	ammonium chloride, 18 mg/ml potassium guaiacolsulfonate, 18 mg/ml	phenylephrine hydrochloride, 1 mg/ml	chlorpheniramine maleate, 0.4 mg/ml	sodium citrate, 12 mg/ml banana flavor
Endotussin-NN (Endo)	dextromethorphan hydrobromide, 2 mg/ml	ammonium chloride, 8 mg/ml	—	pyrilamine maleate, 1.5 mg/ml	alcohol, 4%
Endotussin-NN Pediatric (Endo)	dextromethorphan hydrobromide, 1 mg/ml	ammonium chloride, 12 mg/ml	—	—	alcohol, 4%
Fedahist Expectorant (Dooner/Rorer)	—	guaifenesin, 20 mg/ml	pseudoephedrine hydrochloride, 6 mg/ml	chlorpheniramine maleate, 0.4 mg/ml	—

Product[a] (Manufacturer)	Cough Suppressant	Expectorant	Sympathomimetic	Antihistamine	Other
Fedahist Syrup and Tablets (Dooner/Rorer)	—	—	pseudoephedrine hydrochloride, 6 mg/ml 60 mg/tablet	chlorpheniramine maleate, 0.4 mg/ml 4 mg/tablet	—
Formula 44 (Vicks)	dextromethorphan hydrobromide, 1 mg/ml	—	—	doxylamine succinate, 0.6 mg/ml	sodium citrate, 50 mg/ml alcohol, 10%
Formula 44 Cough Discs (Vicks)	dextromethorphan hydrobromide, 5 mg	—	—	—	benzocaine, 1.25 mg menthol, anethole, peppermint oil } 0.35%
Formula 44-D (Vicks)	dextromethorphan hydrobromide, 2 mg/ml	guaifenesin, 10 mg/ml	phenylpropanolamine hydrochloride, 2.5 mg/ml	—	alcohol, 10%
2/G (Dow)	—	guaifenesin, 20 mg/ml	—	—	alcohol, 3.5% corn derivatives
2/G-DM (Dow)	dextromethorphan hydrobromide, 3 mg/ml	guaifenesin, 20 mg/ml	—	—	alcohol, 5% corn derivatives
GG-Cen Capsules and Syrup (Central Pharmacal)	—	guaifenesin, 200 mg/capsule 20 mg/ml	—	—	alcohol, 10% (syrup)
G G Tussin (Vitarine)	—	guaifenesin, 20 mg/ml	—	—	alcohol, 3.5%
G-Tussin DM (Columbia)	dextromethorphan hydrobromide, 3 mg/ml	guaifenesin, 20 mg/ml	—	—	alcohol, 1.4%
Halls (Warner-Lambert)	dextromethorphan hydrobromide, 1.5 mg/ml	—	phenylpropanolamine hydrochloride, 3.75 mg/ml	—	menthol eucalyptus oil alcohol, 22% glycerin
Histadyl EC (Lilly)	codeine phosphate[b], 2 mg/ml	ammonium chloride, 22 mg/ml	ephedrine hydrochloride, 1 mg/ml	methapyrilene fumarate, 2.7 mg/ml	menthol alcohol, 5%
Histivite-D (Vitarine)	dextromethorphan hydrobromide, 1 mg/ml	ammonium chloride, 17.3 mg/ml	ephedrine sulfate, 0.81 mg/ml	methapyrilene fumarate, 2.5 mg/ml	menthol alcohol, 4.8%
Hold 4 Hour Cough Suppressant (Beecham)	dextromethorphan	—	—	—	benzocaine
Hold Liquid Cough Suppressant (Beecham)	dextromethorphan hydrobromide	—	phenylpropanolamine hydrochloride	—	alcohol
Hydriodic Acid Cough Syrup (Upjohn)	—	hydrogen iodide, 13–15 mg/ml	—	—	—
Hytuss Tablets[c] (Hyrex)	—	guaifenesin, 100 mg	—	—	—
Hytuss 2X Capsules (Hyrex)	—	guaifenesin, 200 mg	—	—	—
Kiddies Pediatric (Vitarine)	—	potassium guaiacolsulfonate, 5.83 mg/ml ammonium chloride, 5.83 mg/ml	—	—	cocillana bark extract menthol alcohol, 2% wild cherry flavor
Kleer Chewable Tablets (Scrip)	dextromethorphan hydrobromide, 2.5 mg	—	phenylephrine hydrochloride, 5 mg	chlorpheniramine maleate, 2 mg	—

Product[a] (Manufacturer)	Cough Suppressant	Expectorant	Sympathomimetic	Antihistamine	Other
Lanatuss[c] (Lannett)	—	guaifenesin, 20 mg/ml	phenylpropanolamine hydrochloride, 1 mg/ml	chlorpheniramine maleate, 0.4 mg/ml	sodium citrate, 39.4 mg/ml citric acid, 12 mg/ml
Mercodol with Decapryn (Merrell-National)	codeine phosphate[b], 2 mg/ml	—	phenylephrine hydrochloride, 1 mg/ml etafedrine hydrochloride, 2 mg/ml	doxylamine succinate, 1.2 mg/ml	alcohol, 5%
Multi-Symptom (Parke-Davis)	dextromethorphan hydrobromide, 2 mg/ml	—	pseudoephedrine hydrochloride, 6 mg/ml	brompheniramine maleate, 0.4 mg/ml	alcohol, 5%
Naldetuss (Bristol)	dextromethorphan hydrobromide, 3 mg/ml	—	phenylpropanolamine hydrochloride, 3.5 mg/ml	phenyltoloxamine citrate, 1.5 mg/ml	acetaminophen, 32.4 mg/ml
Neophiban Tablets (O'Neal, Jones & Feldman)	—	guaifenesin, 50 mg	phenylpropanolamine hydrochloride, 12.5 mg	phenyltoloxamine citrate, 25 mg	acetaminophen, 195 mg
N-N Cough Syrup (Vitarine)	dextromethorphan hydrobromide, 2 mg/ml	potassium guaiacolsulfonate, 13 mg/ml ammonium chloride, 13 mg/ml	—	chlorpheniramine maleate, 0.1 mg/ml	alcohol, 5% glycerin menthol syrup wild cherry flavor
Noratuss (North American)	codeine phosphate[b], 0.67 mg/ml	ammonium chloride, 6.48 mg/ml potassium guaiacolsulfonate, 1.08 mg/ml terpin hydrate, 1.08 mg/ml	—	—	cocillana extract, 0.89 mg/ml sodium benzoate, 0.1% cherry flavor
Nortussin (North American)	—	guaifenesin, 3.33 mg/ml	—	—	alcohol, 3.5% cherry flavor
Novahistine DH (Dow)	codeine phosphate[b], 2 mg/ml	—	phenylpropanolamine hydrochloride, 3.75 mg/ml	chlorpheniramine maleate, 0.4 mg/ml	alcohol, 5%
Novahistine DMX (Dow)	dextromethorphan hydrobromide, 2 mg/ml	guaifenesin, 20 mg/ml	pseudoephedrine hydrochloride, 6 mg/ml	—	alcohol, 10%
Novahistine Expectorant (Dow)	codeine phosphate[b], 2 mg/ml	guaifenesin, 20 mg/ml	phenylpropanolamine hydrochloride, 3.75 mg/ml	chlorpheniramine maleate, 0.4 mg/ml	alcohol, 7.5%
Ornacol Capsules and Liquid (Smith Kline & French)	dextromethorphan hydrobromide, 30 mg/capsule 3 mg/ml	—	phenylpropanolamine hydrochloride, 25 mg/capsule 2.5 mg/ml	—	alcohol, 8% (liquid)
Orthoxicol (Upjohn)	dextromethorphan hydrobromide, 2 mg/ml	—	methoxyphenamine hydrochloride, 3.4 mg/ml	—	—
Pediaquil (Philips Roxane)	—	guaifenesin, 10 mg/ml	phenylephrine hydrochloride, 0.5 mg/ml	—	alcohol, 5% sorbitol corn syrup currant and caramel flavors
Pertussin 8-Hour Cough Formula (Chesebrough-Pond)	dextromethorphan hydrobromide, 1.5 mg/ml	—	—	—	alcohol, 9.5%

Product[a] (Manufacturer)	Cough Suppressant	Expectorant	Sympathomimetic	Antihistamine	Other
Pertussin Cough Syrup for Children (Chesebrough-Pond)	dextromethorphan hydrobromide, 0.7 mg/ml	guaifenesin, 5 mg/ml	—	—	alcohol, 8.5%
Pinex Regular & Concentrate (Roberts)	—	potassium guaiacolsulfonate	—	—	pine tar oil eucalyptus oil grindella extract glycerin
Prunicodeine[c] (Lilly)	codeine sulfate[b], 2 mg/ml	terpin hydrate, 5.83 mg/ml	—	—	wild cherry white pine sanguinaria alcohol
Quelidrine (Abbott)	dextromethorphan hydrobromide, 2 mg/ml	ammonium chloride, 8 mg/ml ipecac fluidextract, 0.001 ml/ml	ephedrine hydrochloride, 1 mg/ml phenylephrine hydrochloride, 1 mg/ml	chlorpheniramine maleate, 0.4 mg/ml	alcohol, 2%
Queltuss Tablets (O'Neal, Jones & Feldman)	dextromethorphan hydrobromide, 15 mg	guaifenesin, 100 mg	—	—	—
Quiet-Nite (Rexall)	dextromethorphan hydrobromide, 0.5 mg/ml	—	ephedrine sulfate, 0.33 mg/ml	chlorpheniramine maleate, 0.06 mg/ml	acetaminophen, 20 mg/ml alcohol, 25%
Rem (Block)	dextromethorphan hydrobromide, 1 mg/ml	ammonium chloride, 1%	—	—	glycerin, 6% alcohol, 1.2% tar, 0.02%
Robitussin (Robins)	—	guaifenesin, 20 mg/ml	—	—	alcohol, 3.5%
Robitussin A-C (Robins)	codeine phosphate[b], 2 mg/ml	guaifenesin, 20 mg/ml	—	—	alcohol, 3.5%
Robitussin-CF (Robins)	dextromethorphan hydrobromide, 2 mg/ml	guaifenesin, 20 mg/ml	phenylpropanolamine hydrochloride, 2.5 mg/ml	—	alcohol, 1.4%
Robitussin DAC (Robins)	codeine phosphate[b], 2 mg/ml	guaifenesin, 20 mg/ml	pseudoephedrine hydrochloride, 6 mg/ml	—	alcohol, 1.4%
Robitussin-DM (Robins)	dextromethorphan hydrobromide, 3 mg/ml	guaifenesin, 20 mg/ml	—	—	alcohol, 1.4%
Robitussin-PE (Robins)	—	guaifenesin, 20 mg/ml	pseudoephedrine hydrochloride, 6 mg/ml	—	alcohol, 1.4% sucrose, 714 mg/ml
Romex (Amer. Pharm.)	dextromethorphan hydrobromide, 2 mg/ml	guaifenesin, 6.6 mg/ml	phenylephrine hydrochloride, 1 mg/ml	chlorpheniramine maleate, 0.2 mg/ml	—
Romilar III (Block)	dextromethorphan hydrobromide, 1 mg/ml	—	phenylpropanolamine hydrochloride, 2.5 mg/ml	—	alcohol, 20% flavor
Romilar Capsules (Block)	dextromethorphan hydrobromide, 15 mg	—	phenylephrine hydrochloride, 5 mg	chlorpheniramine maleate, 1 mg	acetaminophen, 120 mg
Romilar CF (Block)	dextromethorphan hydrobromide, 3 mg/ml	ammonium chloride, 1%	—	—	alcohol, 20% 0.2 ml/ml flavor
Romilar Children's (Block)	dextromethorphan hydrobromide, 1.5 mg/ml	—	—	—	sodium citrate citric acid grape flavor

Product[a] (Manufacturer)	Cough Suppressant	Expectorant	Sympathomimetic	Antihistamine	Other
Ryna-Tussadine Expectorant Liquid and Tablets (Mallinckrodt)	—	guaifenesin, 20 mg/ml 100 mg/tablet	phenylpropanolamine hydrochloride, 1.25 mg/ml 6.25 mg/tablet phenylephrine hydrochloride, 0.75 mg/ml 3.75 mg/tablet	pyrilamine maleate, 1.25 mg/ml 6.25 mg/tablet chlorpheniramine maleate, 0.2 mg/ml 1 mg/tablet	alcohol, 3% (liquid)
Silence Is Golden (Bristol-Myers)	dextromethorphan hydrobromide, 2 mg/ml	—	—	—	honey flavor
Silexin Cough Syrup and Tablets (Otis Clapp)	dextromethorphan hydrobromide	guaifenesin (syrup)	—	—	benzocaine (tablet)
Soltice (Chattem)	dextromethorphan hydrobromide, 2 mg/ml	guaifenesin, 20 mg/ml	phenylpropanolamine hydrochloride, 2.5 mg/ml	—	—
Sorbutuss[c] (Dalin)	dextromethorphan hydrobromide, 2 mg/ml	guaifenesin, 20 mg/ml ipecac fluidextract, 0.0006 ml/ml	—	—	potassium citrate, 17 mg/ml citric acid, 7 mg/ml mint flavor glycerin–sorbitol vehicle
St. Joseph Cough Syrup for Children (Plough)	dextromethorphan hydrobromide, 1.5 mg/ml	—	—	—	sodium citrate menthol alcohol, 0.38%
Sucrets Cough Control Formula (Beecham)	dextromethorphan hydrobromide	—	—	—	benzocaine
Supercitin[c] (Vitarine)	dextromethorphan hydrobromide, 2 mg/ml	—	—	chlorpheniramine maleate, 0.2 mg/ml	acetaminophen, 12 mg/ml
Symptom 1 (Parke-Davis)	dextromethorphan hydrobromide, 2 mg/ml	—	—	—	alcohol, 5%
Toclonol Expectorant[c] (Cenci)	carbetapentane citrate, 1.5 mg/ml	terpin hydrate, 3.33 mg/ml	—	—	sodium citrate, 13.23 mg/ml citric acid, 1.33 mg/ml glycerin, 0.56 ml/ml menthol, 0.166 mg/ml alcohol, 7.2%
Toclonol with Codeine[c] (Cenci)	codeine[b], 2 mg/ml carbetapentane citrate, 1.5 mg/ml	terpin hydrate, 3.33 mg/ml	—	—	sodium citrate, 13.23 mg/ml citric acid, 1.33 mg/ml glycerin, 0.56 ml/ml menthol, 0.166 mg/ml alcohol, 7.2%
Tolu-Sed[c] (First Texas)	codeine phosphate[b], 2 mg/ml	guaifenesin, 20 mg/ml	—	—	alcohol, 10%
Tolu-Sed DM[c] (First Texas)	dextromethorphan hydrobromide, 2 mg/ml	guaifenesin, 20 mg/ml	—	—	alcohol, 10%
Tonecol (A.V.P.)	dextromethorphan hydrobromide, 2 mg/ml	guaifenesin, 5 mg/ml	phenylephrine hydrochloride, 1 mg/ml	chlorpheniramine maleate, 0.2 mg/ml	sodium citrate, 3 mg/ml alcohol, 7% cherry flavor

Product[a] (Manufacturer)	Cough Suppressant	Expectorant	Sympathomimetic	Antihistamine	Other
Triaminic Expectorant (Dorsey)	—	guaifenesin, 20 mg/ml	phenylpropanolamine hydrochloride, 2.5 mg/ml	pheniramine maleate, 1.25 mg/ml pyrilamine maleate, 1.25 mg/ml	alcohol, 5%
Triaminic Expectorant with Codeine (Dorsey)	codeine phosphate[b], 2 mg/ml	guaifenesin, 20 mg/ml	phenylpropanolamine hydrochloride, 2.5 mg/ml	pheniramine maleate, 1.25 mg/ml pyrilamine maleate, 1.25 mg/ml	alcohol, 5%
Triaminicol (Dorsey)	dextromethorphan hydrobromide, 3 mg/ml	ammonium chloride, 18 mg/ml	phenylpropanolamine hydrochloride, 2.5 mg/ml	pheniramine maleate, 1.25 mg/ml pyrilamine maleate, 1.25 mg/ml	—
Tricodene C-V (Pfeiffer)	codeine phosphate[b], 1.6 mg/ml	terpin hydrate	—	pyrilamine maleate, 0.83 mg/ml	sodium citrate menthol glycerin honey syrup
Tricodene DM (Pfeiffer)	dextromethorphan hydrobromide, 2 mg/ml	—	—	—	—
Tricodene Forte (Pfeiffer)	dextromethorphen hydrobromide, 2 mg/ml	—	phenylpropanolamine hydrochloride, 2.5 mg/ml	chlorpheniramine maleate, 0.4 mg/ml	—
Tricodene Pediatric (Pfeiffer)	dextromethorphan hydrobromide, 2 mg/ml	—	phenylpropanolamine hydrochloride, 2.5 mg/ml	—	—
Trind (Mead Johnson)	—	guaifenesin, 10 mg/ml	phenylephrine hydrochloride, 0.5 mg/ml	—	acetaminophen, 24 mg/ml alcohol, 15%
Trind-DM (Mead Johnson)	dextromethorphan hydrobromide, 1.5 mg/ml	guaifenesin, 10 mg/ml	phenylephrine hydrochloride, 1 mg/ml	—	acetaminophen, 24 mg/ml alcohol, 15%
Troutman's (G.E. Labs)	dextromethorphan hydrobromide, 2 mg/ml	—	—	—	alcohol ammonium chloride corn syrup sucrose caramel horehound menthol peppermint
Tussagesic Suspension (Dorsey)	dextromethorphan hydrobromide, 3 mg/ml	terpin hydrate, 18 mg/ml	phenylpropanolamine hydrochloride, 2.5 mg/ml	pheniramine maleate, 1.25 mg/ml pyrilamine maleate, 1.25 mg/ml	acetaminophen, 24 mg/ml
Tussagesic Tablets (Dorsey)	dextromethorphan hydrobromide, 30 mg	terpin hydrate, 180 mg	phenylpropanolamine hydrochloride, 25 mg	pheniramine maleate, 12.5 mg pyrilamine maleate, 12.5 mg	acetaminophen, 325 mg
Tussar-2 (Armour)	codeine phosphate[b], 2 mg/ml carbetapentane citrate, 1.5 mg/ml	guaifenesin, 10 mg/ml	—	chlorpheniramine maleate, 0.4 mg/ml	sodium citrate, 26 mg/ml citric acid, 4 mg/ml methylparaben, 0.1% alcohol, 5%
Tussar DM (Armour)	dextromethorphan hydrobromide, 3 mg/ml	—	phenylephrine, 1 mg/ml	chlorpheniramine maleate, 0.4 mg/ml	methylparaben, 0.2%

Antitussive Products

Product[a] (Manufacturer)	Cough Suppressant	Expectorant	Sympathomimetic	Antihistamine	Other
Tussar-SF[c] (Armour)	codeine phosphate[b], 2 mg/ml carbetapentane citrate, 1.5 mg/ml	guaifenesin, 10 mg/ml	—	chlorpheniramine maleate, 0.4 mg/ml	sodium citrate, 26 mg/ml citric acid, 4 mg/ml methylparaben, 0.1% alcohol, 12%
Tusscapine Suspension and Tablets (Fisons)	noscapine, 3 mg/ml 15 mg/tablet	—	—	—	lime flavor (suspension) raspberry flavor (tablet)
Tussciden Expectorant (Cenci)	—	guaifenesin, 20 mg/ml	—	—	—
Vicks Cough Syrup (Vicks)	dextromethorphan hydrobromide, 0.7 mg/ml	guaifenesin, 5 mg/ml	—	—	sodium citrate, 40 mg/ml alcohol, 5%
Vicks Cough Silencer Tablets (Vicks)	dextromethorphan hydrobromide, 2.5 mg	—	—	—	benzocaine, 1 mg menthol, anethole, peppermint oil } 0.35%

[a] Liquid unless specified otherwise.
[b] Schedule V drug: OTC sale forbidden in some states.
[c] Sugar free.

Lozenge Products

Product (Manufacturer)	Anesthetic	Antibacterial	Other
Axon (McKesson)	benzocaine, 5 mg	cetylpyridinium chloride, 2.5 mg	—
Cépacol (Merrell-National)	—	cetylpyridinium chloride, 1:1500	benzyl alcohol, 0.3%
Cépacol Troches (Merrell-National)	benzocaine, 10 mg	cetylpyridinium chloride, 1:1500	—
Cépastat (Merrell-National)	—	phenol, 1.45%	menthol, 0.12% eucalyptus oil, 0.04% sorbitol
Cherry Chloraseptic (Eaton)	—	phenol, sodium phenolate (total phenol, 1.4%) (these ingredients are also anesthetic)	—
Colrex Troches (Rowell)	benzocaine, 10 mg	—	black currant flavor
Conex (O'Neal, Jones & Feldman)	benzocaine, 5 mg	cetylpyridinium chloride, 0.5 mg	methylparaben, 2 mg propylparaben, 0.5 mg
Creozets (Creomulsion)	—	—	beechwood creosote; white pine; ipecac; menthol; cascara; wild cherry; alcohol, 1%
Hold (Calgon)	benzocaine	—	dextromethorphan hydrobromide
Listerine (Warner-Lambert)	—	hexylresorcinol, 2.4 mg	eucalyptol, menthol
Listerine Cough Control (Warner-Lambert)	benzocaine, 2.5 mg	—	dextromethorphan hydrobromide, 7.5 mg
Meloids Pastilles (Cunningham)	—	—	licorice, 98 mg; sugar, 48 mg; capsicum, 2 mg; menthol, 1.8 mg
Menthol Chloraseptic (Eaton)	—	phenol, sodium phenolate (total phenol, 1.4%) (these ingredients are also anesthetic)	—
Mycinettes (Pfeiffer)	benzocaine, 10 mg	cetylpyridinium chloride, 2.5 mg	terpin hydrate, 10 mg

Product (Manufacturer)	Anesthetic	Antibacterial	Other
Mycinettes Sugar Free (Pfeiffer)	benzocaine, 15 mg	cetylpyridinium chloride, 2.5 mg	terpin hydrate, 10 mg mannitol sorbitol
Oracin (Vicks)	benzocaine, 6.25 mg	—	menthol, sorbitol base
Oradex-C (Commerce)	benzocaine, 10 mg	cetylpyridinium chloride, 2.5 mg	—
Robitussin-DM Cough Calmers (Robins)	—	—	dextromethorphan hydrobromide, 7.5 mg guaifenesin, 50 mg
Semets (Beecham Labs)	benzocaine, 3 mg	cetylpyridinium chloride, 1:1500	—
Sepo (Otis Clapp)	benzocaine	—	—
Silence Is Golden (Bristol-Myers)	—	—	dextromethorphan hydrobromide, 5 mg honey flavor
Spec-T Sore Throat Anesthetic (Squibb)	benzocaine, 10 mg	—	—
Spec-T Sore Throat/Cough Suppressant (Squibb)	benzocaine, 10 mg	—	dextromethorphan hydrobromide, 10 mg
Spec-T Sore Throat/Decongestant (Squibb)	benzocaine, 10 mg	—	phenylephrine hydrochloride, 5 mg phenylpropanolamine hydrochloride, 10.5 mg
Spongiacaine (Otis Clapp)	benzocaine	—	—
Sucrets (Calgon)	—	hexylresorcinol, 2.4 mg	—
Synthaloids (Buffington)	benzocaine	calcium–iodine complex	—
Thantis (Hynson, Westcott & Dunning)	—	meralein sodium, 8.1 mg	salicyl alcohol, 64.8 mg
Throat Discs (Marion)	—	—	capsicum, peppermint, anise, cubeb, glycyrrhiza extract, linseed
Trocaine (North American)	benzocaine, 5 mg	—	—
Trokettes (Vitarine)	benzocaine, 10 mg	cetylpyridinium chloride, 1:3000 cetalkonium chloride, 1:3000	orange flavor
Vicks Medi-trating (Vicks)	benzocaine, 5 mg	cetylpyridinium chloride, 1.66 mg	menthol, camphor, eucalyptus oil
Victors (Vicks)	—	–	menthol, eucalyptus oil

Cold and Allergy Products

Product (Manufacturer)	Dosage Form	Sympathomimetic	Antihistamine	Analgesic	Other
Alka-Seltzer Plus (Miles)	effervescent tablet	phenylpropanolamine bitartrate, 24.08 mg	chlorpheniramine maleate, 2.0 mg	aspirin, 324 mg	—
Allerest (Pharmacraft)	time capsule	phenylpropanolamine hydrochloride, 50 mg	pyrilamine maleate, 15 mg methapyrilene fumarate, 10 mg	—	—
Allerest Regular and Children's (Pharmacraft)	tablet	phenylpropanolamine hydrochloride, 18.7 mg 9.4 mg (children's)	chlorpheniramine maleate, 2 mg 1 mg (children's)	—	—

Product (Manufacturer)	Dosage Form	Sympathomimetic	Antihistamine	Analgesic	Other
Allergesic (Vitarine)	tablet	phenylpropanolamine hydrochloride, 18.7 mg	chlorpheniramine maleate, 2 mg	—	—
Anodynos Forte (Buffington)	tablet	phenylephrine hydrochloride, 10 mg	chlorpheniramine maleate, 2 mg	salicylamide acetaminophen	caffeine
Apcohist Allergy Tablets (Amer. Pharm.)	tablet	phenylpropanolamine hydrochloride, 25 mg	methapyrilene fumarate, 5 mg chlorpheniramine maleate, 1 mg	—	—
Aspirin Free Dristan (Whitehall)	tablet	phenylephrine hydrochloride, 5 mg	chlorpheniramine maleate, 2 mg	acetaminophen	caffeine
Bayer Children's Cold Tablets (Glenbrook)	tablet	phenylpropanolamine hydrochloride, 3.125 mg	—	aspirin, 81 mg	—
Bayer Decongestant (Glenbrook)	tablet	phenylpropanolamine hydrochloride, 12.5 mg	chlorpheniramine maleate, 2 mg	aspirin, 325 mg	—
Cenagesic (Central)	tablet	phenylephrine hydrochloride, 5 mg	pyrilamine maleate, 12 mg	salicylamide, 250 mg phenacetin, 120 mg	ascorbic acid, 30 mg caffeine, 15 mg
Chlor-Trimeton (Schering)	syrup tablet	—	chlorpheniramine maleate, 0.4 mg/ml 4 mg/tablet	—	—
Chlor-Trimeton Decongestant (Schering)	tablet	pseudoephedrine sulfate, 60 mg	chlorpheniramine maleate, 4 mg	—	—
Codimal (Central)	tablet capsule	pseudoephedrine hydrochloride, 30 mg	chlorpheniramine maleate, 2 mg	salicylamide, 150 mg acetaminophen, 150 mg	—
Colrex (Rowell)	capsule	phenylephrine hydrochloride, 5 mg	chlorpheniramine maleate, 2 mg	acetaminophen, 325 mg	—
Conex DA (O'Neal, Jones & Feldman)	tablet	phenylpropanolamine hydrochloride, 50 mg	phenyltoloxamine citrate, 50 mg	—	—
Conex Plus (O'Neal, Jones & Feldman)	tablet	phenylpropanolamine hydrochloride, 25 mg	phenyltoloxamine citrate, 25 mg	acetaminophen, 250 mg	—
Congespirin (Bristol-Myers)	chewable tablet	phenylephrine hydrochloride, 1.25 mg	—	aspirin, 81 mg	—
Contac (Menley & James)	time capsule	phenylpropanolamine hydrochloride, 50 mg	chlorpheniramine maleate, 4 mg	—	belladonna alkaloids, 0.2 mg
Coricidin (Schering)	tablet	—	chlorpheniramine maleate, 2 mg	aspirin, 325 mg	—
Coricidin "D" (Schering)	tablet	phenylpropanolamine hydrochloride, 12.5 mg	chlorpheniramine maleate, 2 mg	aspirin, 325 mg	—
Coricidin Demilets (Schering)	children's chewable tablet	phenylephrine hydrochloride, 2.5 mg	chlorpheniramine maleate, 0.5 mg	aspirin, 80 mg	—
Coricidin Medilets (Schering)	children's chewable tablet	—	chlorpheniramine maleate, 0.5 mg	aspirin, 80 mg	—
Coryban-D (Pfipharmecs)	capsule	phenylpropanolamine hydrochloride, 25 mg	chlorpheniramine maleate, 2 mg	—	caffeine, 30 mg
Co Tylenol (McNeil)	tablet	pseudoephedrine hydrochloride, 30 mg	chlorpheniramine maleate, 2 mg	acetaminophen, 325 mg	—
Co Tylenol Cold Formula for Children (McNeil)	liquid	pseudoephedrine hydrochloride, 1.5 mg/ml	chlorpheniramine maleate, 0.1 mg/ml	acetaminophen, 24 mg/ml	alcohol, 7%

Product (Manufacturer)	Dosage Form	Sympathomimetic	Antihistamine	Analgesic	Other
Covanamine (Mallinckrodt)	liquid	phenylpropanolamine hydrochloride, 1.25 mg/ml phenylephrine hydrochloride, 0.75 mg/ml	pyrilamine maleate, 1.25 mg/ml chlorpheniramine maleate, 0.2 mg/ml	—	—
Covangesic (Mallinckrodt)	liquid tablet	phenylpropanolamine hydrochloride, 1.25 mg/ml 12.5 mg/tablet phenylephrine hydrochloride, 0.75 mg/ml 7.5 mg/tablet	pyrilamine maleate, 1.25 mg/ml 12.5 mg/tablet chlorpheniramine maleate, 0.2 mg/ml 2.0 mg/tablet	acetaminophen, 24 mg/ml 275 mg/tablet	alcohol, 7.5% (liquid)
DayCare (Vicks)	liquid	phenylpropanolamine hydrochloride, 0.83 mg/ml	—	acetaminophen, 20 mg/ml	—
Decapyryn (Merrell-National)	syrup	—	doxylamine succinate, 1.25 mg/ml	—	—
Demazin (Schering)	syrup repetabs	phenylephrine hydrochloride, 0.5 mg/ml 20 mg/tablet	chlorpheniramine maleate, 0.2 mg/ml 4 mg/tablet	—	alcohol, 7.5% (syrup)
D-Feda (Dooner/ Rorer)	syrup	pseudoephedrine hydrochloride, 6 mg/ml	—	—	—
Dristan (Whitehall)	tablet	phenylephrine hydrochloride, 5 mg	chlorpheniramine maleate, 2 mg	aspirin	caffeine aluminum hydroxide magnesium carbonate
Dristan (Whitehall)	time capsule	phenylephrine hydrochloride, 20 mg	chlorpheniramine maleate, 4 mg	—	—
Duadacin (Hoechst-Roussel)	capsule	phenylephrine hydrochloride, 5 mg	pyrilamine resin adsorbate equiv. to pyrilamine maleate, 12.5 mg chlorpheniramine maleate, 1 mg	salicylamide, 200 mg acetaminophen, 120 mg	ascorbic acid, 50 mg caffeine, 30 mg
Duradyne-Forte (O'Neal, Jones & Feldman)	tablet	phenylephrine hydrochloride, 5 mg	chlorpheniramine maleate, 2 mg	salicylamide, 225 mg acetaminophen, 160 mg	caffeine, 30 mg
Emagrin Forte (Otis Clapp)	tablet	phenylephrine hydrochloride, 5 mg	—	acetaminophen salicylamide	atropine sulfate, 0.06 mg caffeine
Endecon (Endo)	tablet	phenylpropanolamine hydrochloride, 25 mg	—	acetaminophen, 325 mg	—
Euphenex (O'Neal, Jones & Feldman)	tablet	—	phenyltoloxamine citrate, 25 mg	acetaminophen, 300 mg	caffeine, 15 mg
Extendac (Vitarine)	extended-action capsule	phenylpropanolamine hydrochloride, 50 mg	pheniramine maleate, 12.5 mg chlorpheniramine maleate, 1 mg	—	belladonna alkaloids, 0.2 mg
Fedahist (Dooner/ Rorer)	tablet syrup	pseudoephedrine hydrochloride, 60 mg/tablet 6 mg/ml	chlorpheniramine maleate, 4 mg/tablet 0.4 mg/ml	—	—
Fedrazil (Burroughs Wellcome)	tablet	pseudoephedrine hydrochloride, 30 mg	chlorcyclizine hydrochloride, 25 mg	—	—
Fendol (Buffington)	tablet	phenylephrine hydrochloride, 10 mg	—	salicylamide acetaminophen	caffeine atropine sulfate, 0.13 mg

Product (Manufacturer)	Dosage Form	Sympathomimetic	Antihistamine	Analgesic	Other
Ginsopan (O'Neal, Jones & Feldman)	tablet	phenylpropanolamine hydrochloride, 25 mg phenylephrine hydrochloride, 2.5 mg	pyrilamine maleate, 12.5 mg chlorpheniramine maleate, 1 mg	—	—
Hista-Compound No. 5 (North American)	tablet	phenylephrine hydrochloride, 4 mg	chlorpheniramine maleate, 2 mg	salicylamide, 227.5 mg phenacetin, 162.5 mg	caffeine, 32.5 mg
Hot Lemon (Rexall)	tablet	phenylephrine hydrochloride, 10 mg	chlorpheniramine maleate, 2 mg	acetaminophen, 600 mg	ascorbic acid, 60 mg
Inhiston (Plough)	tablet	—	pheniramine maleate, 10 mg	—	—
Kiddisan (O'Neal, Jones & Feldman)	chewable tablet	phenylephrine hydrochloride, 1.25 mg	chlorpheniramine maleate, 0.5 mg	salicylamide, 80 mg	ascorbic acid, 30 mg
Midran Decongestant (Columbia Medical)	tablet	phenylephrine hydrochloride, 5 mg	chlorpheniramine maleate, 2 mg	salicylamide, 97.5 mg acetaminophen, 32.5 mg	caffeine, 32.5 mg
Naldegesic (Bristol)	tablet	pseudoephedrine hydrochloride, 15 mg	—	acetaminophen, 325 mg	—
Nazac Timed-Disintegration Decongestant (Columbia Medical)	time capsule	phenylpropanolamine hydrochloride, 50 mg	pheniramine maleate, 12.5 mg chlorpheniramine maleate, 1 mg	—	belladonna alkaloids, 0.16 mg
Neo-Synephrine Compound (Winthrop)	tablet	phenylephrine hydrochloride, 5 mg	thenyldiamine hydrochloride, 7.5 mg	acetaminophen, 150 mg	caffeine, 15 mg
Novafed (Dow)	syrup	pseudoephedrine hydrochloride, 6 mg/ml	—	—	alcohol, 7.5%
Novafed A (Dow)	syrup	pseudoephedrine hydrochloride, 6 mg/ml	chlorpheniramine maleate, 0.4 mg/ml	—	alcohol, 5%
Novahistine Elixir (Dow)	syrup	phenylpropanolamine hydrochloride, 3.75 mg/ml	chlorpheniramine maleate, 0.4 mg/ml	—	alcohol, 5%
Novahistine Sinus Tablets (Dow)	tablet	pseudoephedrine hydrochloride, 30 mg	chlorpheniramine maleate, 2 mg	acetaminophen, 325 mg	—
Novahistine Tablets (Dow)	tablet	phenylpropanolamine hydrochloride, 18.75 mg	chlorpheniramine maleate, 2 mg	—	—
NyQuil (Vicks)	liquid	ephedrine sulfate, 2.67 mg/ml	doxylamine succinate, 2.5 mg/ml	acetaminophen, 20 mg/ml	alcohol, 25%
Ornex (Smith Kline & French)	capsule	phenylpropanolamine hydrochloride, 18 mg	—	acetaminophen, 325 mg	—
Pyrroxate (Upjohn)	capsule tablet	methoxyphenamine hydrochloride, 25 mg	chlorpheniramine maleate, 2 mg	aspirin, 227.5 mg phenacetin, 162.5 mg	caffeine, anhydrous, 32.5 mg
Rhinidrin (Central Pharmacal)	tablet	phenylpropanolamine hydrochloride, 25 mg	phenyltoloxamine citrate, 25 mg	acetaminophen, 150 mg phenacetin, 150 mg	—
Sinacon (Meyer)	tablet	pseudoephedrine hydrochloride, 15 mg	—	acetaminophen, 325 mg	—
Sinapils (Pfeiffer)	tablet	phenylpropanolamine hydrochloride, 12.5 mg	chlorpheniramine maleate, 1.0 mg	acetaminophen, 325 mg	caffeine, 32.4 mg
Sinarest (Pharmacraft)	tablet	phenylephrine hydrochloride, 18.7 mg	chlorpheniramine maleate, 2 mg	acetaminophen, 325 mg	—

Product (Manufacturer)	Dosage Form	Sympathomimetic	Antihistamine	Analgesic	Other
Sine-Aid (McNeil)	tablet	phenylpropanolamine hydrochloride, 25 mg	—	acetaminophen, 325 mg	—
Sine-Off (Menley & James)	tablet	phenylpropanolamine hydrochloride, 18.75 mg	chlorpheniramine maleate, 2 mg	aspirin, 325 mg	—
Sinulin (Carnrick)	tablet	phenylpropanolamine hydrochloride, 37.5 mg	chlorpheniramine maleate, 2 mg	acetaminophen, 325 mg salicylamide, 250 mg	homatropine methylbromide, 0.75 mg
Sinurex (Rexall)	tablet	phenylpropanolamine hydrochloride, 25 mg	chlorpheniramine maleate, 0.5 mg methapyrilene fumarate, 6.25 mg	salicylamide, 300 mg	—
Sinustat (Vitarine)	tablet	phenylpropanolamine hydrochloride, 25 mg	phenyltoloxamine dihydrogen citrate, 22 mg	acetaminophen, 325 mg	—
Sinutab (Warner-Chilcott)	tablet	phenylpropanolamine hydrochloride, 25 mg	phenyltoloxamine citrate, 22 mg	acetaminophen, 325 mg	—
Sinutab Extra Strength (Warner-Chilcott)	tablet	phenylpropanolamine hydrochloride, 25 mg	phenyltoloxamine citrate, 22 mg	acetaminophen, 500 mg	—
Sinutab II (Warner-Chilcott)	tablet	phenylpropanolamine hydrochloride, 25 mg	—	acetaminophen, 325 mg	—
Spantac (North American)	capsule	phenylpropanolamine hydrochloride, 50 mg	chlorpheniramine maleate, 4 mg	—	belladonna alkaloids, 0.2 mg
St. Joseph Cold Tablets for Children (Plough)	chewable tablet	phenylpropanolamine hydrochloride, 3.125 mg	—	aspirin, 81 mg	—
Sudafed (Burroughs Wellcome)	tablet syrup	pseudoephedrine hydrochloride, 30 mg/tablet, 6 mg/ml	—	—	—
Super Anahist (Warner-Lambert)	tablet	phenylpropanolamine hydrochloride, 25 mg	phenyltoloxamine citrate, 6.25 mg thonzylamine hydrochloride, 6.25 mg	acetaminophen, 325 mg aspirin, 227 mg phenacetin, 97.2 mg	caffeine
Super-Decon (Vitarine)	capsule	phenylephrine hydrochloride, 5 mg	methapyrilene hydrochloride, 12.5 mg	salicylamide, 250 mg	ascorbic acid, 50 mg caffeine, 32 mg
Symptom 2 (Parke-Davis)	syrup	pseudoephedrine hydrochloride, 6 mg/ml	—	—	alcohol, 5%
Symptom 3 (Parke-Davis)	syrup	—	brompheniramine maleate, 0.4 mg/ml	—	alcohol, 5%
Timed Cold Capsules (Amer. Pharm.)	time capsule	phenylpropanolamine hydrochloride, 50 mg	chlorpheniramine maleate, 1 mg pheniramine maleate, 12.5 mg	—	belladonna alkaloids, 0.16 mg
Triaminic (Dorsey)	syrup	phenylpropanolamine hydrochloride, 2.5 mg/ml	pheniramine maleate, 1.25 mg/ml pyrilamine maleate, 1.25 mg/ml	—	—
Triaminicin (Dorsey)	tablet	phenylpropanolamine hydrochloride, 25 mg	chlorpheniramine maleate, 2 mg	aspirin, 450 mg	caffeine, 30 mg
Triaminicin Allergy (Dorsey)	tablet	phenylpropanolamine hydrochloride, 37.5 mg	chlorpheniramine maleate, 4.0 mg	—	—
Triaminicin Chewables (Dorsey)	chewable tablet	phenylpropanolamine hydrochloride, 6.25 mg	chlorpheniramine maleate, 0.5 mg	—	—

Cold and Allergy Products

Product (Manufacturer)	Dosage Form	Sympathomimetic	Antihistamine	Analgesic	Other
Tri-Nefrin (Pfeiffer)	tablet	phenylpropanolamine, 25 mg	chlorpheniramine maleate, 1.0 mg methapyrilene fumarate, 4 mg	—	—
Valihist (Otis Clapp)	capsule	phenylephrine hydrochloride, 10 mg	chlorpheniramine maleate, 1 mg	acetaminophen	caffeine
VapoRub (Vicks)	ointment	—	—	—	camphor menthol turpentine spirits eucalyptus oil cedar leaf oil myristica oil thymol
VapoSteam (Vicks)	liquid (for vaporizers)	—	—	—	polyoxyethylene dodecanol, 1.8% eucalyptus oil, camphor, menthol } 12.4% tincture of benzoin, 5% alcohol, 55%
Vasominic TD (A.V.P.)	tablet	phenylpropanolamine hydrochloride, 50 mg	pheniramine maleate, 25 mg pyrilamine maleate, 25 mg	—	—
Viromed (Whitehall)	liquid tablet	pseudoephedrine hydrochloride (liquid) pseudoephedrine (tablet)	chlorpheniramine maleate (tablet)	acetaminophen (liquid) aspirin (tablet)	dextromethorphan hydrobromide alcohol, 16.6% (liquid) guaifenesin (tablet)
Ursinus (Dorsey)	in-lay tablet	phenylpropanolamine hydrochloride, 25 mg	pheniramine maleate, 12.5 mg pyrilamine maleate, 12.5 mg	calcium carbaspirin (equiv. to 300 mg of aspirin)	—
4-Way Cold Tablets (Bristol-Myers)	tablet	phenylephrine hydrochloride, 5 mg	—	aspirin, 324 mg	magnesium hydroxide, 125 mg white phenolphthalein, 15 mg

Topical Decongestant Products

Product (Manufacturer)	Application Form	Sympathomimetic	Preservative	Other
Afrin (Schering)	nasal spray nose drops	oxymetazoline hydrochloride, 0.05%	benzalkonium chloride, 0.2 mg/ml phenylmercuric acetate, 0.02 mg/ml	sorbitol, 57 mg/ml aminoacetic acid, 3.8 mg/ml sodium hydroxide
Afrin Pediatric (Schering)	nose drops	oxymetazoline hydrochloride, 0.25 mg/ml	benzalkonium chloride, 0.02 mg/ml phenylmercuric acetate, 0.02 mg/ml	aminoacetic acid, 3.8 mg/ml sorbitol, 57.1 mg/ml
Alconefrin (Alcon)	nose drops	phenylephrine hydrochloride	—	—
Allerest (Pharmacraft)	nasal spray	phenylephrine hydrochloride, 0.5%	benzalkonium chloride	edetate disodium sodium bisulfite saline phosphate buffer

Product (Manufacturer)	Application Form	Sympathomimetic	Preservative	Other
Benzedrex (Smith Kline & French)	inhaler	propylhexedrine, 250 mg	—	aromatics
Contac Nasal Mist (Menley & James)	nasal spray	phenylephrine hydrochloride, 0.5%	cetylpyridinium chloride, 0.02% thimerosal, 0.011%	methapyrilene hydrochloride, 0.2%
Coricidin (Schering)	nasal spray	phenylephrine hydrochloride, 0.5%	—	—
Dristan (Whitehall)	inhaler nasal spray	propylhexedrine (inhaler) phenylephrine hydrochloride (spray)	benzalkonium chloride (spray) thimerosal (spray)	pheniramine maleate (spray) menthol eucalyptol methyl salicylate
Dristan Long Lasting Nasal Mist (Whitehall)	nasal spray	xylometazoline hydrochloride	benzalkonium chloride thimerosal	—
Dristan Long Lasting Vapor Nasal Mist (Whitehall)	nasal spray	xylometazoline hydrochloride	benzalkonium chloride thimerosal	menthol camphor eucalyptol
Duramist PM (Pfeiffer)	nasal spray	xylometazoline, 0.1% (w/v)	thimerosal, 0.002%	—
Duration (Plough)	nasal spray nose drops	oxymetazoline hydrochloride, 0.05%	phenylmercuric acetate, 0.002%	—
Duration Mentholated Vapor Spray (Plough)	nasal spray	oxymetazoline hydrochloride, 0.05%	phenylmercuric acetate	—
Efedron Nasal Jelly (Hyrex)	jelly	ephedrine hydrochloride, 0.6%	chlorobutanol, 0.85%	cinnamon oil menthol
Hydra (North American)	nasal spray	phenylephrine hydrochloride, 0.25%	cetyltrimethylammonium bromide, 0.25% chlorobutanol, 0.25%	methapyrilene hydrochloride, 0.20%
I-Sedrin Plain (Lilly)	nose drops	ephedrine, 1%	chlorobutanol, 0.5%	glucono delta lactone
Isophrin Hydrochloride (Riker)	nasal spray nose drops	phenylephrine hydrochloride, 0.125, 0.25, 0.5, and 1%	—	—
Nasal Douche Powder (Alvin Last)	powder	—	—	sodium bicarbonate sodium chloride sodium borate menthol eucalyptol
Naso Mist (Vitarine)	nasal spray	phenylephrine hydrochloride, 0.5%	benzalkonium chloride, 0.02%	methapyrilene hydrochloride, 0.15%
Neo-Synephrine Hydrochloride (Winthrop)	nasal spray nose drops nasal jelly	phenylephrine hydrochloride, 0.25 and 0.5% (spray) 0.125, 0.25, 0.5, and 1% (drops) 0.5% (jelly)	benzalkonium chloride, 0.02% (spray) 0.125% (drops) thimerosal, 0.001% methylparaben (drops) propylparaben (drops) sodium bisulfite (drops) phenylmercuric acetate (jelly)	—
Neo-Synephrine II (Winthrop)	nasal spray nose drops	xylometazoline hydrochloride, 0.1% (spray) 0.1% and 0.05% (drops)	benzalkonium chloride, 0.02% thimerosal, 0.001%	—
Newphrine (Vitarine)	nose drops	phenylephrine hydrochloride, 0.25%	methylparaben, 0.02% propylparaben, 0.01%	sodium bisulfite, 0.2%
NTZ (Winthrop)	nose drops nasal spray	phenylephrine hydrochloride, 0.5%	benzalkonium chloride, 1:5000	thenyldiamine hydrochloride, 0.1%
Privine (Ciba)	nose drops nasal spray	naphazoline hydrochloride, 0.05%	benzalkonium chloride, 1:5000	—
Sine-Off Once-A-Day (Menley & James)	nasal spray	xylometazoline hydrochloride, 0.1%	—	menthol eucalyptol camphor methyl salicylate

Product (Manufacturer)	Application Form	Sympathomimetic	Preservative	Other
Sinex (Vicks)	nasal spray	phenylephrine hydrochloride, 0.50%	cetylpyridinium chloride, 0.04% thimerosal, 0.001%	methapyrilene hydrochloride, 0.125% menthol eucalyptol camphor methyl salicylate
Sinex-L.A. (Vicks)	nasal spray	xylometazoline hydrochloride, 0.1%	thimerosal, 0.001%	—
Sinutab (Warner-Chilcott)	nasal spray	xylometazoline, 0.1%	benzalkonium chloride, 0.02%	thonzonium bromide, 0.05%
Soltice (Chattem)	nasal spray	phenylephrine hydrochloride, 0.026 mg/ml	—	methapyrilene hydrochloride, 6 mg/ml
St. Joseph (Plough)	nasal spray nose drops	oxymetazoline hydrochloride, 0.025%	phenylmercuric acetate	—
Super Anahist (Warner-Lambert)	nasal spray	phenylephrine hydrochloride, 0.25%	thimerosal, 0.002%	alcohol, 0.038%
Triaminicin (Dorsey)	nasal spray	phenylpropanolamine hydrochloride, 0.75% phenylephrine hydrochloride, 0.25%	benzalkonium chloride, 1:10,000	pheniramine maleate, 0.125% pyrilamine maleate, 0.125%
Tyrohist (Columbia Medical)	nasal spray	phenylephrine hydrochloride, 0.25%	cetalkonium chloride, 0.04%	pyrilamine maleate, 0.15%
Va-Tro-Nol (Vicks)	nose drops	ephedrine sulfate, 0.35%	thimerosal, 0.001%	methapyrilene hydrochloride, 0.15% menthol eucalyptol camphor methyl salicylate
Vicks (Vicks)	inhaler	levodesoxyephedrine, 50 mg	—	menthol camphor methyl salicylate bornyl acetate
4–Way (Bristol-Myers)	nasal spray	phenylephrine hydrochloride, 0.05% naphazoline hydrochloride, 0.05% phenylpropanolamine hydrochloride, 0.2%	—	pyrilamine maleate, 0.2%

Asthma Products

Lawrence J. Hak

Chapter 8

Questions to Ask the Patient

Has a physician diagnosed the condition as asthma?

How old is the patient?

Are you under the care of a physician?

Do you have heart disease, high blood pressure, hyperthyroidism, or diabetes?

What medications are you taking?

Which asthma products have you used before? Were they effective?

Bronchial asthma is defined as "a disease characterized by an increased responsiveness of the trachea and bronchi to various stimuli and manifested by a widespread narrowing of the airways that changes in severity either spontaneously or as a result of therapy" (1).

The overall incidence of asthma in the United States is about 3% (2). About 50% of asthmatic patients developed the disease before age 10, and another 30% before age 30. However, asthma may develop even in later years. Before age 10 the incidence is twice as common in males as in females; by age 30 the incidence is equal. Although asthma is a common childhood disease, many children "grow out" of it by adulthood. A long-term follow-up study of childhood asthma reported that 20 years later, 70% of the patients were symptom free (3).

Although patients are generally characterized as having either extrinsic or intrinsic asthma, many patients present characteristics of both (Table 1). A history of allergy to environmental allergens, a family history of allergic disorders, seasonal variation in the symptoms, positive skin tests, and elevated circulating immunoglobulin E (IgE) levels characterize extrinsic asthma. Patients with intrinsic asthma usually have a negative family history of allergy, negative skin tests, and normal levels of IgE but may develop nasal polyps and aspirin sensitivity (4–6). About 2–10% of asthmatic patients develop an acute asthma attack after taking as little as 300 mg of aspirin (7). The phrase "asthma triad" has been used in referring to people with intrinsic asthma, nasal polyps, and aspirin intolerance (8).

ORIGINS OF ASTHMA

Asthma attacks generally are precipitated by an allergic response to drugs; inhaled allergens such as pollen, dust, or mold; a respiratory tract infection; inhaled pollutants; exercise; or a psychophysiological response to stress (9). Two or more of these factors may interact in varying degrees to precipitate an attack. An allergic response is the major precipitating factor in about 30% of people who have asthma, and respiratory infections are a major factor in about 40%.

Physiology of the Respiratory System

The respiratory system is a series of airways ending in air sacs. The mouth and nasal passages lead to the pharynx, which branches into the esophagus and the trachea. The trachea divides into two large bronchi, each supplying air to one lung. Each bronchus progressively divides into smaller branches (bronchioles) which give rise to alveolar ducts, alveolar sacs, and alveoli (Figure 1) (10).

When an airway branches, its walls become thinner; at the level of the alveoli, all that remains is a thin layer of cells surrounded by pulmonary capillaries. The process of respiration, which is an exchange of gases, occurs in the alveoli. Oxygen passes across the alveolar walls into the capillaries, and carbon dioxide diffuses in the opposite direction.

The lungs are essentially elastic air sacs suspended in the airtight thoracic cavity. The movable walls of this cavity are formed by the sternum, ribs, and diaphragm. As the thoracic cavity becomes enlarged, the pressure within the cavity becomes less than the atmospheric pressure, and air will enter, expanding the lungs. The process of enlarging the thoracic cavity is accomplished via two simultaneous mechanisms. The diaphragm, when relaxed, is a dome-shaped muscle that extends upward into the thoracic cavity. As the diaphragm contracts, it becomes flattened and moves downward into the abdomen, causing an increase in the longitudinal size of the thoracic cavity. The ribs are attached to the vertebrae and protrude forward and downward to the sternum. Contraction of the external intercostal muscles raises the ribs, causing an elevation and forward movement of the sternum and an increase in the anterior–posterior chest cavity diameter. During inspiration the movement of the

Table 1. Clinical Characteristics of Asthma

	Extrinsic, Atopic	Intrinsic, Nonatopic
Onset of symptoms	childhood	adults over age 35
Family history of allergy	positive	negative
Skin tests	positive	negative
IgE	elevated	normal
Aspirin sensitivity	negative	positive

respiration

characteristics of asthma

airway obstruction

attacks

diaphragm and ribs occurs simultaneously, thus increasing the thoracic cavity size, and the lungs fill with air.

During quiet breathing, relaxation of these processes and recoil of the lungs and abdominal wall provide sufficient pressure to cause expiration. For labored breathing, as occurs with exercise, contraction of the internal intercostal muscles and several abdominal muscles provides sufficient pressure on the thoracic cavity to cause forceful air expiration.

For respiration to function efficiently, inhaled air must be cleaned and humidified before it is delivered to the alveoli. The nasal cavities are lined with highly vascular mucous membranes and ciliated epithelial cells (see Figure 1, Chapter 7). As air passes over these areas, it is warmed, humidified, and filtered. Dust particles, bacteria, and other foreign matter are trapped in the mucus and propelled toward the pharynx by the movement of the nasal cilia. Humidification and filtration continue as air passes through the trachea, bronchi, and bronchioles, which also are lined by a ciliated mucous membrane. Trapped particles are moved upward by the wavelike movement of the cilia and are deposited in the oral cavity, where they are either expelled or swallowed.

Bronchial smooth muscle tone is under neural and humoral control (11). Some β-adrenergic receptors, specifically β_2-receptors, are found in the bronchioles; their stimulation causes bronchodilation. Bronchial smooth muscle is also under the control of the parasympathetic system via the vagus nerve. Stimulation of this system causes bronchoconstriction. Under normal circumstances these two systems are balanced.

Pathophysiology of Asthma

The mechanism by which asthma attacks occur is not completely understood. There are indications that both allergy and an imbalance of autonomic nervous functions are involved (12). Patients with an allergic component (extrinsic asthma) have markedly elevated levels of IgE (13, 14). Plasma cells that produce IgE have been identified in the tonsils, adenoids, bronchial and peritoneal lymph nodes, and mucosa of the respiratory and GI tracts (15). With initial antigenic stimulation, IgE is produced and becomes fixed to histamine-containing mast cells in the pulmonary tissue. These sensitized cells, on subsequent exposure to an antigen, release chemical mediators such as histamine, bradykinin, and slow-reacting substance of anaphylaxis (SRS-A) into surrounding tissue, causing bronchoconstriction.

Patients with intrinsic asthma do not have increased levels of IgE but seem to exhibit an imbalance in autonomic function (7). Although this disorder has not been fully elucidated, the release of chemical mediators which cause bronchoconstriction was shown to be modulated by intracellular concentrations of the cyclic nucleotides, 3′,5′-guanosine monophosphate (cyclic GMP) and 3′,5′-adenosine monophosphate (cyclic AMP) (16). Cyclic GMP enhances release of the mediators, and cyclic AMP inhibits it. The intracellular concentration of these nucleotides seems to be from autonomic control—cholinergic stimulation increases cyclic GMP, and β-adrenergic stimulation increases cyclic AMP. Bronchoconstriction is mediated through reflex cholinergic pathways via the vagus nerve (17). A relative decrease in β-adrenergic activity has been proposed as the mechanism for bronchoconstriction (18, 19). Thus the hypersensitivity of bronchiolar smooth muscle in asthmatics may result from either overactive vagal reflexes or a deficiency in the β-adrenergic control (12).

The hallmark of the asthmatic attack is airway obstruction. However, there is some question whether this condition results from bronchospasm (20). Some studies show that bronchospasm plays little or no role in the pathogenesis of asthma (21). Others name excessive contraction of bronchial smooth muscle and hypersecretion of mucus as the major pathologies (1). Whatever the initiating factor, autopsy findings in patients who have died of asthma include mucus plugs that block terminal bronchioles, increased number and size of goblet cells, thickened basement membrane, hypertrophied smooth muscle of the preterminal bronchioles, and inflammatory infiltration of the bronchiolar submucosa (1).

Signs and Symptoms

Asthma characteristically occurs in episodes lasting from a few minutes to several hours. Between attacks there are often no symptoms. Attacks, which often occur in the middle of the night, usually begin with tightness in the chest; coughing and wheezing occur and become more severe over time. Dyspnea is severe, and expiration is more difficult than inspiration. As a result, in prolonged or severe attacks the lungs become overinflated, and there is audible wheezing and physical exhaustion. The sputum is viscid and difficult to expectorate. Some patients with chronic asthma have shortness of breath and wheezing.

PATIENT ASSESSMENT

It is important that the pharmacist determine whether symptoms of dyspnea, cough, and wheezing are related to asthma or another related disease. The signs and symptoms to look for in a patient experiencing an attack are:

- Tachycardia;
- Perspiration;

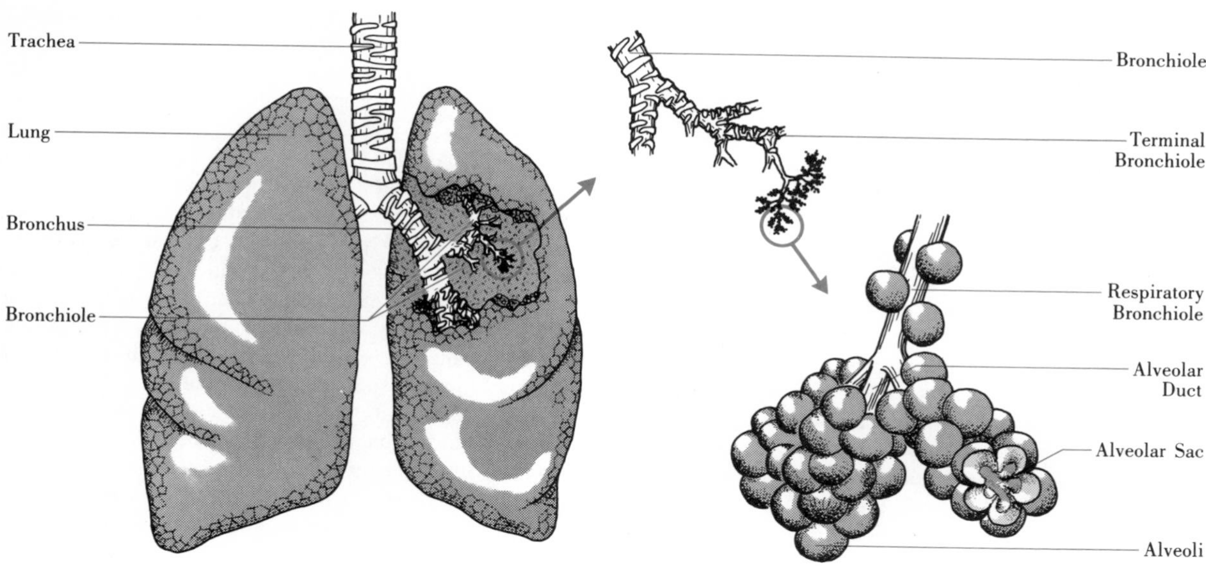

Figure 1. Anatomy of the upper and lower respiratory passages and the bronchial tree.

symptoms

referral or OTC drug

severity of symptoms

- Flushing of the face;
- Dyspnea and wheezing;
- Retraction of the sternocleidomastoid muscle;
- Apprehension;
- Chest distention;
- Tenacious sputum;
- Flaring nostrils.

Sinus tachycardia with a pulse rate up to 120/minute is a very common finding (22). Sternocleidomastoid muscle retraction is a consistent finding in patients with severely impaired pulmonary function (23).

Although it is not the pharmacist's responsibility to make a differential diagnosis, certain information may help determine whether to recommend an OTC product or physician referral. If the symptoms are new and the patient has not been diagnosed by a physician as having asthma, physician referral for evaluation is essential. OTC medication for asthma relief should never be used unless a diagnosis of asthma has been established by a physician. Diagnosis is important to rule out other causes of pulmonary symptoms, establish a baseline for the disease's severity, explore the etiology of the patient's asthma so that the causative factor may be removed, and avoid OTC medications that may worsen other conditions.

If a patient with new pulmonary symptoms describes a history of hypertension or heart disease, physician referral is again essential, since patients with congestive heart failure may awaken in the middle of the night with dyspnea and cough resulting from pulmonary edema. Shortness of breath and chest pain in women taking oral contraceptives may be signs of pulmonary emboli rather than asthma, and the patient should be referred to a physician.

People with chronic bronchitis and emphysema have symptoms similar to asthma. However, these symptoms are continuous, not episodic, and should not be treated with OTC drugs except under a physician's care.

If a diagnosis of asthma has been established previously, it is important to determine how severe the symptoms are and which self-treatment approaches already have been tried. If a bronchodilator (aerosol, oral, or both) is being used but the dyspnea is becoming worse, a severe attack is imminent, and the patient should see a physician immediately. In this situation, OTC products are useless. If, on the other hand, the dyspnea is mild, occurs intermittently, and does not worsen, recommendation of an OTC asthma product is appropriate.

TREATMENT

Products for treatment of asthmatic symptoms are manufactured in various oral dosage forms and as OTC inhalants. The pharmacist should have the patient consult a physician if symptoms are not relieved within 20 minutes after epinephrine is administered by aerosol or within 1 hour after oral bronchodilators are administered.

Ingredients in OTC Products

There is general agreement that the quantity of chemical mediators released is modulated by the intracellular concentration of cyclic AMP and that increased levels of cyclic AMP result in bronchial smooth muscle relaxation. Therefore agents that augment the intracellular cyclic AMP concentration are useful in asthma therapy (12, 16, 17). Two main classes of pharmacological agents have this effect—the sympathomimetic agents (β-adrenergic stimulators) and the methylxanthines. The β-adrenergic agents, by stimulating β-receptors, increase production of cyclic 3′,5′-AMP. Phosphodiesterase, a normally occurring intracellular enzyme, rapidly destroys cyclic AMP (Figure 2). The methylxanthines exert their activity by inhibiting phosphodiesterase, thereby allowing intracellular concentrations of cyclic AMP to accumulate.

Until the introduction of adrenergic agents that have mainly β_2-activity (e.g., metaproterenol and terbutaline), asthma had to be treated with drugs that had mixed α- and β-activity (e.g., ephedrine and epinephrine). Although this older therapy is effective, it also is the source of many side effects. For example, epinephrine stimulates β_1-, β_2-, and α-adrenergic receptors. Thus parenteral administration of epinephrine produces not only bronchodilation, but also tachycardia and increased blood pressure, which may be detrimental to asthmatic patients with cardiovascular disease. It should be noted that repeated use of sympathomimetic amines at shorter intervals than those recommended reduces the receptor's ability to respond to subsequent stimulation; tolerance to the drug action may develop. The methylxanthines, by virtue of their ability to increase intracellular concentrations of cyclic AMP, also may cause undesired effects including cardiac, CNS, and skeletal muscle stimulation.

therapeutic agents
mechanisms of action
dosages
side effects

Ephedrine

Since the mid-1920's, ephedrine has been widely used in asthma therapy (24–28). It is effective orally and is partially metabolized by the liver, but about 75% of the dose is excreted unchanged in the urine (29). Its onset of action occurs in 30–60 minutes and lasts 2–3 hours (26, 30–32). Ephedrine has direct α- and β-adrenergic receptor stimulating activity (29, 33). It also acts indirectly by causing norepinephrine to be released from peripheral sympathetic fibers. Ephedrine is used for asthma because of its β-stimulating activity, which results in bronchodilation. As with most sympathomimetic amines, tolerance develops with rapidly repeated doses.

Because ephedrine crosses the blood–brain barrier, it often causes tenseness, nervousness, tremors, and sleeplessness (33, 34). Peripheral effects include tachycardia, palpitations, and systolic and diastolic blood pressure elevation. Urinary retention also may occur, especially in older male patients with prostatic hypertrophy (29, 33, 34). Overdosage exaggerates these side effects. Normal doses may produce a significant and potentially dangerous rise in blood pressure if they are taken concurrently with monoamine oxidase (MAO) inhibitors because these agents also increase blood pressure by inhibiting norepinephrine metabolism.

Because of its oral effectiveness, slow onset, prolonged action, and decreased potency as compared to epinephrine, ephedrine (alone or in combination with theophylline) has been used to prevent attacks in patients with milder forms of asthma rather than as acute therapy for moderate to severe asthma (5, 35). For adults, doses of 12.5–25 mg of ephedrine, not more often than every 4 hours and not to exceed 150 mg in 24 hours, are effective in relieving bronchoconstriction (36). If symptoms are not relieved within 1 hour after taking a dose, additional ephedrine should not be taken; a physician should be consulted immediately. For children 12 or under, who should be under a physician's direct supervision, the FDA OTC Panel on Cold, Cough, Allergy, Bronchodilator, and Antiasthmatic Products recommends that no dosage be included in OTC labeling. The panel does recommend professional labeling which states that for children 6–12 years old the dosage is 6.25–12.5 mg, not more often than every 4 hours and not to exceed 75 mg in 24 hours; for children 2–6 it is 0.3–0.5 mg/kg in 24 hours (36).

Administering sympathomimetic amines systemically may affect glucose metabolism, resulting in increased serum glucose levels. Diabetics should be reminded of this possibility by reference to the label warning and should be instructed to monitor urine sugars closely while taking ephedrine-containing products. People with heart disease, high blood pressure, or hyperthyroid disease should use ephedrine only as directed by a physician.

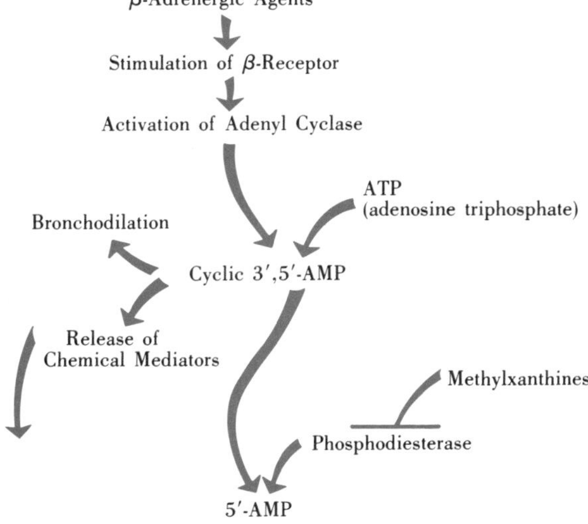

Figure 2. β-Adrenergic agents.

Methoxyphenamine

Methoxyphenamine hydrochloride is a sympathomimetic amine structurally related to ephedrine. It is most effective used chronically to relieve or prevent mild symptoms. Acute attacks should be treated with more potent agents. Methoxyphenamine hydrochloride produces antiasthmatic effects similar to those of ephedrine but may exhibit fewer side effects (37–39). Symptomatic improvement begins about 1 hour after oral administration and continues 2–3 hours (32, 34, 37).

The most common side effects of methoxyphenamine hydrochloride are dry mouth and, occasionally, mild anorexia, nausea, lightheadedness, dizziness, and drowsiness. The drug causes little or no CNS stimulation and no increase in blood pressure or heart rate (37, 38). In an oral dose of 200 mg it is therapeutically equivalent to 30 mg of ephedrine. No data are available on methoxyphenamine hydrochloride use in children under 12; in this age group it should be used only on a physician's advice. The usual adult dose is 100 mg every 4–6 hours, not to exceed 600 mg in 24 hours (40).

Epinephrine

Epinephrine is effective only when given parenterally or via inhalation because of its instability in gastric fluids and metabolism by enzymes in the gut wall (29). Because it has a profound effect on the cardiovascular system, it is given parenterally (0.2–0.3 ml of 1:1000 solution) in severe attacks only after other means of therapy have failed. All OTC aerosol products used for asthma contain epinephrine or one of its salt forms. Used correctly, these products deliver a small quantity of epinephrine directly to the bronchioles, where the drug exerts its effect. There are few side effects because significant systemic absorption does not occur. However, aerosol overuse may cause enough systemic absorption to produce side effects.

Epinephrine exerts α-, β_1-, and β_2-stimulating effects that cause both vasoconstriction of the vessels that supply the bronchial mucosa and bronchodilation. Vasoconstriction probably causes a decrease in bronchial mucosal edema and a decrease in systemic drug absorption (5, 33). Relief usually occurs within 5–10 minutes after epinephrine is administered, but because of its short duration of action (about 30–40 minutes), relapse frequently occurs within a few hours (5, 32, 33, 35).

As with all sympathomimetics, frequent use leads to tolerance. This effect is a problem especially with epinephrine inhalation; patients with moderate to severe attacks increase epinephrine use, delaying the time before seeking professional help and often precipitating a serious attack that could lead to status asthmaticus (life-threatening asthma attack). Patients should therefore be advised not to continue epinephrine use if symptoms are not relieved within 20 minutes or become worse, but to seek medical assistance immediately. Although epinephrine administration rapidly relieves airway obstruction, hypoxemia (deficient oxygenation of the blood) may persist as long as 1 hour, even though the patient is breathing comfortably (41). This result probably stems from poor perfusion of lung areas by blood despite the improved ventilation the patient may experience. For this reason it is advisable for patients to refrain from exercise for at least 1 hour after an attack.

Epinephrine's main side effects are tremors, nervousness, restlessness, insomnia, and palpitations (33). Dry mouth and throat and gastric irritation also are common, probably resulting from vasoconstriction caused by a local effect of the drug reaching these areas. These effects may be alleviated by gargling after each use of an aerosol epinephrine preparation (33, 35). Tilting the head back to form a straight passageway for the inhaled drug also has been suggested to improve delivery of the active ingredient and to prevent dryness.

One to three inhalations of a 1% aqueous solution via nebulizer or an equivalent amount of aerosolized epinephrine may be used not more than once every 3 hours except on a physician's advice. The same dosage may be used in children over 4, if they are able to use aerosol dosage forms and access to use is supervised by an adult (36). Epinephrine by inhalation should not be used by people with congestive heart failure, cardiac arrhythmias, or high blood pressure except on a physician's advice. As with ephedrine, monoamine oxidase inhibitors should not be taken concurrently except under a physician's supervision. Epinephrine also should not be used to treat symptoms of asthma unless a diagnosis of asthma has been made by a physician.

Epinephrine by inhalation has been used for many years without question concerning its safety. In the early 1960's, aerosol products containing isoproterenol and metaproterenol (orciprenaline) became widely used also with little concern for their safety. In the United Kingdom there were reports of a rapidly rising mortality rate from asthma, especially in children 10–14 years old (42, 43). Deaths were sudden and unexpected, and patients often were found clasping an empty aerosol container (42). The first researchers to suggest that sympathomimetic aerosols may have been the causative agent wrote: "We suspect that patients with asthma may be killing themselves by the excessive use of sympathomimetic agents in the form of metered or pressurized aerosols containing isoprenaline, orciprenaline, or adrenaline" (43). These reports prompted investigators to examine drug use patterns and mortality rates in England and Wales (44–48).

epinephrine mechanism

tolerance development

side effects

doses

isoproterenol use and mortality

The investigations brought forward several interesting observations. During this period, aerosols containing sympathomimetic agents were available as OTC products in the United Kingdom. Between 1961 and 1967 the following percentage of total aerosolized sympathomimetic sales in England was estimated: isoetharine, 1%; epinephrine, 4%; metaproterenol, 8%; isoproterenol in doses of 0.2 mg or less, 59%; and isoproterenol in doses of more than 0.2 mg, 28%. Thus 87% of total sales contained isoproterenol. After the possible hazards of these products were published in both professional and lay literature in 1966 and 1967, a significant downward mortality trend began. Between 1967 and 1968, epinephrine, metaproterenol, and isoetharine sales changed little. However, isoproterenol sales declined by about 30% in 1968 alone. In December 1968, new poison regulations in England became effective, eliminating the OTC sale of isoproterenol.

Although these data are subject to varying interpretations (many factors may affect mortality in asthma), the evidence strongly implicates isoproterenol use as a causative factor. There are no such reports implicating epinephrine. Although increasing mortality rates were reported in England, no such increases occurred in the United States, possibly because the English preparations contained as much as 5 times the isoproterenol concentration of the American products.

As was noted previously, epinephrine stimulates α-receptors, causing constriction of the mucosal bronchiolar blood vessels. This property may allow for a decreased epinephrine absorption rate into the systemic circulation, causing less toxicity. Isoproterenol (predominantly a β-stimulator) is expected to produce vasodilation, which may increase its own absorption rate. The significance of this hypothesis, although not firmly established, may be inferred by the rapid onset of tachycardia upon isoproterenol inhalation. The evidence seems to indicate that epinephrine by inhalation, used according to instructions, is a safe and effective OTC preparation.

Theophylline

With the exception of dyphylline, which exerts its own action, theophylline is the pharmacologically active xanthine derivative used in asthma therapy (33). It is also the most potent xanthine with respect to its effects on the bronchi and cardiovascular system. Its main effects are skeletal muscle stimulation, smooth muscle and bronchiolar relaxation, coronary artery dilation, and decreased peripheral vascular resistance (49). A transient increase in cardiac output also occurs, resulting in an increase in glomerular filtration rate and a diuresis of short duration.

theophylline use in asthma therapy

therapeutic plasma levels

side effects

dosages

barbiturates in combination products

Theophylline's half-life is highly variable among patients (2.5–9.5 hours, average about 6) (50–52). Doses of 400–3200 mg/day may be necessary to maintain therapeutic plasma concentrations—10–20 μg/ml (50). Toxicity often occurs at plasma levels of more than 20 μg/ml, and there is seldom toxicity at less than 13 μg/ml. Absorption is slowed by food, but in chronic use, accumulation occurs, and therapeutic levels are maintained even when the drug is taken with food. The xanthines are partly metabolized and excreted as methyluric acids or methylxanthines. None is completely metabolized to uric acid; therefore their use in patients with gout is not contraindicated (5).

The main side effects (early signs of toxicity) of theophylline are anorexia, nausea, headaches, and vomiting. Severe toxicity involving CNS stimulation leading to convulsions, coma, and cardiovascular collapse has been reported in children (54) and occasionally in adults. Most of these cases occurred in pediatric patients receiving suppositories in combination with oral or parenteral theophylline preparations. Pharmacists therefore should advise patients not to take (or administer) two theophylline-containing products in different dosage forms except under a physician's advice and supervision and to discontinue their use if nausea, vomiting, or restlessness occurs. Usual adult theophylline doses are 100–200 mg orally every 6 hours, not to exceed 800 mg in 24 hours; theophylline should not be used in children under 12 except on a physician's advice. For other derivatives the dosage should be calculated according to the amount of theophylline base present: aminophylline (85%), theophylline olamine (75%), choline oxtriphylline (65%), and dyphylline (70%).

Theophylline became popular as an oral bronchodilator in the 1930's, and pharmaceutical manufacturers began to produce a multitude of dosage forms and fixed combination products. A historical study of the subject stated (55): "This plethora of preparations may have been either a cause or a result of the irrational use of theophylline."

Early theophylline use resulted in nausea and GI irritation; thus enteric-coated tablets and rectal suppositories were introduced. However, the GI side effects occurred with greater frequency when "trough" (lowest) plasma levels were above 20 μg/ml (50). Some mechanism mediated centrally through the medullary chemoreceptor trigger zone rather than direct irritation of the gastric mucosa may be responsible for these symptoms. Significantly lower blood levels due to poor absorption were reported with enteric-coated tablets than with uncoated tablets (56). Rectal suppositories containing aminophylline also have been shown to be slowly and erratically absorbed as compared to oral tablets and liquid (53, 56). The use of theophylline olamine as a retention enema produces reliable therapeutic levels, although they are somewhat lower than those expected with oral uncoated tablets (57).

Several investigators demonstrated that theophylline in hydroalcoholic solution provides equivalent or slightly higher blood levels than oral tablets (58, 59). The rapid absorption from hydroalcoholic solutions may allow the use of oral therapy for moderately severe attacks, making hospital admission unnecessary (60). Although this reasoning has some merit in acute situations, such rapid absorption offers no advantage and may actually be undesirable when chronic sustained levels are the goal (61). Usual doses of hydroalcoholic elixirs range from 30 to 60 ml, so that carrying a day's supply of medication is cumbersome. The amount of alcohol present should be carefully considered in evaluating the medication profile. The evidence indicates that oral, uncoated tablets are the dosage form of choice.

Many pharmaceutical manufacturers have introduced combination products usually containing theophylline (100–130 mg), ephedrine (24 mg), and phenobarbital (8 mg). For states that have placed all drug products containing barbiturates under prescription control, some manufacturers have replaced the barbiturates with antihistamines, which are thought to have sedative effects. The merits of barbiturates or antihistamines in such combinations have not been established. The theophylline dose in these combinations and ephedrine is present in therapeutic concentrations. Phenobarbital is added to decrease the CNS stimulation caused by ephedrine; however, with chronic use, CNS effects are minimal, and 8 mg of phenobarbital probably is of no benefit. Barbiturates may depress the respiratory center and potentially cause underventilation. In studies of theophylline alone, in combination with ephedrine, and in conventional fixed dose combinations, theophylline in individualized doses provided control of asthmatic symptoms; the addition of ephedrine provided no additional benefit; however, the combination caused an increase in the incidence of insomnia, nervousness, and GI complaints (62, 63). Fixed dose combinations were relatively ineffective in these studies.

Other Agents

Antihistamines

Some combination asthma products have contained antihistamines to antagonize the histamine effects. However, they have no effect on bradykinin and slow-reacting

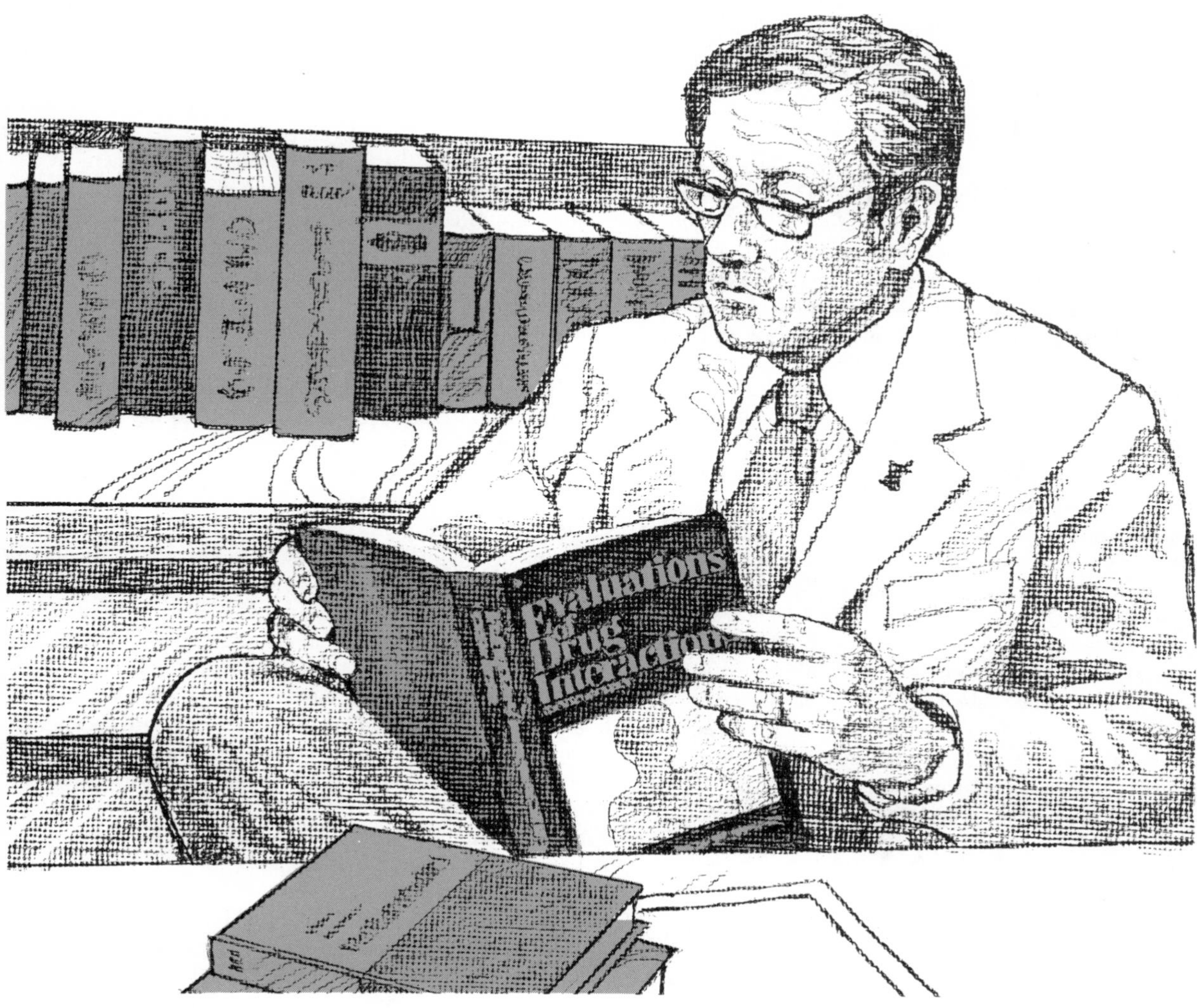

other ingredients in asthma products

water as a therapeutic agent

substance of anaphylaxis and thus are ineffective as therapeutic agents for asthma. Antihistamines also have anticholinergic activity, causing watery secretions in the bronchi to be reduced and resulting in the formation of thicker mucus that is more difficult to expectorate. Because mucus plugs are a main cause of airway obstruction, antihistamines may actually worsen an asthmatic attack.

Expectorants

Many asthma products contain expectorants, especially guaifenesin and potassium iodide. These agents probably are not more effective as expectorants than an adequate hydration of the patient. Therefore their use in asthma is questionable. Also, because of the concern for iodide toxicity the FDA OTC Panel recommended that iodide-containing, i.e., expectorant, products be restricted to prescription status.

Antitussives

Antitussives such as codeine and dextromethorphan hydrobromide are used occasionally in asthma products. Coughing is the major mechanism for removing bronchial secretions and mucus plugs. Therefore antitussives generally should not be used for asthma, since the cause of the cough should be given priority in treatment.

Water

Water remains a major therapeutic agent in asthma treatment, a fact that should be stressed with all patients. Adequate hydration increases the watery secretions in the bronchioles and thins mucus secretions. This thinning allows for easier mucus removal and decreased mucus plug formation. Effective delivery of water to the lungs depends on adequate oral intake. Additional benefit may be gained from vaporizers, cool mist humidifiers, and showers. Care should be taken to keep the cool mist humidifier clean to prevent mold on the atomizing mechanism. Home furnace humidifiers should be considered as important adjuncts to therapy. Unhumidified heated winter air may have as little as 4–10% relative humidity.

Specialized Dosage Forms

Administering bronchodilators via inhalation provides rapid and effective treatment of acute asthmatic symptoms. The drug is delivered directly to its site of action (the bronchioles), eliminating delays in absorption and distribution found with other administration routes. Commercially available aerosolized units provide additional advantages in that the contents remain in a stabilized form and are protected from contamination by organisms, atmospheric gases, and sunlight. The small compact units also allow patients to carry the drug without difficulty.

aerosols

advice for the patient

Proper aerosol formulation and use constitute the key to effective therapy and prevention of complications. For the inhaled mist to be deposited in the bronchioles, the particle size must be 0.5–5 μm (64, 65). Particles larger than 5 μm are deposited in the upper airways; those smaller than 0.5 μm do not settle out and thus are exhaled. Most commercially available aerosol preparations provide particle size in the range 0.5–5.0 μm. Conventional nebulizers, although somewhat less reliable than aerosols in their ability to deliver an accurate dose of appropriate particle size, are adequate when used properly but do not provide the easy use, drug stability, and protection from contamination.

PRODUCT SELECTION GUIDELINES

Before recommending an OTC product for asthma it is important that the pharmacist have a good understanding of the patient's condition. A complete patient profile alerts the pharmacist to conditions such as heart disease, diabetes, hypertension, aspirin sensitivity, and prescription medications being taken that can duplicate or interact with OTC products. It also may provide an indication concerning the patient's compliance with drug regimens. Regular dosing with oral agents to maintain therapeutic blood levels is necessary to prevent asthma symptoms. Patients who consistently forget to take oral medications may do better by treating symptoms as they occur with an aerosolized product.

It must also be remembered that the patient is usually the best judge of whether a particular agent is effective or not. After recommending an agent the pharmacist should alert the patient to the caution: "Do not continue to take this product but seek medical assistance if symptoms are not relieved within 1 hour or become worse." There is nothing gained by continuing ineffective therapy. When OTC medications do not provide sufficient relief without bothersome side effects, physician referral is the necessary next step.

Education in asthma medication use is as important as drug choice. Improper use of aerosol agents may decrease effectiveness and increase side effects. The patient should be instructed to hold the aerosol upside down, close the lips and teeth around the mouthpiece, forcefully exhale as much air as possible, then inhale deeply through the mouthpiece. Shortly after inhalation begins, the bottle should be pressed down to activate the spray, and inhalation should continue. The patient should then pause a few seconds and slowly exhale. An alternative method is for the patient not to close the teeth and lips around the mouthpiece but to hold the mouthpiece at the level of the lips, with the mouth open. It is important to position the tongue away from the mainstream of the mist; otherwise the medication will be deposited in the oral cavity and upper airways. If symptoms are not relieved in 20 minutes, a physician should be consulted. If headache, nervousness, or palpitations occur, the medication should be discontinued. The mouthpiece should be washed daily with warm water to prevent clogging, and it should always be kept free of particles. Gargling after each use prevents dry mouth and throat irritation.

Doses of oral sympathomimetics or xanthines should be spaced evenly throughout the day; the last dose should be taken at bedtime because many attacks tend to occur during the night. The pharmacist should stress that these oral medications should be taken regularly to prevent asthma symptoms and will probably be of little value in treating an acute attack. Patients should be informed that nervousness or insomnia may occur during the initiation of therapy with these agents but usually disappears in a few days with adaptation, despite continued dosing. If these symptoms persist beyond a few days, the patient should consult a physician. Patients with aspirin sensitivity should be cautioned that some asthma combination drug preparations contain aspirin. However, the FDA Panel has recommended that no aspirin be included in products used for asthma (66). If nausea, vomiting, or restlessness occurs after taking OTC xanthine preparations, the dosage should be reduced. OTC combination xanthine medications should not be taken with prescription medication containing theophylline salts or with theophylline rectal suppositories. Adequate hydration and humidification of room air, rest, and avoidance of allergens and stressful situations are also important considerations that should be discussed. When stressful situations, e.g., exercise, are unavoidable, prophylactic use of an aerosol prior to exposure may prevent an asthmatic attack. Cold air may precipitate an asthmatic attack in some individuals.

SUMMARY

Although asthma has been studied intensively, its pathogenesis is not completely understood. Evidence indicates that several factors interrelate in variable degrees to precipitate an attack. These factors include allergy, genetics, infection, autonomic nervous system balance, and psychophysiological response to stress. Patients should not self-treat any wheezing symptom unless a proper diagnosis has been made.

The choice of agents in asthma therapy is also complex. The severity of the disease, existence of other diseases, previous response to therapy, and current medications for both asthma and other diseases are important considerations that should be known before recommendations for OTC asthma products are made. Continuous oral therapy should be used for the prevention and control of asthmatic symptoms. In mild cases, ephedrine (12.5–25 mg) or methoxyphenamine hydrochloride (100 mg) every 4–6 hours may provide adequate protection. Theophylline or one of its derivatives is the oral therapy of choice in individuals with more severe asthma. However, unless appropriate plasma levels are obtained, this agent may provide unsatisfactory results. Because individuals vary in their ability to metabolize theophylline, individualized dosage regimens give the best results. Usual adult doses are 100–200 mg every 6 hours, not to exceed 800 mg in 24 hours. Appropriate plasma theophylline levels are highly effective with relatively little toxicity. Levels below 10 μg/ml are relatively ineffective, and those above 20 μg/ml are often toxic. Theophylline should be used correctly as a single-entity preparation, which under present FDA regulations is limited to prescription by a physician.

If exacerbation of the disease occurs, oral therapy should be supplemented with aerosol bronchodilator inhalation. In patients who have mild asthma without concurrent cardiovascular disease, OTC products that contain epinephrine may provide adequate therapy. In severe asthma, treatment may include glucocorticoids (e.g., prednisone), antibiotics, xanthine derivatives, and the prescription-only bronchodilators, such as isoproterenol or metaproterenol inhalers. Patients should be cautioned that overuse of aerosol bronchodilators and prescription aerosols may lead to tolerance, cardiovascular toxicity, or progression of the attack to life-threatening severity by delaying the time before a physician is consulted.

Water provides a major therapeutic modality in treating all asthmatic patients. It is important that patients be instructed in maintaining an adequate oral fluid intake and a relative humidity in the home or office as high as is tolerable.

therapy considerations

summary

REFERENCES

(1) American Thoracic Society, *Am. Rev. Respir. Dis., 85,* 762 (1962).

(2) "Prevalence of Selected Chronic Respiratory Conditions in the United States—1970," Vital and Health Statistics, Series 10, No. 84, DHEW Publication No. (HRA) 74-1511, National Center for Health Statistics, Health Resources Administration, Rockville, Md., Sept. 1973.

(3) F. M. Rackemann and M. C. Edwards, *N. Engl. J. Med., 246,* 815, 858 (1952).

(4) A. L. Sheffer and M. D. Valentine, *Med. Clin. North Am., 53,* 239 (1969).

(5) R. P. McCombs, *N. Engl. J. Med., 286,* 1186 (1972).

(6) D. A. Mathison, D. D. Stevenson, E. M. Tan, and J. H. Vaughan, *J. Am. Med. Assoc., 224,* 1134 (1973).

(7) R. F. Lockey, D. L. Rucknagel, and N. E. Vanselow, *Ann. Intern. Med., 78,* 57 (1973).

(8) R. D. Snyder and G. L. Siegel, *Ann. Allergy, 25,* 377 (1967).

(9) "Harrison's Principles of Internal Medicine," 8th ed., G. W. Thorn, R. D. Adams, E. Braunwald, K. J. Isselbacher, and R. G. Petersdorf, Eds., McGraw-Hill, New York, N.Y., 1977, pp. 1349–1354.

(10) P. M. Penna, *J. Am. Pharm. Assoc., NS13,* 690 (1973).

(11) G. N. Beall, D. C. Heiner, D. P. Tashkin, and B. J. Whipp, *Ann. Intern. Med., 78,* 405 (1973).

(12) W. A. Mahon, *Can. Med. Assoc. J., 110,* 376 (1974).

(13) T. Berg and S. G. Johansson, *Int. Arch. Allergy Appl. Immunol., 36,* 219 (1969).

(14) K. Ishizaka and T. Ishizaka, *J. Immunol., 99,* 1187 (1967).

(15) "Pathogenic Basis of Disease," S. L. Robbins, Ed., Saunders, Philadelphia, Pa., 1974, p. 803.

(16) M. Kaliner, *Can. Med. Assoc. J., 110,* 431 (1974).

(17) W. M. Gold, G. F. Kessler, and D. Y. Yu, *J. Appl. Physiol., 3,* 719 (1972).

(18) A. Szentivanyi, *J. Allergy, 42,* 203 (1968).

(19) A. Szentivanyi, *Ann. Allergy, 24,* 253 (1966).

(20) A. S. Rebuck, *Drugs, 7,* 344 (1974).

(21) M. S. Dunnill, *J. Clin. Pathol., 13,* 27 (1960).

(22) A. S. Rebuck and J. Read, *Am. J. Med., 51,* 788 (1971).

(23) E. R. McFadden, Jr., R. Kiser, and W. J. deGroot, *N. Engl. J. Med., 288,* 221 (1973).

(24) T. G. Miller, *Am. J. Med. Sci., 170,* 157 (1925).

(25) W. S. Middleton and K. K. Chen, *Arch. Intern. Med., 39,* 385 (1927).

(26) K. K. Chen and C. F. Schmidt, *Medicine, 9,* 339 (1930).

(27) K. K. Chen and C. F. Schmidt, *J. Pharmacol. Exp. Ther., 24,* 339 (1924).

(28) K. K. Chen, *Arch. Intern. Med., 39,* 404 (1927).

(29) "The Pharmacological Basis of Therapeutics," L. S. Goodman and A. Gilman, Eds., Macmillan, New York, N.Y., 1970, pp. 507–513.

(30) A. H. Beckett, J. W. Gorrod, and D. C. Taylor, *J. Pharm. Pharmacol.,* suppl., *24,* 65P (1972).

(31) G. R. Wilkinson and A. H. Beckett, *J. Pharm. Sci., 57,* 1933 (1968).

(32) E. Bresnick, J. F. Beaky, L. Levinson, and M. S. Segal, *J. Clin. Invest., 28,* 1182 (1949).

(33) C. G. Blumstein, *Semin. Drug. Treat., 2,* 385 (1973).

(34) M. C. S. Kennedy and S. L. O. Jackson, *Br. Med. J., 2,* 1506 (1963).

(35) F. Sadik, C. T. Bauguess, and J. H. Fincher, *J. Am. Pharm. Assoc., NS15,* 247 (1975).

(36) *Federal Register, 41,* 38371 (1976).

(37) J. J. Curry, J. E. Fuchs, and S. Leard, *J. Allergy, 20,* 104 (1949).

(38) R. S. B. Pearson, *Br. Med. J., 2,* 905 (1958).

(39) E. C. Roy, J. H. Seaburg, and L. E. Johns, *J. Allergy, 20,* 364 (1949).

(40) *Federal Register, 41,* 38372 (1976).

(41) H. A. Rees, J. S. Millar, and K. W. Donald, *Lancet, 2,* 1164 (1967).

(42) J. M. Smith, *Lancet, 1,* 1042 (1966).

(43) M. J. Greenberg and A. Pines, *Br. Med. J., 1,* 563 (1967).

(44) P. J. D. Heaf, *Br. Med. Bull., 26,* 245 (1970).

(45) W. H. W. Inman and A. M. Adelstein, *Lancet, 2,* 279 (1969).

(46) F. E. Speizer, R. Doll, and P. Heaf, *Br. Med. J., 1,* 335 (1968).

(47) F. E. Speizer and R. Doll, *Br. Med. J., 3,* 245 (1968).

(48) F. E. Speizer, R. Doll, P. Heaf, and L. B. Strong, *Br. Med. J., 1,* 339 (1968).

(49) T. G. Tong, *Drug Intell. Clin. Pharm., 7,* 156 (1973).

(50) J. J. Jenne, E. Wyze, F. S. Rood, and F. M. MacDonald, *Clin. Pharmacol. Ther., 13,* 349 (1972).

(51) P. A. Mitenko and R. I. Ogilvie, *Clin. Pharmacol. Ther., 14,* 509 (1973).

(52) P. A. Mitenko and R. I. Ogilvie, *Clin. Pharmacol. Ther., 13,* 329 (1972).

(53) L. P. Lillehei, *J. Am. Med. Assoc., 205,* 530 (1968).

(54) H. L. Bacal, K. Linegar, R. L. Denton, and R. Gourdeau, *Can. Med. Assoc. J., 80,* 6 (1959).

(55) M. Weinberger and S. Riegelman, *N. Engl. J. Med., 291,* 151 (1974).

(56) S. H. Waxler and J. A. Schack, *J. Am. Med. Assoc., 143,* 736 (1950).

(57) J. W. Yunginger, M. Shigeta, I. Smith, M. Green, and H. Keitel, *Ann. Allergy, 24,* 469 (1966).

(58) J. T. McGinn, *Curr. Ther. Res., 7,* 110 (1965).

(59) J. Schluger, J. T. McGinn, and D. J. Hennessy, *Am. J. Med. Sci., 233,* 296 (1957).

(60) H. Herxheimer, *N. Engl. J. Med., 291,* 1192 (1974).

(61) M. Weinberger and S. Riegelman, *N. Engl. J. Med., 291,* 1193 (1974).

(62) M. Weinberger and E. Bronsky, *Clin. Pharmacol. Ther., 17,* 585 (1975).

(63) M. M. Weinberger and E. A. Bronsky, *J. Pediatr., 84,* 421 (1974).

(64) "The Theory and Practice of Industrial Pharmacy," L. Lachman, H. A. Lieberman, and J. L. Kanig, Eds., Lea and Febiger, Philadelphia, Pa., 1970, p. 614.

(65) M. Lippmann and R. E. Albert, *Am. Ind. Hyg. Assoc. J., 30,* 257 (1969).

(66) *Federal Register, 41,* 38326 (1976).

Product (Manufacturer)	Dosage Form	Ephedrine	Epinephrine	Theophylline	Other
Amodrine (Searle)	tablet	25 mg (as racemic hydrochloride)	—	—	aminophylline, 100 mg phenobarbital, 8 mg
Asma-Lief (Columbia Medical)	tablet	24 mg (as hydrochloride)	—	130 mg	phenobarbital, 8 mg
AsthmaHaler (Norcliff Thayer)	oral inhalant	—	7 mg/ml (as bitartrate)	—	—
AsthmaNefrin (Norcliff Thayer)	inhalant solution	—	2.25% (epinephrine base as racemic hydrochloride)	—	chlorobutanol, 0.5%
Breatheasy (Pascal)	inhalant	—	2.2% (as hydrochloride)	—	benzyl alcohol, 1% isotonic salts, 0.5%
Bronitin (Whitehall)	tablet	24 mg	—	130 mg	guaifenesin, 100 mg pyrilamine maleate, 16 mg
Bronitin Mist (Whitehall)	inhalant	—	bitartrate	—	—
Bronkaid (Winthrop)	tablet	24 mg (as sulfate)	—	100 mg (anhydrous)	guaifenesin, 100 mg magnesium trisilicate, 74.52 mg
Bronkaid Mist (Winthrop)	inhalant	—	0.5%	—	ascorbic acid, 0.07% alcohol, 34% hydrochloric and nitric acid buffers
Bronkotabs (Breon)	tablet	24 mg (as sulfate)	—	100 mg	guaifenesin, 100 mg phenobarbital, 8 mg
Phedral (North American)	tablet	24.3 mg	—	129.6 mg	phenobarbital, 8.1 mg
Primatene M (Whitehall)	tablet	24 mg (as hydrochloride)	—	130 mg	pyrilamine maleate, 16 mg
Primatene Mist (Whitehall)	inhalant	—	NS[a]	—	alcohol, 34%
Primatene P (Whitehall)	tablet	24 mg (as hydrochloride)	—	130 mg	phenobarbital, 8 mg
Tedral (Warner-Chilcott)	tablet elixir suspension	24 mg/tablet 1.2 mg/ml (elixir) 2.4 mg/ml (suspension) (all as hydrochloride)	—	130 mg/tablet (anhydrous) 6.5 mg/ml (elixir) 13 mg/ml (suspension)	phenobarbital, 8 mg/tablet 0.4 mg/ml (elixir) 0.8 mg/ml (suspension)
Thalfed (Beecham Labs)	tablet	25 mg (as hydrochloride)	—	120 mg (hydrous)	phenobarbital, 8 mg
Vaponefrin Solution (Fisons)	inhalant	—	2.25% (epinephrine base as racemic hydrochloride)	—	chlorobutanol, 0.5%
Verquad (Knoll)	tablet suspension	24 mg/tablet 2.4 mg/ml (both (as hydrochloride)	—	130 mg/tablet 13 mg/ml (both as calcium salicylate)	guaifenesin, 100 mg/tablet 10 mg/ml phenobarbital, 8 mg/tablet 0.8 mg/ml

[a] Not stated.

Internal Analgesic Products

W. Kent Van Tyle

Chapter 9

Questions to Ask the Patient

What type of pain do you have, and how long have you had it?

Do you have any other symptoms which you feel might be associated with the pain you have?

Do you have a fever? How high? How long have you had it?

Have you ever had an allergic reaction to aspirin?

Do you have or have you ever had asthma, other allergic diseases, or ulcers?

Are you taking medication for gout, arthritis, or diabetes? If so, what?

Are you taking any medication which affects the clotting of your blood? Have you ever had any problem with your blood being slow to clot?

Internal analgesics are used to relieve pain. Although classification as analgesics would seem to exclude their use for other purposes, certain compounds in this group also possess pharmacological activities that make them valuable for reducing elevated body temperature and for ameliorating various inflammatory conditions.

Even though pain is a common experience, it is not a simple condition to define. Pain is a sensation, but it is also an interpretation of that sensation that can be influenced by many factors. Fatigue, anxiety, fear, and the anticipation of more pain all affect the perception of and reaction to pain. Studies show that various personality types experience pain differently; the introverted personality has a lower pain threshold than the extrovert (1). In addition, the perception of pain may be modified significantly by suggestion. Studies indicate that approximately 35% of patients suffering pain from a variety of causes report their pain as being "satisfactorily relieved" by placebo (2).

ETIOLOGY

Pain is usually a protective mechanism, occurring when tissue is damaged or when cells are altered by pain stimuli which threaten to produce tissue damage. Pain resulting from a functional disturbance or pathology is called "organic" pain. In contrast, "psychogenic" pain is a symptom of an underlying behavioral disturbance and is not a consequence of organic pathology. Organic pain is the type of pain usually presented to the pharmacist when advice is sought on nonprescription analgesics and is amenable to treatment with internal analgesics.

Origin and Perception of Pain

Pain is categorized, according to its origin, as either somatic or visceral. Somatic pain arises from the musculoskeletal system or skin; visceral pain originates from the organs or viscera of the thorax and abdomen.

Free nerve endings serve as pain receptors to initiate nerve impulses which travel via specialized pain fibers through the spinal cord and/or brain stem to specific receiving areas of the brain. These receptors are found throughout the superficial skin layers and in certain deeper tissues such as membranous bone covering, arterial walls, muscles, tendons, joint surfaces, and membranes lining the skull (3). Pain-evoking stimuli have in common the ability to injure cells and to cause the release of a proteolytic enzyme which produces polypeptides from the globulins found in intercellular fluid. Polypeptides produced in this way stimulate nerve endings at the injury or trauma site and thus initiate the pain impulse (4).

Pain fibers enter the dorsal roots of the spinal cord and interconnect with other nerve cells which cross to the opposite side of the cord and ascend to the brain. A pain impulse terminates in the thalamus, where conscious perception of pain appears to be localized, or in well-defined areas of the cerebral cortex, where recognition and interpretation of the nature and location of the pain impulse occur.

Pain initiation, transmission, and perception are essentially the same for both visceral and somatic pain. One important distinction, however, is that highly localized visceral damage rarely causes severe pain. Diffuse stimulation of nerve endings throughout an organ is required to produce significant visceral pain. Conditions producing visceral pain include ischemia of organ tissue, chemical destruction of visceral tissue, spasm of visceral smooth muscle, and physical distention of an organ or stretching of its associated mesentery (3).

In evaluating the etiology and therapy of pain it is important to recognize the potential for referred pain, or pain seeming to be in a part of the body that is not the actual body part initiating the pain signal. Unlike somatic pain, visceral pain cannot be localized by the brain as coming from a specific organ. Instead, most visceral pain is interpreted by the brain as coming from various skin segments, or it is "referred" to various body surface areas (Table 1).

When a pharmacist is advising as to the need of or potential benefit to be derived from nonprescription analgesic products, an appreciation of the sites of referred visceral pain is invaluable. Failure to recognize the possibility of referred visceral pain could mean that a serious visceral pathology might go undiagnosed and untreated while ineffective self-medication with nonprescription analgesics is attempted.

Pain Responsive to OTC Analgesics

referred visceral pain

intracranial and extracranial headaches

migraine

tension

sinus

The analgesic products available for self-medication are more effective in treating musculoskeletal, or somatic, pain than visceral pain (5). Nonprescription analgesic therapy is used most frequently for headache or for pain associated with peripheral nerves (neuralgia), joints (arthralgia), or muscles (myalgia).

Table 1. Areas Associated With Referred Visceral Pain

Origin	Localization on Body Surface
Appendix	around umbilicus localizing in right lower quadrant of abdomen
Bladder	lower abdomen over bladder
Esophagus	pharynx, lower neck, arms, midline chest region
Gallbladder	upper central portion of abdomen; lower right shoulder
Heart	base of neck, shoulders, and upper chest; down arms (left side involvement more frequent than right)
Kidney and ureters	regions of lower back over site of affected organ; anterior abdominal wall below and to the side of umbilicus
Stomach	anterior surface of chest or upper abdomen
Uterus	lower abdomen

Summarized from A. C. Guyton, *Textbook of Medical Physiology*, 4th ed., Saunders, Philadelphia, Pa., 1971, pp. 577–591, and L. Zetzel, in *Textbook of Medicine*, Vol. 1, 13th ed., P. B. Beeson and W. McDermott, Eds., Saunders, Philadelphia, Pa., 1971, p. 1327.

Headache

The most common form of pain is headache. Estimates are that, each week, 15% of the population experiences headache pain (6). Headache may be classified as either intracranial or extracranial, depending on the area of initiation of the pain (7). Intracranial headache results from inflammation or traction of sensitive intracranial structures, primarily vascular. Its etiology includes tumor, abscess, hematoma, and infection. Intracranial headache is an uncommon situation, but because of the potential seriousness of its underlying causes it requires immediate medical attention.

Because headache may be a symptom of a serious underlying pathology, the pharmacist should evaluate the potential for intracranial headache and should be prepared to recommend medical attention when appropriate. Intracranial headache produced by tumor or meningeal traction is "deep, aching, steady, dull, and seldom rhythmic or throbbing" (8). The pain may be continuous, is generally more intense in the morning, and may be associated with nausea and vomiting. Pain location cannot be used to differentiate headache of intracranial origin. Concomitant disturbances in sensory function such as blurred vision, dizziness, or hearing loss or changes in personality, behavior, speech patterns, or memory are signals to seek immediate medical attention.

The more common headache forms are extracranial and of diverse etiology. Migraine headache is characterized by intense, throbbing, hemicranial pain lasting from several hours to 1–2 days. The pain often is preceded by visual disturbances, numbness and tingling in the lips, face, or hands, and dizziness and confusion; as the pain increases in intensity, it is often accompanied by nausea and vomiting (3, 8, 9). A hereditary association is seen in 60–80% of patients with migraine; however, the exact cause of the condition is not known. Abnormalities in platelet aggregation resulting in increased plasma serotonin levels are seen in patients with migraine. Increased platelet aggregation occurs during the preheadache phase and parallels increased plasma serotonin levels (10–12). Preheadache vasoconstriction occurs in migraine possibly in response to the increased plasma serotonin levels and is followed by both intracranial and extracranial vasodilation (13). Because of the resulting vascular tone loss, the arteries begin to pulsate with the rising and falling intravascular pressure, and intense pain results from the distention and traction of the affected arteries. Preliminary research suggests that drugs that inhibit platelet aggregation (e.g., aspirin) and the associated serotonin release may be of value in reducing the intensity and frequency of migraine attacks (14).

The "tension" headache is the result of spasms of the somatic musculature of the neck and scalp. Symptoms include a feeling of tightness or pressure at the base of the head or in the muscles of the back of the neck. Pain with a tension headache is often located in the forehead or at the base of the skull and is usually bilateral.

The "sinus" headache may be distinguished characteristically from headache of other etiology because its location is restricted to the frontal areas of the head and behind or around the eyes. Sinus headaches often recur and subside at the same times each day, and the pain often is intensified by bending over. For example, sinus pain may be present on awakening and may subside after a few hours with facilitated sinus drainage. Accompanying symptoms include rhinorrhea, nasal congestion, and a feeling of pressure in the sinuses. The underlying cause is irritation and edema of the nasal and sinusoidal mucous membranes with resultant pressure placed on pain-sensitive sinus walls. Infection or allergy is the usual cause, and short-term decongestant therapy often is helpful in facilitating sinus drainage and reducing intrasinus pressure.

In addition to being a symptom of sinus headache, pain around or behind the eyes may be caused by uncorrected visual problems associated with difficulty in focusing on near or far objects. Tonic ciliary muscle contraction as an attempt to gain clear vision may result in extraocular muscle spasm and referred retro-orbital pain. If retro-orbital headache recurs persistently, referral for ophthalmic examination is indicated. Similarly, recurrent facial or mandibular pain may indicate the need for professional dental examination and treatment.

Neuralgia

Pain in the distribution of a sensory nerve is called neuralgia. The trigeminal nerve frequency is affected, and trigeminal neuralgia is characterized by sharp, stabbing pain in the face or jaw region occurring in brief, agonizing episodes. The cause of trigeminal neuralgia is unknown, but it apparently is not the result of organic damage to the nerve (15, 16). Because of the intense pain of trigeminal neuralgia, therapy with drugs more potent than those available in nonprescription medications is required.

Dull, aching facial pain localized in the trigeminal nerve area may occur in association with or during recovery from an upper respiratory tract infection. Although the pain often is described as "neuralgia," the exact etiology usually is unknown. Nevertheless, nonprescription analgesics frequently are helpful in alleviating this type of facial pain.

Myalgia

Pain from skeletal muscle, or myalgia, is common. The most frequent cause is strenuous exertion by the untrained person. However, prolonged tonic contraction produced by tension or by maintaining a certain body position for extended periods also may produce muscle pain (7). Myalgia responds well to nonprescription analgesics and adjunctive treatment with rubefacients, counterirritants, and heat. (See Chapter 25 for further information on these products.)

Arthralgia

The most frequent cause of joint pain is inflammation of the synovial membrane (arthritis) or the associated bursa (bursitis). Joints that require free movement between two bones are constructed to maintain the articulating ends of the bones bathed in a lubricating synovial fluid. The two opposing bone ends are held in position by tough, fibrous tissue which forms an enclosure around the bone ends. The inner lining of this fibrous enclosure is the synovial membrane, which produces the lubricating synovial fluid (17). Bursae are saclike structures that contain fluid formed at sites of joint friction, e.g., where a tendon passes over a bone.

Rheumatoid arthritis is a chronic inflammation of synovial membranes, often occurring at multiple sites throughout the body and having a predilection for smaller joints such as those of the hands, fingers, wrists, feet, and toes. Characteristic symptoms include joint stiffness, especially pronounced after arising in the morning, pain with joint motion, and swelling and tenderness of affected joints. Studies indicate that approximately 2.5–3% of the adult population is afflicted with this condition, the highest incidence occurring in people over 40 (18). Although the cause of rheumatoid arthritis is obscure, hereditary influence has been demonstrated, and an immunological mechanism has been proposed.

pain associated with peripheral nerves, joints, and muscles

Because of the slow, subtle nature of the onset of rheumatoid arthritis, many people attempt self-medication in the initial stages on the premise that advancing age inevitably brings aches and pains. As the disease progresses, it is a common practice to increase the dosage of nonprescription analgesics voluntarily to maintain relief from arthritic pain. The pharmacist should caution about the potential for chronic toxicity or drug interaction and should be on guard for symptoms that indicate overmedication. Also, because rheumatoid arthritis is a progressive, degenerative disease, medical attention must be encouraged to institute physical therapy and exercise to maintain the maximum possible mobility of affected joints.

Osteoarthritis, or degenerative joint disease, is the most common form of arthritis. It develops when joint cartilage repair does not keep pace with its degeneration. Onset is gradual and usually localized to a few joints. Pain and stiffness are the major symptoms. Pain is usually greatest after exercise.

bursa inflammation

Bursitis

This condition may be caused by trauma, gout, infection, or rheumatoid arthritis. Although the most common site of bursa inflammation is the shoulder, the knee (housemaid's knee) and the elbow (tennis elbow) also may be affected. Common symptoms include pain and limited motion of the affected joint; depending on the severity, the pain usually will respond to analgesic therapy. Limiting motion of the affected joint often hastens recovery (19, 20).

fever

Normal Thermoregulation and Fever

In a normothermic individual the internal body temperature is maintained within 1°F of its normal mean temperature by a complex thermoregulatory system. Although the normal mean body temperature is 98.6°F (37°C) measured orally, normal body temperature may range from approximately 97°F (36.1°C) to higher than 99°F (37.2°C). Measured rectally, these normal values are 1°F higher (18).

To maintain a constant body temperature, the ther-

causes of fever
mechanisms
role of prostaglandins
activity of salicylates

moregulatory system must balance heat production with heat loss. Thermoregulation is accomplished by keeping the temperature control center in the hypothalamus continually apprised of body temperature. Temperature-sensitive neurons located in the hypothalamus and skin relay body temperature information to the hypothalamus. Responding to this information, the hypothalamus initiates responses either to conserve heat and to increase heat production or to increase heat loss.

The skin is the primary site of heat loss from the body. Heat is carried by the blood from internal structures to the body surface where it is lost to the surroundings by processes of radiation, conduction, and evaporation. The rate of heat loss from the skin is directly related to the cutaneous blood flow rate, which in turn is a reflection of the degree of tone in the cutaneous vasculature. Consequently, the hypothalamic thermoregulatory center can change the rate of heat loss by altering the degree of vasoconstriction in the cutaneous vasculature. It also facilitates cooling by stimulating sweating, which increases the rate of evaporative heat loss from the skin. Heat production can be enhanced by hormonally mediated increases in cellular metabolism and by increased muscle tone and shivering.

Fever, or the elevation of body temperature above normal, may occur as the result of infection by various organisms including both gram-negative and gram-positive bacteria, viruses, fungi, yeasts, and protozoa (21). Other causes of fever include drugs, dehydration, tissue damage, antigen–antibody reactions, and malignancies. Pyrogens, or fever-producing substances, are categorized as either exogenous or endogenous. Exogenous pyrogens are not produced by the body; for example, the endotoxins are produced by gram-negative bacteria. Endogenous pyrogen is produced and released within the body by liver and spleen cells, blood monocytes, and neutrophils. Pyrogen release occurs as a consequence of the phagocytosis of the infectious agent or in response to stimulation by bacterial endotoxin (21, 22). The production and release of endogenous pyrogens constitute the common mediator of fever produced by infectious agents.

Experimental evidence in animals strongly suggests that prostaglandins of the E series are produced in response to circulating endogenous pyrogen and that the E prostaglandins act on the anterior hypothalamus to elevate the set point above normal, producing fever. Endogenous pyrogen increases the concentration of E prostaglandins in cerebrospinal fluid, and drugs that inhibit the synthesis of E prostaglandins in response to endogenous pyrogen have antipyretic activity (23–30).

In response to E prostaglandins the hypothalamus directs the re-establishment of body temperature to correspond to the new elevated set point. Within hours the body temperature reaches this new set point, and a febrile condition results. During the period of upward temperature readjustment, symptoms of chills, shivering, and feeling cold are experienced, even though the body temperature is elevated above normal. These are manifestations of peripheral heat conservation and production mechanisms, e.g., vasoconstriction and increased skeletal muscle tone with shivering.

Fever produces a clouding of intellectual function, disorientation, and possibly delirium. Headache is common in a febrile individual and is thought to be the result of dilation and stretching of the larger arteries at the base of the brain. Tachycardia often occurs concomitantly with fever and is usually of little concern unless there is a history of impaired cardiovascular function (31).

Fever itself does not require therapy unless there is a possibility of CNS damage, cardiovascular insufficiency, or significant discomfort to the patient. Temperatures as high as 105°F (40.6°C) usually are tolerated by adults. However, children are more prone to convulsions with temperatures in this range. When body temperature rises above 106°F (41.1°C), tissue damage begins. The brain is acutely sensitive to temperatures in this range because brain tissue does not regenerate. Body temperatures above 110°F (43.3°C) are fatal within hours (32, 33).

TREATMENT

On the basis of careful patient history evaluation, the pharmacist should decide whether the pain can be self-medicated or physician referral is necessary. If the pain is amenable to self-medication with an analgesic, the pharmacist should recommend an appropriate product.

Ingredients in OTC Products

Salicylates

By virtue of their historical significance, extent of use, and spectrum of pharmacological activity, the salicylates represent the standard prototype of non-narcotic analgesics. They produce their pharmacological effects through the production of salicylate ion in the body. Salicylic acid, sodium salicylate, methyl salicylate, and aspirin (acetylsalicylic acid) are all salicylates. However, only aspirin and sodium salicylate are used internally. Although it is chemically related, salicylamide is not a salicylate (34).

The salicylates have analgesic, antipyretic, and anti-inflammatory activity and are most effective in treating mild to moderate pain of the dull, aching type that originates in somatic structures. In doses of 325–650 mg, "controlled experiments have repeatedly shown aspirin to be superior to placebo in pathologic pain of a wide variety of etiologies" (34). Salicylates produce analgesia both centrally, by acting on hypothalamic structures, and peripherally, by inhibiting pain impulse production in pain receptors (5, 35). Recent studies suggest that prostaglandin synthesis inhibition by aspirin is involved in this peripheral mechanism. Prostaglandin E_1 sensitizes peripheral pain receptors, making them more sensitive to chemical or mechanical initiation of pain impulses (36). Aspirin inhibits prostaglandin synthesis and desensitizes pain receptors to the initiation of pain impulses by decreasing prostaglandin production at inflammation and trauma sites (37).

Therapeutic aspirin doses effectively reduce elevated body temperature. Aspirin therapy for fever reduction is initiated most frequently in children because of their propensity for fever-induced convulsions. Salicylates reduce elevated body temperature by causing the hypothalamic thermoregulatory center to re-establish a normal set point. Heat production is not inhibited, but rather, heat loss is augmented by increasing cutaneous blood flow and sweating (5). Recent studies suggest that prostaglandins are involved in the production of fever and that aspirin exerts its antipyretic effect by inhibiting prostaglandin synthesis (5, 38).

The FDA OTC Panel on Internal Analgesic, Antipyretic, and Antirheumatic Products recommends that the adult oral aspirin dose should be 325–650 mg every 4 hours while symptoms persist, not to exceed 4000 mg in 24 hours. On the basis of pharmacokinetic considerations, the Panel recommends that the maximum single dose should be 975 mg (39). This dose is to be administered only once as a single dosage or as the initial (loading) dosage in a multiple-dose regimen. These dose recommendations apply to aspirin used either as an analgesic or as an antipyretic. The Panel recommendations for pediatric aspirin dosage are summarized in Table 2.

Although aspirin's efficacy in treating inflammatory conditions such as rheumatic fever, and rheumatoid arthritis is well established, the mechanism by which these beneficial effects are produced is not. Studies show that anti-inflammatory effect of salicylates is the result of their inhibiting prostaglandin synthesis (37, 40). Prostaglandins of the E type are formed at inflammation sites where they produce vasodilation and potentiate plasma exudate formation produced by other mediators such as histamine and bradykinin (41, 42). Research in animals shows a correlation between potentiation of plasma exudate formation and the vasodilator activity of prostaglandins and suggests that prostaglandins probably do not increase vascular permeability and plasma exudate formation directly in inflammation (43). Therefore at least part of aspirin's anti-inflammatory effect is attributable to decreased prostaglandin synthesis at inflammation sites, with a resultant decrease in vasodilation and plasma exudate formation.

Aspirin doses in the range 4–6 g/day are effective in managing rheumatoid arthritis. Proposed nonprescription labeling regulations for aspirin direct the patient not to exceed 4 g in a 24-hour period. Consequently, self-medication with aspirin for arthritis is inadequate therapy because the aspirin dose required for efficacy is greater than that deemed safe for self-medication (39). Pain of osteoarthritis may be relieved by 2.5–4 g of aspirin per day in four divided doses.

Contraindications

Aspirin may compromise hemostasis by inhibiting platelet aggregation and by reducing plasma prothrombin levels. In a normal individual, a single 650-mg (10 gr) dose of aspirin approximately doubles the mean bleeding time for 4–7 days (5, 44). This increase in bleeding time is due not primarily to hypoprothrombinemia but rather to inhibited platelet aggregation. Although the exact mechanism remains unclear, decreased platelet aggregation may be the result of aspirin-induced inhibition of prostaglandin synthesis in the platelet (45–47). Salicylate doses of more than 6 g/day are required to reduce plasma prothrombin levels, and the minimal prolongation of prothrombin time that occurs with these doses is rarely clinically significant (5, 44). Salicylates reduce plasma prothrombin levels by interfering with the use of vitamin K for prothrombin synthesis (48).

recommended aspirin doses

effects on bleeding time

pediatric doses

Table 2. Recommended Pediatric Single Dosage Schedule for Aspirin and Acetaminophen

Age of Child, Years	Number of 80-mg Pediatric Dosage Units to Be Taken Every 4 Hours[a]	Dosage Every 4 Hours, mg	Maximum Total 24-Hour Dosage, mg
<2[b]	—	—	—
2 to <4	2	160	800
4 to <6	3	240	1200
6 to <9	4	320	1600
9 to <11	5	400	2000
11 to <12	6	480	2400

Summarized from the Report of the FDA OTC Panel on Internal Analgesic, Antipyretic, and Antirheumatic Products, *Federal Register*, *42*, 35368 (1977).

[a] Not to exceed 5 single dosages in 24 hours or to be used for more than 5 days except under the advice and supervision of a physician.

[b] There is no recommended dosage except under the advice and supervision of a physician.

cautions concerning aspirin use

GI bleeding

hypersensitivity reactions

effects on other drugs

Platelet aggregation is an important hemostatic mechanism, especially in capillaries and other small blood vessels. When small vessel damage occurs, platelets adhere to exposed collagen fibers and aggregate to form a plug. A fibrin network forms, and a clot develops to stop bleeding from the damaged vessel. Platelet aggregation is an extremely important mechanism for controlling the oozing type of capillary bleeding. Aspirin may potentiate capillary bleeding from the GI tract (49), post-tonsillectomy tonsillar bed (50), and tooth sockets following dental extractions (39). Consequently, aspirin therapy should be discontinued at least 1 week prior to surgery, and aspirin should be used to relieve the pain of tonsillectomy or dental extraction only under the advice and supervision of a physician or dentist. The FDA OTC Panel on Internal Analgesic, Antipyretic, and Antirheumatic Products recommends the following warning on all oral aspirin products to be chewed (chewable tablets or gums) (39): "Do not take this product for at least 7 days after tonsillectomy or oral surgery except under the advice and supervision of a physician."

Aspirin use should be avoided by individuals with hypoprothrombinemia, vitamin K deficiency, hemophilia, or history of other clotting disorders and by those with a history of peptic ulcer or GI bleeding. In contrast to aspirin, acetaminophen does not affect platelet aggregation and bleeding time (44, 49). A recent study demonstrated that in both normal patients and hemophiliacs a 6-week course of acetaminophen (1950 mg/day) had no effect on bleeding time or platelet aggregation (51). Therefore acetaminophen may be useful in patients where concern about hemostasis contraindicates aspirin use.

Salicylates affect uric acid secretion and reabsorption by the renal tubules. In low doses of 1–2 g/day, salicylates inhibit tubular uric acid secretion without affecting reabsorption. Consequently, low salicylate doses reduce urate excretion by the kidney, elevate plasma urate levels, and may precipitate an acute gout attack. For this reason, self-medication with salicylates by individuals with a history of gout should be discouraged.

Dyspepsia with heartburn, epigastric distress, and nausea or vomiting occurs in approximately 5% of patients taking aspirin (52). More common than dyspepsia is mild GI bleeding following aspirin ingestion in 40–70% of patients. GI blood loss usually is in the range of 2–6 ml/day, but as much as 10 ml/day has been reported (53, 54). GI blood loss usually is not clinically significant, but prolonged aspirin use may result in continued blood loss and a persistent iron-deficient anemia (55, 56). Gastroscopic examination in salicylate-treated patients often reveals ulcerative and hemorrhagic lesions of the gastric mucosa, although lesions are not always visible in those experiencing blood loss (5, 6, 57).

Massive GI bleeding characterized by the vomiting of blood (hematemesis) or the presence of large amounts of digested blood in the stools (melena) has been linked to aspirin ingestion. Approximately 30–40% of hospital admissions for hematemesis and/or melena are attributable to prior salicylate use (58–60). Individuals who take aspirin at least 4 days per week during a 12-week period have a significantly greater likelihood of suffering major GI bleeding than the less frequent user or nonuser of aspirin. The incidence rate of hospital admissions for major upper GI bleeding attributable to regular aspirin use is estimated to be about 15/100,000/year (61). Aspirin is contraindicated in individuals having a history of peptic ulcer disease or GI bleeding because it may activate latent ulcers or aggravate existing ones. In addition, ingesting alcohol with aspirin increases GI bleeding, and patients taking aspirin daily should be advised of the potential hazards of alcohol ingestion (62, 63).

In predisposed individuals, aspirin may produce a hypersensitivity reaction characterized by any of the following symptoms: shortness of breath, skin rash and edema, hives (urticaria), severe asthma attack, anaphylaxis with laryngeal edema, bronchoconstriction, and shock. Aspirin hypersensitivity occurs most frequently in persons having a history of asthma or chronic urticaria. Up to 20% of such persons may exhibit aspirin hypersensitivity (64–67). In contrast, the incidence of aspirin hypersensitivity in the general population is estimated to be 0.2–0.9% (5).

It has been suggested that there are at least two major types of aspirin hypersensitivity, which differ in mechanism, type of response, and cross-sensitivities (39). One type usually exhibits shortness of breath or asthmalike symptoms in response to aspirin. Current evidence suggests that asthmalike symptoms are related to prostaglandin synthesis inhibition by aspirin, and cross-sensitivity has been demonstrated with other prostaglandin synthesis inhibitors including flufenamic acid, ibuprofen, indomethacin, mefenamic acid, and phenylbutazone (68–70). Acetaminophen does not usually show cross-sensitivity in this group (68).

The second aspirin-hypersensitive group usually exhibits skin reactions such as edema, rash, or hives. The mechanism for this reaction may be immunological, and this group may be more susceptible to cross-sensitivity with acetaminophen (71).

A history of asthma or aspirin allergy contraindicates aspirin use for self-medication. In addition, a history of asthmalike reactions to the prostaglandin synthesis inhibitors also contraindicates self-medication with aspirin. Limited studies on cross-sensitivity suggest that in persons exhibiting asthmalike symptoms with aspirin, acetaminophen may be an acceptable analgesic/antipyretic drug. Finally, persons with known aspirin hypersensitivity should be cautioned about using other nonprescription medications which may contain aspirin.

Drug Interactions

Uricosuric agents such as probenecid and sulfinpyrazone are effective in treating gout because they block the tubular reabsorption of uric acid. Salicylates inhibit the uricosuric effects of both drugs by blocking this inhibitory effect on uric acid reabsorption (72, 73). Consequently, the concurrent administration of salicylates with either probenecid or sulfinpyrazone should be avoided because of the possibility of precipitating acute gouty attacks, hyperuricemia, or urate stone formation.

Because of their effects on hemostasis and GI mucosa, salicylates have the potential for producing hemorrhaging if administered with oral anticoagulants. The effect of oral anticoagulants on bleeding time may be enhanced by the salicylates, and the severity of salicylate-induced GI bleeding may be augmented as a result of hemostasis impairment by anticoagulant drugs (74). It is advised that the concurrent administration of aspirin and oral anticoagulants be avoided. For analgesic/antipyretic activity, acetaminophen is recommended for self-medication in patients receiving oral anticoagulant therapy (75).

Several reports suggest that the lowering of blood glucose levels by the sulfonylurea oral hypoglycemics may be enhanced when aspirin is administered concurrently. Salicylates displace tolbutamide and chlorpropamide from plasma protein binding sites and have intrinsic hypoglycemic activity when taken by diabetics (5, 76). Controlled clinical studies documenting the significance of this interaction are lacking. However, in view of existing evidence, it is advisable to monitor closely diabetics who are receiving both salicylates and a sulfonylurea hypoglycemic agent. In recommending a nonprescription analgesic for concurrent administration, the pharmacist should take into consideration that acetaminophen seems to have less potential for interaction than the salicylates.

All anti-inflammatory drugs used to treat arthritis and other inflammatory diseases are potentially ulcerogenic. Because of possible enhanced GI erosion when these agents are used in combination with aspirin, it is recommended that persons taking prescription anti-inflammatory drugs should not self-medicate concurrently with salicylates (39).

Salicylate Toxicity

Mild salicylate toxicity may occur in adults after repeated administration of large doses or in young children as a result of therapeutic overdosage. Symptoms consist of dizziness, ringing in the ears, difficulty in hearing, nausea, vomiting, diarrhea, mental confusion, and lassitude (5). Skin eruptions may appear if salicylates are continued for a week or longer, and more pronounced CNS symptoms may develop, e.g., incoherent speech, delirium, or hallucinations.

The mean lethal aspirin dose in adults is 20–30 g, and the toxic dose for children is 0.15 g/kg (77, 78). Symptoms of salicylate poisoning include those cited for mild toxicity along with hyperventilation, dimness of vision, mental confusion, delirium, hallucinations, convulsions, and coma. Acid–base disturbances are prominent and vary from respiratory alkalosis to metabolic acidosis. Initially, salicylate effects on the respiratory center in the medulla produce hyperventilation and respiratory alkalosis. In severely intoxicated adults and in most children under 5, respiratory alkalosis rapidly changes to metabolic acidosis (5, 78).

Salicylate poisoning affects other physiological functions. Metabolic rate is increased, resulting in increased heat production and fever. Children are more prone than adults to develop high fever in salicylate poisoning (77). Hypoglycemia results from increased tissue glucose use and may be especially serious in children (5). Bleeding may occur from the GI tract due to erosion of the mucosal lining, or hemorrhaging from other sites may occur as a consequence of aspirin inhibition of platelet aggregation (77, 78).

Emergency management of aspirin poisoning is designed to delay drug absorption and to remove it from the stomach. If the person is conscious and able to swallow, one or two glasses of milk should be given to dilute the drug, delay gastric emptying, and slow absorption. However, the volume of liquid given to children should not exceed 50 ml/10 kg (79).

Activated charcoal (50 g in 400 ml of water) may be given orally in a dose of 5 ml/kg and is very effective in delaying aspirin absorption from the stomach. However, syrup of ipecac is not effective used in combination with activated charcoal. Because of the rapid absorption of salicylates from the GI tract, emptying the stomach at home or en route to an emergency medical facility is advised. Vomiting should be induced even if the patient has vomited spontaneously. An emetic of 1 tbsp (15 ml) of syrup of ipecac followed by half a glass of water should be given. If emesis does not occur in 30 minutes, the process should be repeated with the same ipecac dose. For children under 1 year of age, the dose should be 2 tsp (10 ml) of syrup of ipecac. Administering fluids to a person convulsing or to one who is not completely conscious is absolutely contraindicated (77–79).

Biopharmaceutics of Aspirin-Containing Products

The rate-limiting step for achieving therapeutic blood levels with solid dosage forms of aspirin is dissolution into rather than absorption from GI fluids (80). Factors affecting dissolution rate include the degree of GI motility, the gastric fluid pH, and the diffusion layer pH (the region of high salicylate concentration surrounding the dissolving aspirin particles). Aspirin's dissolution rate is increased by raising the pH of the surrounding medium (81). Including alkaline buffering agents in the tablet formulation produces an elevated pH in the diffusion layer, increasing the aspirin's dissolution rate. If formulated properly, buffered aspirin has significantly greater dissolution and absorption rates than nonbuffered aspirin (39, 82, 83). However, there is no evidence from controlled clinical studies that buffered aspirin provides a more rapid onset or greater degree of pain relief than nonbuffered aspirin (39, 82).

The degree of salicylate-induced gastric irritation and erosion is a function of the salicylate concentration and the duration of exposure at the gastric mucosal surface. Although aspirin solutions also may produce GI erosion, undissolved aspirin particles are thought to be primarily responsible for gastric mucosal damage because they produce high salicylate concentrations at mucosal surfaces in the region of their diffusion layer (84). Buffered aspirin tablets produce less GI bleeding than nonbuffered tablets, presumably because they dissolve more rapidly, reducing the exposure time of the gastric mucosa to the offending aspirin particles (82, 85).

Aspirin is absorbed more rapidly in solution than from either buffered or nonbuffered tablets because the dissolution factor is eliminated (83). Highly buffered aspirin solutions with a neutralizing capacity of at least

drug interactions
toxicity
emergency overdose treatment
dissolution factors
buffered aspirin

20 mEq of hydrochloric acid significantly decrease the amount of gastric bleeding (86, 87). However, the effervescent-type buffered aspirin solutions achieve their buffering action at the expense of a high sodium content. For this reason their use by patients whose sodium intake is restricted should be avoided. In addition, there is no valid evidence that highly buffered aspirin solutions produce more rapid or effective analgesia than either plain or buffered aspirin tablets (82).

Enteric-coated aspirin is specially formulated to prevent tablet dissolution until it reaches the more alkaline pH of the small intestine, preventing the gastric distress associated with dissolution in the stomach. However, aspirin absorption from enteric-coated tablets may be highly erratic. Tablets sometimes dissolve prematurely in the stomach or possibly not at all (88). The variable aspirin absorption from enteric-coated tablets also is caused by differences in the tablets' gastric retention time (89, 90).

biopharmaceutic considerations

formulation factors

other salicylates

dosage regimen

liquid salicylate preparation

aspirin use during pregnancy

Timed-release aspirin is a formulation using encapsulation techniques attempting to prolong the product's duration of action. Such products are not useful for rapid pain relief because their absorption is delayed. However, the prolonged absorption may make timed-release aspirin useful as a bedtime medication. Studies show that 6–8 hours after ingestion of a single 1300-mg aspirin dose the total serum salicylate concentration is significantly higher with the timed-release product tested than with regular tableted aspirin (91). Timed-release aspirin has been implicated in hemorrhagic gastritis (92), but definitive clinical studies are not available (93).

Other Aspirin and Salicylate Dosage Forms

Carbaspirin calcium is a complex of urea and calcium acetylsalicylate which is hydrolyzed in the GI tract to aspirin, calcium, and urea (94). Although it may be absorbed more rapidly, there is no evidence that it offers a clinically significant advantage over aspirin in the rate at which analgesia is achieved (95). Because it is a larger molecule than aspirin, 414 mg is required to produce the same pharmacological effect as 325 mg of aspirin. The recommended adult dose is 414–828 mg every 4 hours while symptoms persist, not to exceed 4968 mg in 24 hours (39).

Choline salicylate is the only liquid salicylate preparation currently available. It is absorbed from the stomach more rapidly than aspirin in tablet form, but this property has little clinical significance (39, 95). Evidence suggests that choline salicylate is less potent than aspirin as an analgesic/antipyretic; however, it may produce less GI bleeding and distress (34, 39, 95). A dose of 435 mg of choline salicylate is equivalent to 325 mg of sodium salicylate. The recommended adult dose is 435–870 mg every 4 hours, not to exceed 5220 mg in 24 hours (39).

Magnesium salicylate is equivalent to sodium salicylate in analgesic/antipyretic potency. Claims remain to be proven that it might be indicated when aspirin cannot be tolerated (39). In addition, the possibility of systemic magnesium toxicity exists in persons with renal insufficiency who take maximum daily doses of magnesium salicylate. The recommended adult dose is 325–650 mg every 4 hours, not to exceed 4000 mg in 24 hours (39).

Sodium salicylate produces blood salicylate levels as high as equimolar doses of aspirin; however, it is probably less effective than aspirin as an analgesic/antipyretic (96). The sodium content of the maximum daily sodium salicylate dose (25 mEq) is sufficient to contraindicate its use in persons on sodium-restricted diets. The recommended adult dose of sodium salicylate is 325–650 mg every 4 hours, not to exceed 4000 mg in 24 hours (39).

Aspirin and Pregnancy

Recent evidence from studies in laboratory animals and from retrospective studies in humans suggests that aspirin use during the later months of pregnancy has adverse effects on both the mother and the fetus. The administration of 200 mg/kg/day of aspirin to rats during the last 6 days of pregnancy produced a prolongation of labor, a prolongation of parturition time, and increased in utero fetal death (97).

A 20-year retrospective study of 103 women who took aspirin doses greater than 3250 mg/day during the last 6 months of pregnancy suggests that aspirin has detrimental effects on pregnancy. In comparison with control groups of women, those using aspirin had significantly ($p < 0.05$) longer gestation periods, longer labor periods, and greater blood loss at delivery. These effects on pregnancy may be related to its inhibition of prostaglandin synthesis, platelet aggregation, and prothrombin synthesis (98).

Studies of 144 Australian women who used aspirin-containing OTC analgesic preparations during pregnancy reached similar conclusions (99, 100). The major effects reported for regular aspirin use during pregnancy included an increased frequency of anemia during pregnancy, a prolonged gestation period, an increased incidence of complicated deliveries, a high incidence of antepartum and postpartum hemorrhage, increased perinatal mortality, and decreased neonate birth weight.

Interpretation of these results is complicated, however, by a higher incidence of smoking in the aspirin-using group and by the fact that the OTC analgesic products used by these women were combinations of either aspirin, salicylamide, and caffeine or aspirin, phenacetin, and caffeine. Smoking has been established to have numerous detrimental effects on pregnancy including lower birth weight of the neonate, increased perinatal mortality, and increased spontaneous abortion (101). In addition, a study of 1515 mother–child pairs exposed to aspirin for at least 8 days per month during at least 6 months of the pregnancy found "no evidence that aspirin as used by pregnant women in the United States is related to perinatal mortality or low birth weight" (102). It is possible therefore that the differences in perinatal mortality and birth weight reported in the Australian studies (99, 100) are due to confounding factors such as smoking rather than totally to aspirin use.

In attempting to reconcile the Australian (99, 100) and U.S. (102) reports, the amount and frequency of aspirin use also must be considered. In the Australian study the group of women showing the greatest incidence of detrimental aspirin effect on pregnancy admitted taking OTC analgesic preparations every day during the pregnancy. This dosage represented a higher frequency of aspirin use than that evaluated in the U.S. study.

Aspirin readily traverses the placenta and often is found in higher concentration in the blood of the neonate than in that of the mother (100, 103, 104). Normal analgesic aspirin doses taken by the mother prior to delivery may decrease platelet aggregation in the neonate (105) and possibly produce clinical bleeding (106). As a consequence of these observations, the FDA OTC Panel on Internal Analgesic, Antipyretic, and Antirheumatic Products has recommended that aspirin-containing products not be used during the last 3 months of pregnancy except under the advice and supervision of a physician (39).

The *p*-Aminophenols

Analgesic compounds in this class include acetaminophen and phenacetin. These compounds are analgesic/antipyretic and are effective in treating mild to moderate pain such as headache, neuralgia, and pain of musculoskeletal origin (34, 107). The major part of a phenacetin dose is biotransformed to acetaminophen, which is thought to be primarily responsible for the compound's analgesic/antipyretic activity (108). However, phenacetin also has been shown to have intrinsic analgesic/antipyretic activity in laboratory animals (108, 109). The mechanism and site of analgesic action of these compounds have not been definitely established (5).

Dosage Considerations

Studies document the analgesic efficacy of phenacetin and acetaminophen in doses of 300–600 mg (110–113). The recommended adult dose of acetaminophen is 325–650 mg every 4 hours, not to exceed a total of 3900 mg in 24 hours. Table 2 gives the recommended acetaminophen pediatric dosage. Although comparative analgesic effectiveness is difficult to establish because of the nature of existing clinical testing procedures, acetaminophen and phenacetin are about as potent as aspirin as analgesics and antipyretics (34). However, a single 1000-mg acetaminophen dose is less effective than 600 mg of aspirin in relieving pain associated with rheumatoid arthritis when it is given as an analgesic supplement to regular anti-inflammatory drug therapy (114).

Both phenacetin and acetaminophen are effective antipyretic agents, and both reduce fever by acting on the hypothalamic thermoregulatory center to increase body heat dissipation. Acetaminophen reduces fever by inhibiting the action of endogenous pyrogen on the hypothalamus, probably by inhibiting prostaglandin synthesis (38, 115, 116). In febrile individuals, both compounds begin to reduce body temperature about 30 minutes after administration and produce their peak effect in 2–4 hours (110). Clinical studies indicate that acetaminophen and aspirin are equally effective as antipyretics (117–119).

Although there are reports of minimal anti-inflammatory activity with acetaminophen, the *p*-aminophenols have no therapeutic use as anti-inflammatory drugs in rheumatoid arthritis treatment (5, 34, 107, 120).

Toxicity of *p*-Aminophenols

Although methemoglobin production contributes to phenacetin toxicity in acute overdose, therapeutic phenacetin doses in the range 1–2 g/day cause only minimal methemoglobinemia, which is usually of no clinical significance (5). Phenacetin-induced hemolytic anemia has been associated most frequently with chronic drug ingestion; however, clinically significant hemolysis may occur with the administration of a single dose of phenacetin. Phenacetin produces hemolytic anemia in an individual deficient in glucose-6-phosphate dehydrogenase or in an immunologically sensitive individual (121). Glucose-6-phosphate dehydrogenase deficiency is a genetically transferable enzyme deficiency which predisposes a person to acute, drug-induced hemolytic episodes. This deficiency occurs rarely in Americans of West European genetic origin but has an incidence of about 13% in American Negroes (122). In contrast, acetaminophen rarely produces hemolytic anemia and produces almost no methemoglobin formation (123–125).

acetaminophen

phenacetin

Because it lacks many undesirable effects produced by aspirin, acetaminophen is gaining favor in this country as the "common household analgesic" (5, 126). However, there is also growing concern that increasing household availability and the public's lack of recognition of acetaminophen's acute toxicity will produce a new health hazard (127–130). Acetaminophen poisoning may produce fatal hepatic necrosis (131–133).

In adults, symptoms of acute toxicity may occur following the ingestion of more than 7 g (134); however, reversible liver damage has been reported in a 16-year-old woman after ingestion of a single 5.85-g dose (135). A single oral ingestion of 15–25 g is seriously hepatotoxic and potentially fatal (136–138). Estimates of the ingested acetaminophen dose are not reliable predictors of potential hepatotoxicity. Plasma acetaminophen levels should be determined following ingestion of a potentially toxic amount, and nomograms have been established to relate plasma acetaminophen levels to the likelihood of hepatotoxicity (139, 140). The plasma acetaminophen half-life is prolonged in cases of hepatotoxicity and is a valuable predictor of hepatic necrosis. If the plasma acetaminophen half-life exceeds 4 hours, hepatic necrosis is likely to occur (141).

The progression of symptoms with acetaminophen poisoning include: vomiting within a few hours; anorexia, nausea, and stomach pain within 24 hours; evidence of liver injury in 2–4 days with jaundice; and death at any time in 2–7 days (5, 134). In addition, kidney damage, disturbances in clotting mechanisms, metabolic acidosis, hypoglycemia, and myocardial necrosis may occur (5, 128, 129). In nonfatal cases the hepatic damage is usually reversible (142). Emergency first aid treatment of acetaminophen poisoning should include emesis with syrup of ipecac (142). Activated charcoal will reduce acetaminophen absorption significantly but is most effective if given within the first 30 minutes following acetaminophen ingestion (143). The dose and contraindication considerations for syrup of ipecac and activated charcoal previously discussed for salicylate poisoning also apply to acetaminophen overdose. The oral administration of a solution of acetylcysteine (Mucomyst) has been reported to be beneficial in preventing the hepatic necrosis of acetaminophen poisoning (144, 145) and is currently being evaluated for this purpose. The oral dose of acetylcysteine recommended by the Rocky Mountain Poison Center for acetaminophen poisoning is: loading dose of 140 mg/kg, followed in 4 hours with a maintenance dosage regimen of 70 mg/kg every 4 hours for 17 doses. Dilute the commercially available product with Coca Cola, Pepsi, Fresca, or unsweetened grapefruit juice to a 5% solution (146).

acetaminophen poisoning treatment

Salicylamide

Although it is structurally similar to salicylates, salicylamide is not converted to salicylate in the body, and its pharmacological activity resides in the salicylamide molecule itself (147). Salicylamide's unusual pharmacokinetic character complicates interpretation of the compound's efficacy and formulation factors. Oral salicylamide doses below 600 mg are almost completely metabolized to inactive metabolites during transit through the GI mucosa and hepatic circulation before ever reaching the systemic circulation. Consequently, "breakthrough doses" greater than 300–600 mg are required to saturate the intestinal and hepatic enzyme systems and to achieve effective systemic concentrations (39, 148).

Salicylamide has been shown to have greater analgesic effects in animals than aspirin (149, 150); however, studies in humans with pathological pain have shown that salicylamide has no superiority over aspirin in doses below 600 mg and is indistinguishable from placebo (34, 39). Salicylamide has been proven consistently inferior to aspirin as an antipyretic in both animal and human studies and is currently estimated to be about half as potent as aspirin as an antipyretic (34, 39, 151, 152). Persons allergic to aspirin usually have no cross-sensitivity to salicylamide, and salicylamide does not increase prothrombin time (39, 153). The FDA OTC Panel on Internal Analgesic, Antipyretic, and Antirheumatic Products concluded (39) that salicylamide is "ineffective in the currently recommended doses of 300–600 mg."

analgesic nephropathy

Analgesic Renal Toxicity

Reports first appeared in the 1950's linking chronic analgesic use to renal papillary necrosis and interstitial nephritis (154–157). The syndrome is characterized by asymptomatic sloughing of renal papillary tissue, sometimes with the elimination of "brown lumps" of necrotic tissue in the urine. Tissue necrosis may be accompanied by oliguria, nausea and vomiting, massive diuresis, or hematuria. Anemia may be present as the syndrome progresses, and final stages include renal insufficiency, hypertension, and death (158).

Analgesic nephropathy has been linked most consistently to the use of phenacetin-containing analgesic combination products. Current opinion suggests that aspirin alone is not an initiator of nephropathy but that it may worsen or perpetuate the progression of papillary necrosis and renal dysfunction (159–165). Aspirin-induced inhibition of prostaglandin synthesis has been suggested to contribute to the nephrotoxicity of aspirin–phenacetin combinations by causing ischemic changes in the ascending loop of Henle predisposing to phenacetin-induced tissue necrosis (39, 166).

Phenacetin appears to be used chronically not for analgesia but to elicit stimulant and euphoric effects. In the United States, data indicate that phenacetin-containing products are involved in almost all reported cases of analgesic-induced kidney disease (39). Numerous epidemiological studies suggest temporal and dose relationships between phenacetin ingestion and renal dysfunction (167–173), and follow-up studies in countries after complete removal of phenacetin from nonprescription use support the causality assumption (167, 173). Prolonged use of phenacetin-containing analgesics also has been associated with cancer of the renal pelvis and urinary bladder (174–177).

PRODUCT SELECTION GUIDELINES

In evaluating the relative merits of nonprescription internal analgesic products, the choices are aspirin or acetaminophen and the formulation of the product. Aspirin is the most frequently used nonprescription analgesic except when specifically contraindicated because of its effects on hemostasis or GI erosion or in cases of allergic hypersensitivity. Buffered aspirin has the advantage of producing less GI distress but retains the other contraindications of aspirin. Highly buffered aspirin solutions produce less GI erosion, but they contain large amounts of sodium and should not be used by individuals on low-sodium diets. Enteric-coated aspirin products may reduce the likelihood of GI erosion but have a longer onset of action due to their delayed and possibly incomplete absorption. The delayed onset of such products precludes their use in acute pain when prompt relief is desired.

In many cases, acetaminophen is the drug of choice. It is less likely to trigger asthmalike symptoms in asthmatics, but hypersensitivity reactions to the drug have been reported (178). Because acetaminophen does not cause gastric mucosal erosion and does not affect platelet function, it may be recommended for individuals with a history of peptic ulcer disease (179). Although acetaminophen in a dose of 650 mg four times per day for a 2-week period significantly increases prothrombin time, two 650-mg doses 4 hours apart do not (180, 181). In addition, a 6-week course of acetaminophen (1950 mg/day) does not affect bleeding time or platelet aggregation (51). Consequently, the intermittent use of acetaminophen by individuals receiving oral anticoagulant therapy should present no serious interaction. Because of its lack of anti-inflammatory activity, acetaminophen is not an acceptable substitute for aspirin in treating rheumatoid arthritis and similar inflammatory conditions. Acetaminophen is the nonprescription analgesic of choice for patients taking uricosuric drugs because it does not antagonize the uricosuric effect (178). In addition, acetaminophen's stability in liquid dosage forms provides a convenient and palatable pediatric analgesic/antipyretic preparation.

The rationale for including caffeine in many analgesic combinations remains obscure. According to the FDA Panel (39), "There is some inconclusive evidence to suggest that caffeine may exert additional analgesia when used in combination with other analgesics." An evaluation of analgesic combinations in treating cancer pain showed that 65 mg of caffeine did not increase significantly the analgesic efficacy of 650 mg of aspirin (182).

Recent claims promoting "extra-strength pain relievers" require clarification. Such products are usually combinations of several analgesic ingredients and may include acetaminophen, salicylamide, and aspirin. Because the total analgesic ingredients may be more than 325 mg, or 5 gr, the implication in these products' promotional materials is that they are "stronger" and hence more effective. These claims only confuse the consumer because combinations have not been proven more effective than the sum of their individual ingredients. In most controlled clinical trials, pain relief provided by analgesic combinations has not been superior to that of aspirin alone (5).

SUMMARY

The appropriate choice of an analgesic agent involves a consideration of both patient and drug factors. In determining the drug of choice for recommendation, the pharmacist must consider the following factors: the condition being treated; the nature and origin of the pain or fever; accompanying symptoms; a history of asthma or other allergic disease, hypersensitivity reactions, peptic ulcer, or clotting disorders; and the concomitant use of other medication. In addition, product selection must include evaluation of the product's proven efficacy, formulation factors, and the potential for adverse effects.

REFERENCES

(1) D. R. Haslam, *Br. J. Psychol.*, *58*, 139 (1967).
(2) H. K. Beecher, in "Nonspecific Factors in Drug Therapy," K. Rickels, Ed., Charles C Thomas, Springfield, Ill., 1968, p. 27.
(3) A. C. Guyton, "Textbook of Medical Physiology," 5th ed., Saunders, Philadelphia, Pa., 1976, pp. 662–677.
(4) V. B. Mountcastle, "Medical Physiology," Vol. 1, 13th ed., Mosby, St. Louis, Mo., 1974, pp. 348–381.
(5) "The Pharmacological Basis of Therapeutics," 5th ed., L. S. Goodman and A. Gilman, Eds., Macmillan, New York, N.Y., 1975, pp. 325–358.
(6) M. L. Tainter and A. J. Ferris, "Aspirin in Modern Therapy," Sterling Drug Inc., New York, N.Y., 1969, p. 43.
(7) H. G. Wolff, "Headache and Other Head Pain," 2nd ed., Oxford University Press, New York, N.Y., 1963.
(8) "Textbook of Medicine," 14th ed., P. B. Beeson and W. McDermott, Eds., Saunders, Philadelphia, Pa., 1975, pp. 614–619.
(9) "Harrison's Principles of Internal Medicine," 8th ed., G. W. Thorn, R. D. Adams, E. Braunwald, K. J. Isselbacher, and R. G. Petersdorf, Eds., McGraw-Hill, New York, N.Y., 1977, pp. 20–28.
(10) S. V. Deshmukh and J. S. Meyer, *Stroke*, *7*, 11 (1976).
(11) J. R. Couch, *Neurology*, *26*, 348 (1976).
(12) S. V. Deshmukh and J. S. Meyer, *Headache*, *17*, 101 (1977).
(13) J. Edmeads, *Headache*, *17*, 148 (1977).
(14) D. J. Dalessio, *J. Am. Med. Assoc.*, *239*, 52 (1978).
(15) "Textbook of Medicine," 13th ed., P. B. Beeson and W. McDermott, Eds., Saunders, Philadelphia, Pa., 1971, pp. 149–154.
(16) "The Merck Manual," 12th ed., Merck Sharp & Dohme Research Laboratories, Rahway, N.J., 1972, p. 1304.
(17) W. S. Gilmer, Jr., in "Concepts of Disease," J. B. Brunson and E. A. Gall, Eds., Macmillan, New York, N.Y., 1971, p. 746.
(18) "Textbook of Medicine," 14th ed., P. B. Beeson and W. McDermott, Eds., Saunders, Philadelphia, Pa., 1975, p. 142.
(19) "The Merck Manual," 12th ed., Merck Sharp & Dohme Research Laboratories, Rahway, N.J., 1972, p. 1222.
(20) "Textbook of Medicine," 14th ed., P. B. Beeson and W. McDermott, Eds., Saunders, Philadelphia, Pa., 1975, p. 161.
(21) A. S. Milton, *J. Pharm. Pharmacol.*, *28*, 393 (1976).
(22) L. Weinstein and M. N. Swartz, in "Pathologic Physiology—Mechanisms of Disease," 5th ed., W. A. Sodeman, Jr., and W. A. Sodeman, Eds., Saunders, Philadelphia, Pa., 1974, pp. 473–488.
(23) W. Feldberg and K. P. Gupta, *J. Physiol. (London)*, *228*, 41 (1973).
(24) W. Feldberg, K. P. Gupta, A. S. Milton, and S. Wendlandt, *J. Physiol. (London)*, *234*, 279 (1973).
(25) W. Feldberg and P. N. Saxena, *J. Physiol. (London)*, *217*, 547 (1971).
(26) W. Feldberg and P. N. Saxena, *J. Physiol. (London)*, *219*, 739 (1971).
(27) C. A. Harvey and A. S. Milton, *J. Physiol. (London)*, *250*, 18P (1975).
(28) C. A. Harvey, A. S. Milton, and D. W. Straughan, *J. Physiol. (London)*, *248*, 26P (1975).
(29) A. S. Milton and S. Wendlandt, *J. Physiol. (London)*, *207*, 76P (1970).
(30) A. S. Milton, *J. Pharm. Pharmacol.*, *28*, 393 (1976).
(31) F. Allison, Jr., in "Concepts of Disease," J. G. Brunson and E. A. Gall, Eds., Macmillan, New York, N.Y., 1971, p. 443.
(32) A. C. Guyton, "Textbook of Medical Physiology," 5th ed., Saunders, Philadelphia, Pa., 1976.
(33) "Manual of Medical Therapeutics," 20th ed., M. G. Rosenfeld, Ed., Little, Brown, Boston, Mass., 1971, p. 236.
(34) W. T. Beaver, *Am. J. Med. Sci.*, *250*, 577 (1965) and *251*, 576 (1966).
(35) R. K. Lim, F. Guzman, D. W. Rodgers, K. Goto, C. Braun, G. D. Dickerson, and R. J. Engle, *Arch. Intern. Pharmacodyn. Ther.*, *152*, 25 (1964).
(36) S. H. Ferreira, *Nature New Biol.*, *240*, 200 (1972).
(37) J. R. Vane, *Nature New Biol.*, *231*, 232 (1971).
(38) R. J. Flower, *Am. Heart J.*, *86*, 844 (1973).
(39) *Federal Register*, *42*, 35368 (1977).
(40) S. H. Ferreira and J. R. Vane, *Annu. Rev. Pharmacol.*, *14*, 57 (1974).
(41) A. Willis, *J. Pharm. Pharmacol.*, *21*, 126 (1969).
(42) T. J. Williams and M. J. Peck, *Nature*, *270*, 530 (1977).
(43) T. J. Williams, *Br. J. Pharmacol.*, *56*, 341P (1976).
(44) J. H. Weiss, in "Aspirin, Platelets and Stroke," W. S. Fields and W. K. Hass, Eds., W. H. Green, St. Louis, Mo., 1971, p. 54.
(45) J. R. O'Brien, *Br. J. Haematol.*, *29*, 523 (1975).
(46) J. B. Smith and A. L. Willis, *Nature*, *231*, 235 (1971).
(47) H. J. Weiss, *Am. Heart J.*, *92*, 86 (1976).
(48) K. P. Link, R. S. Overman, W. R. Sullivan, C. F. Huebner, and L. D. Scheel, *J. Biol. Chem.*, *147*, 463 (1943).
(49) C. Pochedly and G. Ente, *Pediatr. Clin. North Am.*, *19*, 1104 (1972).
(50) S. H. Reuter and W. W. Montgomery, *Arch. Otolaryngol.*, *80*, 214 (1964).
(51) C. H. Mielke, D. Heiden, A. F. Britten, J. Ramos, and P. Flavell, *J. Am. Med. Assoc.*, *235*, 613 (1976).
(52) A. Muir, in "Salicylates—An International Symposium," A. St. J. Dixon, B. K. Martin, M. J. H. Smith, and P. H. N. Wood, Eds., J. & A. Churchill, London, England, 1963, p. 230.
(53) L. T. Stubbe, *Br. Med. J.*, *2*, 1062 (1958).
(54) M. I. Grossman, K. K. Matsumoto, and R. J. Lichter, *Gastroenterology*, *40*, 383 (1961).
(55) W. H. J. Summerskill and A. S. Alvarez, *Lancet*, *2*, 925 (1958).
(56) H. Heggarty, *Br. Med. J.*, *1*, 491 (1974).
(57) H. E. Paulus and M. W. Whitehouse, *Annu. Rev. Pharmacol.*, *13*, 107 (1973).
(58) A. Muir and I. A. Cossar, *Br. Med. J.*, *2*, 7 (1955).
(59) H. F. Lange, *Gastroenterology*, *33*, 778 (1957).
(60) A. S. Alvarez and W. H. J. Summerskill, *Lancet*, *2*, 920 (1958).
(61) M. Levy, *N. Engl. J. Med.*, *290*, 1158 (1974).
(62) K. Goulston and A. R. Cooke, *Br. Med. J.*, *4*, 664 (1968).
(63) C. D. Needham, J. Kyle, P. F. Jones, S. J. Johnson, and D. F. Kerridge, *Gut*, *12*, 819 (1971).
(64) G. A. Settipane and F. H. Chafee, *J. Allergy Clin. Immunol.*, *53*, 200 (1974).
(65) B. Giraldo, M. N. Blumenthal, and W. W. Spink, *Ann. Intern. Med.*, *71*, 479 (1969).
(66) B. T. Fein, *J. Allergy*, *29*, 598 (1971).
(67) M. Moore-Robinson and R. P. Warin, *Br. Med. J.*, *4*, 262 (1967).
(68) A. Szczeklik, R. J. Gryglewski, and G. Czerniawska-Mysik, *Br. Med. J.*, *1*, 67 (1975).
(69) A. Szczeklik and G. Czerniawska-Mysik, *Lancet*, *1*, 488 (1976).
(70) A. Szczeklik, R. J. Gryglewski, G. Czerniawska-Mysik, and A. Zmuda, *J. Allergy Clin. Immunol.*, *58*, 10 (1976).
(71) J. A. M. Phills, L. Perelmutter, and A. Liakopoulou, *J. Allergy Clin. Immunol.*, *49*, 97 (1972).
(72) T. F. Yü, P. G. Dayton, and A. B. Gutman, *J. Clin. Invest.*, *42*, 1330 (1963).
(73) "Evaluations of Drug Interactions," 2nd ed., APhA, Washington, D.C., 1976, p. 226.

(74) *Ibid.*, p. 270.
(75) *Ibid.*, p. 263.
(76) H. Wishinsky, E. J. Glasser, and S. Perkal, *Diabetes*, suppl., *11*, 18 (1962).
(77) R. E. Gosselin, H. C. Hodge, R. P. Smith, and M. N. Gleason, "Clinical Toxicology of Commercial Products," 3rd ed., Williams and Wilkins, Baltimore, Md., 1969, pp. 209–214.
(78) H. B. Andrews, *Am. Fam. Physician*, *8*, 102 (1973).
(79) H. R. Dreisbach, "Handbook of Poisoning: Diagnosis and Treatment," 9th ed., Lange Medical, Los Altos, Calif., 1977, pp. 14–21, 285–290.
(80) G. Levy and J. R. Leonards, in "The Salicylates—A Critical Bibliographic Review," M. J. H. Smith and P. K. Smith, Eds., Interscience, New York, N.Y., 1966, pp. 5–47.
(81) G. Levy, in "Salicylates—An International Symposium," A. St. J. Dixon, B. K. Martin, M. J. H. Smith, and P. H. N. Wood, Eds., J. & A. Churchill, London, England, 1963, pp. 9–16.
(82) *Medical Letter on Drugs and Therapeutics*, *16*, 57 (1974).
(83) J. R. Leonards, *Clin. Pharmacol. Ther.*, *4*, 476 (1963).
(84) K. W. Anderson, in "Salicylates—An International Symposium," A. St. J. Dixon, B. K. Martin, M. J. H. Smith, and P. H. N. Wood, Eds., J. & A. Churchill, London, England, 1963, pp. 217–223.
(85) J. R. Leonards and G. Levy, *Arch. Intern. Med.*, *129*, 457 (1972).
(86) J. R. Leonards and G. Levy, *Clin. Pharmacol. Ther.*, *10*, 571 (1969).
(87) P. H. Wood, E. A. Harvey-Smith, and A. S. Dixon, *Br. Med. J.*, *1*, 669 (1962).
(88) L. Stubbe, J. H. Pietersen, and C. van Heulen, *Br. Med. J.*, *1*, 675 (1962).
(89) E. Nelson, *Clin. Pharmacol. Ther.*, *4*, 283 (1963).
(90) J. R. Leonards and G. Levy, *J. Am. Med. Assoc.*, *193*, 99 (1965).
(91) L. E. Hollister, *Clin. Pharmacol. Ther.*, *13*, 1 (1972).
(92) J. R. Hoon, *J. Am. Med. Assoc.*, *229*, 841 (1974).
(93) R. John, *J. Am. Med. Assoc.*, *230*, 823 (1974).
(94) "Merck Index," 8th ed., Merck and Co., Rahway, N.J., 1968, p. 189.
(95) "Drugs of Choice 1978–1979," W. Modell, Ed., Mosby, St. Louis, Mo., 1978, pp. 210–211.
(96) "AMA Drug Evaluations," 3rd ed., Publishing Sciences Group, Littleton, Mass., 1977, p. 345.
(97) H. Tuchmann-Duplessis, D. Hiss, G. Mottot, and I. Rosner, *Toxicology*, *3*, 207 (1975).
(98) R. B. Lewis and J. D. Schulman, *Lancet*, *2*, 1159 (1973).
(99) E. Collins and G. Turner, *Lancet*, *2*, 335 (1975).
(100) G. Turner and E. Collins, *Lancet*, *2*, 338 (1975).
(101) J. E. Fielding, *N. Engl. J. Med.*, *298*, 337 (1978).
(102) S. Shapiro, R. R. Monson, D. W. Kaufman, V. Siskin, O. P. Heinonin, and D. Slone, *Lancet*, *1*, 1375 (1976).
(103) G. Levy and L. K. Garrettson, *Pediatrics*, *53*, 201 (1974).
(104) P. A. Palmisano and G. Cassady, *J. Am. Med. Assoc.*, *209*, 556 (1969).
(105) W. A. Bleyer and R. T. Breckenridge, *J. Am. Med. Assoc.*, *213*, 2049 (1970).
(106) R. R. Haslam, H. Ekert, and G. L. Gillam, *J. Pediatr.*, *84*, 556 (1974).
(107) L. O. Randall, in "Physiological Pharmacology," Vol. 1, W. S. Root and F. G. Hofmann, Eds., Academic, New York, N.Y., 1963, pp. 356–369. 356–369.
(108) B. B. Brodie and J. Axelrod, *J. Pharmacol. Exp. Ther.*, *97*, 58 (1949).
(109) A. H. Conney, M. Sansur, F. Soroko, R. Koster, and J. J. Burns, *J. Pharmacol. Exp. Ther.*, *151*, 133 (1966).
(110) P. K. Smith, "Acetophenetidin—A Critical Bibliographic Review," Interscience, New York, N.Y., 1958.
(111) F. B. Flinn and B. B. Brodie, *J. Pharmacol. Exp. Ther.*, *94*, 76 (1948).
(112) S. L. Wallenstein and R. W. Houde, *Fed. Proc. Fed. Am. Soc. Exp. Biol.*, *13*, 414 (1954).
(113) D. R. L. Newton and J. M. Tanner, *Br. Med. J.*, *2*, 1096 (1956).
(114) E. C. Huskisson, *Br. Med. J.*, *4*, 196 (1974).
(115) W. G. Clark and S. G. Moyer, *J. Pharmacol. Exp. Ther.*, *181*, 183 (1972).
(116) R. J. Flower and J. R. Vane, *Nature*, *240*, 410 (1972).
(117) A. N. Eden, *Am. J. Dis. Child.*, *114*, 284 (1967).
(118) M. T. Colgan and A. A. Mintz, *J. Pediatr.*, *50*, 552 (1957).
(119) L. Tarlin, P. Landrigan, R. Babineau, and J. J. Alpert, *Am. J. Dis. Child.*, *124*, 880 (1972).
(120) J. Hajnal, J. Sharp, and A. J. Popert, *Ann. Rheum. Dis.*, *18*, 189 (1959).
(121) M. Swanson, *Drug Intell. Clin. Pharm.*, *7*, 6 (1973).
(122) P. A. Parks and J. Banks, *Ann. N.Y. Acad. Sci.*, *123*, 198 (1965).
(123) "AMA Drug Evaluations," 3rd ed., Publishing Sciences Group, Littleton, Mass., 1977, pp. 346–347.
(124) L. O. Boreus and F. Sandberg, *Acta Physiol. Scand.*, *28*, 261 (1953).
(125) E. Manor, A. Marmor, S. Kaufman, and H. Leiba, *J. Am. Med. Assoc.*, *236*, 2777 (1976).
(126) E. E. Czapek, *J. Am. Med. Assoc.*, *235*, 636 (1976).
(127) J. R. DiPalma, *Am. Fam. Physician*, *13*, 142 (1976).
(128) E. Sutton and L. F. Soyka, *Clin. Pediatr. (Philadelphia)*, *12*, 692 (1973).
(129) H. Matthew, *Clin. Toxicol.*, *6*, 9 (1973).
(130) R. Goulding, *Pediatrics*, *52*, 883 (1973).
(131) D. G. Davidson and W. N. Eastham, *Br. Med. J.*, *2*, 497 (1966).
(132) P. G. Rose, *Br. Med. J.*, *1*, 381 (1969).
(133) R. Clark, V. Borirakchanyavat, A. R. Davidson, R. P. H. Thompson, B. Widdop, R. Goulding, and R. Williams, *Lancet*, *1*, 66 (1973).
(134) A. T. Proudfoot and N. Wright, *Br. Med. J.*, *3*, 557 (1970).
(135) E. Fernandez and A. C. Fernandez-Brito, *N. Engl. J. Med.*, *296*, 577 (1977).
(136) J. Koch-Weser, *N. Engl. J. Med.*, *295*, 1297 (1976).
(137) J. Ambre and M. Alexander, *J. Am. Med. Assoc.*, *238*, 500 (1977).
(138) B. McJunkin, K. W. Barwick, W. C. Little, and J. B. Winfield, *J. Am. Med. Assoc.*, *236*, 1874 (1976).
(139) B. Rumack and H. Matthew, *Pediatrics*, *55*, 871 (1975).
(140) L. F. Prescott, G. R. Sutherland, J. Park, I. J. Smith, and A. T. Proudfoot, *Lancet*, *2*, 109 (1976).
(141) L. F. Prescott, P. Roscoe, N. Wright, and S. S. Brown, *Lancet*, *1*, 519 (1971).
(142) E. P. Krenzelok, L. Best, and A. S. Manoguerra, *Am. J. Hosp. Pharm.*, *34*, 391 (1977).
(143) G. Levy and J. B. Houston, *Pediatrics*, *58*, 432 (1976).
(144) L. Lyons, J. S. Studdiford, and A. M. Sommaripa, *N. Engl. J. Med.*, *296*, 174 (1977).
(145) R. G. Peterson and B. H. Rumack, *J. Am. Med. Assoc.*, *237*, 2406 (1977).
(146) R. D. Scalley and C. S. Conner, *Am. J. Hosp. Pharm.*, *35*, 964 (1978).
(147) D. C. Brodie and I. J. Szekely, *J. Am. Pharm. Assoc. Sci. Ed.*, *40*, 414 (1951).
(148) L. Fleckenstein, J. M. Mazzullo, G. R. Mundy, R. A. Horvitz, and L. Lasagna, *Clin. Pharmacol. Ther.*, *17*, 233 (1975).
(149) E. R. Hart, *J. Pharmacol. Exp. Ther.*, *89*, 205 (1947).
(150) E. M. Bavin, F. J. Macrae, D. E. Seymour, and P. D. Waterhouse, *J. Pharm. Pharmacol.*, *4*, 872 (1952).
(151) A. J. Vignec and M. Gasparik, *J. Am. Med. Assoc.*, *167*, 1821 (1958).
(152) M. P. Borovsky, *Am. J. Dis. Child.*, *100*, 23 (1960).
(153) A. J. Quick, *J. Pharmacol. Exp. Ther.*, *128*, 95 (1960).
(154) O. Spuhler and H. N. Zollinger, *Z. Klin. Med.*, *151*, 1 (1953).
(155) L. F. Prescott, *J. Pharm. Pharmacol.*, *18*, 331 (1966).
(156) J. H. Shelley, *Clin. Pharmacol. Ther.*, *8*, 427 (1967).
(157) M. H. Gault, T. C. Rudwal, W. D. Engles, and J. B. Dossetor, *Ann. Intern. Med.*, *68*, 906 (1968).
(158) B. Koch, A. H. Irvine, J. R. McIver, and E. Liepa, *Can. Med. Assoc. J.*, *98*, 8 (1968).
(159) L. F. Prescott, *Scott. Med. J.*, *14*, 82 (1969).
(160) P. Kincaid-Smith, B. M. Saker, I. F. McKenzie, and K. Muriden, *Med. J. Aust.*, *1*, 203 (1968).
(161) M. A. McIver and J. B. Hobbs, *Med. J. Aust.*, *1*, 197 (1975).
(162) U. C. Dubach, B. Rosner, A. Müller, P. S. Levy, H. R. Baumeler, A. Peier, and T. Ehrensperger, *Lancet*, *1*, 539 (1975).
(163) R. D. Emkey and J. Mills, *J. Rheumatol.*, *1*, 126 (1974).
(164) A. F. Macklon, A. W. Craft, M. Thompson, and D. N. S. Kerr, *Br. Med. J.*, *1*, 597 (1974).
(165) R. J. Bulger, L. A. Healey, and P. Polinsky, *Ann. Rheum. Dis.*, *27*, 339 (1968).
(166) R. S. Hanra and P. Kincaid-Smith, *Br. Med. J.*, *3*, 559 (1970).
(167) K. Grimlund, *Acta Med. Scand.*, *174*, 3 (1963).
(168) A. F. Burry, P. DeJersey, and D. Weedon, *Med. J. Aust.*, *1*, 873 (1966).
(169) N. R. Eade and L. Lasagna, *J. Pharmacol. Exp. Ther.*, *155*, 301 (1967).
(170) U. Bengtsson, *Acta Med. Scand.*, *388*, 5 (1962).
(171) H. H. Pearson, *Med. J. Aust.*, *2*, 308 (1967).
(172) D. Bell, D. N. S. Kerr, J. Swinney, and W. K. Yeates, *Br. Med. J.*, *3*, 378 (1969).
(173) D. R. Wilson, *Can. Med. Assoc. J.*, *107*, 752 (1972).
(174) N. Hultengren, C. Lagergren, and A. Ljungqvist, *Acta Chir. Scand.*, *130*, 314 (1965).
(175) U. Bengtsson, L. Angevall, H. Ekman, and L. Lehman, *Scand. J. Urol. Nephrol.*, *2*, 145 (1968).
(176) G. Hoybye and O. E. Nielson, *Scand. J. Urol. Nephrol.*, *5*, 190 (1971).
(177) R. A. Mannion and D. Susmano, *J. Urol.*, *106*, 692 (1971).
(178) *Medical Letter on Drugs and Therapeutics*, *13*, 74 (1971).
(179) C. H. Mielke, Jr., and A. F. Britten, *N. Engl. J. Med.*, *282*, 1270 (1970).
(180) A. M. Antlitz, J. A. Mead, Jr., and M. A. Tolentino, *Curr. Ther. Res.*, *10*, 501 (1968).
(181) A. M. Antlitz and L. F. Awalt, *Curr. Ther. Res.*, *11*, 360 (1969).
(182) C. G. Moertel, D. L. Ahmann, W. F. Taylor, and N. Schwartau, *J. Am. Med. Assoc.*, *229*, 55 (1974).

Product[a] (Manufacturer)	Aspirin	Phenacetin	Salicylamide	Acetaminophen	Caffeine	Other
Actamin (Buffington)	—	—	—	NS[b]	—	—
Alka-Seltzer Effervescent Pain Reliever and Antacid (Miles)	324 mg	—	—	—	—	sodium bicarbonate, 1.904 g citric acid, 1.0 g
Amphenol (O'Neal, Jones & Feldman)	—	—	—	325 mg	—	—
Anacin (Whitehall)	400 mg	—	—	—	32.5 mg	—
Anodynos (Buffington)	NS[b]	—	NS[b]	NS[b]	NS[b]	—
Apamide (Dome)	—	—	—	300 mg	—	—
Arthralgen (Robins)	—	—	250 mg	250 mg	—	—
Arthritis Pain Formula (Whitehall)	486 mg (micronized)	—	—	—	—	aluminum hydroxide magnesium hydroxide
Arthritis Strength Bufferin (Bristol-Myers)	486 mg	—	—	—	—	magnesium carbonate, 145.8 mg aluminum glycinate, 72.9 mg
Arthropan Liquid (Purdue Frederick)	—	—	—	—	—	choline salicylate, 174 mg/ml (equivalent to 130 mg of aspirin)
A.S.A. Compound Capsules (Lilly)	227 mg	160 mg	—	—	32.5 mg	—
A.S.A. Enseals (Lilly)	325 and 650 mg	—	—	—	—	enteric coating
Ascriptin (Rorer)	325 mg	—	—	—	—	magnesium hydroxide, 75 mg aluminum hydroxide gel, dried, 75 mg
Ascriptin A/D (Rorer)	325 mg	—	—	—	—	magnesium hydroxide, 150 mg aluminum hydroxide gel, dried, 150 mg
Aspergum (Plough) (chewing gum)	228 mg	—	—	—	—	—
Asphal-G (Central Pharmacal)	250 mg	120 mg	—	—	15 mg	—
Aspirin Free Anacin-3 (Whitehall)	—	—	—	500 mg	32 mg	—
B-A (O'Neal, Jones & Feldman)	325 mg	—	—	—	—	aluminum hydroxide, 100 mg magnesium hydroxide, 30 mg
Bancap Capsule (O'Neal, Jones & Feldman)	—	—	200 mg	300 mg	—	—
Bayer Aspirin (Glenbrook)	325 mg	—	—	—	—	—
Bayer Children's Aspirin (Glenbrook)	81 mg	—	—	—	—	—
Bayer Timed-Release Aspirin (Glenbrook)	650 mg	—	—	—	—	—
BC Tablet and Powder (Block)	467 mg/tablet 810 mg (powder)	—	—	—	—	potassium chloride, 84 mg (powder)
Bromo-Seltzer (Warner-Lambert) (granules)	—	130 mg/capful	—	325 mg/capful	32.5 mg/ capful	sodium bicarbonate and citric acid to yield 2.8 g of sodium citrate/capful
Buffaprin (Buffington)	NS[b]	—	—	—	—	magnesium oxide

Product[a] (Manufacturer)	Aspirin	Phenacetin	Salicylamide	Acetaminophen	Caffeine	Other
Bufferin (Bristol-Myers)	324 mg	—	—	—	—	magnesium carbonate, 97.2 mg aluminum glycinate, 48.6 mg
Buffinol (Otis Clapp)	NS[b]	—	—	—	—	magnesium oxide
Calurin (Dorsey)	—	—	—	—	—	calcium carbaspirin equivalent to 300 mg of aspirin
Cama (Dorsey) (in-lay tablet)	600 mg	—	—	—	—	magnesium hydroxide, 150 mg aluminum hydroxide gel, dried, 150 mg
Capron Capsules (Vitarine)	227 mg	162 mg	—	65 mg	32 mg	—
Congespirin Chewable (Bristol-Myers)	81 mg	—	—	—	—	phenylephrine hydrochloride, 1.25 mg
Cope (Glenbrook)	421.2 mg	—	—	—	32 mg	magnesium hydroxide, 50 mg aluminum hydroxide, 25 mg methapyrilene fumarate, 12.5 mg
Cystex (Smith, Miller & Patch)	—	—	NS[b]	—	—	methenamine sodium salicylate benzoic acid
Datril (Bristol-Myers)	—	—	—	325 mg	—	—
Datril 500 (Bristol-Myers)	—	—	—	500 mg	—	—
Doan's Pills (Purex)	—	—	—	—	32 mg	magnesium salicylate, 325 mg
Dolcin (Dolcin Corp.)	240.5 mg	—	—	—	—	calcium succinate monohydrate, 182 mg
Dolor (Geriatric Pharmaceutical)	230 mg	—	—	230 mg	30 mg	calcium carbonate, 100 mg dry skim milk powder, 50 mg
Dularin Syrup (Dooner/Rorer)	—	—	—	24 mg/ml	—	—
Duradyne (O'Neal, Jones & Feldman)	230 mg	150 mg	—	30 mg	15 mg	—
Duragesic (Meyer)	325 mg	—	—	—	—	salicylsalicylic acid, 162.5 mg
Ecotrin (Smith Kline & French)	300 mg	—	—	—	—	enteric coating
Emagrin (Otis Clapp)	NS[b]	—	NS[b]	—	NS[b]	—
Empirin Compound (Burroughs Wellcome)	227 mg	162 mg	—	—	32 mg	—
Excedrin (Bristol-Myers)	194.4 mg	—	129.6 mg	97 mg	64.8 mg	—
Excedrin P.M. (Bristol-Myers)	194.4 mg	—	129.6 mg	162 mg	—	methapyrilene fumarate, 25 mg
Febrinol (Vitarine)	—	—	—	325 mg	—	—
Felsol Powder (American Felsol)	—	—	—	—	—	antipyrine, 975 mg (powder)
Fendon Tablets and Elixir (Amer. Pharm.)	—	—	—	324 mg/tablet 24 mg/ml	—	alcohol, 10% (elixir)

Product [a] (Manufacturer)	Aspirin	Phenacetin	Salicylamide	Acetaminophen	Caffeine	Other
Fizrin Powder (Glenbrook)	325 mg/packet	—	—	—	—	sodium bicarbonate, 1.825 g/packet citric acid, 1.449 g/packet sodium carbonate, 400 mg/packet
Goody's Headache Powder (Goody's)	455 mg	325 mg	—	—	32.5 mg	—
Liquiprin Suspension (Norcliff Thayer)	—	—	—	48 mg/ml	—	—
Measurin (Breon) (timed-release)	660 mg	—	—	—	—	—
Meadache (Organon)	—	—	150 mg	150 mg	32 mg	phenyltoloxamine dihydrogen citrate, 44 mg
Momentum (Whitehall)	162.5	—	—	—	—	salicylsalicylic acid, 325 mg phenyltoloxamine citrate
Neocylate (Central Pharmacal)	—	—	—	—	—	potassium salicylate, 280 mg aminobenzoic acid, 250 mg
Nilain (A.V.P.)	325 mg	—	—	162.5 mg	32.5 mg	—
Nilprin 7½ (A.V.P.)	—	—	—	486 mg	—	—
Pabirin (Dorsey)	300 mg	—	—	—	—	aminobenzoic acid, 300 mg aluminum hydroxide gel, dried, 100 mg
PAC (Upjohn)	228 mg	163 mg	—	—	32 mg	—
Panodynes Analgesic (Keystone)	260 mg	—	64.8 mg	64.8 mg	16.2 mg	—
Percogesic (Endo)	—	—	—	325 mg	—	phenyltoloxamine citrate, 30 mg
Persistin (Fisons)	160 mg	—	—	—	—	salicylsalicylic acid, 485 mg
S-A-C (Lannett)	—	—	230 mg	150 mg	30 mg	—
Sal-Fayne Capsules (Smith, Miller & Patch)	228 mg	166 mg	—	—	32 mg	—
Sinarest (Pennwalt)	—	—	—	325 mg	—	phenylpropanolamine hydrochloride, 18.7 mg chlorpheniramine maleate, 2 mg
Sine-Aid (McNeil)	—	—	—	325 mg	—	phenylpropanolamine hydrochloride, 25 mg
Sinu-Lets (Columbia Medical)	—	—	—	325 mg	—	phenylpropanolamine hydrochloride, 25 mg phenyltoloxamine citrate, 22 mg
SK-APAP Tablets and Elixir (Smith Kline & French)	—	—	—	325 mg/tablet 24 mg/ml	—	alcohol, 8% (elixir)
S.P.C. (North American)	—	130 mg	195 mg	—	16.25 mg	—
Stanback Tablets and Powder (Stanback)	324 mg/tablet 648 mg (powder)	—	97 mg/tablet 194 mg (powder)	—	16 mg/tablet 32 mg (powder)	—
Stanco (Stanback)	325 mg	—	—	—	—	—
St. Joseph Aspirin (Plough)	325 mg	—	—	—	—	—
St. Joseph Aspirin for Children Chewable Tablets (Plough)	81 mg	—	—	—	—	—

Product[a] (Manufacturer)	Aspirin	Phenacetin	Salicylamide	Acetaminophen	Caffeine	Other
Tempra Syrup, Tablets, and Drops (Mead Johnson)	—	—	—	24 mg/ml (syrup) 325 mg/tablet 100 mg/ml (drops)	—	alcohol, 10% (syrup and drops)
Tenol (North American)	—	—	—	325 mg	—	—
Trigesic (Squibb)	230 mg	—	—	125 mg	30 mg	—
Tylaprin Elixir (Cenci)	—	—	—	24 mg/ml	—	alcohol, 7%
Tylenol Extra Strength (McNeil)	—	—	—	500 mg/tablet 33.3 mg/ml	—	alcohol, 8.5%
Tylenol Tablets, Chewable Tablets, Drops, and Liquid (McNeil)	—	—	—	325 mg/tablet 80 mg/chewable tablet 100 mg/ml (drops) 24 mg/ml (liquid)	—	alcohol, 7% (drops and liquid)
Uracel (North American)	—	—	—	—	—	sodium salicylate, 324 mg
Valadol Tablets and Liquid (Squibb)	—	—	—	325 mg/tablet 24 mg/ml	—	alcohol, 9% (liquid)
Valorin (Otis Clapp)	—	—	—	NS[b]	—	—
Vanquish Caplet (Glenbrook)	227 mg	—	—	194 mg	33 mg	magnesium hydroxide, 50 mg aluminum hydroxide gel, dried, 25 mg
Zarumin (J. B. Williams)	—	—	260 mg	—	—	potassium salicylate, 228 mg

[a] Tablet unless specified otherwise.
[b] Quantity not specified.

Nutritional Supplement, Mineral, and Vitamin Products

Marianne Ivey

Chapter 10

Questions to Ask the Patient

What are your age and weight?

Do you participate regularly in sports?

Do you suffer from any chronic illnesses (e.g., diabetes)?

Are you currently taking any medication (prescription or OTC)?

Are you menstruating now?

Do you eat meats, vegetables, dairy products, and grain products every day?

Why are you requesting a nutritional supplement/vitamin/mineral? What are your symptoms? Have they appeared suddenly or gradually?

American consumers are convinced that they need more and better nutrients than their diets provide—they spend $350 million per year on vitamin products and $300–$500 million per year on health foods (1, 2). The health science professions frequently have associated health with nutrition. Actually, there is much to learn about adequate nutrition, and much that has been learned has not been communicated effectively to the general public. In many cases the average American diet does not need supplementation (3). Misconceptions about the value of supplementation were shown in a survey in which 75% of those interviewed believed that supplemental vitamins furnish energy (4).

Marketing practices may confuse the issue further. The label "organic" is misleading because all foods are organic. Organically grown foods are foods grown without the use of agricultural chemicals and processed without chemicals or additives. However, no laws exist that enforce the label "organically grown" to comply with the definition. There is no evidence that organically grown food is more nutritious than foods grown using chemical fertilizers (5), although valid questions have been raised concerning the safety of chemicals such as fertilizers, pesticides, and preservatives.

Frequently, "natural" vitamins are supplemented with the synthetic vitamin. For example, the amount of ascorbic acid acquired from rose hips (the fleshy fruit of a rose) is relatively small, and synthetic ascorbic acid is added to prevent an unreasonable tablet size (6). However, this addition is not indicated on the label, and such products often cost considerably more than the synthetic, equally effective vitamin.

The pharmacist as a public adviser should realize that one of the greatest dangers of food fads is that they sometimes are used in place of sound medical care. The false hope of superior health or freedom from disease may attract individuals with cancer, heart disease, arthritis, or other serious illnesses, and the pharmacist should be aware of the therapeutic value, if any, of these fads.

The Food and Drug Administration has issued bans against several claims and statements regarding food and food supplements. Claims cannot be made that foods or diet supplements alone can prevent, cure, or treat illness or that ingredients such as rutin, inositol, bioflavonoids, and aminobenzoic acid have nutritional value. Another FDA rule requires that all nutrients (caloric, protein, carbohydrate, and fat) as well as the percentage of the recommended daily dietary allowance (RDA) of vitamins and minerals be listed on the container of all food shipped interstate. Also, it has been proposed that products containing more than 50% of the RDA of certain ingredients must be called dietary supplements rather than foods and that those containing more than 150% of the RDA of a nutrient must be classified and labeled as drugs. Further guidelines for nutritional advice may come from the FDA OTC Panel on Vitamin, Mineral, and Hematinic Drug Products, but the Panel's final report has not yet been published.

Recommended daily allowances were developed by the Food and Nutrition Board of the National Academy of Sciences/National Research Council (Table 1). They have replaced the minimum daily requirement (MDR). The values of the RDA's should be interpreted as goals at which to aim in providing nutritional needs—they are not absolute nutritional standards or recommendations for an ideal diet, nor are they required for all individuals. The RDA is not designed to meet the needs of ill patients, nor does it account for the nutrients lost in cooking and other handling procedures. The individual RDA depends on age, sex, body size, and activity level as well as

Table 1. Recommended Daily Dietary Allowances

	Age, years	Weight, lbs.	Height, in.	Energy, kcal	Protein, g	Vitamin A Activity RE[a]	Vitamin A Activity IU[b]	Vitamin D, IU	Vitamin E Activity[c], IU	Ascorbic Acid, mg	Folic Acid[d], μg
Children	1–3	28	34	1300	23	400	2000	400	7	40	100
	4–6	44	44	1800	30	500	2500	400	9	40	200
	7–10	66	54	2100	36	700	3300	400	10	40	300
Males	11–14	97	63	2800	44	1000	5000	400	12	45	400
	15–18	134	69	3000	54	1000	5000	400	15	45	400
	19–22	147	69	3000	54	1000	5000	400	15	45	400
	23–50	154	69	2700	56	1000	5000		15	45	400
	51+	154	69	2400	56	1000	5000		15	45	400
Females	11–14	97	62	2400	44	800	4000	400	12	45	400
	15–18	119	65	2100	48	800	4000	400	12	45	400
	19–22	128	65	2100	46	800	4000	400	12	45	400
	23–50	128	65	2000	46	800	4000		12	45	400
	51+	128	65	1800	46	800	4000		12	45	400
Pregnant[e]				+300	+30	1000	5000	400	15	60	800
Lactating				+300	+20	1200	6000	400	15	80	600

Excerpted from Food and Nutrition Board, National Academy of Sciences/National Research Council Recommended Daily Dietary Allowances, Revised 1974. The allowances are intended to provide for individual variations among most normal persons as they live in the United States under usual environmental stresses. Diets should be based on a variety of common foods in order to provide other nutrients for which human requirements have been less well defined.

[a] Retinol equivalents.

[b] All intakes are assumed to be half as retinol and half as β-carotene when calculated from international units (IU). As retinol equivalents, three-fourths are as retinol and one-fourth as β-carotene.

[c] Total vitamin E activity, estimated to be 80% as tocopherol and 20% as other tocopherols.

recommended daily allowances

assessing nutritional status

undernourished groups

environmental and physical conditions (e.g., whether a person is pregnant, lactating, or ill).

NUTRITIONAL SUPPLEMENTS

Often, patients requesting a nutritional supplement self-diagnose their condition. By careful evaluation the pharmacist can determine the patient's nutritional status. If the evidence indicates a nutritional deficiency or any serious illness, the pharmacist should refer the patient to a physician for further diagnosis and treatment. Patients purchasing an OTC dietary supplement should be instructed as to use, storage, and possible side effects.

Determining Nutritional Status

The assessment of nutritional status is very difficult. Clinical impressions about nutrition are often erroneous because the stages between the well-nourished and the poorly nourished states are not well defined. Only when emaciation from disease, economics, or climatic conditions are obvious are clinical impressions reliable.

There are guidelines, however, by which the pharmacist can gain a more objective impression of a patient's nutritional status. Knowing the population groups that are most often poorly nourished, exercising good observation skills, and knowing what questions may yield helpful information are valuable indicators. Frequently undernourished groups in the United States include infants, preschool children, lactating or pregnant women, and the elderly. School children, factory workers, businesspersons, and farmers are less likely to be poorly nourished.

The pharmacist may observe the patient's physical condition to help guide in diet supplementation. The texture, amount, and appearance of the hair may suggest nutritional status. The eyes, particularly the conjunctiva, may indicate vitamin A and iron deficiencies, and the mouth may show stomatitis, glossitis, or hypertrophic or pale gums. The number and general condition of the teeth may reflect the patient's choice of food. Visible goiter, skin color and texture, the presence of edema, and obesity or thinness relative to bone structure also may be indications of malnutrition.

The more specific the information from the patient, the more helpful the pharmacist can be in determining the need for nutritional supplementation. Questions regarding foods generally not included in the diet may give the pharmacist more information. Previous treatment for similar symptoms also may be important.

Nutritional deficiencies cannot always be corrected at the pharmacy level. Although nutritional deficiencies may lead to disease, disease may lead to nutritional deficiencies. It is the pharmacist's responsibility to refer patients with a suspected serious illness to a physician for a definitive assessment. Guidelines for the clinical appraisal of nutritional status include evaluation of medical and dietary history; growth, development, and fitness; signs consistent with deficiencies; and biochemical assessment. The self-treated nutritional deficiencies, e.g., ascorbic acid deficiency (scurvy), niacin deficiency, (pellagra), and protein deficiency (kwashiorkor), seldom

Niacin, mg[e]	Riboflavin, mg	Thiamine, mg	Vitamin B_6[f], mg	Vitamin B_{12}[g], μg	Calcium, mg	Phosphorus, mg	Iodine, μg	Iron, mg	Magnesium, mg	Zinc, mg
9	0.8	0.7	0.6	1.0	800	800	60	15	150	10
12	1.1	0.9	0.9	1.5	800	800	80	10	200	10
16	1.2	1.2	1.2	2.0	800	800	110	10	250	10
18	1.5	1.4	1.6	3.0	1200	1200	130	18	350	15
20	1.8	1.5	2.0	3.0	1200	1200	150	18	400	15
20	1.8	1.5	2.0	3.0	800	800	140	10	350	15
18	1.6	1.4	2.0	3.0	800	800	130	10	350	15
16	1.5	1.2	2.0	3.0	800	800	110	10	350	15
16	1.3	1.2	1.6	3.0	1200	1200	115	18	300	15
14	1.4	1.1	2.0	3.0	1200	1200	115	18	300	15
14	1.4	1.1	2.0	3.0	800	800	100	18	300	15
13	1.2	1.0	2.0	3.0	800	800	100	18	300	15
12	1.1	1.0	2.0	3.0	800	800	80	10	300	15
+2	+0.3	+0.3	2.5	4.0	1200	1200	125	18[h]	450	20
+4	+0.5	+0.3	2.5	4.0	1200	1200	150	18	450	25

[d] The folic acid allowances refer to dietary sources as determined by *Lactobacillus casei* assay. Pure forms of folic acid may be effective in doses less than one-fourth of the recommended dietary allowance.
[e] Although allowances are expressed as niacin, it is recognized that on the average, 1 mg of niacin is derived from each 60 mg of dietary tryptophan.
[f] Pyridoxine hydrochloride.
[g] Cyanocobalamin.
[h] This increased requirement cannot be met by ordinary diets; therefore the use of supplemental iron is recommended.

are severe conditions but rather are milder forms of malnutrition.

Protein and Calorie (Energy) Deficiency

protein–calorie malnutrition

In developing nations, protein–calorie malnutrition (PCM) is fairly common. In the United States it is quite uncommon, except in certain disease states; in fact, an excess intake of protein and energy is more common. The RDA for protein is 44–56 g for adults, and for energy it is 1800–3000 cal. In most cases, excess protein intake (to as much as 300 g) does not lead to disease conditions. Excess calorie intake leads to obesity, the degree of overweight that prevents the body from functioning normally.

causes

In developing nations, protein–calorie malnutrition may be caused by a food supply shortage or by inadequate information and understanding of nutrition or disease. Kwashiorkor is a protein deficiency; marasmus is caused by the inadequacy of all nutrients. In the United States, protein–calorie malnutrition is more commonly caused by conditions such as Crohn's disease; malabsorption syndromes; short bowel syndromes caused by surgery, trauma, or radiation; severe burns; jaw fractures; neoplastic diseases; and renal disease. Protein and calorie intake in some very active people, e.g., athletes, dancers, and manual laborers, may not be adequate to meet their needs. However, in the United States, high activity levels are very infrequent for much of the population.

Several products are available for use as dietary supplements or tube feedings (oral, nasogastric, or gastrostomy tubes). The pharmacist's role regarding these products may be more as a consultant to other health professionals and less as a primary therapist for the self-treating patient. The pharmacist should first establish why the patient believes a dietary supplement, vitamin–mineral supplement, tonic, or health food is needed. Weight loss or failure to gain weight in a highly active, otherwise healthy individual may safely indicate the recommendation of a product with a high protein and calorie concentration. Patients with a history of weight loss without apparent cause should be referred to a physician. The concern is the possibility of neoplastic disease for which expedient referral to a qualified practitioner or diagnostic clinic may be crucial.

Types of Formulas

dietary adjuncts

Supplementary formula products are used as dietary adjuncts to a regular diet; they should not be used as the sole dietary product because they are not nutritionally complete. Some (Mull-Soy and Nutramigen) are milk free and can be used by individuals who have milk allergy disease. (See Chapter 12 for additional information.) One product (Controlyte) is restricted in its protein content and in electrolytes. It is appropriate for people with acute or chronic renal failure, where the diet must be carefully controlled. Many supplementary formula products may be combined with special recipes to make preparations such as desserts, malts, and shakes that still maintain the controlled intake.

Complete formulas can be used orally or as tube

feedings, and they may be used as the sole dietary intake if the patient's electrolytes are monitored (7). They also may be used as supplementation to a regular diet. The complete formulas contain various ingredients that make them appropriate for special needs. Several (Instant Breakfast, Sustacal, and Meritene) are milk based; others (Compleat-B and Gerber Meat Base Formula) have a mixed food base. A third type has a synthetic, not a natural, food as a base for proteins and carbohydrates. This type supplies the protein in the form of crystalline amino acids or protein hydrolysate (the carbohydrate in the form of oligosaccharide or disaccharide) and the vitamins and minerals as the individual chemicals. These formulas are also called "elemental diets." Examples of chemically defined products are Vivonex and Jejunal. Some complete supplementary products (Precision LR, Flexical, and Portagen) are only partly chemically defined. The differences in their formulation make the products appropriate for different needs.

complete formulas
special uses
available forms
precautions
mineral deficiencies
anemia

Nearly all chemically defined diets have a very low fat content and contain electrolytes, minerals, trace elements, and water-soluble and fat-soluble vitamins. All the chemically based products require little or no digestion, are absorbed by a small part of the intestine, and have a low residue. The low residue reduces the number and volume of the stools, making these products appropriate for patients with ileostomies or colostomies who wish also to decrease fecal output. The low-residue products also may be appropriate for patients with brain damage from strokes, congenital defects, or retardation or for elderly persons with stool incontinence. More commonly, they are used in postoperative care, in GI diseases, and in neoplastic disease where tissue breakdown is extensive.

Formulation and Dosage

Supplementary and complete formulas are available in several forms. Some are powders that must be diluted with water or milk, some are liquids that must be diluted further, and some are ready-to-use liquids. The extent of dilution is based on the amount of nutrients needed and the amount that can be tolerated. Most often, adults will not tolerate preparations of more than 25% weight/volume (w/v), which generally delivers 1.0 cal/ml, and infants, 12% w/v, which generally delivers 0.5 cal/ml. (Infants should be started on a concentration of 7–7.5% w/v, increasing to 12% over 4–5 days.) For children over 10 months, 15% w/v may be initiated, with gradual increases to 25%. Higher concentrations may cause diarrhea because the sugar in the preparations acts as an osmotic diarrheal.

If the preparations are taken orally, 100–150 ml should be ingested at one time. Over the course of a day, 2000 ml (about 2 qt) of most preparations provides about 2000 cal. If the product is tube fed, 40–60 ml/hour may be given initially. The container should be kept cold to prevent bacterial growth, and all prepared products remaining after 24 hours should be discarded. The tubing should be rinsed three times per day with sterile water. If diarrhea, nausea, or distention occurs, the diet should be withheld for 24 hours, then gradually resumed. In elderly or unconscious patients or patients who recently have had surgery, elevating the head of the bed is advisable during administration of the preparation to avoid aspiration.

Cautions

Many formulas are relatively new, and complete indications for use and instructions on storage, preparation, and use are not available. Pharmacists should take care not to store products as they come from the manufacturer in areas with temperatures higher than 75°F (23.8°C) and should check expiration dates before dispensing.

Because all formulas are excellent media for bacterial growth, they should be prepared each day and refrigerated until used. If they become bacterially contaminated, they may cause diarrhea. Diarrhea also may occur from the osmolar carbohydrate load, especially simple sugars, or from fat intolerance (however, some elemental diets are fat free).

Patients must be monitored to detect biochemical abnormalities of electrolyte values and to ensure adequate nutrition and hydration. Urine and blood glucose concentrations should be measured; diabetics may require increased insulin doses. Edema may be precipitated or aggravated in patients with protein–calorie malnutrition or cardiac, renal, or hepatic disease because of the relatively high sodium content of the chemically defined diets. Frequently, hospital dieticians prepare formulas so that the electrolytes may be tailored to the individual patient.

MINERALS

Most normal diets in the United States supply the necessary amount of iron, calcium, and trace elements. The pharmacist should be able to recognize signs of mineral deficiencies in patients so that prompt physician referral may be made.

Iron

Iron deficiency anemia is a widespread problem. Although it causes few deaths, it contributes to the poor health and suboptimal performance of many people. Milder iron deficiencies that do not lead to anemia but are probably very common no doubt present clinical manifestations, but they are less often recognizable. Iron plays an important role in oxygen and electron transport. In the body it is either functional or stored. Functional iron is found in hemoglobin, myoglobin, heme enzymes, and cofactor and transport iron. The rest is stored in the form of ferritin and hemosiderin. Ferritin is a micelle of ferric hydroxyphosphate surrounded by 24 identical protein units (8). Hemosiderin consists of aggregated ferritin molecules and additional components (9). The storage sites of ferritin and hemosiderin are the liver, spleen, and bone marrow.

Normally, adult males have about 50 mg of iron/kg; females have about 35 mg/kg (10). Hemoglobin is about 0.34% iron. Normal hemoglobin in adult males is about 14–17 g/100 ml of blood; in adult females, it is 12–14 g/100 ml. The RDA for iron is 10–18 mg for all adults.

About 10% of oral iron in food or as an iron supplement is absorbed. In an iron-deficient person, about 20% is absorbed. Ingested iron is solubilized in gastric juice and is reduced to the ferrous form. It is then chelated with substances such as ascorbic acid, sugars, and amino acids. These chelates have low molecular weights and may be solubilized and absorbed before they reach the alkaline medium of the distal small intestine, where precipitation occurs. Iron is probably absorbed passively into the mucosal layer, then transferred actively to transferrin and used in the bone marrow for incorporation into red blood cells or incorporated into all of the other body cells. Some of the transferrin iron is stored in the spleen, liver, and bone marrow. Iron is released from the body by the flaking of skin cells; in the urine, sweat, and feces; and by blood loss.

Etiology of Iron Deficiency

Iron deficiency may result from inadequate diet, malabsorption, pregnancy and lactation, or blood loss. Because the amount of normal iron excretion through the urine, feces, and skin is very small, iron deficiency caused by poor diet or malabsorption may develop very slowly and manifest itself only after a period of years. Unless it is proven otherwise, iron deficiency in an adult male or postmenopausal female is caused by blood loss. Blood loss may occur with conditions such as hiatus hernia, peptic ulcers, esophageal varices, diverticulitis, intestinal parasites (especially hookworm), regional enteritis, and ulcerative colitis. The pharmacist should be aware of the possibility of these various illnesses.

Blood loss also may occur from drug ingestion. Many drugs directly irritate the gastric mucosa or have an indirect effect on the GI tract. These drugs include the salicylates, nonsalicylate analgesics (e.g., indomethacin and phenylbutazone), reserpine, steroids, and most drugs used in the treatment of neoplasms, such as fluorouracil, mithramycin, and dactinomycin.

Menstrual blood losses may contribute to iron deficiency. Normally, the blood lost during a menstrual period is 60–80 ml; in 95% of women this volume represents about 1.4 mg or less of iron lost (11). Normal loss in addition to menstrual iron loss indicates a total daily iron need of 7–23 mg. Average U.S. diets contain about 5–7 mg of iron/1000 cal, and women on restricted diets may need supplemental iron. Some women who consider their menses normal actually lose 100–200 ml of blood per period. To make up this loss would require as much as 40 mg/day of iron in the diet (about 10% of food iron is absorbed). Clearly, for these women, supplemental iron is desirable.

Another source of blood loss is blood donation. A donation is usually about 500 ml of blood. If the hemoglobin is normal, about 250 mg of iron is lost.

Iron deficiency may be caused by not eating enough animal protein and cereal food made with iron-fortified flour. Clay eating (geophagia) leads to iron deficiency by the chelation or precipitation of iron in the gut (12). Chronic diarrhea commonly leads to iron deficiency. Achlorhydria and partial or total gastrectomy cause decreased iron absorption.

Evaluation

Early symptoms of iron deficiency frequently are vague and are related to other disease states. Easy fatigability, weakness, and lassitude cannot be related easily to iron deficiency. Often, patients without obvious symptoms have iron deficiency anemia, discovered during a routine medical examination. Other symptoms of anemia include pallor, dyspnea on exertion, palpitation, and a feeling of exhaustion. Coldness and numbness of extremities may be reported.

The pharmacist may ascertain the cause of the patient's disease by consulting the medication record. The patient might have been treated for ulcers or hemorrhoids, conditions that could cause blood loss. Checking the medication record for previous use of drugs such as phenylbutazone, reserpine, or warfarin might yield another reason for blood loss. Medications, such as aspirin, that may cause blood loss are bought without a prescription and often are not included on a medication record. In these cases the pharmacist must question the patient. A patient who indicates blood loss should be referred to a physician. In any indication of blood loss, time is very important. Abnormal blood loss may be indicated by any of the following symptoms:

iron deficiency

indications and symptoms

blood loss

therapy

- Vomiting blood;
- Bright red blood in the stool or dark, tarry stools;
- Large clots or an abnormally large flow (200 ml or more) during the menstrual period;
- Cloudy or pink/red appearance of the urine (ruling out dyes in drugs which may cause urine discoloration).

Blood loss, particularly through the stool, is not always obvious to the patient. Before suggesting self-treatment, the pharmacist must consider the patient's medication history and overall appearance.

Other questions may be asked for indications of iron deficiency: Do you eat balanced meals on a regular basis? Do you have cravings for clay or ice (13)? Have you given blood recently? The pharmacist should ascertain the chronicity of the patient's problem and whether medical care has been sought. Depending on the answers, the pharmacist might suggest iron supplementation with self-monitoring to check for improvement. Generally, iron supplementation should be considered when food intake is restricted or when the patient is pregnant, lactating, or menstruating.

Treatment

If iron supplementation can be suggested safely, the pharmacist must determine which iron product is best. The choice of an iron preparation should be based on how well it is absorbed, how well it is tolerated in therapeutic doses, and price. Because ferrous salts are more soluble than ferric salts, it seems reasonable to choose an iron product of the ferrous group. Ferrous sulfate has been the standard against which other salts of iron—ferrous succinate, ferrous lactate, ferrous fumarate, ferrous glycine sulfate, ferrous glutamate, and ferrous gluconate—have been compared. All are absorbed about as well as ferrous sulfate. Ferrous citrate, ferrous tartrate, ferrous pyrophosphate, and some ferric salts are not absorbed as well (14). A cost table on iron preparations published recently (15) shows that ferrous salts are also the least costly per gram of iron. Considering absorption data and prices on timed-release products, it can be seen that patients purchasing such products may be getting "less for more."

Ferrous salts have been given in combination with ascorbic acid. At a ratio of 200 mg of ascorbic acid to 30 mg of elemental iron the increased amount of iron absorbed validated this practice (14). Some experts feel that the cost of the iron–ascorbic acid combination does not warrant its use for the moderate increase in iron absorption (16). If cost is a factor, ascorbic acid tablets may be used, not in a combination product. This type of therapy is probably more appropriate for people with iron store deficiencies in addition to plasma deficiencies.

various iron salts
formulations
side effects
interactions
overdose

In a 320-mg hydrated ferrous sulfate tablet, 20% (about 60 mg) is elemental iron. In patients with iron deficiencies, 20% of the elemental iron is absorbed. If three tablets per day are taken, 36 mg of iron is absorbed; if four tablets are taken, 48 mg is absorbed. Between 36 and 48 mg of iron is enough to support maximum incorporation into red blood cells (0.3 g of hemoglobin/100 ml of blood).

Enteric-coated or delayed-release iron preparations are not pharmacologically advantageous. Because progressively less iron is absorbed as it moves from the duodenum to the ileum, these products decrease the overall iron absorption by delaying the time of release. These products generally are more expensive than other iron preparations, and no advantage (except, perhaps, patient compliance) is derived from their use.

All iron products tend to irritate the GI mucosa. The symptoms are nausea, GI pain, and diarrhea. These symptoms may be decreased by decreasing the dosage, by using other ferrous salts such as succinate, lactate, gluconate, or fumarate, or by giving iron with meals. Although giving iron with food is less irritating, food decreases the amount of iron absorbed by 40–50% (14). Periodically, physicians recommend iron with instructions for between-meal dosing. It is advantageous for absorption if the patient is able to tolerate the iron taken in this manner. If nausea or diarrhea is a problem, the pharmacist should be consulted; it usually is better to suggest taking the iron with food or decreasing the number of tablets than for the patient to decide to stop taking the supplement entirely.

Constipation, a frequent side effect of iron therapy, has prompted the formulation of medications that contain iron and a stool softener. If iron and a stool softener do, in fact, prevent constipation, such a preparation is indicated. However, not all patients become constipated with iron therapy. In one study, adverse effects of iron were believed to be psychological (17). Therefore pharmacists might consider de-emphasizing side effects.

Another observation with iron therapy is that stools become black and tarry. Usually, this effect is caused by unabsorbed iron, but it also may be caused by occult blood, if the patient has indicated GI bleeding in the past. If the stools do not darken during iron therapy, it may be that the iron tablet did not break up.

Iron chelates with many substances. Its interaction with antacids is therapeutically significant (18). The mechanism is probably related to the relative alkalinization of the stomach contents. Therefore the chelate of iron with the antacid (e.g., magnesium trisilicate) is even more insoluble in the alkaline medium. Iron appears to chelate with several of the tetracyclines, resulting in decreased tetracycline and iron absorption (19). The manufacturers of allopurinol recommend that iron and allopurinol not be given together. In animals, allopurinol may increase hepatic uptake of iron; however, this effect has not been shown in humans.

Iron deficiency anemia is diagnosed by a physician or in a diagnostic clinic, on the basis of tests such as hemoglobin, hematocrit, serum iron, and iron-binding capacity. To monitor the effect of iron therapy, the pharmacist and physician may inquire about the patient's own perception of well-being. The physician generally uses the hemoglobin to measure the effect of iron therapy. The pharmacist might remind the patient who has a prescription for iron to have a blood test to check for the appropriate response in 1–2 months. Usually, hemoglobin is corrected in this time; correction of plasma iron takes 3–4 months.

Most healthy patients who self-medicate probably should not be taking more than one iron tablet per day. The usual dose for iron deficiency is one to four tablets per day. The iron should be taken between meals or, in cases of gastric pain or irritation, with food. Patients should be cautioned that the stool may darken from the iron. If antacids or tetracyclines are taken, iron should be taken at a separate time. One month of therapy is probably reasonable for self-medication with iron. If the patient has no response after this period, a physician should be consulted.

Iron Toxicity

Accidental poisoning with iron occurs most frequently in children. The sugar-coated, brown iron tablets look like chocolate and attract children. About 50% of iron poisoning cases are fatal. As few as 15 tablets of 0.3 g of ferrous sulfate have been lethal, but the ingestion of as many as 70 tablets has been followed by recovery. Outcome depends on speed of appropriate treatment.

The symptoms of acute iron poisoning are reflected by several organ systems. Because iron salts in large doses are corrosive to the gastric mucosa, pain, vomiting (the vomitus may contain blood and particles of the iron tablets), and diarrhea occur (ribbons of mucosa may be seen in the watery diarrhea) (20). These symptoms may lead to electrolyte imbalances and shock. In later phases of what may seem like recovery, pneumonitis (if the vomitus is aspirated) and acidosis may occur, and cardiovascular collapse may ensue. Autopsies frequently show liver damage, and there may be pyloric stenosis. Renal damage usually does not occur.

The treatment for iron overdose may be started at home by inducing vomiting immediately and then administering milk and eggs. The remainder of the therapy, which should be carried out in an appropriately equipped hospital, includes gastric lavage, the administration of deferoxamine mesylate (5–10 g), and supportive care such as oxygen or antibiotics, as the condition requires.

A more insidious kind of iron toxicity may occur during prolonged therapy with iron. In the treatment of refractory anemia, oral iron may be excessively absorbed, leading to iron overload. Alcoholic patients also become iron overloaded. Wine contains iron, and alcohol increases ferric iron absorption. Patients with chronic liver disease and chronic pancreatic disease absorb more iron than normal from the gut. Iron overload also may occur when individuals who do not need iron take it for prolonged periods. The pharmacist should be aware of this possibility and should discourage the use of iron when there is no evidence to indicate its need.

Calcium

Calcium is a major component of bones and teeth. It is necessary for blood clotting and the integrity of many cells, especially those of the neuromuscular system. The present RDA of calcium is 800–1200 mg for adults and 240–800 mg for infants and children. (The methods of calculating these values are being reviewed.) The small intestine controls the amount of calcium absorbed. Thus patients taking relatively low amounts of calcium absorb more, and some taking large amounts excrete more as fecal calcium. Calcium requirements also appear to increase as protein consumption increases (21, 22).

A dietary deficiency disease caused by insufficient calcium intake is not known. The major pathological conditions that may lead to skeletal mineral depletion are the malabsorption syndromes and uremia. In uremic patients the kidney is unable to convert vitamin D to its most active form; thus calcium absorption is impaired when adaptation mechanisms cannot compensate for low calcium intake. Various disturbances, including neuromuscular irritability, may occur and may progress to tetany or major seizures. Other manifestations include osteomalacia and bone deformities. Therapy consists of 4–12 g/day of calcium, and patients require monitoring. Serum calcium should be maintained at 9–11 mEq/1000 ml of blood. Urine calcium levels are not an accurate reflection of serum calcium levels.

Calcium may be toxic. Large amounts taken as dietary supplementation or as antacids may lead to high calcium levels in the urine and renal stones. The latter may result in renal damage.

The most common calcium salts available without a prescription are calcium carbonate, calcium gluconate, and calcium lactate. Of these, calcium carbonate is preferred because it provides more elemental calcium per given weight of calcium salt.

Trace Elements

Trace elements, found combined in minute quantities in plant and animal tissue, are considered essential in the physiological process. RDA's for zinc, copper, and other minerals have been established. Many multiple-vitamin products contain trace elements in addition to the "essential" vitamins and minerals.

Zinc

The 1974 RDA for zinc is 15 mg for adults—more for pregnant (20 mg) and lactating (25 mg) women—and 3–10 mg for infants and children. Zinc is necessary for wound healing, and impaired taste and smell acuity may be improved with zinc supplementation (23, 24). Poor appetite and poor growth may occur in children with low zinc intake. Zinc supplementation is most important for people with chronic wounds and with wounds following surgery and trauma. Patients on chemically defined diets as a sole nutritional source must be observed for zinc deficiency. Zinc and copper seem to have a relationship; in some patients, administration of copper increases zinc levels (25). Some OTC multiple vitamins contain zinc.

Copper

Copper is needed to maintain adequate blood cell production. It also seems required for the use of iron. Intake of 2–5 mg/day is adequate to prevent copper deficiencies. Copper deficiency states are rare except in patients whose sole nutritional intake is a chemically defined source, e.g., patients fed intravenously with total parenteral nutrition (26).

iron overload

calcium RDA, deficiency, and available salts

essential trace elements

Selenium

Selenium has been identified as an essential trace element in humans (27, 28). Although cases of selenium deficiency are not common in the general population, there appears to be an association between selenium deficiency and protein malnutrition disease (kwashiorkor) (29) and multiple sclerosis (30). Moreover, epidemiological studies suggest that cancer and heart disease are most common in areas of low ambient selenium availability (31).

A statistically significant inverse relationship was found between blood selenium levels in adult males and the total cancer mortality in 10 U.S. cities (32). Female human breast cancer mortalities in the United States are lower in areas in which grain and forage crops are high in selenium (33). A study of serum selenium levels of 110 cancer patients found that lower selenium levels were usually associated with distant metastasis, multiple primary tumors, multiple recurrences, and a short survival time (34). As selenium levels reached or exceeded the mean value for the carcinoma group, the tumor was usually confined to the region of origin, distant metastasis occurred less frequently, and multiple primary lesions and recurrences seldom appeared.

Excess selenium does not produce the same signs in humans as those observed in animals. However, excess selenium does produce growth retardation, muscular weakness, infertility, focal hepatic necrosis (35), dysphagia, dysphomia, bronchopneumonia, and respiratory failure (36). Selenium has been implicated in four cases of amyotrophic lateral sclerosis in west central South Dakota, where naturally occurring toxication is endemic in livestock (36).

Others

Fluorine, iodine, and chromium are needed in humans and are generally available through the diet.

Other species need cobalt, manganese, molybdenum, nickel, tin, vanadium, and silicon (37). Further observations in humans on long-term, chemically defined diets may indicate that these elements also are essential to good health.

Some OTC protein products (Gevral Protein, Meritene, and Sustagen) contain trace minerals such as magnesium, zinc, manganese, copper, and iodide. The same trace metals also are commonly found in multiple-vitamin and mineral combinations. Some trace metals (e.g., zinc, manganese, and copper) are available as single-entity products.

VITAMINS

Vitamins generally are supplied adequately through most diets, and vitamin deficiencies that are diagnosed early usually can be corrected easily by administering large doses of the missing vitamin. The pharmacist should be aware of physical, environmental, or social conditions (e.g., following a vegetarian diet) that may be conducive to inadequate vitamin intake.

sources of vitamin A

retinol

causes of deficiency

signs and symptoms

retinol equivalents

Fat-Soluble Vitamins

Vitamins A, D, and E are fat soluble. Severe deficiencies of any of these vitamins may result in conditions as serious as blindness or bone deformity. Excessive doses also may be harmful.

Vitamin A

Vitamin A is needed to prevent night blindness and xerosis (drying) of the conjunctiva, the first symptoms of vitamin A deficiency. Drying of the epithelium on other sites of the body, nerve lesions, and increased pressure in the cerebrospinal fluid also may occur. Pregnant women must have an adequate vitamin A intake to avoid malformation of the fetus. Vitamin A is consumed as preformed vitamin A from animal sources and as carotenoids, of which the most active is carotene, from plant sources. Particularly good sources are kidney, milk products, eggs, fish liver oil, and palm oil. If skim milk is used, it should be fortified with vitamin A or supplemented in another way. The term "vitamin A" designates several biologically active compounds. Vitamins A (retinol) and A_2 (3-dehydroretinol) are alcohols. Retinol is the major naturally occurring form. Because the vitamin is fat soluble, it is stored in the body, mainly in the liver. Deficiencies rarely occur in well-nourished populations, and when they do occur, they develop slowly. Serum levels usually remain normal until the liver reserve becomes very small.

There are several etiologies of vitamin A deficiency. Before 1968 there was an epidemic of vitamin A deficiency in Brazil due to the provision of skim milk to Brazilian children without a supplementary vitamin A capsule. The skim milk was the sole diet. Diseases such as cancer, tuberculosis, pneumonia, chronic nephritis, urinary tract infections, and prostatic diseases may cause massive excretion of vitamin A (38). Conditions in which there is fat malabsorption, such as GI diseases of sprue, obstructive jaundice, cystic fibrosis, and cirrhosis of the liver, also may cause very low or absent vitamin A stores. In the United States, vitamin A deficiency occurs more frequently because of diseases of fat malabsorption than because of malnutrition.

The signs and symptoms of vitamin A deficiency related to the eye are drying, wrinkling, and hazing of the cornea. Lack of tears may be caused by obstruction of the tear duct. Bitot spots (small patches of bubbles that resemble tiny drops of meringue) may appear. The conjunctiva may look dry and opaque, and photophobia may occur. The cornea may become ulcerous, and infection may then destroy it. If corneal destruction occurs, there may be loss of vision. This process occurs more rapidly in children than in adults.

The most recent revision of the RDA for vitamin A uses a new unit of measurement—retinol equivalents (RE). It incorporates vitamin A and its provitamin, carotene (39). The RDA for adult males is 5000 international units (IU), or 1000 RE. For adult females it is 4000 IU (800 RE); pregnant women need 1000 RE, and lactating women, 1200 RE. Doses of vitamin A for infants receiving unfortified or skim milk formulas should be 1500 IU/day. Patients with corneal lesions due to hypovitaminosis A should take 25,000–50,000 IU/day of a water-dispersible vitamin A preparation. The FDA had ruled that products containing more than 10,000 IU of vitamin A per dose could not be sold without a prescription, but this ruling has been reversed (40). The duration of therapy should be assessed by clinical evaluation.

If the pharmacist establishes that the patient has poor dietary habits (e.g., the patient is an alcoholic), an OTC multiple vitamin that contains the RDA of vitamin A should be recommended. The incidence of hypervitaminosis has been increasing, particularly among food faddists. Doses as low as 18,500 IU of vitamin A given to infants 3–6 months old for 1–3 months have been toxic (41). Toxicity usually occurs at 20–30 times the RDA (20,000–30,000 RE; 100,000–150,000 IU). Fatigue, malaise, and lethargy are the common signs. Abdominal upset, bone and joint pain, throbbing headaches, insomnia, restlessness, night sweats, loss of body hair, brittle nails, exophthalmus, rough and scaly skin, peripheral edema, mouth fissures, and hepatomegaly also are common. Constipation, menstrual irregularity, and emotional liability have been reported in some cases (42). Single doses of 2,000,000 IU (400,000 RE) may precipitate acute toxicity 4–8 hours after ingestion. Headache is predominant, but it may be accompanied by diplopia, nausea, vomiting, vertigo, or drowsiness (43). Treatment consists of discontinuing ingestion of the vitamin A. The prognosis is good.

The systemic use of vitamin A for treating acne and preventing infection and its topical use in wound healing are not warranted by clinical evidence. A topical product incorporating retinoic acid has shown positive clinical response in the treatment of mild to moderately severe acne.

The pharmacist should advise patients about vitamin A supplementation to avoid deficiency (if the diet is not adequate), discourage excessive dosage, and refer patients who seem to have clinical vitamin A deficiency to a physician. This last point is made because of the speed of disastrous consequences and because diagnosis, treatment, and follow-up require laboratory assessment.

Vitamin D

Vitamin D is a collective name for several structurally similar chemicals and their metabolites—ergocalciferol (vitamin D_2) is derived from ergosterol, cholecalciferol (vitamin D_3) is derived from cholesterol, and dihydrotachysterol (vitamin D_1) is a synthetic reduction product of vitamin D_2. Some very active metabolites of vitamin D_3 have been identified. One metabolite, 25-hydroxycholecalciferol, is formed in the liver, carried on protein to the kidneys, and further converted to several more active metabolites, of which the most active is 1,25-dihydroxycholecalciferol (1,25-DHCC) (44). Vitamin D is needed to stimulate calcium absorption from the small intestine and to mobilize bone calcium. It is closely involved with parathyroid hormone, phosphate, and calcitonin in the homeostasis of serum calcium.

Vitamin D has properties of both hormones and vitamins. If there is sufficient exposure to sunlight, sterol in the skin is irradiated, and vitamin D is synthesized. If sun exposure is not sufficient, vitamin D must be obtained from the diet. If an adequate amount of vitamin D is not consumed or is not activated by sunlight, rickets, tetany, or osteomalacia may occur. Although diets in the United States rarely are deficient in vitamin D to the extent that rickets occurs, vitamin D deficiencies caused by renal disease (the kidney is less capable of forming 1,25-dihydroxycholecalciferol), malabsorption syndromes, short bowel syndromes due to many causes, hypoparathyroid disease, chronic use of anticonvulsants, and hypophosphatemia are common.

Food sources of vitamin D are fish liver oils and irradiated yeast. Many foods are fortified with vitamin D, particularly milk products and cereals. The RDA for vitamin D is 400 IU for infants and adults, including pregnant and lactating women. An FDA ruling that doses of vitamin D above 400 IU could be available to consumers only with a physician's prescription has been reversed by Congress. Doses of vitamin D above 400 IU may be made available as OTC products and as dietary supplements (40).

The signs and symptoms of vitamin D deficiency diseases are reflected as calcium abnormalities, specifically those involved with the bone formation. As serum calcium and inorganic phosphate decrease, compensatory mechanisms attempt to increase the calcium. Increased parathyroid hormone secretion may lead to secondary hyperparathyroidism. If physiological mechanisms fail to make the appropriate adjustments in calcium and phosphorus levels, rickets or osteomalacia develops. Rickets is a failure of bone matrix mineralization. The epiphyseal plate may widen owing to failure of calcification. As a result, rickets is manifested by soft bones and deformed joints. The diagnosis is made radiologically by observing the bone deformities.

sources of vitamin D

RDA

signs and symptoms of vitamin D deficiency

Large doses of vitamin D are prescribed for rickets. For children, 1000–4000 IU per dose is given; for adults with osteodystrophy of renal disease, the dose range is 50,000–5,000,000 IU. Smaller doses of 0.25–1.0 μg/day are given when 1,25-dihydroxycholecalciferol is used.

The monitoring procedure for therapy, regardless of the particular vitamin D entity used, is extremely important. Urine and blood calcium levels must be checked to avoid hypercalcemia. Because phosphate binds with

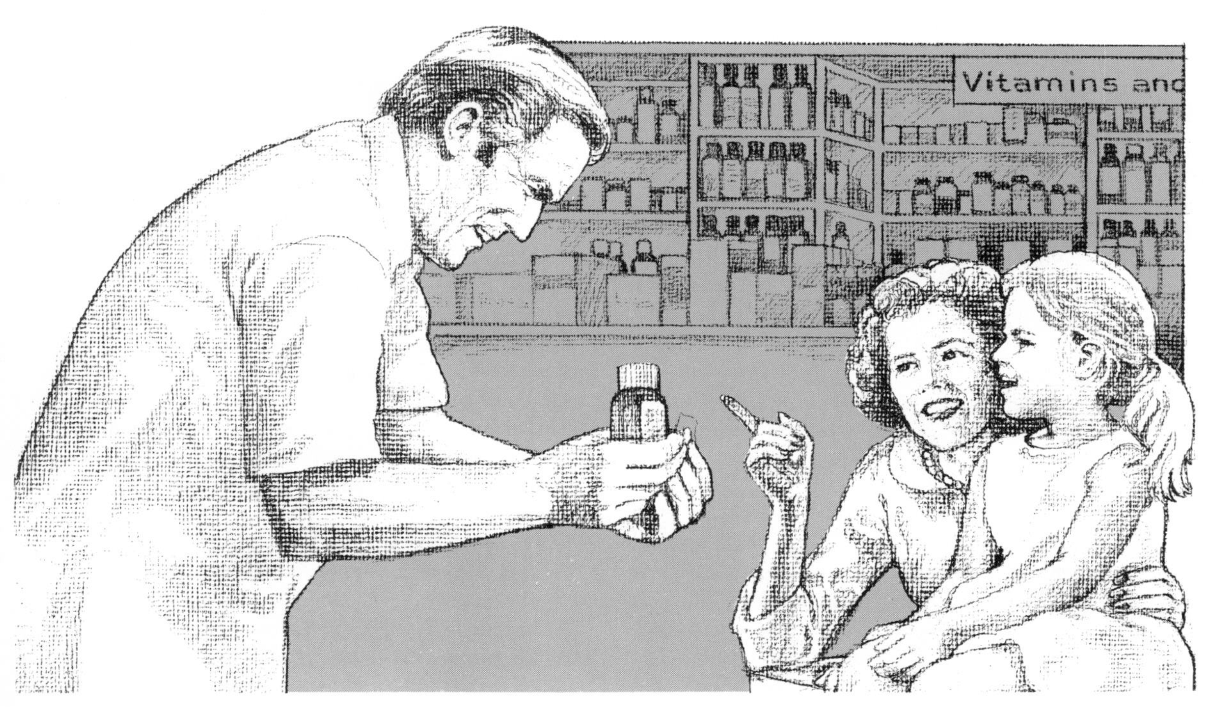

calcium and may be deposited in soft tissue such as brain, eyes, heart, and kidney, phosphate in the serum also must be regulated.

Concurrent drug therapy must be monitored closely. Phosphate in chronically used drugs such as certain laxatives may lower the calcium level and contribute to a vitamin D deficiency. Patients who have vitamin D deficiency caused by renal problems should use caution in taking antacids. The pharmacist should point out to patients with renal problems that antacids should be chosen for the specific ingredients they contain; e.g., aluminum antacids may be chosen because they bind phosphates, and magnesium antacids avoided because of their toxicity in renal disease. A calcium antacid may be used to help increase serum calcium levels.

vitamin D interactions

toxicity

Vitamin D is toxic when taken in large doses for long periods. Hypervitaminosis D may occur with 4000 IU/day. Doses of 50,000–100,000 IU/day are dangerous to adults and children. Doses of 1380–2370 IU have not been shown to be detrimental to children, but doses exceeding 1000 IU are not advisable (45, 46).

The signs and symptoms of hypervitaminosis D are anorexia, nausea, weakness, weight loss, polyuria, constipation, vague aches, stiffness, soft tissue calcification, nephrocalcinosis, hypertension, anemia, hypercalcemia, acidosis, and irreversible renal failure. The pharmacist should check the medication profile for a possible cause of the problem. For example, if a patient complained of bone pain and stiffness and the medication record showed therapy with vitamin D, the pharmacist might suspect hypervitaminosis. If a recent blood test has not been taken to measure serum calcium, a physician should be consulted.

Most people obtain the RDA of vitamin D in dietary sources and by exposure to sunlight. If a patient asks for a vitamin D supplement and the pharmacist determines that the need is based on poor dietary intake or indoor confinement, a multiple-vitamin supplement may be recommended. Patients who request therapeutic doses of vitamin D should be referred to a physician when the pharmacist ascertains that a need exists.

calcitriol

Liquid preparations that contain vitamin D should be measured carefully, particularly when given to infants. Patients using prescription vitamin D products should be encouraged to see a physician regularly. The vitamin D product of choice—1,25-dihydroxycholecalciferol metabolite—is now available commercially as calcitriol (Rocaltrol, Roche). Presently, vitamins D_2 and D_3 probably are interchangeable. Dihydrotachysterol may be the drug of choice in renal disease and hypoparathyroidism because it is active in its present state and needs no further metabolism for vitamin D activity and because it is less expensive than calcitriol.

Vitamin E

tocopherols

Vitamin E is the most potent of the eight natural alcohol compounds called tocopherols; specifically, it includes α-tocopherol and salts. The American diet now includes more soybean products, which have a considerable amount of γ-tocopherol. Although γ-tocopherol is less potent, it may contribute as much as 20% of the ingested vitamin E. Future RDA revisions may list vitamin E as a tocopherol equivalent.

Vitamin E has become an extremely controversial nutrient in the last few years through claims for its therapeutic effect as a drug. As a nutrient in humans, vitamin E seems necessary in preventing problems involving the musculature and the nervous and vascular systems. Many of its effects found in animals, particularly the induction of fertility, have not been shown in humans.

vitamin E RDA, toxicity, and dosages

The RDA for adults is 12–15 IU/day and less for infants (4 IU/day) and children. It is dependent on the amount of polyunsaturated fatty acids (PUFA) consumed. The need for vitamin E increases as polyunsaturated fatty acid consumption increases. The ratio is 0.4–0.5 mg of vitamin E per gram of polyunsaturated fatty acids consumed. Foods high in polyunsaturated fats also have a high vitamin E content. The richest natural sources of vitamin E are vegetable oils, particularly safflower oil. Nuts and cereals also contain vitamin E. The refining process of oils and cereals may diminish the vitamin E content greatly.

Vitamin E deficiency rarely occurs. Reported cases involved premature infants fed commercial formulas that contained relatively low ratios of vitamin E to polyunsaturated fatty acids and adults and children with fat malabsorption diseases (sprue, cystic fibrosis, pancreatitis, biliary cirrhosis, and idiopathic conditions). In infants the signs and symptoms were edema, anemia, reticulocytosis, and thrombocytosis (47). The cause was low vitamin E levels. Signs and symptoms in adults included decreased red blood cell survival time and muscle lesions. With vitamin E deficiency, creatine excretion in the urine may be very high, and enzymes reflecting muscle damage may be increased in the plasma.

The therapeutic dosage of vitamin E for infants is 75–100 IU/day. In adults the dose of vitamin E required to return blood levels of tocopherol to normal was 60–80 IU/day for several weeks (48). However, higher doses have been used.

It is unlikely that the pharmacist would see distinguishable vitamin E deficiency in the pharmacy. Infants with edema should be referred to a physician because edema may be a symptom of heart disease, renal disease, or other serious diseases and its cause cannot be distinguished without laboratory tests.

Patients with intermittent claudication and angina pectoris were reported to improve with daily doses of 400–3200 IU of vitamin E (49, 50). More studies are needed, particularly with angina, because the beneficial effects were small and not statistically significant. Clinical trials have failed to show that vitamin E protects against miscarriages, sterility, menopausal abnormalities, muscular dystrophies, cystic fibrosis, ulcers, or diabetes. As part of the antioxidant theory of vitamin E it has been suggested that large doses retard the aging process. This theory suggests that aging is a buildup of cellular components that have been destroyed by their exposure to oxygen, cosmic rays, or pollution. Vitamin E as an antioxidant is claimed to protect against this reaction. The theory has not been proven or disproven clinically, and research continues in this area.

Vitamin E has been ingested in large quantities without apparent pharmacological toxicity. Thus long-term use at high doses cannot be discouraged on the basis of toxicity. In advising patients on vitamin E the pharmacist should stress the following points:

- The average American diet adequately protects against vitamin E deficiency;
- The FDA requires that all infant formulas contain adequate amounts of vitamin E (human and cow's milk contain enough vitamin E to protect against vitamin E deficiency in infants);
- High doses of vitamin E are a waste of money;
- Attempting to self-treat a potentially serious symptom such as chest pain with vitamin E only delays proper medical treatment.

If vitamin E has been prescribed, iron should not be taken at the same time. Studies with supplementation of infant formulas containing iron and vitamin E show that blood tocopherol levels do not increase (51).

Water-Soluble Vitamins

Water-soluble vitamins include ascorbic acid, thiamine hydrochloride, riboflavin, niacin, pyridoxine hydrochloride, cyanocobalamin, folic acid, pantothenic acid, biotin, bioflavonoids, choline, and inositol. RDA's have been established for most of these vitamins. The value of inositol in human nutrition is unknown.

Ascorbic Acid (Vitamin C)

As a nutrient, ascorbic acid is necessary to prevent scurvy. Humans and a few other species must consume ascorbic acid because it is not produced by the body. Today, scurvy is rare and develops only when psychiatric illness, alcoholism, age, GI disease, food fads, or ignorance causes inadequate nutritional consumption; infants fed artificial formulas without vitamin supplements also may develop scurvy. In adults, scurvy occurs 4–5 months after all ascorbic acid consumption is stopped.

Ascorbic acid is involved in the formation of connective tissue, osteoid, and dentin. A deficiency causes impairment of wound healing and reopening of old wounds. Early manifestations include anorexia, weakness, neurasthenia, and joint and muscle aches. Another early sign is prominent hair follicles on the thighs and buttocks due to plugging with keratin. The hair is coiled in the hair follicle and looks like a corkscrew, or it may be fragmented after it erupts. Bleeding abnormalities, such as hemorrhaging in the skin, muscles, joints, GI mucosa, and major organs, also occur. The gingiva of the teeth become swollen, hemorrhagic, infected, and sometimes necrotic, and, if the condition is untreated, the teeth fall out. Death may occur suddenly in untreated scurvy. In infants with ascorbic acid deficiency, growth and development are retarded, skin and gum hemorrhaging occur, bone development is impaired, and anemia may develop.

Because only 10 mg/day of ascorbic acid prevents scurvy and a normal diet containing fresh fruits and vegetables contains many times this amount, pharmacists rarely are confronted with symptoms of ascorbic acid deficiency. The most common early symptom of the deficiency is prominent hair follicles. Rough skin is likely to be a problem, most often in winter, when fresh fruits and vegetables are not as plentiful. The pharmacist should find out the sites of the roughness and appearance of the hairs. If answers to questions indicate a deficiency, the pharmacist should determine whether more serious signs and symptoms exist, such as easy bruisability, spontaneous petechiae, or purpura (blood spots just under the skin). If they do not exist and if the patient does not take a multiple-vitamin product or an ascorbic acid supplement, a multiple-vitamin product may be recommended. Most of these products contain 40 mg or more of ascorbic acid per dose.

symptoms of ascorbic acid deficiency

Because the 1974 RDA for ascorbic acid in adults is 45 mg, the pharmacist also may recommend daily dosing (e.g., a 50-mg tablet) with ascorbic acid. If the patient is already taking a daily vitamin supplement, additional vitamin C probably is not helpful. If hemorrhagic signs are present, the pharmacist should refer the patient to a physician: many serious diseases may cause similar problems, the diagnosis for which cannot be determined by a pharmacist.

treatment

In the treatment of severely scorbutic patients, 300 mg/day of ascorbic acid for 5 days is recommended to build up the body store, followed by a daily allowance of 45 mg in the food or by a supplement in addition to food (52). Infants who do not have vitamin C supplements in their formula should receive 35–50 mg/day; those who are breast-fed receive a sufficient amount.

role in common cold

Doses of ascorbic acid recommended for prevention (1–4 g/day) and treatment (as much as 15 g/day) of the common cold are pharmacological doses. Since Pauling's (53, 54) writings on ascorbic acid and the common cold, much literature has appeared. The question of ascorbic acid's efficacy has been reviewed by the Department of Drugs of the American Medical Association, and the studies indicate (55) that there is "little convincing evidence to support claims of clinically important efficacy." The results of one study showing a positive correlation between ascorbic acid in high doses and amelioration of cold symptoms was nonreproducible by the same investigators (56, 57).

drug interactions

Drug interactions may occur with ascorbic acid. The most frequent ones occur with warfarin sodium or dicumarol. The clinical evidence is sketchy, however, and pharmacists aware of the concurrent administration of either of these drugs with ascorbic acid should discuss the possible interaction with the patient and the physician and suggest that prothrombin times be measured regularly. Because ascorbic acid acidifies the urine, other drug interactions may occur. Ascorbic acid is used to acidify the urine of patients taking methenamine compounds, although a study suggests that ascorbic acid may not routinely acidify the urine (58). The acid converts the compounds to formaldehyde to produce their antibacterial activity. Patients with spine injuries and neurogenic bladders often take ascorbic acid to prevent urinary tract infections. Acidic drugs (e.g., salicylates) are resorbed to a greater extent in the renal tubules with acidified urine (59). Basic drugs (e.g., tricyclic antidepressants and the amphetamines) are excreted more rapidly in acidified urine, and therefore their effect is antagonized (60–62). Ascorbic acid forms a soluble chelate with iron to improve iron absorption.

Urine glucose tests are affected by large quantities of ascorbic acid in the urine. The TesTape and Clinistix tests may read false negative, and Clinitest tablets and Benedict's solution may be false positive (63, 64). The pharmacist may instruct the patient on how to modify the technique to avoid the interaction with the tape method. TesTape may be dipped in the urine, and the color correlation made at the moving front of the liquid on the tape, where different diffusion rates allow the glucose to separate chromatographically from the ascorbic acid on the tape.

The pharmacist should ascertain whether the patient is diabetic or uses other medications whose effects are antagonized or increased by ascorbic acid. The unproven efficacy, possible adverse effects, and interactions do not lend themselves to the recommendation of ascorbic acid doses larger than the RDA.

RDA for thiamine

signs and symptoms of thiamine deficiency

toxicity

RDA for riboflavin

riboflavin deficiency

Ascorbic acid tablets and liquid concentrations are available in many sizes as ascorbic acid and sodium ascorbate. Sodium ascorbate is the soluble salt for parenteral use.

Thiamine Hydrochloride (Vitamin B_1)

Thiamine is a coenzyme in several enzyme-catalyzed reactions in humans. Several of these reactions are important in providing energy. The RDA for thiamine is 1.0–1.5 mg for adults, 0.7–1.2 mg for children, and 0.3–0.5 mg for infants. The amount needed increases with increased caloric consumption. The most familiar natural thiamine source is the hull of rice grains. Other good sources are pork, beef, fresh peas, and beans. It was in animals and humans whose diets consisted largely of polished rice that thiamine deficiency disease (beriberi) first was observed. Today, beriberi caused by nutritional deficiency rarely occurs in the Western world, unless it is precipitated by economic or medical conditions. Thiamine deficiency is most common in alcoholics, whose nutrition is severely or entirely neglected.

Signs and symptoms of thiamine hydrochloride deficiency are evident 12–14 days after thiamine intake is stopped. The abnormalities center in the cardiovascular and neurological systems. The deficiency causes cardiac failure possibly accompanied by edema, tachycardia on only minimal exertion, enlarged heart, and electrocardiographic abnormalities. The patient may have pain in the precordial or epigastric area. Neuromuscular symptoms are paresthesia of the extremities of maximal use, weakness, and atrophy. An acute form of thiamine hydrochloride deficiency occurs in alcoholics and other patients who have been vomiting for extended periods. The neurological signs (Wernicke's encephalopathy) are particularly evident. Nystagmus occurs when the patient is asked to gaze up and down along a horizontal plane. Administration of glucose solutions without thiamine administration may precipitate symptoms that range from mild confusion to coma. Death is common if treatment is withheld. Damage to the cerebral cortex may occur in patients who survive and may lead to Korsakoff's psychosis. The symptoms of the psychosis are impaired retentive memory and cognitive function: the patient commonly confabulates when given a piece of information or when asked a question.

Beriberi may develop in infants whose mothers are on a polished rice diet and in the Orient in regions where thiamine hydrochloride supplements are not used. The signs and symptoms of infantile beriberi also are neurological. Aphonia, or silent crying, may occur, and the signs of meningitis may be mimicked. Death ensues if treatment is not initiated with thiamine.

The thiamine dosage for treating heart failure symptoms caused by this deficiency is 5–10 mg three times per day. At this dose the failure is corrected rapidly, but the neurological signs correct much more slowly. The thiamine dosage for neurological deficits is 30–100 mg given parenterally for less than a week or until an oral diet can be started. The pharmacist may wish to recommend multiple-vitamin supplements to patients known to have poor dietary habits due to alcoholism.

Thiamine's toxicity is relatively mild. The oral dosage must exceed 200–300 mg before toxicity occurs. Most of the excess dose, i.e., more than 2–3 mg, is excreted in the urine. After parenteral administration, symptoms of itching, tingling, and pain may be noticed. There have been rare reports of anaphylactic reactions occurring after parenteral injections.

Thiamine is available as an elixir, an injectable solution, a powder, and a tablet. If it is mixed in a solution, the solution should be acidic.

Riboflavin (Vitamin B_2)

Riboflavin is a constituent of two coenzymes that are essential to oxidative enzyme systems involved in electron transport. Cellular growth cannot occur without riboflavin. The RDA for riboflavin is 1.1–1.8 mg for adults (more for pregnant and lactating women), 0.8–1.2 mg for children, and 0.4–0.6 mg for infants. It appears that the need for riboflavin increases during periods of increased cell growth, e.g., during pregnancy and wound healing. Natural sources of riboflavin are eggs, meat, milk, fish, and liver.

Riboflavin deficiency caused by inadequate nutrition is rare, found among the poor and in alcoholics. It usually accompanies other vitamin deficiencies. The signs and symptoms of riboflavin deficiency are angular stomatitis, cheilosis, and sore throat. In later stages there may be seborrheic dermatitis of the face and generalized dermatitis. Photophobia may occur, and the eyes may itch and burn. Folic acid utilization may depend on riboflavin; thus anemia may accompany riboflavin deficiency. The signs and symptoms of riboflavin deficiency may indicate other very serious conditions, such as blood dyscrasia.

A complete dietary history should be obtained from the patient. In some cases a therapeutic trial of riboflavin may be carried out before diagnosis is made. The therapeutic dose is 10 mg orally. Larger doses are not harmful but provide no additional benefit. The patient should be monitored to assess symptomatic improvement.

Riboflavin is not very soluble. If its absorption is a problem, 25 mg of the soluble riboflavin salt may be given intramuscularly. Riboflavin also is given intravenously as a component of injectable multivitamins, but the dosage is relatively low (about 10 mg per dose). Intravenous doses of 50 mg of riboflavin may decrease pulse rates in adults. Excess riboflavin is excreted in the urine. It has a yellow fluorescence.

Most OTC multiple-vitamin products contain 1–5 mg of riboflavin per dose; some products contain as much as 10 mg.

Niacin (Nicotinic Acid)

Niacin and niacinamide are constituents of the coenzymes nicotinamide adenine dinucleotide (NAD) and nicotinamide adenine dinucleotide phosphate (NADP). These enzymes are electron transfer agents; i.e., they accept or donate hydrogen in the respiratory mechanism of all body cells. Niacin results from the biological transformation of the amino acid tryptophan and is converted to niacinamide. Both niacin and niacinamide are effective in treating niacin deficiency (pellagra). Niacinamide produces less flushing than niacin.

RDA for niacin

The RDA for niacin is 12–20 mg for adults. More is needed during physiological stress (e.g., pregnancy, lactation, burns, and hyperthyroidism). The RDA depends somewhat on caloric intake—1000 cal provide 4.4 mg of niacin. Foods rich in niacin and/or tryptophan are beef, cow's milk, and whole eggs.

niacin deficiency, signs and symptoms

Pellagra is rare, occurring most frequently in alcoholics, the elderly, and individuals on bizarre diets. It also occurs in areas where much corn is eaten because, although corn contains enough niacin to prevent pellagra, the niacin is bound to indigestible constituents, making it unavailable. The main systems affected are the nervous system, the skin, and the GI tract. Symptoms affecting the nervous system are peripheral neuropathy, myelopathy, and encephalopathy. Mania may occur, and seizures and coma precede death. Before the cause was discovered, many psychiatric admissions were due to the symptoms of niacin deficiency. There is a characteristic rash in niacin-deficient patients. Skin over the face and on pressure points may be thickened and hyperpigmented, may appear as a severe burn, and may become secondarily infected. The entire GI tract is affected, including angular fissures around the mouth, atrophy of the epithelium of the tongue, and hypertrophy of the papillae. Inflammation of the small intestine also may occur in association with episodes of bleeding and/or diarrhea. A summary of niacin deficiency symptoms in the various systems is called the "3 D's"—diarrhea, dementia, and dermatitis.

The diagnosis is clear if all systems are affected. However, if the skin is unaffected, the diagnosis is much more difficult. A complete dietary history with subsequent calculation of niacin consumption may point to the disease. Treatment involves the ingestion of 300–500 mg/day of niacinamide in divided doses. Because other nutritional deficiencies often are present, the therapy should include the other B vitamins, vitamin A, and iron.

Niacin in much higher doses has been used for other therapeutic purposes such as lowering lipids in the blood. Its side effects at these dosages prevent it from being the drug of choice. Niacinamide is ineffective as a lipid-lowering agent. Niacin also is used for patients with peripheral vascular disease, but the clinical results of its use in these patients are varied. Dosages suggested by the manufacturer are 150 mg/day in divided doses.

side effects

High niacin dosages cause significant and potentially life-threatening side effects. Because of the effects on the GI tract, high niacin doses are contraindicated in patients with gastritis or peptic ulcer. Niacin may release histamine, and its use in patients with asthma should be undertaken carefully. It also may impair liver function, causing cholestatic jaundice, and may disturb glucose tolerance and cause hyperuricemia. If niacin and niacinamide are used in high doses, laboratory parameters, suggested by the potential side effects, should be followed.

Niacin and niacinamide are available as tablets of many strengths, as injectable powders, and as elixirs (50 mg/0.5 ml). Doses of niacin in supplemental products usually are 10–20 mg; products containing 20 mg usually are used as prenatal vitamins. Products containing 100 mg of niacinamide are classified by the FDA as drugs rather than as dietary supplements and are available without a prescription.

Pyridoxine Hydrochloride (Vitamin B_6)

RDA for pyridoxine

Pyridoxine hydrochloride, pyridoxal hydrochloride, and pyridoxamine are all equally effective in nutrition. Pyridoxine hydrochloride is the form most frequently used in vitamins. The RDA is 1.6–2 mg for adults and 0.3–1.2 mg for infants and children; for pregnant and lactating women it is 2.5 mg. Foods rich in pyridoxine hydrochloride are meats, cereals, lentils, nuts, and some fruits and vegetables such as bananas, avocados, and potatoes. Cooking destroys some of the vitamin. The average U.S. diet provides the RDA; certain restricted diets and haphazard diets do not. Artificial infant formulas are required to contain pyridoxine hydrochloride.

symptoms of deficiency

The symptoms of pyridoxine hydrochloride deficiency in infants are convulsive disorders and irritability. Treatment with pyridoxine hydrochloride (e.g., 2 mg/day for infants) brings the encephalogram back to normal. Symptoms in adults whose diets are deficient in pyridoxine hydrochloride or who have been given a pyridoxine hydrochloride antagonist are indistinguishable from those of niacin and riboflavin deficiencies. They include pellagralike dermatitis, oral lesions, peripheral neuropathy, and dulling of mentation. Other conditions or circumstances also may be related to pyridoxine hydrochloride requirements. Treatment of sideroblastic anemia requires 50–200 mg/day of pyridoxine hydrochloride to aid in producing hemoglobin and erythrocytes. Because these amounts are more than physiological requirements, the anemia is not a nutritional deficiency.

interactions

Several drugs affect pyridoxine hydrochloride utilization. Isoniazid and cycloserine (antitubercular drugs) seem to antagonize pyridoxine hydrochloride. Hydralazine appears to have this effect as well (65). Perioral numbness resulting from peripheral neuropathy is a clinical manifestation of this antagonism, occurring most frequently in patients with poor diets. Psychotic behavior or seizures, both produced by cycloserine, may be prevented with increased pyridoxine hydrochloride intake. To overcome the antagonism, 50 mg/day of pyridoxine hydrochloride with isoniazid and as much as 200 mg/day with cycloserine should be used. Penicillamine may bind with pyridoxine hydrochloride, causing pyridoxine hydrochloride responsive neurotoxicity.

Estrogen seems to increase significantly the amount of tryptophan excreted in the urine. Thus women taking oral contraceptives have shown increased tryptophan metabolite excretion (66–68). Pyridoxine hydrochloride corrects this abnormality. A multivitamin product has been formulated that contains more than 10 times the RDA of pyridoxine hydrochloride. It also contains 0.1 mg of folic acid and vitamin E, both of which are depleted with the use of contraceptive steroids (69).

Pyridoxine hydrochloride may act as an antagonist to the pharmacological action of levodopa. Because it facilitates the transformation of levodopa to dopamine before the levodopa can cross into the CNS, pyridoxine hydrochloride should be avoided by patients taking levodopa. However, it may be useful for patients who have taken an overdose of levodopa. The pharmacist should inform patients taking levodopa of the effects of pyridoxine hydrochloride. A vitamin product that does not contain pyridoxine hydrochloride has been formulated for parkinsonian patients taking levodopa. A carbidopa and levodopa combination product is not affected by the concurrent administration of pyridoxine hydrochloride. Pyridoxine hydrochloride is available as a tablet in varying strengths and as injectable solutions.

Cyanocobalamin (Vitamin B_{12})

Cyanocobalamin is involved with folic acid in many body cell activities, and it is necessary for the incorporation of folic acid into cells. It also is involved in fat and carbohydrate metabolism as a constituent of a coenzyme system. The RDA for cyanocobalamin is 3 μg for adults and 0.3–2 μg for infants and children. More is needed by pregnant and lactating women because of cyanocobalamin drain by the fetus and by milk production. Cyanocobalamin is produced almost exclusively by microorganisms, hence its presence in animal protein. It also may be found in the root nodules of legumes because of the presence of organisms.

Cyanocobalamin deficiency may be caused by inadequate ingestion, absorption, utilization, or increased requirement or excretion of this vitamin (70). Vegetarian diets may need supplementation with cyanocobalamin. Because cyanocobalamin is so well conserved by the body through enterohepatic cycling, the deficiency requires decades to develop. In patients whose deficiency is related to malabsorption the reabsorption phase of the enterohepatic cycle is affected, and the deficiency occurs in 3–6 years. In healthy individuals who have not restricted their diets, adequate cyanocobalamin levels are maintained by the body. Some people lack the glycoprotein (intrinsic factor) necessary for cyanocobalamin absorption and develop pernicious anemia.

cyanocobalamin deficiency, signs and symptoms

Because cyanocobalamin is important in cell production, the signs and symptoms of a deficiency are manifested in organ systems with rapidly duplicating cells. Thus an effect on the hematopoietic system results in anemia. The GI tract also is affected, glossitis and epithelial changes occurring along the entire tract. Because of cyanocobalamin's importance in myelin production, deficiency states cause many neurological symptoms and signs, such as paresthesia (manifested as tingling and numbness in the hands and feet), progressing to unsteadiness, poor muscular coordination, mental slowness, confusion, agitation, optic atrophy, hallucinations, and overt psychosis. Surgical removal of portions of the stomach and small intestine often result in cyanocobalamin deficiency. Regional enteritis, tropical sprue, idiopathic steatorrhea, and celiac disease impair cyanocobalamin absorption.

Certain drugs may impair cyanocobalamin absorption. Neomycin reduces the absorption, and malabsorption is increased if colchicine is also a part of therapy (71, 72).

treatment

Treatment of cyanocobalamin deficiency used to involve the administration of crude liver extracts orally and parenterally. Because crystalline cyanocobalamin is now readily available, this is the preferred form. Treatment of pernicious anemia or permanent gastric or ileal damage with cyanocobalamin is lifelong.

dosage forms

Cyanocobalamin is available in tablet and injectable dosage forms. Oral forms may be used if the deficiency is nutritionally based; intramuscular or subcutaneous administration is necessary for deficiencies caused by malabsorption. Hydroxycobalamin is a long-acting form equal in hematopoietic effect to cyanocobalamin. Because it is bound to blood proteins, it remains in the body for a longer period. However, this advantage is not great enough to justify the cost and pain of injecting it. There are a few OTC products that contain more than 1.5 times the RDA of cyanocobalamin. These products are no longer classified as dietary supplements but as drugs. Cyanocobalamin has no therapeutic value beyond that of correcting cyanocobalamin deficiencies, unless its placebo effect is considered. The deficiency may be corrected with 1 μg of oral cyanocobalamin daily or 100 μg given parenterally each month. Doses larger than needed do not cause toxicity because excretion through the urine occurs when tissue and plasma binding sites are saturated.

Folic Acid

RDA for folic acid

In its function in the body, folic acid (pteroylglutamic acid) is closely related to cyanocobalamin. Folates must be converted enzymatically before they can be absorbed, and in the body, folate coenzymes are involved in the transfer of one-carbon units in protein synthesis. The RDA for folic acid is 400 μg for adults and 50–300 μg for infants and children, depending on age. During pregnancy, 800 μg is required, and during lactation, 600 μg.

The folate content of food is subject to destruction depending on how it is processed. Canning, long exposure to heat, and refining destroy 50–100% of the folates.

Generally, foods richest in folates are fresh green vegetables. Yeast and liver and other organ meats also contain folates.

The requirement for folic acid is related to metabolic rate and cell turnover. Thus increased amounts of folic acid are needed during pregnancy (especially with twin or multiple fetuses), during infections, in hemolytic anemias and blood loss where red blood cell production attempts to meet the increased needs, in infancy, and in cases of increased metabolic rates such as hyperthyroidism. Rheumatoid arthritis, perhaps because of the proliferation of synovial membranes or the possible salicylate-induced blood loss, also increases folate requirements. Certain hematopoietic malignancies also cause an increased need for folic acid.

It is fairly easy for individuals to become folate deficient, particularly if fresh vegetables and fruits are not eaten. The symptoms of deficiency are much the same as those of cyanocobalamin deficiency—sore mouth, diarrhea, and CNS symptoms such as irritability and forgetfulness. A common sign of folic acid deficiency is megaloblastic anemia.

The causes of folic acid deficiency are similar to those of B vitamin deficiencies. Nutritionally, the diet must include foods that need little cooking because folates are heat labile. Alcoholics frequently have folic acid deficiency, as do individuals with malabsorption diseases. Conditions that cause rapid cell turnover may induce potentially life-threatening folic acid deficiency.

Several drugs taken chronically may increase the need for folic acid. Phenytoin and possibly other related anticonvulsants may cause an inhibition of folic acid absorption, leading to megaloblastic anemia (73). This problem is complicated further by the fact that folic acid supplementation may decrease serum phenytoin levels, decreasing seizure control (74). With this consideration in mind, when dispensing folic acid to patients whose medication record indicates concurrent phenytoin use, the pharmacist should ask whether seizure activity is controlled. Another possible drug interaction occurs with oral contraceptive drugs, which may cause folic acid deficiencies (75). This effect is extremely rare and probably is not a significant side effect (76–83). Trimethoprim may act as a folic acid antagonist in humans. Megaloblastic anemia may be precipitated in patients who had a relatively low folate level at the onset of trimethoprim therapy; short-term therapy, however, does not lead to megaloblastic anemia. Pyrimethamine, which is related to trimethoprim, in large doses may induce megaloblastic anemia. Folinic acid may be administered to reverse the anemia because the mechanism of pyrimethamine's folic acid antagonism is inhibition of active tetrahydrofolate production (79). Methotrexate also causes folic acid antagonism.

Folic acid given without cyanocobalamin to patients with pernicious anemia may correct the anemia but has no effect on the damage to the nervous system. The symptoms of the damage include incoordination, impaired sense of position, and a spectrum of mental disturbances. Because of this effect of folic acid, OTC vitamin preparations are not permitted to contain more than 0.4 mg of folic acid; vitamins for pregnant or lactating women can contain as much as 0.8 mg (80). Including cyanocobalamin in the oral preparation is, of course, not helpful if the patient has pernicious anemia. Cyanocobalamin must be given parenterally to these patients, who must be monitored carefully.

The dose of folic acid for correction of a deficiency is usually 100 μg. If the deficiency occurs with conditions that may increase the folate requirement or suppress red blood cell formation (e.g., pregnancy, hypermetabolic states, alcoholism, or hemolytic anemia), the dose is 0.5–1 mg. Doses larger than 1 mg are excreted in the urine and, except in some life-threatening hematologic diseases, are not beneficial. Maintenance therapy for deficiencies may be stopped after 1–4 months if the diet contains at least one fresh fruit or vegetable daily (81). For chronic malabsorption diseases, folic acid may be required for a long period, and parenteral doses are needed in severe cases. Folic acid toxicity is nearly nonexistent because of its water solubility and water excretion—15 mg can be given daily without toxic effect.

folic acid deficiency, signs and symptoms

drug interactions

symptoms of biotin deficiency

Pantothenic Acid

Pantothenic acid is a precursor to coenzyme A, a product active in many biological reactions in the body. Although its RDA has not been established, it is contained in many foods which make it easily available. Intake of 5–10 mg/day of pantothenic acid satisfies the need. Pantothenic acid deficiency is very hard to detect. In malabsorption syndromes it is difficult to separate pantothenic acid deficiency symptoms from many other ones. Pantothenic acid has been withheld experimentally, and the resulting symptoms are abdominal pain, vomiting, and cramps. Later, muscle tenderness, weakness, paresthesia, and insomnia occur. Administration of large doses of pantothenic acid reverses these symptoms.

Pantothenic acid is not known to have any therapeutic use. It frequently is incorporated into oral multiple-vitamin preparations. As much as 20 g has been administered, and the toxicity is minimal, appearing as diarrhea.

Biotin

Although biotin is one of the B-complex vitamins, the RDA has not yet been established. Biotin is distributed widely in animal tissue and appears necessary for the formation of protein from amino acids. In rats, biotin also seems necessary for appropriate glucose utilization, and some of its effects are similar to those of insulin. In humans, biotin is synthesized by gut flora. Serum biotin levels in normal subjects are 213–404 ng/ml. Biotin deficiency in humans may be caused by the ingestion of a large number of egg whites. Egg whites contain avidin, a protein that inactivates biotin; this inactivation causes a dermatitis, a grayish skin color, anorexia, anemia, hypercholesterolemia, and lassitude (82). In pregnant women, blood biotin levels decrease as gestation progresses.

In rats a combination of oxytetracycline and succinylsulfathiazole inhibited the intestinal synthesis of biotin. A similar effect might be expected in humans after using gut-sterilizing antibiotics, but it has not been reported.

Biotin has been incorporated into several multiple-vitamin preparations. It has been used therapeutically in infants and children to treat seborrheic dermatitis and propionic acidemia. There was slight improvement in muscle tone with oral doses (5 mg for 5 days) (83).

Bioflavonoids

The term "bioflavonoids" has been used to designate flavones and flavonols. Bioflavonoids were called vitamin P ("P" for permeability), but this designation is no longer used because no vitamin activity has been documented. This group of agents includes rutin and hesperidin, which have stimulated controversy in the medical literature. The controversy stems from their proposed use in the treatment of vascular bleeding disorders such as vascular purpura, retinal hemorrhages, cerebrovascular accidents, and lymphedema. Deficiency states have not been induced or discovered in humans or animals. There appears to be no clinical use for the agents. Studies involving rutin as a pharmacological entity continue, particularly in Europe (84, 85).

flavones and flavonols

use of large vitamin doses

Choline

Choline is a precursor of acetylcholine, which is an important donator of a methyl group used in the formation of other biological substances. It may be formed from methionine by the donation of a methyl group from the methionine. Choline is a component of several phospholipids. No choline deficiency disease in humans has been reported. Rats, hamsters, dogs, chickens, and pigs develop choline deficiency diseases including fatty liver, cirrhosis, anemia, renal lesions, and hypertension. These findings have been the basis for treating alcoholics with choline, although the literature reports no therapeutic value. Although choline is found in egg yolks, cereal, fish, and meat, it is also synthesized in the body; therefore it is doubtful that it is a vitamin.

Choline is available as a tablet, powder, or syrup and in combination with other nutritional ingredients. Its stated use is the decrease of fatty liver.

Inositol

Inositol is a sugar found in large amounts in muscle and brain tissues. It is widely distributed in nature and is synthesized in the body, but its biological value and metabolism are unknown. In cell culture, inositol appears necessary for amino acid transport and for the movement of potassium and sodium. As a sugar it is approximately one-third as effective as glucose in correcting diabetic ketosis. Inositol is available as a tablet, powder, or syrup. Its value in human nutrition has not been documented.

Megadose Vitamin Therapy

The toxicity of individual vitamins ranges from nearly no observable side effects to life-threatening side effects. Because the life-threatening side effects are insidious and because a wide range of supposed health benefits are attributed to vitamins, individual or multiple vitamins are often consumed in large doses. However, no beneficial effects from megavitamin therapy have been found (86). In addition, large doses often have serious side effects.

Megadoses of vitamin A used in treating minimal brain dysfunction and psychiatric conditions have led to toxicity (87). The Committee on Nutrition of the American Academy of Pediatrics concludes that there is no place for the use of megavitamin therapy in the treatment of neuropsychiatric disorders (88).

Megadoses of ascorbic acid may be harmful. There are indications of increased danger of developing urinary tract stones, interference with the completion of a normal pregnancy (with doses of 6 g/day for 3 days), diarrhea (with doses of 1 g/day or more), and a rebound phenomenon in infants born of mothers who had taken 400 mg/day of ascorbic acid before delivering (these infants required more than the usual amount of ascorbic acid to prevent scurvy) (89–92). However, more clinical evidence is needed to confirm these observations.

Niacin and niacinamide, in doses of as much as 3000 mg/day, have been used in megavitamin therapy for schizophrenia. Most controlled studies do not show significantly different results when compared with placebo (93).

The occurrence and degree of side effects are sometimes related to other variables such as concurrent medications the patient is consuming and the patient's ethnic background. Large vitamin doses may be necessary to correct deficits caused by cancer chemotherapy, certain genetic diseases, or malabsorption syndromes.

An advertising approach used by at least one pharmaceutical manufacturer is to suggest that certain prescription drugs or human conditions require greater vitamin consumption. The patients included in these claims are those who receive long-term antibiotic therapy, are elderly, are taking oral contraceptives, are pregnant, have had recent surgery, or have had a bone fracture. Many of these claims can be substantiated to some degree by existing studies. It should be remembered, however, that generalization about certain populations is often inappropriate.

SUMMARY

By being familiar with recommended dietary daily allowances of the various vitamins and minerals and knowing which natural sources provide these RDA's, the pharmacist can supply a valuable patient service. In addition, the pharmacist should be able to recognize symptoms of vitamin and mineral deficiencies; prompt physician referral often is crucial in these cases. A patient's cultural or socioeconomic background and physical condition are guidelines in helping the pharmacist determine nutritional status. Pregnant and lactating women require more nutrients than normal healthy adults.

Supplementary formula products should be used as adjuncts to a regular diet and not as a substitute for food. Although dietary products can be obtained without a prescription, they are complex agents with specific indications. Medical assessment must precede their use. The pharmacist should review dilution, preparation technique, storage, and administration of these products with the patient and should offer to discuss with the patient unusual effects, such as diarrhea, that may be caused by the formulas. An antidiarrheal may be indicated or merely a change in administration or storage procedures. The pharmacist should not be reluctant to consult a dietician or physician (especially a gastroenterologist, oncologist, or surgeon, who often deals with nutrition problems) concerning nutritional supplementation and should refer patients when necessary.

The pharmacist should stress to patients that "fad" diets are no substitute for sound medical care. For example, although megadose vitamin therapy has been used with success in certain patient populations, there is no evidence to indicate that large doses ensure good health. Indeed, serious side effects have been reported. The FDA OTC Panel on Vitamin, Mineral, and Hematinic Drug Products is reviewing this aspect and other areas of nutrition.

REFERENCES

(1) *Chemical Engineering News, 51,* 9 (1973).
(2) B. Wolnak, *Food Drug Cosmet. Law J., 27,* 453 (1972).
(3) D. Coldsmith, *Mod. Med., 43,* 121 (1975).
(4) "A Study of Health Practices and Opinions," Final Report, Conducted for FDA, HEW, Contract No. FDA 66-193, June 1972, and FDA Talk Paper, Oct. 6, 1972.
(5) *Nutrition Reviews Supplement, 32,* 53 (1974).
(6) A. Kamil, *J. Nutr., 4,* 92 (1972).
(7) R. M. Kark, *J. Am. Diet Assoc., 64,* 476 (1974).
(8) R. R. Crichton, *N. Engl. J. Med., 284,* 1413 (1971).
(9) T. H. Bothwell and C. A. Finch, "Iron Metabolism," Little, Brown, Boston, Mass., 1962.
(10) Committee on Iron Deficiency, *J. Am. Med. Assoc., 203,* 407 (1968).
(11) L. Hallberg, H. G. Harwerth, and A. Vannatti, "Iron Deficiency Pathogenesis, Clinical Aspects, Therapy," Academic, New York, N.Y., 1970. p. 169.
(12) V. Minnich, A. Okcuoglu, Y. Tarçon, A. Arcasoy, S. Cin, O. Yörükoglu, F. Renda, and B. Demirag, *Am. J. Clin. Nutr., 21,* 78 (1968).
(13) W. H. Crosby, *J. Am. Med. Assoc., 235,* 2765 (1976).
(14) H. Brise and L. Hallberg, *Acta Med. Scand. Suppl., 376,* 23 (1962).
(15) *Medical Letter, 20,* 46 (1978).
(16) "Modern Nutrition in Health and Disease: Dietotherapy," 5th rev., R. S. Goodheart and M. E. Shils, Eds., Lea and Febiger, Philadelphia, Pa., 1973, p. 316.
(17) D. N. S. Kerr and L. S. P. Davidson, *Lancet, 2,* 489 (1958).
(18) G. J. L. Hall and A. E. Davis, *Med. J. Aust., 2,* 95 (1969).
(19) P. J. Neuvonen, G. Gothoni, R. Hackman, and K. Bjorksten, *Br. Med. J., 4,* 532 (1970).
(20) M. N. Gleason, R. Gosselin, H. Hodge, and R. Smith, "Clinical Toxicology of Commercial Products," 3rd ed., Williams and Wilkins, Baltimore, Md., 1969, p. 108.
(21) S. Margen and D. H. Calloway, *Fed. Proc., 26,* 629 (1967).
(22) R. M. Walker and H. M. Linkswiler, *J. Nutr., 102,* 1297 (1972).
(23) C. F. Mills, "Trace Element Metabolism in Animals," Livingstone, Edinburgh, Scotland, 1970, p. 75.
(24) H. H. Sandstead, *Am. J. Clin. Nutr., 26,* 1251 (1973).
(25) R. W. Vilter, *N. Engl. J. Med., 291,* 188 (1974).
(26) M. F. Ivey, W. Mueller, M. Riella, and B. Scribner, *Am. J. Hosp. Pharm., 32,* 1032 (1975).
(27) H. A. Schroeder, D. V. Frost, and J. J. Balassa, *J. Chronic Dis., 23,* 227 (1970).
(28) H. A. Schroeder and A. D. Nason, *Clin. Chem., 17,* 461 (1971).
(29) K. Schwarz, *Fed. Proc., 20,* Part 1, 665 (1961).
(30) J. Wilstrom, T. Westermarck, and J. Palo, *Acta Neurol. Scand., 54,* 287 (1976).
(31) D. V. Frost and D. Ingvoldstad, *Chem. Scr., A8,* 96 (1975).
(32) R. J. Shamberger and D. V. Frost, *Can. Med. Assoc. J., 100,* 682 (1969).
(33) G. N. Schrauzer and D. Ishmael, *Ann. Clin. Lab. Sci., 4,* 441 (1974).
(34) W. L. Broghamer, K. P. McConnell, and A. L. Blotcky, *Cancer, 37,* 1384 (1976).
(35) R. S. Shakman, *Arch. Environ. Health, 28,* 105 (1974).
(36) A. W. Kilness and F. H. Hochberg, *J. Am. Med. Assoc., 237,* 2843 (1977).
(37) W. Mertz, *J. Am. Diet Assoc., 64,* 163 (1974).
(38) T. Moore, "Vitamin A," Elsevier, Amsterdam, Netherlands, 1957, p. 355.
(39) J. Bieri, *J. Am. Diet Assoc., 64,* 171 (1974).
(40) P. L. White, *J. Am. Med. Assoc., 238,* 1762 (1977).
(41) National Academy of Sciences/National Research Council Food and Nutrition Board, "Recommended Dietary Alowances," Publ. No. 1694, 7th ed., Washington, D.C., 1968.
(42) "Modern Nutrition in Health and Disease: Dietotherapy," 5th rev., R. S. Goodheart and M. E. Shils, Eds., Lea and Febiger, Philadelphia, Pa., 1973, p. 152.
(43) "Harrison's Principles of Internal Medicine," 8th ed., G. W. Thorn, R. D. Adams, E. Braunwald, K. J. Isselbacher, and R. G. Petersdorf, Eds., McGraw-Hill, New York, N.Y., 1977, p. 464.
(44) J. Myrtle and A. Norman, *Science, 171,* 79 (1971).
(45) S. Fomon, M. Youroszar, and L. Thomas, *J. Nutr., 89,* 345 (1966).
(46) D. Fraser and R. Slater, *Pediatr. Clin. North Am., 5,* 417 (1958).
(47) J. Ritchie, M. Fish, V. McMasters, and M. Grossman, *N. Engl. J. Med., 279,* 1185 (1968).
(48) M. Horwitt, *Am. J. Clin. Nutr., 8,* 451 (1960).
(49) J. T. B. Williams, D. Fenna, and R. A. McBeth, *Surg. Gynecol. Obstet., 662,* 132 (1971).
(50) T. W. Anderson, *Can. Med. Assoc. J., 10,* 40 (1974).
(51) L. A. Barness, F. A. Oski, M. Williams, G. Marrow, and S. Arnaud, *Am. J. Clin. Nutr., 21,* 40 (1968).
(52) "Modern Nutrition in Health and Disease: Dietotherapy," 5th rev., R. S. Goodheart and M. E. Shils, Eds., Lea and Febiger, Philadelphia, Pa., 1973, p. 253.
(53) L. Pauling, *Proc. Nat. Acad. Sci. (USA), 67,* 1643 (1970).
(54) L. Pauling, *Am. J. Clin. Nutr., 24,* 1294 (1971).
(55) M. Dykes and P. Meier, *J. Am. Med. Assoc., 231,* 1073 (1973).
(56) T. Anderson, D. Reid, and G. Beaton, *Can. Med. Assoc. J., 107,* 503 (1972).
(57) T. Anderson, G. Suranyi, and G. Beaton, *Can. Med. Assoc. J., 111,* 31 (1974).
(58) D. C. McLeod and M. C. Nahata, *N. Engl. J. Med., 296,* 1413 (1977).
(59) G. Levy and J. Leonards, *J. Am. Med. Assoc., 217,* 81 (1971).
(60) F. Sjoqvist, *Clin. Pharmacol. Ther., 10,* 826 (1969).
(61) L. Gram, B. Kofod, J. Christiansen, and O. Rafaelsen, *Clin. Pharmacol. Ther., 12,* 239 (1971).
(62) M. Rowland, *J. Pharm. Sci., 58,* 408 (1969).
(63) J. Feldman, W. Kelley, and H. Lebovitz, *Diabetes, 19,* 337 (1970).
(64) J. Mayson, O. Schumaker, and R. Nakamura, *Am. J. Clin. Pathol., 58,* 297 (1972).
(65) N. H. Raskin, *N. Engl. J. Med., 273,* 1182 (1965).
(66) M. Baumblatt and F. Winston, *Lancet, 1,* 832 (1970).
(67) A. Lubby, P. Davis, M. Murphy, M. Gordon, M. Brin, and H. Spiegel, *Lancet, 2,* 1083 (1970).
(68) A. Lubby, P. Davis, M. Murphy, M. Gordon, M. Brin, and H. Spiegel, *Am. J. Clin. Nutr., 24,* 684 (1971).
(69) T. Necheles and L. Snyder, *N. Engl. J. Med., 282,* 858 (1970).
(70) "Modern Nutrition in Health and Disease: Dietotherapy," 5th rev., R. S. Goodheart and M. E. Shils, Eds., Lea and Febiger, Philadelphia, Pa., 1973, p. 225.
(71) W. Faloon and R. Chodos, *Gastroenterology, 56,* 1251 (1969).
(72) E. Jacobson, R. Chodos, and W. Faloon, *Am. J. Med., 28,* 524 (1960).
(73) C. Gerson, *Gastroenterology, 63,* 246 (1972).
(74) H. Kutt, J. Kaynes, and F. McDowell, *Arch. Neurol. (Chicago), 14,* 489 (1966).
(75) T. Necheles and L. Snyder, *N. Engl. J. Med., 282,* 858 (1970).
(76) N. Elgee, *Ann. Intern. Med., 72,* 409 (1970).
(77) R. Swerdloff, W. Odell, G. Bray, R. Fiser, A. Wolfsen, D. Fisher, and M. Sperling, *West. J. Med., 122,* 22 (1975).
(78) A. Bingel and P. Benoit, *J. Pharm. Sci., 62,* 179 (1973).
(79) "The Pharmacological Basis of Therapeutics," 5th ed., L. S. Goodman and A. Gilman, Eds., Macmillan, New York, N.Y., 1975, p. 1058.
(80) *Federal Register, 41,* 46172 (1976).
(81) "Modern Nutrition in Health and Disease: Dietotherapy," 5th rev., R. S. Goodheart and M. E. Shils, Eds., Lea and Febiger, Philadelphia, Pa., 1973, p. 242.
(82) V. Sydenstricker, S. Singal, A. Briggs, and H. Isbell, *J. Am. Med. Assoc., 118,* 1199 (1942).
(83) N. Barnes, D. Hull, L. Balgobin, and D. Gompertz, *Lancet, 2,* 244 (1970).
(84) E. Foldi-Borcsok and M. Foldi, *Am. J. Clin. Nutr., 26,* 185 (1973).
(85) R. Eastham, T. Perham, and P. Pocock, *Br. Med. J., 4,* 491 (1972).
(86) V. D. Herbert, *J. Am. Pharm. Assoc., NS17,* 764 (1977).
(87) B. A. Shaywitz, N. J. Siegel, and H. A. Pearson, *J. Am. Med. Assoc., 238,* 1749 (1977).
(88) Committee on Nutrition, American Academy of Pediatrics, *Pediatrics, 58,* 910 (1976).
(89) M. Briggs, P. Garcia-Webb, and P. Davies, *Lancet, 2,* 201 (1973).
(90) E. Samborskaja and T. Ferdman, *Nutr. Abstr. Rev., 37,* 73 (1967).
(91) G. A. Goldsmith, *J. Am. Med. Assoc., 216,* 337 (1971).
(92) W. A. Cochrane, *Can. Med. Assoc. J., 93,* 893 (1965).
(93) T. Ban, *Can. Psychiatr. Assoc. J., 16,* 413 (1971).

Product* (Manufacturer)	Vitamin A, IU	Vitamin D, IU	Vitamin E, IU	Ascorbic Acid (C), mg	Thiamine (B_1), mg	Riboflavin (B_2), mg	Niacin, mg
Abdec Baby Drops[a] (Parke-Davis)	5,000[b]	400	—	50	1.0[c]	1.2	10[d]
Abdec Kapseal (Parke-Davis)	10,000[q]	400	5	75	5.0[f]	3.0	25[d]
Abdec Teens Tablets (Parke-Davis)	7,500[q]	400	30[q]	180	4.5[f]	5.1	60[d]
Abdec Teens with Iron Tablets (Parke-Davis)	7,500[q]	400	30[q]	180	4.5[f]	5.1	60[d]
Abdol c̄ Minerals (Parke-Davis)	5,000[b]	400	—	50	2.5[f]	2.5	20[d]
A.C.N. (Person & Covey)	25,000[b]	—	—	250	—	—	25[d]
Adabee (Robins)	10,000	—	—	250[e]	15.0[f]	10.0	50[d]
Adabee c Minerals (Robins)	10,000	—	—	250[e]	15.0[f]	10.0	50[d]
Allbee-T (Robins)	—	—	—	500	15.5[f]	10.0	100[d]
Allbee with C (Robins)	—	—	—	300	15.0[f]	10.0	50[d]
Aprisac (North American)	—	—	5	—	—	—	—
AVP Natal (A.V.P.)	5,000	—	—	100	—	—	—
B-C-Bid Capsules (Geriatric Pharm.)	—	—	—	300	15.0[f]	10.0	50[d]
B-Complex Capsules (North American)	—	—	—	—	1.5[c]	2.0	10[d]
B Complex Tablets (Squibb)	—	—	—	—	0.7	0.7	9
B Complex with Vitamin C (Squibb)	—	—	—	300	10.0	10.0	100[d]
Beminal 500 (Ayerst)	—	—	—	500	25.0	12.5	100.0[d]
Beminal Forte with Vitamin C (Ayerst)	—	—	—	250	25.0	12.5	50.0[d]
Beta-Vite Liquid[n] (North American)	—	—	—	—	10.0[c]	—	—
Beta-Vite w/Iron Liquid[n] (North American)	—	—	—	—	10.0[c]	—	—
Bewon Elixir[n] (Wyeth)	—	—	—	—	0.25[c]	—	—
B Nutron (Nion)	—	—	—	—	2.0	3.0	10[d]
Brewers Yeast (North American)	—	—	—	—	0.06	0.02	0.15
Calcicaps (Nion)	—	400	—	—	—	—	—
Calcicaps with Iron (Nion)	—	400	—	—	—	—	—
Calcium, Phosphate, and Vitamin D (Squibb)	—	180	—	—	—	—	—
Calciwafers (Nion)	—	—	66.7	—	—	—	—
Cal-Prenal (North American)	4,000[q]	400	—	50	2.0[c]	2.0	10[d]
C-B Vone Capsules (USV)	—	—	—	250	25.0[f]	10.0	74[d]
Cebefortis (Upjohn)	—	—	—	150	5.0[f]	5.0	50[d]
Cebetinic (Upjohn)	—	—	—	25	2.0[f]	2.0	10[d]
Cecon Solution[a] (Abbott)	—	—	—	60	—	—	—
Ceebec (Person & Covey)	—	—	—	300	25.0	15	100[d]
Centrum (Lederle)	5,000	400	30	90	2.25	2.6	20[d]
Cevi-Bid (Geriatric Pharm.)	—	—	—	500	—	—	—
Ce-Vi-Sol Drops[a] (Mead Johnson)	—	—	—	35	—	—	—
Cherri-B Liquid[a] (North American)	—	—	—	—	1.5[c]	0.3	6[d]
Chew-E (North American)	—	—	200	—	—	—	—
Chew-Vite (North American)	5,000	400	—	50	3.0	2.5	20[d]

Pyridoxine Hydrochloride (B_6), mg	Cyanocobalamin (B_{12}), μg	Folic Acid, μg	Pantothenic Acid, mg	Iron, mg	Calcium, mg	Phosphorus, mg	Magnesium, mg	Other
1.0	—	—	5.0[e]	—	—	—	—	—
1.5	2.0[g]	—	10.0[h]	—	—	—	—	—
6	6	—	—	—	—	—	—	—
6	6	—	—	18[m]	—	—	—	—
0.5	1.0[g]	100	2.5[i]	15[j]	44[k]	34[k]	1.0[j]	potassium, 5.0 mg[j] manganese, 1.0 mg[j] zinc, 0.5 mg[j] others[z]
—	—	—	—	—	—	—	—	—
5.0	—	—	—	—	—	—	—	—
5.0	—	—	—	15	103	80	—	—
10.0	5.0	—	23.0	—	—	—	—	desiccated liver, 150 mg
5.0	—	—	10.0[i]	—	—	—	—	—
—	—	—	—	75[o]	58[k]	45[k]	—	manganese, 2.5 mg[j] zinc, 0.1 mg[j] copper, 0.1 mg[j]
10.0	—	—	—	66[m]	—	—	—	purified veal bone ash, 500 mg
5.0	5.0	—	—	—	—	—	—	—
0.1	—	—	1.0[i]	—	—	—	—	dried yeast, 100 mg desiccated liver, 70 mg
0.9	2.0	—	—	—	—	—	—	—
2.0	4.0	—	20.0[i]	—	—	—	—	—
10.0	5.0	—	—	—	20.0	—	—	saccharin, 0.15 mg
3.0	2.5	—	—	—	10.0	—	—	—
—	25.0	—	—	—	—	—	—	—
—	25.0	—	—	75[o]	—	—	—	—
—	—	—	—	—	—	—	—	—
0.2	1.0[g]	20	0.2[i]	8[p]	—	—	—	brewers yeast, 150 mg manganese sodium citrate, 16 mg
0.007	—	—	0.05	—	—	—	—	—
—	—	—	—	—	750	360	—	—
—	—	—	—	46[p]	750	360	—	—
—	—	—	—	—	255	156	—	—
—	—	—	—	—	171.1[k] 35.3[p]	136.7[k]	—	—
1.0	2.0[r]	100	—	50[m]	230	—	—	iodine, 150 μg[l]
1.5	5.0	—	7.5	—	—	—	—	choline, 25 mg
1.0	2.0	—	10.0[i]	—	—	—	—	—
0.5	5.0	—	—	38[p]	—	—	—	—
—	—	—	—	—	—	—	—	—
5.0	10.0	—	—	—	10	—	—	—
3	9	400	10	27	162	125	100	biotin, 150 μg iodine, 150 μg copper, 3 mg zinc, 22.5 mg manganese, 7.5 mg potassium, 7.5 mg
—	—	—	—	—	—	—	—	—
—	—	—	—	—	—	—	—	alcohol, 5%
0.09	—	—	0.12[h]	—	—	—	—	—
—	—	—	—	—	—	—	—	—
1.0	1.0[r]	—	—	—	—	—	—	—

Product* (Manufacturer)	Vitamin A, IU	Vitamin D, IU	Vitamin E, IU	Ascorbic Acid (C), mg	Thiamine (B_1), mg	Riboflavin (B_2), mg	Niacin, mg
Chocks (Miles)	2,500	400	15	60	1.05	1.2	13.5
Chocks-Bugs Bunny (Miles)	2,500	400	15	60	1.05	1.2	13.5
Chocks-Bugs Bunny Plus Iron (Miles)	2,500	400	15	60	1.05	1.2	13.5
Chocks Plus Iron (Miles)	2,500	400	15	60	1.05	1.2	13.5
Clusivol 130 (Ayerst)	10,000	400	0.5	150.0	10.0 [f]	5.0	50.0 [d]
Clusivol Syrup (Ayerst)	25,000	400	—	15.0	1.0	1.0	5.0 [d]
Cod Liver Oil Concentrate Capsules (Schering)	10,000	400	—	—	—	—	—
Cod Liver Oil Concentrate Tablets (Schering)	4,000	200	—	—	—	—	—
Cod Liver Oil Tablets with Vitamin C (Schering)	4,000	200	—	50	—	—	—
Combex Kapseals (Parke-Davis)	—	—	—	—	2.25 [f]	2.6	30
Combex Kapseals c̄ Vitamin C (Parke-Davis)	—	—	—	90	2.25 [f]	2.6	30
Dayalets (Abbott)	5,000	400	30	60	1.5 [c]	1.7	20 [d]
Dayalets plus Iron (Abbott)	5,000	400	30	60	1.5 [c]	1.7	20 [d]
De-Cal (North American)	—	125	—	—	—	—	—
Di-Calcium Phosphate Capsules (North American)	—	333	—	—	—	—	—
Dical-D (Abbott)	—	133	—	—	—	—	—
Dical-D with Vitamin C Capsules (Abbott)	—	133	—	15	—	—	—
Drisdol (Winthrop)	—	200	—	—	—	—	—
Duo-CVP Capsules (USV)	—	—	—	—	—	—	—
Dura-C 500 Graduals (Amfre-Grant)	—	—	—	500	—	—	—
Engran-HP (Squibb)	8,000	400	30	60	1.7	2.0	20
Epsilan-M (Warren-Teed)	—	—	100	—	—	—	—
Feminaid (Nion)	5,000	400	10	200	2.0	3.0	15 [d]
Feminins (Mead Johnson)	5,000	400	10	200	1.5 [c]	3.0	15
Femiron with Vitamins (J. B. Williams)	5,000	400	—	60	1.5	1.7	20 [d]
Ferritrinsic (Upjohn)	—	—	—	50	2.0 [f]	2.0	10 [d]
Ferrolip Plus (Flint)	—	—	—	50	2.5 [f]	1.0	5 [d]
Filibon Tablets (Lederle)	5,000 [q]	400	30	60 [i]	1.5	1.7	20 [d]
Flintstones (Miles)	2,500	400	15	60	1.05	1.2	13.5
Flintstones Plus Iron (Miles)	2,500	400	15	60	1.05	1.2	13.5
Folbesyn (Lederle)	—	—	—	180	10.0	5.0	50.0 [d]
Ganatrex [a] (Merrell-National)	5,000 [b]	400	30	60	1.5 [c]	1.7	20 [d]
Geralix Liquid [y] (North American)	—	—	—	—	3.3 [c]	1.7	—
Geriamic (North American)	—	—	—	75	15.0 [c]	5.0	30 [d]
Gerilets (Abbott)	5,000	400	45	90 [e]	2.25 [c]	2.6	30 [d]
Geriplex (Parke-Davis)	5,000 [q]	—	5	50 [e]	5.0 [f]	5.0	15 [d]

Pyridoxine Hydrochloride (B_6), mg	Cyanocobalamin (B_{12}), μg	Folic Acid, μg	Pantothenic Acid, mg	Iron, mg	Calcium, mg	Phosphorus, mg	Magnesium, mg	Other
1.05	4.5	300	—	—	—	—	—	—
1.05	4.5	300	—	—	—	—	—	—
1.05	4.5	300	—	15	—	—	—	—
1.05	4.5	300	—	15	—	—	—	—
0.5	2.5	—	—	15.0[j]	120.0[t]	—	3.0[j]	panthenol, 1.0 μg zinc, 0.6 mg[j] manganese, 0.5 mg[j]
0.6	2.0	—	3.0[h]	—	—	—	0.03	manganese, 0.5 mg zinc, 0.5 mg saccharin, 3.8 mg
—	—	—	—	—	—	—	—	—
—	—	—	—	—	—	—	—	—
—	—	—	—	—	—	—	—	—
3	9	0.4	15	—	—	—	—	—
3	9	0.4	15	—	—	—	—	—
2.0	6.0	400	—	—	—	—	—	—
2.0	6.0	400	—	18	—	—	—	—
—	—	—	—	—	250	—	—	—
—	—	—	—	—	75[k] 14[p]	58[k]	—	—
—	—	—	—	—	147[k] 295[k]	114[k] 228[k]	—	—
—	—	—	—	—	147[k]	114[k]	—	—
—	—	—	—	—	—	—	—	—
—	—	—	—	—	—	—	—	citrus bioflavonoid compound, 200 mg
—	—	—	—	—	—	—	—	—
2.5	8.0	800	—	18	650	—	100	iodine, 150 μg
—	—	—	—	—	—	—	—	—
25	10.0	100	10.0	18	126	—	—	zinc, 10.0 mg potassium, 10.0 mg
25	10.0	100	10.0	18	—	—	—	zinc, 10.0 mg
2.0	5.0	100	10.0[i]	20[m]	—	—	—	—
—	—	33	—	60[j]	—	—	—	intrinase, ⅓ NF XI unit desiccated liver, 100 mg
1.0	10.0	—	—	28[s]	—	—	—	—
2	6	400	—	18[m]	125[t]	—	100[u]	iodine, 150 μg others[z]
1.05	4.5	300	—	—	—	—	—	—
1.05	4.5	300	—	15	—	—	—	—
3.0	9.0	400	—	—	—	—	—	—
2.0	6.0	—	—	—	—	—	—	alcohol, 15% invert sugar
0.7	—	—	—	—	33[w]	—	0.33	alcohol, 15% choline bitartrate, 100 mg inositol, 100 mg others[z]
0.5	3.0	—	2.0[i]	50	—	—	—	brewers yeast, 50 mg choline bitartrate, 25 mg methionine, 25 mg inositol, 20 mg
3.0	9.0	400	15	27	—	—	—	biotin, 0.45 mg
—	2.0[g]	—	—	30[j]	59[k]	46[k]	—	aspergillus oryzae enzymes, 162.5 mg choline dihydrogen citrate, 20 mg others[z]

Product* (Manufacturer)	Vitamin A, IU	Vitamin D, IU	Vitamin E, IU	Ascorbic Acid (C), mg	Thiamine (B_1), mg	Riboflavin (B_2), mg	Niacin, mg
Geriplex-FS Kapseals (Parke-Davis)	5,000 [q]	—	5	50 [e]	5.0 [f]	5.0	15 [d]
Geriplex-FS Liquid [x] (Parke-Davis)	—	—	—	—	1.2 [c]	1.7 [k]	15 [d]
Geritinic (Geriatric Pharm.)	—	—	—	—	1.0 [c]	1.0	10 [d]
Geritol Junior Liquid [n] (J. B. Williams)	8,000 [b]	400	—	—	5.0	5.0	100 [d]
Geritol Junior Tablets (J. B. Williams)	5,000	100	—	30	2.5	2.5	20 [d]
Geritol Liquid [n] (J. B. Williams)	—	—	—	—	5.0	5.0	100 [d]
Geritol Tablets (J. B. Williams)	—	—	—	75	5.0	5.0	30 [d]
Gerix Elixir [x] (Abbott)	—	—	—	—	6.0 [c]	6.0	100 [d]
Gerizyme [y] (Upjohn)	—	—	—	—	3.3 [c]	3.3	33.3 [d]
Gevrabon [x] (Lederle)	—	—	—	—	5.0	2.5	50 [d]
Gevral (Lederle)	5,000 [q]	—	30	60	1.5 [f]	1.7	20 [d]
Gevral Protein (Lederle)	2,167 [b]	217	4.3	22	2.2	2.2	6.5 [d]
Gevral T Capsules (Lederle)	5,000 [q]	400	45	90	2.25	2.6	30 [d]
Gevrite (Lederle)	5,000 [b]	—	—	60	1.5	1.7	20 [d]
Golden Bounty B Complex with Vitamin C (Squibb)	—	—	—	100	4.0	4.8	4.67
Golden Bounty Multivitamin Supplement with Iron (Squibb)	5,000	400	15	60	1.5	1.7	20 [d]
Hi-Bee W/C Capsules (North American)	—	—	—	300	15.0 [f]	10.0	50 [d]
Iberet (Abbott)	—	—	—	150 [e]	6.0 [c]	6.0	30 [d]
Iberet-500 (Abbott)	—	—	—	500 [e]	6.0 [c]	6.0	30 [d]
Iberet Oral Solution [n] (Abbott)	—	—	—	37.5	1.5 [c]	1.5	7.5 [d]
Iberet-500 Oral Solution [n] (Abbott)	—	—	—	75	0.9 [c]	0.9	4.5 [d]
Iberol (Abbott)	—	—	—	75 [e]	3.0 [c]	3.0	15 [d]
Incremin with Iron Syrup [n] (Lederle)	—	—	—	—	10.0 [c]	—	—
Iodine Ration (Nion)	—	—	—	—	—	—	—
K-Forte Potassium Supplement with Vitamin C Chewable (O'Connor)	—	—	—	10	—	—	—
Lederplex Capsules (Lederle)	—	—	—	—	2.0	2.0	10 [d]

Pyridoxine Hydrochloride (B_6), mg	Cyanocobalamin (B_{12}), µg	Folic Acid, µg	Pantothenic Acid, mg	Iron, mg	Calcium, mg	Phosphorus, mg	Magnesium, mg	Other
—	2.0[g]	—	—	30[j]	59[k]	46[k]	—	aspergillus oryzae enzymes, 162.5 mg dioctyl sodium sulfosuccinate, 100 mg others[z]
1.0	5.0[g]	—	—	15[v]	—	—	—	poloxamer 188, 200 mg alcohol, 18%
0.1	3.0	—	—	35[v]	10[w]	8[w]	1.0[j]	yeast concentrate, 125 mg potassium, 1.0 mg[j] iodine, 20 µg[l] others[z]
1.0	3.0	—	4.0[h]	100[v]	—	—	—	—
1.0	2.5	—	2.0[i]	25[j]	—	—	—	—
1.0	3.0	—	4.0[h]	100[v]	—	—	—	methionine, 75 mg/oz. choline bitartrate, 100 mg
0.5	3.0	—	2.0[i]	50[j]	—	—	—	—
1.64	6.0	—	—	15	—	—	—	—
1.0	3.3	—	3.3[h]	5[p]	100[w]	—	3.5[j]	inositol, 100 mg potassium, 10.0 mg[j] alcohol, 18% others[z]
1.0	1.0	—	10.0	15	—	—	2.0	manganese, 2 mg alcohol, 18% zinc, 2 mg inositol, 100 mg choline, 100 mg iodine, 100 µg[l] others[z]
2.0	6	400	—	18[m]	162[k]	125[k]	100[u]	iodine, 150 µg
0.22	0.87	—	2.2[i]	4.3[m]	359	52.8[k]	0.4	choline, 21 mg inositol, 22 mg lysine monohydrate, 1.1 g iodine, 40 µg[l] copper, 400 µg[u] zinc, 220 µg[u] manganese, 400 µg[u] potassium, 13 mg
3.0	9.0	400	—	27[m]	162[k]	125[k]	100[u]	potassium, 5.0 mg[j] zinc, 22.5 mg iodine, 225 µg[l] copper, 1.5 mg others[z]
2.0	—	—	—	18[m]	230[t]	—	—	—
—	25.0[r]	—	—	—	—	—	—	—
2.0	6.0	400	—	18	—	—	—	—
5.0	—	—	10.0[i]	—	—	—	—	—
5.0	25.0	—	10.0[i]	105	—	—	—	—
5.0	25.0	—	10.0[i]	105	—	—	—	—
1.25	6.25	—	2.5[h]	26.25	—	—	—	—
0.75	3.8	—	1.5[h]	16	—	—	—	—
1.5	12.5	—	3.0[i]	105	—	—	—	—
5.0	25.0	—	—	30[o]	—	—	—	sorbitol, 3.5 g lysine monohydrochloride, 300 mg
—	—	—	—	—	—	—	—	iodine (kelp), 150 µg
—	—	—	—	—	—	—	—	potassium, 39 mg[p] (also citrate and chloride)
0.2	1.0	3.0[i]	—	—	—	—	—	liver fraction and desiccated liver, 340 mg choline, 20 mg inositol, 10 mg

Product* (Manufacturer)	Vitamin A, IU	Vitamin D, IU	Vitamin E, IU	Ascorbic Acid (C), mg	Thiamine (B_1), mg	Riboflavin (B_2), mg	Niacin, mg
Lederplex Liquid[n] (Lederle)	—	—	—	—	2.5	2.5	12.5[d]
Lederplex Tablets (Lederle)	—	—	—	—	2.0	2.0	10[d]
Lipoflavonoid Capsules (Smith, Miller & Patch)	—	—	—	100	0.33[c]	0.33	3.33[d]
Lipotriad Capsules (Smith, Miller & Patch)	—	—	—	—	0.33[c]	0.33	3.33[d]
Lipotriad Liquid[n] (Smith, Miller & Patch)	—	—	—	—	1.0[c]	1.0	10[d]
Liquid Geritonic[n] (Geriatric Pharm.)	5,000	400	—	60	3.0[f]	3.0	10[d]
Livitamin Capsules (Beecham Labs)	—	—	—	100	3.0[f]	3.0	10[d]
Livitamin Chewable (Beecham Labs)	—	—	—	100[j]	3.0[f]	3.0	10[d]
Livitamin Liquid[y] (Beecham Labs)	—	—	—	—	3.0[c]	3.0	10[d]
Lofenalac (Mead Johnson)	1,600	400	10	52	0.5	0.6	8.0
Lufa Capsules (USV)	—	—	4	—	2.0[f]	2.0	5.0[d]
Methischol Capsules (USV)	—	—	—	—	3.0[f]	3.0	10[d]
Monster Vitamins (Bristol-Myers)	3,500	400	—	40	1.1	1.2	15[d]
Monster Vitamins & Iron (Bristol-Myers)	3,500	400	—	40	1.1	1.2	15[d]
Mucoplex (Stuart)	—	—	—	—	—	1.5	—
Multicebrin (Lilly)	10,000	400	6.6	75	3[c]	3	25
Multiple Vitamins (North American)	5,000	400	—	50	3.0[f]	2.5	20[d]
Multiple Vitamins with Iron (North American)	5,000	400	—	50	2.0[f]	2.5	20[d]
Mulvidren Softabs (Stuart)	4,000	400	—	25 56[e]	2.0[f]	2.0	10[d]
Multivitamins (Rowell)	5,000	400	10	50	2.5[f]	2.5	20[d]
M.V.M. Liquid (Amfre-Grant)	10,000	400	4.5	150	6.0[c]	3.0	60[d]
Myadec (Parke-Davis)	10,000	400	30	250	10.0[f]	10.0	100[d]
Nap Tabs (North American)	—	—	—	150	5.0[c]	5.0	50[d]
Natabec (Parke-Davis)	8,000[q]	400	30	60	1.7[f]	2.0	20[d]
Natalins Tablets (Mead Johnson)	8,000	400	30	90	1.7	2.0	20
Natural Theratab (North American)	10,000[b]	400	25	150	25.0[c]	25.0	100[d]

Pyridoxine Hydrochloride (B_6), mg	Cyanocobalamin (B_{12}), μg	Folic Acid, μg	Pantothenic Acid, mg	Iron, mg	Calcium, mg	Phosphorus, mg	Magnesium, mg	Other
0.25	6.25	—	2.5 [h]	—	—	—	—	liver fraction and desiccated liver, 590 mg choline, 25 mg inositol, 5 mg
0.1	1.0	—	3.0 [i]	—	—	—	—	liver fraction and desiccated liver, 250 mg choline, 50 mg inositol, 25 mg
0.33	1.67	—	0.33 [i]	—	—	—	—	choline bitartrate, 233 mg lemon–bioflavonoid complex, 100 mg
0.33	1.67	—	0.33 [i]	—	—	—	—	choline bitartrate, 233.3 mg
1.0	5.0	—	1.0 [i]	—	—	—	—	sugar free
0.1	5.0	—	1.0 [i]	63 [j]	—	—	—	aminoacetic acid, 30 mg potassium, 30 mg [q] choline bitartrate, 30 mg others [z]
3.0	5.0	—	2.0 [i]	33 [m]	—	—	—	desiccated liver, 150 mg copper, 0.66 mg [j]
3.0	3.0	5.0	—	2.0 [i]	17 [m]	—	—	copper, 0.33 mg [u]
3.0	5.0	—	2.0 [h]	36	—	—	—	liver fraction 1, 500 mg copper, 0.66 mg [j]
0.4	2.0	100	3.0	12	600	450	70	potassium, 650 mg zinc, 4.0 mg iodine, 45 μg others [z]
2.0	1.0	—	1.0 [h]	—	—	—	—	unsaturated fatty acids, 423 mg choline bitartrate, 233 mg desiccated liver, 87 mg methionine, 66 mg inositol, 40 mg
2.0	2.0 [r]	—	2.0 [h]	—	—	—	—	choline bitartrate, 240 mg methionine, 110 mg inositol, 83 mg others [z]
1.2	5	100	5.0	—	—	—	—	—
1.2	5	100	5.0	10 [m]	—	—	—	—
—	5.0	—	—	—	—	—	—	liver fraction A, 375 mg liver fraction 2, 375 mg
1.2	3	—	—	—	—	—	—	—
1.0	1.0	—	1.0 [i]	—	—	—	—	—
1.0	1.0	—	1.0	15 [m]	—	—	—	—
1.2	3.0	—	3.0 [i]	—	—	—	—	—
0.5	2.0	—	5 [i]	—	—	—	—	—
1.0	—	—	6.0 [i]	—	38	29	6.0	potassium, 5.0 mg manganese, 1.0 mg
5.0	6.0	400	20	20 [m]	—	—	100 [u]	copper, 2.0 mg [j] zinc, 20 mg [j] manganese, 1.25 mg [j] iodine, 150 μg [l]
5.0	12.5 [r]	—	25.0 [r]	30 [m]	—	—	—	choline bitartrate, 50 mg inositol, 50 mg aminobenzoic acid, 15 mg biotin, 12.5 μg
2.5	8.0	800	—	30	125 [t]	—	100 [u]	iodine, 150 μg [l]
4.0	8.0	800	—	45	200	—	100	iodine, 150 μg
25.0	100.0	100	50.0 [i]	50 [p]	—	—	7.2 [p]	inositol, 250 mg choline bitartrate, 150 mg zinc, 0.18 mg others [z]

Product* (Manufacturer)	Vitamin A, IU	Vitamin D, IU	Vitamin E, IU	Ascorbic Acid (C), mg	Thiamine (B_1), mg	Riboflavin (B_2), mg	Niacin, mg
Neo-Calglucon[n] (Dorsey)	—	—	—	—	—	—	—
Neofol B-12 (Nion)	—	—	—	—	—	—	—
Norimex Capsules (North American)	—	—	—	—	0.183[f]	0.170	0.895[d]
Norimex-Plus Capsules (North American)	3,333	133	—	25	1.67[f]	0.83	6.67[d]
Norlac (Rowell)	8,000	400	30	90	2	2	20
Obron-6 (Pfipharmecs)	5,000	400	—	50	3.0	2.0	20
One-A-Day (Miles)	5,000	400	15	60	1.5	1.7	20
One-A-Day Plus Iron (Miles)	5,000	400	15	60	1.5	1.7	20
One-A-Day Vitamins Plus Minerals (Miles)	5,000	400	15	50	1.5	1.7	20
Optilets-500 (Abbott)	10,000	400	30	500[e]	15.0[c]	10.0	100[d]
Optilets-M-500 (Abbott)	10,000	400	30	500[e]	15.0[c]	10.0	100[d]
Orexin Softabs (Stuart)	—	—	—	—	10.0[f]	—	—
Ostrex Tonic Tablets (Commerce)	—	—	—	—	5.0[c]	—	—
Paladac[n] (Parke-Davis)	5,000	400	—	50	3.0[c]	3.0[k]	20[d]
Paladac c̄ Minerals (Parke-Davis)	4,000[q]	400	10	50[e]	3.0[f]	3.0	20[d]
Pals (Bristol-Myers)	3,500	400	—	60	0.8	1.3	14
Pals with Iron (Bristol-Myers)	3,500	400	—	60	0.8	1.3	14
Peritinic (Lederle)	—	—	—	200	7.5	7.5	30[d]
Poly-Vi-Sol (Mead Johnson)	2,500	400	15	60	1.05	1.2	13.5
Poly-Vi-Sol with Iron (Mead Johnson)	2,500	400	15	60	1.05	1.2	13.5
Probec-T (Stuart)	—	—	—	67	15.0[f]	10.0	100[d]
Ray-D (Nion)	—	400	—	—	1.0[f]	2.0	10
Roeribec (Pfipharmecs)	—	—	—	500	10.0	10.0	100[d]
Simron Plus (Merrell-National)	—	—	—	50	—	—	—
Spancap C Capsules (North American)	—	—	—	500	—	—	—
S.S.S. Tonic[y] (S.S.S.)	—	—	—	—	1.7	0.8	0.7[d]
Stresscaps Capsules (Lederle)	—	—	—	300	10.0	10.0	100[d]
Stresstabs 600 (Lederle)	—	—	30	600	15.0	15.0	100[d]
Stresstabs 600 with Iron (Lederle)	—	—	30	600	15	15	100[d]
Stresstabs 600 with Zinc (Lederle)	—	—	45	600	20	10	100[d]
Stuart Formula (Stuart)	5,000[b]	400	15	60	1.5[f]	1.7	20[d]
Stuart Formula Liquid[n] (Stuart)	3,333[b]	333	0.1	—	1.33[c]	1.33	10[d]
Stuart Hematinic (Stuart)	—	—	—	25	1.7[f]	1.7	25[d]
Stuart Hematinic Liquid[n] (Stuart)	—	—	—	—	1.7[c]	1.7	10[d]

Pyridoxine Hydrochloride (B_6), mg	Cyanocobalamin (B_{12}), μg	Folic Acid, μg	Pantothenic Acid, mg	Iron, mg	Calcium, mg	Phosphorus, mg	Magnesium, mg	Other
—	—	—	—	—	—	—	—	calcium glubionate, 115 mg formic acid, 19.0 mg butylparaben, 0.6 mg
—	10.0[r]	100	—	—	—	—	—	brewers yeast
0.120	—	—	—	—	—	—	—	dried yeast, 368 mg lysine monohydrochloride, 15.6 mg desiccated liver, 5.0 mg
0.167	—	—	—	3	29	22	—	protein hydrolysate, 215 mg choline, 100 mg inositol, 20 mg others[z]
4	8	400	—	60	0.2	—	100	iodine, 150 μg copper, 2 mg zinc, 15 mg
8.2	2.0	—	0.92	33	242	—	1	potassium, 1.7 mg zinc, 0.4 mg manganese, 0.33 mg
2.0	6.0	400	—	—	—	—	—	—
2.0	6.0	400	—	18	—	—	—	—
2.0	6.0	400	10.0	18	100	100	100	zinc, 15 mg copper, 2.0 mg iodine, 150 μg
5.0	12.0	—	20.0[i]	—	—	—	—	—
5.0	12.0	—	20.0[i]	20	—	—	80	copper, 2.0 mg zinc, 1.5 mg manganese, 1 mg iodine, 150 μg
5.0	25.0	—	—	—	—	—	—	—
—	—	—	—	84[j]	750	375	—	copper, 0.061 mg
1.0	5.0[g]	—	5.0[e]	—	—	—	—	—
1.0	5.0[g]	—	5.0[i]	5[k]	23[k]	17[k]	1.0[u]	potassium, 2.5 mg[j] iodine, 50 μg[l]
1.0	2.5	50	5	—	—	—	—	—
1.0	2.5	50	5	12	—	—	—	—
7.5	50.0	50	15.0	100[m]	—	—	—	dioctyl sodium sulfosuccinate, 100 mg
1.05	4.5	300	—	—	—	—	—	—
1.05	4.5	300	—	12	—	—	—	—
5.0	5.0	—	20.0[i]	—	—	—	—	—
—	—	—	—	—	375	300	—	iodine (kelp), 100 μg brewers yeast
8.2	4.0	—	18.0[i]	—	—	—	—	—
1.0	3.33	100	—	10[p]	—	—	—	polysorbate 20, 400 mg
—	—	—	—	—	—	—	—	—
—	0.2	—	—	15[v]	—	—	—	—
2.0	4.0	—	20.0[i]	—	—	—	—	—
5.0	12.0	—	20.0[i]	—	—	—	—	—
25	12	400	20[i]	27[m]	—	—	—	copper, 3 mg
10	25	400	25[m]	115[m]	—	—	—	zinc, 23.9 mg[j] dioctyl sodium sulfosuccinate, 50 mg
2.0	6.0	400	—	18	160	125	100	iodine, 150 μg
0.067	—	—	1.43[h]	5[j]	—	—	—	manganese, 0.33 mg[j]
0.34	2.0	—	1.7[i]	22[m]	—	—	—	—
0.5	—	—	1.43[h]	22[p]	—	—	—	liver fraction 1, 54.0 mg

Product* (Manufacturer)	Vitamin A, IU	Vitamin D, IU	Vitamin E, IU	Ascorbic Acid (C), mg	Thiamine (B_1), mg	Riboflavin (B_2), mg	Niacin, mg
Stuartinic (Stuart)	—	—	—	300 225[e]	6.0[f]	6.0	20[d]
Stuart Prenatal Formula (Stuart)	8,000[q]	400	30	60	1.7[f]	2.0	20[d]
Super Calcicaps (Nion)	—	133	—	—	—	—	—
Super D Cod Liver Oil[n] (Upjohn)	4,000	400	—	—	—	—	—
Super D Perles[n] (Upjohn)	10,000	400	—	—	—	—	—
Super Hydramin (Nion)	4,000	400	—	30	1	1.2	10
Super Plenamins (Rexall)	8,000	400	1.8	56	2.3[c]	2.35	18
Surbex (Abbott)	—	—	—	—	6.0[c]	6.0	30[d]
Surbex-T (Abbott)	—	—	—	500[e]	15.0[c]	10.0	100[d]
Surbex with C (Abbott)	—	—	—	250[e]	6.0[c]	6.0	30[d]
Surbex 750 with Iron (Abbott)	—	—	30	750	15	15	100[d]
Surbex 750 with Zinc (Abbott)	—	—	30	750	15	15	100[d]
Taka-Combex Kapseals (Parke-Davis)	—	—	—	30	10.0[f]	10.0	10[d]
Tega-C Caps (Ortega)	—	—	—	500	—	—	—
Tega-C Syrup[n] (Ortega)	—	—	—	500	—	—	—
Tega-E Caps (Ortega)	—	—	400 1,000	—	—	—	—
Thera-Combex Kapseals (Parke-Davis)	—	—	—	250	25.0[f]	15.0	100[d]
Thera-Combex H-P Kapseals (Parke-Davis)	—	—	—	500	25.0[f]	15.0	100[d]
Theragran (Squibb)	10,000	400	15	200	10.0	10.0	100[d]
Theragran Liquid[n] (Squibb)	10,000	400	—	200	10.0	10.0	100[d]
Theragran-M (Squibb)	10,000	400	15	200	10.0	10.0	100[d]
Therapeutic Vitamins (North American)	1,000[b]	400	15	200	10.0[f]	10.0	100[d]
Therapeutic Vitamins and Minerals (Nion)	10,000	400	15	200	10	10	100
Thera-Spancap (North American)	10,000	400	—	150	6.0[f]	6.0	60[d]
Theron (Stuart)	10,000[q]	400	—	34 300[e]	15.0[f]	10.0	100[d]
Tonebec (A.V.P.)	—	—	—	300	15.0[f]	10.0	5[d]
Tri-Vi-Sol Chewable (Mead Johnson)	2,500	400	—	60	—	—	—
Tri-Vi-Sol Drops[a] (Mead Johnson)	900	240	—	21	—	—	—
Tri-Vi-Sol with Iron Drops[a] (Mead Johnson)	1,500	400	—	35	—	—	—
Unicap (Upjohn)	5,000	400	15	60	1.5[c]	1.7	20
Unicap Chewable (Upjohn)	5,000	400	15	60	1.5[f]	1.7	20[d]
Unicap T (Upjohn)	5,000	400	15	300	10.0[f]	10.0	100[d]
Vastran (Wallace)	—	—	—	100	10.0[c]	5.0	50
Venthera (Amfre-Grant)	10,000	400	50	200	12.5[c]	12.5	100[d]
Vi-Aqua (USV)	5,000	400	1.0	50.0	5.0	5.0	20[d]
Vicon (Meyer)	2,000	—	25	75	5.0[f]	2.5	12.5[d]

Pyridoxine Hydrochloride (B_6), mg	Cyanocobalamin (B_{12}), μg	Folic Acid, μg	Pantothenic Acid, mg	Iron, mg	Calcium, mg	Phosphorus, mg	Magnesium, mg	Other
1.0	25.0	—	10.0[i]	100[m]	—	—	—	—
4.0	8.0	800	—	60[m]	200[j]	—	100[u]	iodine, 150 μg[l]
—	—	—	—	—	334	41.7	—	—
—	—	—	—	—	—	—	—	—
—	—	—	—	—	—	—	—	—
1.5	3	—	2.8	10	483	375	—	protein, 41 g iodine, 0.1 mg
1.0	1.5	—	—	—	—	—	—	—
2.5	5.0	—	10.0[i]	—	—	—	—	—
5.0	10.0	—	20.0[i]	—	—	—	—	—
2.5	5.0	—	10.0[i]	—	—	—	—	—
25	12	400	20	27	20	—	—	—
25	12	400	20	—	20	—	—	zinc, 22.5 mg
0.5	1.0[g]	—	6.0[h]	—	—	—	—	liver concentrate, 340 mg aspergillus oryzae enzymes, 162.5 mg
—	—	—	—	—	—	—	—	—
—	—	—	—	—	—	—	—	—
—	—	—	—	—	—	—	—	—
1.0	5.0[g]	—	20.0[h]	—	—	—	—	aspergillus oryzae enzymes, 162.5 mg
10.0	5.0[g]	—	20.0[h]	—	—	—	—	—
5.0	5.0	—	20.0[i]	—	—	—	—	—
5.0	5.0	—	20.0[h]	—	—	—	—	—
5.0	5.0	—	20.0[i]	12	—	—	65	copper, 2.0 mg zinc, 1.5 mg manganese, 1.0 mg iodine, 150 μg
5.0	5.0[r]	—	20.0[i]	—	—	—	—	—
5	5	—	18.4	12	—	—	65	iodine, 150 μg copper, 2 mg manganese, 1 mg zinc, 1.5 mg
6.0	6.0[r]	—	6.0[i]	—	—	—	—	—
5.0	5.0	—	20.0[i]	15[m]	100[j]	—	—	zinc, 1.5 mg[j] manganese, 1.0 mg[j]
5.0	—	—	10.0[i]	—	—	—	—	—
—	—	—	—	—	—	—	—	—
—	—	—	—	—	—	—	—	—
—	—	—	—	10	—	—	—	—
2.0	6.0	400	—	—	—	—	—	—
2.0	6.0	400	—	—	—	—	—	—
6.0	18.0	400	10.0[i]	18.0	—	—	—	potassium, 5.0 mg[j] copper, 2.0 mg[j] manganese, 1.0 mg[j] iodine, 150 μg[l] zinc, 15.0 mg
1.0	2.0	—	5.0[i]	—	—	—	—	—
5.0	10.0	—	20.0[i]	15[m]	105	80	6.0	potassium, 5.0 mg zinc, 1.5 mg iodine, 150 μg others[z]
0.5	1.0	—	5.0[h]	—	—	—	—	—
1.0	—	—	5.0[i]	—	—	—	35[u]	zinc, 10 mg[u] manganese chloride, 2 mg

Product* (Manufacturer)	Vitamin A, IU	Vitamin D, IU	Vitamin E, IU	Ascorbic Acid (C), mg	Thiamine (B_1), mg	Riboflavin (B_2), mg	Niacin, mg
Vicon-C (Meyer)	—	—	—	300	20.0[f]	10.0	100[d]
Vicon Plus (Meyer)	4,000[q]	—	50	150	10.0[f]	5.0	25[d]
Vigran (Squibb)	5,000	400	30	60	1.5	1.7	20
Vigran Chewable (Squibb)	2,500	400	10	40	0.7	0.8	9
Vigran plus Iron (Squibb)	5,000	400	30	60	1.5	1.7	20
Vi-Magna (Lederle)	5,000	400	—	56	2.8[c]	2.8	18
Vio-Bec (Rowell)	—	—	—	500	25.0[f]	25.0	100[d]
Vio-Geric (Rowell)	5,000	400	30	60	5	5	20
Vi-Penta Infant Drops[a] (Roche)	5,000	400	2	50	—	—	—
Vi-Penta Multivitamin Drops[a] (Roche)	5,000[b]	400	2	50	1.0[c]	1.0	10[d]
Vi-Syneral One-Caps (Fisons)	5,000[b]	—	30	60[e]	1.5[f]	1.7	20[d]
Vitagett (North American)	5,000[b]	400	3	50	3.0[f]	2.5	20[d]
Vita-Kaps Tablets (Abbott)	5,000	400	—	50[e]	3.0[c]	2.5	20[d]
Vita-Kaps-M Tablets (Abbott)	5,000	400	—	50[e]	3.0[c]	2.5	20[d]
Vitamin-Mineral Capsules (North American)	5,000[b]	400	—	50[e]	3.0[f]	2.5	20[d]
Viterra (Pfipharmecs)	5,000	400	3.7	50	3.0	3.0	25
Viterra High Potency (Pfipharmecs)	10,000	400	5	150	10.0	10.0	100
Vi-Zac (Meyer)	5,000	—	50	500	—	—	—
VM Preparation[x] (Roberts)	—	—	—	—	3.0[c]	2.0	20[d]
Z-Bec (Robins)	—	—	45	600	15	10.2	100
Zincaps (Ortega)	—	—	—	—	—	—	—
Zymacap Capsules (Upjohn)	5,000	400	15	90	2.25	2.6	30[d]
Zymalixir Syrup[n] (Upjohn)	—	—	—	—	1.0[c]	1.0	8.0[d]
Zymasyrup[n] (Upjohn)	5,000	400	—	60	1.0[c]	1.0	10[d]

* Vitamin formulations change frequently; therefore, the product label should be consulted before dispensing.
[a] Quantities given are per 0.6 ml.
[b] Palmitate.
[c] Hydrochloride.
[d] Niacinamide.
[e] Sodium salt.
[f] Mononitrate.
[g] Crystalline.
[h] Panthenol.
[i] Calcium salt.
[j] Sulfate.
[k] Phosphate.
[l] Potassium iodide.
[m] Fumarate.
[n] Quantities given are per 5 ml.
[o] Pyrophosphate.
[p] Gluconate.
[q] Acetate.
[r] Concentrate.
[s] Ferrocholinate.
[t] Carbonate.
[u] Oxide.
[v] Ammonium citrate.
[w] Glycerophosphate.
[x] Quantities given are per 30 ml.
[y] Quantities given are per 15 ml.
[z] Also contains other vitamins and/or minerals.

Pyridoxine Hydrochloride (B_6), mg	Cyanocobalamin (B_{12}), μg	Folic Acid, μg	Pantothenic Acid, mg	Iron, mg	Calcium, mg	Phosphorus, mg	Magnesium, mg	Other
5.0	—	—	20.0[i]	—	—	—	70[j]	zinc, 80 mg[j]
2.0	—	—	10.0[i]	—	—	—	70[j]	zinc, 80 mg[j] manganese chloride, 4 mg
2.0	6.0	400	—	—	—	—	—	—
0.7	3.0	200	—	—	—	—	—	—
2.0	6.0	400	—	27	—	—	—	—
0.2	0.5	—	1.0[i]	—	—	—	—	—
25.0	—	—	40.0[i]	—	—	—	—	—
2.4	8	400	—	18	220	125	100	iodine, 150 μg copper, 2 mg zinc, 15 mg
—	—	—	—	—	—	—	—	—
1.0	—	—	10.0[h]	—	—	—	—	biotin, 30 μg
2.0	6.0	400	—	18[j]	—	—	—	—
1.5	2.5	—	5.0[i]	13[j]	215[k]	166[k]	7.5[j]	potassium, 5.0 mg[j] manganese, 1.5 mg[j] zinc, 1.4 mg[j]
0.5	2.0	—	5.0[i]	—	—	—	—	—
0.5	2.0	—	5.0[i]	10	—	—	5.0	zinc, 1.5 mg copper, 1.0 mg manganese, 1.0 mg iodine, 150 μg
1.0	2.0	—	2.0[i]	13[j]	46[k]	35[k]	1.0[j]	potassium, 5.0 mg[j] manganese, 1.5 mg[j] zinc, 1.4 mg[j]
0.82	2.0	—	4.6	10	140	70	5.0	zinc, 1.2 mg copper, 1.0 mg manganese, 1.0 mg iodine, 150 μg
1.6	5.0	—	4.6	10	50	—	5.0	zinc, 1.2 mg copper, 1.0 mg manganese, 1.0 mg iodine, 150 μg
—	—	—	—	—	—	—	—	zinc, 80 mg[j]
—	—	—	—	50	94	94	—	manganese, 2 mg
10.0	6.0	—	25.0	—	—	—	—	zinc, 22.5 mg
—	—	—	—	—	—	—	—	zinc, 25 mg[j]
3.0	9.0	400	15.0	—	—	—	—	—
0.5	2.0	—	—	15[p]	—	—	—	liver concentrate, 65 mg alcohol, 1.5%
0.5	3.0	—	3.0[h]	—	—	—	—	alcohol, 2%

Product (Manufacturer)	Dosage Form[a]	Calories	Protein, g	Carbohydrate, g	Fat, g	Vitamins, Minerals	Indicated Use
Amin-Aid (McGaw)	powder (diluted to 340 ml)	696/340 ml	2.0%	35%	6.5%	—	nitrogen-restricted diets
Bran Fiber Wafer (Nion)	wafer	—	—	—	—	wheat bran, 1000 mg	—
Casec (Mead Johnson)	powder, 1 tbsp	17	4.0	trace	0.1	various[b,c]	sodium restriction cholesterol restriction
Citrotein (Doyle)	powder, 33.4 g	127	7.67	23.3	0.33	various[b,c]	supplementary nourishment
Compleat-B (Doyle)	liquid, 250 mg/bottle	267	10.7	32	10.7	various[b,c]	tube feeding
Controlyte (Doyle)	powder, 100 g	504	0.04	72	24	sodium, 10 mg potassium, 4 mg calcium, 4 mg phosphorus, 8 mg	protein restriction electrolyte restriction high-calorie dietary supplement
Ensure (Ross)	liquid, 240 ml	250	8.8	34.3	8.8	various[b,c]	full liquid diet liquid supplement tube feeding
Ensure Plus (Ross)	liquid, 240 ml	355	13.0	47.3	12.6	various[b,c]	high-calorie liquid food
Flexical (Mead Johnson)	powder	250	5.6	38.1	8.5	various[b,c]	supplementary nourishment tube feeding
Gevral Protein (Lederle)	powder, 26 g	95.3	15.6	7.05	<0.52	various[b,c]	supplementary nourishment
Heatrol (Otis Clapp)	tablet	—	—	—	—	sodium, 249 mg potassium, 21 mg calcium, 12 mg magnesium, 2.5 mg phosphate, 20 mg chloride, 420 mg	electrolyte replenishment for perspiration losses
Instant Breakfast (various)	powder, 3.66 g	130	8.0	23	1.0	various[b,c]	supplementary nourishment
Isocal (Mead Johnson)	liquid, 240 ml	250	8.1	31.2	10.5	various[b,c]	supplementary nourishment tube feeding
Meritene (Doyle)	powder, 32.4 g liquid, 10 fl. oz./can 8 fl. oz./can	277 300 240	18 18 14.4	31 34.5 27.6	9 10 8	various[b,c]	supplementary nourishment tube feeding
Nutrament (Drackett)	liquid, 12 oz./can	360	16	52	10	various[b,c]	supplementary nourishment
Polycose (Ross)	liquid, 120 ml	2 cal/ml	—	50/100 ml	—	—	supplementary nourishment
Precision High Nitrogen Diet (Doyle)	powder, 83 g	300	12.5	62	0.36	various[b,c]	low residue high protein requirement oral tube feeding
Precision Isotonic Diet (Doyle)	powder, 58.4 g	250	7.5	37.5	7.8	various[b,c]	food intolerance tube feeding supplementary nourishment
Precision LR Diet (Doyle)	powder, 85 g	317	7.5	71	0.45	various[b,c]	low residue supplementary nourishment tube feeding
Prototabs (North American)	tablet	—	0.25[d]	—	—	—	amino acid deficiency

Product (Manufacturer)	Dosage Form[a]	Calories	Protein, g	Carbo-hydrate, g	Fat, g	Vitamins, Minerals	Indicated Use
Scott's Emulsion (Beecham)	liquid	—	—	—	—	cod liver oil sodium hypo-phosphite sodium citrate	tonic food supplement
Sustacal (Mead Johnson)	liquid, 360 ml	360	21.7	49.6	8.3	various[b,c]	supplementary nourishment tube feeding
Sustagen (Mead Johnson)	liquid, 240 ml	390	23.5	3.5	66.5	various[b,c]	supplementary nourishment tube feeding
Vivonex (Norwich-Eaton)	powder, 80 g	300	6.167[d]	69.0	0.435	various[b,c]	maintenance elemental diet tube feeding
Vivonex High Nitrogen (Norwich-Eaton)	powder, 80 g	300	13.0[a]	63.1	0.261	various[b,c]	anabolic elemental diet tube feeding

[a] One serving. Powder must be added to liquid as package directs.
[b] Includes vitamins A, D, E, ascorbic acid, thiamine, riboflavin, niacin, pyridoxine hydrochloride, cyanocobalamin, and/or various other substances having vitamin activity.
[c] Includes iron, calcium, phosphorus, iodine, magnesium, copper, zinc, potassium, sodium, and manganese.
[d] Amino acids, including leucine, lysine, phenylalanine, threonine, methionine, arginine, isoleucine, valine, histidine, tryptophan, and/or others.

Iron Products

Product (Manufacturer)	Iron	Vitamins	Other
Arne Timesules (Haag)	ferrous sulfate, 150 mg	—	—
Cefera (Haag)	ferrous fumarate, 200 mg	ascorbic acid, 100 mg	—
Chel-Iron Liquid and Tablets (Kinney)	ferrocholinate, 83.4 mg/ml 330 mg/tablet	—	—
Chel-Iron Pediatric Drops (Kinney)	ferrocholinate, 208 mg/ml	—	—
C-Ron (Rowell)	ferrous fumarate, 200 mg	ascorbic acid, 100 mg	—
C-Ron Forte (Rowell)	ferrous fumarate, 200 mg	ascorbic acid, 600 mg	—
C-Ron Freckles (Rowell)	ferrous fumarate, 100 mg (elemental iron, 33 mg)	ascorbic acid, 50 mg	—
Cytoferin (Ayerst)	ferrous sulfate, 200 mg (elemental iron, 64 mg)	ascorbic acid, 150 mg	—
Dical-D with Iron Capsules (Abbott)	10 mg (as ferric pyrophosphate)	ergocalciferol, 132 IU	dibasic calcium phosphate, 500 mg
Femiron (J. B. Williams)	ferrous fumarate, 20 mg	—	—
Feosol Spansules and Tablets (Smith Kline & French)	ferrous sulfate, 250 mg/spansule 325 mg/tablet	—	—
Ferancee (Stuart)	elemental, 67 mg (as ferrous fumarate)	sodium ascorbate, 114 mg ascorbic acid, 49 mg	—
Ferancee-HP (Stuart)	elemental, 110 mg (as ferrous fumarate, 330 mg)	sodium ascorbate, 281 mg ascorbic acid, 350 mg	—
Fergon Capsules and Tablets (Breon)	ferrous gluconate, 435 mg/capsule 320 mg/tablet	—	—
Fergon c̄ C Caplets (Breon)	ferrous gluconate, 450 mg	ascorbic acid, 200 mg	—
Fer-In-Sol Drops, Syrup, and Capsules (Mead Johnson)	ferrous sulfate, 125 mg/ml (drops) 30 mg/ml (syrup) 190 mg/capsule	—	—

Product (Manufacturer)	Iron	Vitamins	Other
Fermalox Tablets (Rorer)	ferrous sulfate, 200 mg	—	magnesium hydroxide, 100 mg aluminum hydroxide gel, dried, 100 mg
Fero-Grad-500 Tablets (Abbott)	105 mg (as ferrous sulfate)	sodium ascorbate, 500 mg	—
Fero-Gradumet Tablets (Abbott)	105 mg (as ferrous sulfate)	—	—
Ferrobid (Meyer)	ferrous fumarate, 225 mg	ascorbic acid, 100 mg	copper sulfate, 8 mg
Ferrolip Tablets and Syrup (Flint)	ferrocholinate, 333 mg/tablet 83.4 mg/ml	—	—
Ferronord (Cooper)	ferroglycine sulfate complex	—	—
Ferro-Sequels (Lederle)	ferrous fumarate, 150 mg	—	dioctyl sodium sulfosuccinate, 100 mg
Ferrous Sulfate Tablets (Upjohn)	ferrous sulfate, 325 mg	—	—
Fuma Drops (North American)	ferrous fumarate, 20 mg/ml	—	cherry flavor
Fumaral Elixir and Spancaps (North American)	ferrous sulfate, 32.5 mg/ml ferrous fumarate, 330 mg/capsule	ascorbic acid, 200 mg/capsule	alcohol, 5% (elixir)
Hytinic Capsules and Elixir (Hyrex)	elemental, 150 mg/capsule 20 mg/ml (as polysaccharide–iron complex)	—	—
Iron with Vitamin C (Squibb)	50 mg (as ferrous carbonate)	ascorbic acid, 25 mg	—
Ironized Yeast (Glenbrook)	ferrous sulfate, 56.9 mg/tablet	thiamine, 0.33 mg/tablet	—
Laud-Iron (Amfre-Grant)	ferrous fumarate, 324 mg/tablet 20 mg/ml	—	—
Laud-Iron Plus Chewing Tablets (Amfre-Grant)	ferrous fumarate, 100 mg	cyanocobalamin, 5 μg	—
L-Glutavite Capsules (Cooper)	1.7 mg	niacin pyridoxine thiamine mononitrate riboflavin cyanocobalamin	monosodium L-glutamate
Mol-Iron Chronsule Capsules (Schering)	ferrous sulfate, 390 mg	—	—
Mol-Iron Liquid and Tablets (Schering)	ferrous sulfate, 48.7 mg/ml 195 mg/tablet	—	alcohol, 4.75% (liquid)
Mol-Iron with Vitamin C (Schering)	ferrous sulfate, 195 mg	ascorbic acid, 75 mg	—
Mol-Iron with Vitamin C Chronsule Capsules (Schering)	ferrous sulfate, 390 mg	ascorbic acid, 150 mg	—
Niferex Elixir, Capsules, and Tablets (Central Pharmacal)	elemental, 20 mg/ml 150 mg/capsule 50 mg/tablet (as polysaccharide–iron complex)	—	alcohol, 10% (elixir)
Niferex with Vitamin C Tablets (Central Pharmacal)	elemental, 50 mg (as polysaccharide–iron complex)	sodium ascorbate, 168.75 mg ascorbic acid, 100 mg	—
Recoup Tablets (Lederle)	ferrous fumarate, 150 mg	ascorbic acid, 300 mg	dioctyl sodium sulfosuccinate, 50 mg
Simron Capsules (Merrell-National)	ferrous gluconate, 85 mg	—	polysorbate 20, 400 mg
Toleron Suspension and Tablets (Mallinckrodt)	ferrous fumarate, 20 mg/ml 200 mg/tablet	—	—
Tri-Tinic Capsules (North American)	ferrous fumarate, 110 mg	ascorbic acid, 75 mg folic acid, 0.5 mg cyanocobalamin, 7.5 μg	liver–stomach concentrate, 240 mg
Vitron-C (Fisons)	ferrous fumarate, 200 mg	ascorbic acid, 125 mg	—

Diabetes Care Products

R. Keith Campbell

Chapter 11

Questions to Ask the Patient

Is there diabetes in your family?

When were you last tested for diabetes? What were the results of those tests?

How long have you been a diabetic?

Do you take insulin?

What kind of diet has your doctor prescribed? Explain how you test your urine using TesTape, Clinitest tablets, or Diastix.

If you take insulin, where do you inject it? How much do you inject?

How do you feel about being a diabetic? Do members of your family understand the condition and the factors that affect control?

Do you have a regular schedule for exercise?

What drugs have been prescribed for you? Are you taking anything for diabetes?

Do you use "fad" diets?

Are you taking any drugs for pain?

Are you allergic to sulfa drugs?

Do you use alcohol? How much?

What do you think has affected the control of your diabetes? Are you eating differently? Are you exercising more or less? Have you had any infections? Is there anything that is emotionally upsetting you?

Do you belong to the local diabetes association?

Diabetes mellitus is a disease that requires a total health team effort if it is to be managed successfully. The physician must diagnose the condition accurately, classify properly the type of diabetes, and motivate the patient to learn to control and monitor the condition. The dietician explains the importance of diet control and the food exchange system. The nurse helps the patient develop a positive attitude, learn how to perform laboratory tests, monitor control, inject insulin, and keep records of the factors that affect diabetic control. The pharmacist's easy access to the patient offers a unique opportunity to help the patient maintain a proper therapeutic regimen. The pharmacist can answer patient questions about the disease, urine testing, drug therapy, diet, and proper foot care, stress the importance of complying with the physician's, nurse's, and dietician's instructions (1, 2), and monitor the control of diabetic patients, particularly in relation to the use of drugs.

Approximately 4.5 million diabetics (2% of the population) are being treated in the United States. Another 2 million have undiagnosed diabetes (mild symptoms or asymptomatic). Another 5 million will develop diabetes sometime during their lives. The prevalence of diabetes is approximately 10% of the population. Roughly 25% of the population (50 million people) either have diabetes, will develop diabetes, or have had a diabetic relative. It is the third leading cause of death (3) and is responsible for approximately 5% of hospital admissions.

The incidence of diabetes is increasing at a 6% annual rate (4). Diabetes kills nearly 40,000 people each year in this country, and about 300,000 more die of its side effects (5). It is now the number one cause of new blindness in this country; more than half the heart attacks are related to diabetes; five of every six amputations for gangrene today are a result of diabetes; diabetic kidney disease is common and often fatal; neurological complications are remarkably frequent; and complications of pregnancy due to diabetes are well recognized. Coronary artery disease is seven times more prevalent in diabetic women than in normal women (6). Women are 50% more likely to have diabetes than men; nonwhites are 20% more likely to have it than whites; low-income people (with incomes under $5000 per year) are three times more likely to have it than middle- and upper-income people; and the chance of developing it doubles with every 20% of excess weight and decade of life (3).

Some of the reasons for the increase in the number of diabetics include a sharp increase in the number of older people who are more prone to develop the disease, more sophisticated methods of diagnosis, increased efficiency of detection efforts, and third-generation diabetics who never would have been born without the discovery of insulin (6).

Unfortunately, the diabetic is neglected by manufacturers of pharmaceuticals, health and beauty aids, food, drinks, and candy. Diabetics are offered a bewildering selection of products that are not properly formulated or clearly labeled safe to use (5). The pharmacist has an excellent opportunity to help these patients by reiterating instructions and warning signs and by assessing patient ability to carry out self-help measures. The pharmacist also can serve as a consultant to both physician and patient by learning about the disease and the drugs and devices used in its treatment (7).

CLASSIFICATION OF DIABETES

Diabetes mellitus is a difficult condition to define because it is really a variety of conditions that have hyperglycemia as the common physiological problem that needs to be brought under control. Diabetes is a chronic disease characterized by disorders in carbohydrate (and associated fat and protein) metabolism due to an absolute or relative deficiency in the action of insulin and possibly abnormally high amounts of glucagon and other insulin-antagonizing substances such as growth hormone, sympathomimetic amines, and corticosteroids (8). Insulin secretion in diabetes may progress from nearly normal capabilities to a totally deficient state (9).

Some diabetes experts state that there is also a disorder in the structure and function of blood vessels (10). Over the years there has been considerable debate on whether the lesions that develop within the diabetic's retina, kidneys, nerves, and vascular system (commonly referred to as the late complications of diabetes) are due to a disorder in the structure and function of blood vessels or whether they are a consequence of prolonged hyperglycemia caused by inadequate metabolic control (11). Diabetologists who believe that microvascular complications occur independently of hyperglycemia and insulin deficiency and that control of metabolic events is not a factor in their progress are in a minority. The weight of evidence supports the concept that the microvascular complications of diabetes are decreased by reduction of blood glucose concentrations (11). Because of these findings there is a renewed emphasis on strict, but reasonable, control to prevent severe diabetic complications.

types of diabetes
various classifications
contributory factors
major causes

Properly classifying a diabetic into one of several categories in which hyperglycemia is a clinical finding is critical in developing a treatment protocol to bring the patient under control. Diabetics may be classified in several ways: according to degree of glucose tolerance (1), age (12), and other data such as genetic or acquired background, age of onset (juvenile or adult), body weight, degree of hyperglycemia or glucosuria or both, presence or absence of ketone bodies, insulin dependency, degree of severity and stability, treatment priorities, and the presence or absence of large and small blood vessel lesions (13–16). Table 1 is a composite of most of these factors. Table 2 shows features in classification according to age of onset.

Table 3 shows a clinical classification of diabetes (17). This method uses specific radioimmunoassay techniques for measuring circulating insulin levels and divides diabetics into two subgroups. Insulinopenic diabetes, a severe form, occurs most often in juveniles but also occasionally in nonobese elderly adults. Insulinotardic diabetes, a milder form of the insulinopenic condition, occurs predominantly in (usually nonobese) adults. About 10% of diabetics in the United States are classified as insulinopenic, and 15% as insulinotardic (17).

The remaining 75% are insulinoplethoric diabetics. This mild, nonketotic condition usually is seen in frankly obese adults (usually 40–65 years old and often female) and occasionally in children. The obesity is a result of excessive caloric intake, possibly facilitated by hunger resulting from mild postprandial hypoglycemia after excess insulin release.

ETIOLOGY

The most common contributory factors in diabetes are heredity, obesity, age, stress, and vasculitis in certain tissues of the body that are highly perfused with capillaries, such as the retina of the eye, the beta cells in the pancreas, and the kidney (1).

The three major causes center around a genetic (hereditary) tendency, environmental factors (viruses and obesity), and autoimmune responses of the body (18).

Insulinopenic diabetes due to a defect in pancreatic

Table 1. Composite of Various Classifications of Diabetes

Age at Onset, years	Background	Body Weight	Hyperglycemic Symptoms	Fasting Blood Glucose	Ketoacidosis Prone[a]	Insulin Dependent	Glucose Tolerance Sum	Insulin Response to Glucose	Treatment Priorities
≧40 (onset in later decades)	occasionally acquired	obese	often absent	increased or normal	rare	rare	≧800, <800 frequently	normal or delayed	diet, weight loss, sulfonylureas, insulin, education
20–40 (young adult onset)	occasionally acquired	nonobese	usually	usually increased	often	often	≧800, <800 occasionally	decreased	education, diet, insulin, sulfonylureas
0–20 (juvenile onset)	always genetic	nonobese	almost always	usually increased	usual	usual	≧800, <800 rare	decreased or zero	education, insulin, diet

Includes diabetes following pancreatectomy and pancreatitis and diabetes occurring during pregnancy or in association with conditions such as acromegaly, Cushing's syndrome, pheochromocytoma, or mucoviscidosis. [a]Also ketone bodies.

beta cell function may have many causes. Genetic defects in production of certain macromolecules may interfere with proper insulin synthesis, packaging, or release, or the beta cells may be unable to recognize glucose signals or even to replicate normally (19). Extrinsic factors that affect beta cell function include damage caused by viruses such as mumps or Coxsackie B_4 virus, by destructive cytotoxins and antibodies released by sensitized immunocytes, or by autodigestion in the course of an inflammatory disorder involving the adjacent exocrine pancreas.

An underlying genetic defect in beta cell replication or function may predispose to development of beta cell failure after viral infection. Specific HLA genes may increase susceptibility to a diabetogenic virus, or certain immune-response genes may predispose patients to a destructive autoimmune response against their own islet cells. In the severe form of insulinopenic diabetes, circulating islet cell antibodies have been detected in as many as 80% of cases tested in the first few weeks of the diabetes (19). HLA linkage and islet cell antibodies are not features of insulinoplethoric diabetes (19). In insulinotardic patients, as in severe insulinopenic diabetics, the patient may inherit a response to a viral infection that causes a beta cell defect as a consequence of viral stress.

In insulinoplethoric diabetics who have excess insulin and are always obese, hyperinsulinism and insulin resistance may be correlated with a decrease in insulin receptors (20). Studies also have shown that insulin-re-

origins of diabetes

juvenile and maturity onset diabetes

Table 2. Common Classification of Diabetes Mellitus

	Juvenile Onset (Growth) Ketosis Prone	**Maturity Onset (Adult) Ketosis Resistant**
Age of onset	usually, but not always, during childhood or puberty	frequently over 35
Type of onset	abrupt	usually gradual
Family history of diabetes	frequently positive	commonly positive
Nutritional status at time of onset	usually undernourished	obesity usually present
Symptoms	polydipsia, polyphagia, and polyuria	maybe none
Hepatomegaly	rather common	uncommon
Stability	blood sugar fluctuates widely in response to small changes in insulin dose, exercise, and infection	blood sugar fluctuations are less marked
Control of diabetes	difficult	easy, especially if patient adheres to proper diet
Ketosis	frequent, especially if treatment program is insufficient in food and/or insulin	uncommon except in the presence of unusual stress or moderate to severe sepsis
Plasma insulin (endogenous)	negligible to zero	plasma insulin response may be either adequate but delayed so that postprandial hypoglycemia may be present when diabetes is discovered, or diminished but not absent
Vascular complications of diabetes and degenerative changes	infrequent until diabetes has been present for ~5 years	frequent
Diet	mandatory in all patients	if diet is utilized fully, hypoglycemic therapy may not be needed
Insulin	necessary for all patients	necessary for 20–30% of patients
Oral agents	rarely efficacious	efficacious
Incidence	<10%	>75%

Table 3. Clinical Classification of Diabetes Mellitus

Type	Primary Cause	Age at Onset	Postglucose Plasma or Serum Insulin, μU/ml[a]	Treatment
Insulinopenic				
Severe	pancreatic beta cell deficiency	juveniles (nonobese adult)	absent	insulin, diet, education, exercise
Mild to moderate (insulinotardic)		nonobese adults	<50 at 1 hour	eucaloric diet alone, education, and exercise diet plus insulin or sulfonylureas
Insulinoplethoric				
(mild to moderate)	end organ unresponsiveness to insulin action (insulin receptors)	obese adults	>100 at 2 hours	weight reduction diet diet plus insulin or sulfonylureas for symptomatic control

Adapted from J. H. Karam, in *Current Medical Diagnosis and Treatment, 1978,* M. A. Krupp and M. J. Chatton, Eds., Lange Medical, Los Altos, Calif., 1978, p. 738.
[a] Normal response is between 50 and 135 μU/ml at 60 minutes and less than 100 μU/ml at 120 minutes after 100 g oral glucose.

clinical classification of diabetes

mechanisms of carbohydrate metabolism

carbohydrate metabolism in diabetics

gluconeogenesis

glucosuria

sistant, obese patients' tissues exhibit reduced insulin binding. A reduction in the number of insulin receptors is the basic, and possibly genetic, defect in insulin-resistant patients (20).

Normal Carbohydrate Metabolism

The important carbohydrate metabolism sites sensitive to insulin are the liver, where glycogen is formed, stored, and broken down; skeletal muscle, where glucose is oxidized to produce energy; and adipose tissue, where glucose may be converted to fatty acids, glyceryl phosphate, and triglycerides. Some of the important effects of insulin on carbohydrate metabolism in these tissues are increased glucose uptake by tissues, increased glucose oxidation by all pathways, increased energy production from glucose, increased muscle and liver glycogen levels, decreased hepatic glucose output, increased synthesis of fatty acids and triglycerides, decreased lipolysis, decreased production of ketone bodies, and stimulation of the incorporation of amino acids into proteins.

In the normal patient, insulin—in concert with glucagon, somatostatin, growth hormone, corticosteroids, epinephrine, and other chemicals—maintains the blood glucose between 40 and 160 mg/100 ml (mg %) at all times. The major point to keep in mind with reference to all hormones and other chemicals that affect insulin and carbohydrate metabolism is that if any are increased or decreased (as by drug therapy), they can cause a person either to become diabetic or to lose diabetic control.

Diabetic Carbohydrate Metabolism

Insulinopenic

With an understanding of carbohydrate metabolism in the nondiabetic, it is relatively easy to imagine what occurs in an insulinopenic diabetic unable to utilize glucose in muscle and adipose tissue. When a meal is ingested, blood glucose levels increase. With no insulin available to facilitate glucose transport into the fat or muscle tissue, hyperglycemia results. Amino acids are changed into glucose, and liver glycogen is broken down to glucose, which tissues are unable to utilize, increasing the hyperglycemia even more. This process is called gluconeogenesis.

Once blood glucose reaches 180 mg/100 ml, glucose begins to spill into the urine (glucosuria). (This is an average threshold in nondiabetics; the threshold for diabetics may increase to well over 250 mg/100 ml.) This condition in turn leads to an increased frequency of urination (polyuria). The resulting water loss causes a compensatory increase in thirst (polydipsia) and may cause significant hypovolemia and electrolyte loss. Since fats rather than carbohydrates are being metabolized, weight loss occurs over a period of time. The tissue cells, being "hungry" for carbohydrates, signal the person to eat (polyphagia), and eating continues to increase the blood glucose level.

Figure 1 shows the clinical manifestations that result in an untreated insulinopenic diabetic. Note the signs of insulin lack that result in abnormal urine and blood values. A properly trained diabetic patient can learn to test for these abnormalities in the urine and blood to monitor how well the diabetes is being controlled.

Insulin also has a direct inhibitory effect on the enzyme lipase which degrades body fat (lipolysis). Hormones such as glucocorticoids or epinephrine enhance lipolysis. When there is a shortage of insulin, lipase activity is enhanced, and fat is mobilized by conversion to free fatty acids which circulate through the blood. The ketone bodies that result from the breakdown of free fatty

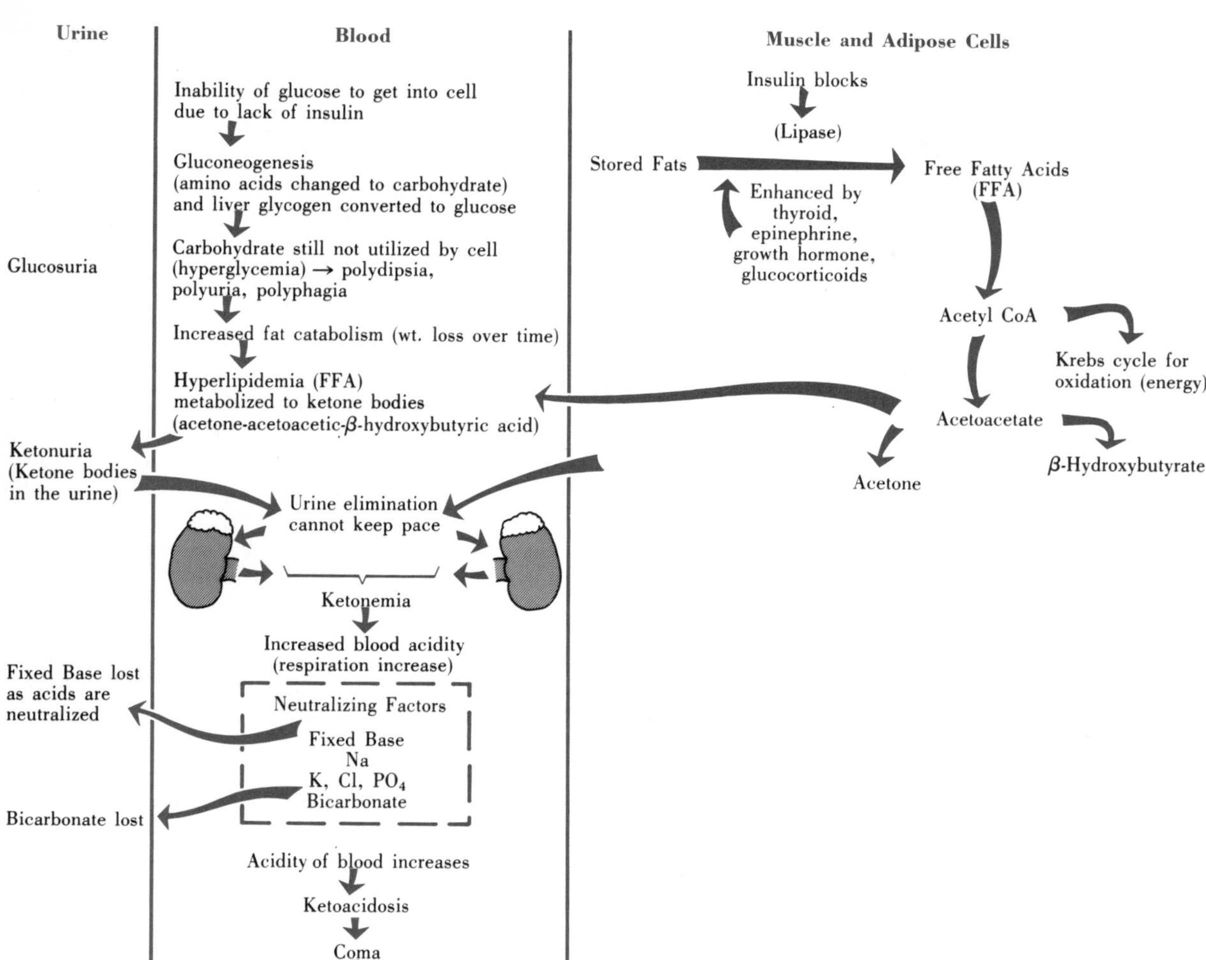

Figure 1. Clinical manifestations in untreated insulinopenic diabetics.

acids eventually lead to acidosis because the ketone bodies are naturally acidic. Ketones also depress the CNS, resulting in coma and death if insulin is not administered.

Insulinotardic/Insulinoplethoric

carbohydrate metabolism in insulinotardic and insulinoplethoric diabetics

Whereas insulinopenic diabetes typically has a rapid onset with the usual signs of polyuria, polyphagia, polydipsia, weakness, weight loss, and dry skin, insulinoplethoric diabetes frequently is unaccompanied by any symptoms (21). Insulinoplethoric diabetes (Figure 2) is discovered most often when sugar is found in the urine or when elevated blood sugar is found on a routine examination. Careful study of this older, obese group of diabetics reveals glucosuria, proteinuria, postprandial hyperglycemia, microaneurisms, and even retinal exudates.

The most interesting abnormal finding in insulinoplethoric diabetics is that they have normal or even greater than normal blood insulin levels. Glucose is transported into muscle and fat cells, and therefore these patients are not ketosis prone and seldom develop ketoacidosis. However, because of their high blood glucose levels, they may develop nonketotic hyperosmolar coma. Increased obesity in these patients may cause hyperinsulinemia, resulting in fewer insulin receptors and thus producing the clinical finding of hyperglycemia. If the disease's progressive nature can be stopped by weight reduction to an ideal body weight, the blood glucose levels of most insulinoplethoric patients will return to normal (21).

late complications of diabetes

Diabetics frequently develop kidney failure (nephropathy), lesions of the eye (retinopathy), and atrophy of the peripheral nerves (neuropathy). Generally, these processes occur because the walls of the capillaries that supply these areas with blood and nutrients thicken. The molecular mechanisms leading to these late complications of diabetes have not been established conclusively (11).

Recent studies have implicated disturbances in polyol and glycoprotein metabolism in diabetic neuropathy.

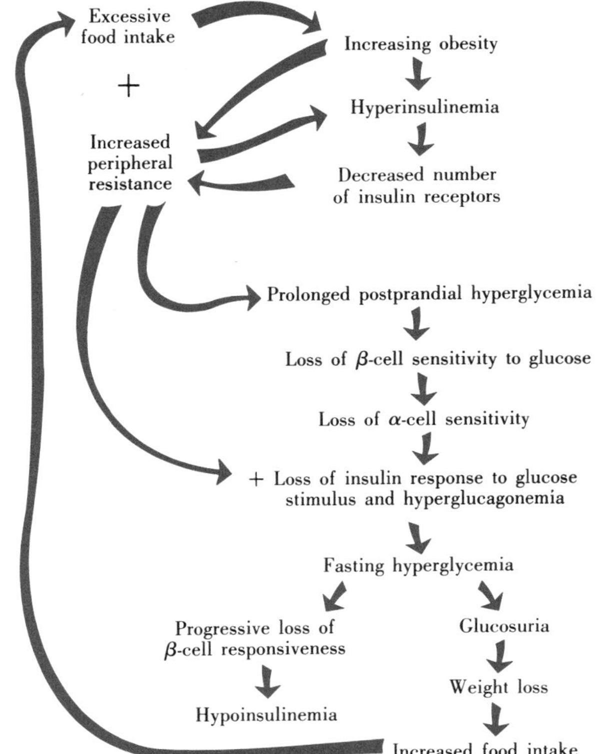

Figure 2. Pathogenesis of insulinoplethoric diabetes mellitus.

polyol pathway
microangiopathy
pharmacist involvement
diabetes screening

During periods of hyperglycemia, neuronal intracellular glucose concentrations rise because nerve tissue does not require insulin for glucose uptake. The enzymes normally involved in glucose metabolism become saturated with glucose, and other metabolic pathways, such as the polyol pathway, metabolize the excess glucose, thus increasing sorbitol levels. Aldose reductase and sorbitol dehydrogenase are two of the enzymes utilized in this noninsulin-dependent pathway of metabolizing glucose that produces abnormally high amounts of fructose and sorbitol.

Both sorbitol and fructose have been found in increased amounts in nerves of hyperglycemic diabetic animals. The accumulation of these polyols could produce osmotic injury to the nerve with myoinositol depletion. Recently, it has been demonstrated that either elimination of hyperglycemia by insulin or exogenous repletion of myoinositol prevents the development of diabetic neuropathy in experimental diabetic animals. It also has been found clinically in diabetic patients that when blood glucose levels are at a normal level, problems of neuropathy often disappear (11).

The basic morphological lesion of diabetic microangiopathy is a widespread thickening of capillary basement membranes. The direct cause of this thickening is unknown; however, since basement membranes are composed of collagenlike glycoproteins, with the synthesis controlled by both posttranscriptional and genetic factors, environmental influences could be very important. Increased capillary permeability, which occurs early in the course of human diabetes, may be normalized by control of hyperglycemia and worsens with deterioration of control. Other abnormalities of glycoprotein metabolism have been found in both insulinopenic and insulinoplethoric diabetics. These findings include increased levels of a minor hemoglobin component, hemoglobin A_1c, which is now used clinically to monitor control of diabetes. Capillary basement membrane thickening may represent only one facet of a generalized abnormality in glycoprotein metabolism due to hyperglycemia or other sequelae of insulin lack.

Atherosclerotic lesions in the diabetic appear to be the same as those in the nondiabetic, but they develop earlier, occur more often, and are generally more severe. Besides the vascular and nerve changes that can take place in diabetics with prolonged hyperglycemia, diabetics frequently experience difficulty in eradicating bacterial infections. Hyperglycemia may impair the phagocytic activity of the body's white blood cells. Most chronic adverse conditions in the diabetic can be traced to an inadequate blood supply to the area (22).

Insulinoplethoric and insulinopenic diabetics also suffer from occlusive vascular changes in the lower extremities as a result of both atherosclerosis and damage to smaller arteries (microangiopathies). This change is one of the reasons that, after age 40, the incidence of gangrene in the feet is 20 times greater in diabetics than in nondiabetics (22).

In insulinotardic diabetics, hyperglycemia results after food ingestion. As with insulinoplethoric diabetics, prolonged hyperglycemia may result in serious complications. However, in insulinotardic diabetics the beta cells eventually do respond and release insulin, and thus the symptoms that bring the insulinotardic patient to the physician are often symptoms of hypoglycemia, e.g., fatigue, weakness, nervousness, anxiety, trembling, headache, sweating, hunger, dizziness, nausea, visual disturbances, tingling of the tongue or lips, unsteadiness, drowsiness, and mental confusion.

EVALUATION

The sooner diabetes is detected, the easier it is to control, and the fewer complications result. The pharmacist's role in promoting and supporting diabetes detection programs cannot be overstressed. During the screening program, as well as at other times, the pharmacist should be able to answer any questions that the diabetic patient may have. In a 3-week period the pharmacist may see up to 70% of the community residents; this contact provides an excellent opportunity to screen patients for diabetes. Possible diabetics then can be referred to physicians for a more complete physical examination and history and for laboratory analysis (23).

Screening for Diabetes

If all pharmacists set aside 1 day per month to screen patients for diabetes, they would have a substantial impact on detecting the more than 2 million undiagnosed diabetics in this country. The actual screening itself is quite simple. Dextrostix, cotton swabs, alcohol lancets, literature, and an analyzing machine to test Dextrostix color changes are all that is needed. Pharmacy students at the University of California at San Francisco have developed a procedure for screening patients as well as a sample release form that can be used by pharmacists, a diabetes screening interview form, and a form that gives the patient the test results.

The program involves taking a blood sample from the subject's finger or ear lobe. The drop of blood is placed on a Dextrostix reagent strip for 60 seconds, then washed off with a water bottle. The color on the reagent strip is then analyzed instrumentally, using an Ames Eyetone.

In some states, only licensed medical technicians, registered nurses, or physicians may withdraw blood from patients legally. Contact with a volunteer nurses association may be of value to launch a screening program (23).

Patients with all types of cardiac problems, including high blood pressure, stroke, congestive heart failure, and angina, have a higher incidence of diabetes. Diabetes also is more common in patients who have suffered from hyperthyroidism, Addison's disease, and Cushing's syndrome. At least 75% of all diabetics have relatives with diabetes (24). Approximately 80% of diabetics are overweight individuals in the 40- to 65-year-old age group.

Signs and Symptoms

The pharmacist should obtain a careful patient history before attempting an evaluation. Some diagnostic hints or signs of diabetes other than the more publicized polydipsia, polyphagia, and polyuria that could be used by the pharmacist to help discover potential diabetics are listed below. Pharmacists who detect these medical problems should refer the patient to a physician who specializes in treating diabetes.

Weight Loss

Weight loss when eating regular meals is a sign of diabetes. The only other condition that causes this phenomenon is hyperthyroidism.

Recurrent Monilial Infections

This condition is common in diabetics, especially fungal infections of the vulva and anus in women. Chronic skin infections, carbuncles, furuncles, and eczema also are more common in diabetics.

Gout

The percentage of patients with gout who have diabetes (5–10%) is higher than the norm. Thus patients with gout should be screened for diabetes.

Prolonged Wound Healing

Minor cuts and scratches take at least twice as long to heal in a diabetic.

Visual Disturbances

These may be the only symptoms the diabetic expresses early in the disease; patients who wear glasses may notice that increasingly stronger lenses are required at relatively short time intervals. Ophthalmologists detect a large number of diabetic patients (22). Cataracts and open-angle glaucoma in older diabetics are common.

Psychological Changes

Fatigue and extreme physical depression occur more often in diabetics. Frequent emotional flare-ups may signal that the body's biochemistry is not normal, possibly because of diabetes. Some of the first symptoms of hypoglycemia affecting the nervous system are irritability, nervousness, and anxiety.

Laboratory Diagnosis

If a patient has glucose in the urine or a higher than normal glucose in the blood or presents one or more of the signs and symptoms of diabetes, the physician should administer an oral glucose tolerance test (OGTT) or other appropriate screening test. Table 4 summarizes the various methods used to diagnose diabetes from this test (12, 21). Patients with borderline oral glucose tolerance tests should be rechecked periodically, especially when they become symptomatic.

importance of patient history

diagnostic signs

tests for diabetes

objectives of diabetic control

therapeutic agents

Other tests used as diagnostic or screening tests for diabetes include the fasting blood sugar (FBS), the 2-hour postprandial (2HPP) blood glucose test, and the hemoglobin A_1c.

Nondiabetic causes of glucose intolerance include liver disease, prolonged physical inactivity, acute stress, fever, trauma, surgery, heart attack, starvation, hypokalemia, renal disease, and endocrine diseases. A positive test for glucose in the urine is not necessarily diagnostic for diabetes; rather, it is an indication for more definitive testing. Glucosuria is symptomatic of many other conditions (e.g., pregnancy or faulty renal function). Glucosuria generally occurs when the mean blood glucose level is 180 mg/100 ml or greater and rarely occurs when this level is less than 130 mg/100 ml (25). The renal threshold for glucose increases with age, so that older diabetics may not show evidence of glucosuria despite a high blood glucose level.

TREATMENT

In order of importance, the objectives of diabetic control are relief of diabetic symptoms, avoidance of hypoglycemic reactions, maintenance of optimal weight, maintenance of blood glucose between 130 and 180 mg/100 ml before meals, and production of little or no glucosuria (26). These objectives can be met only through the combined efforts of the physician, nurse, pharmacist, and patient. Sulfonylureas and insulin are used to control the condition, and OTC products formulated especially for use by the diabetic patient are helpful. Diet, exercise, education, and insulin need to be delicately balanced. Multiple injections create tighter control with fewer complications, improve retinopathy, and result in less glucosuria and a longer life (27–31).

Diabetic Medications

The medications used to treat diabetes can be categorized into two broad areas: oral hypoglycemic agents and insulin. The use of oral hypoglycemic agents is controversial, not only because their effectiveness is questionable, but also because long-term side effects may occur. Pharmacists should monitor patients using oral hypoglycemic agents for reactions with products that can

Table 4. Oral Glucose Tolerance Tests—Diagnostic Criteria for Diabetes Mellitus

Wilkerson Point System[a]			Fajans-Conn Criteria		
Time	mg/100 ml	Points	Time	mg/100 ml	University Group Diabetes Program
Fasting	≧110[b] (130)[c]	1	1 hour	≧160[b] (185)[c]	summation of blood or plasma glucose values at 0, 1, 2, and 3 hours
1 hour	≧170 (195)	0.5	1.5 hours	≧140 (165)	
2 hours	≧120 (140)	0.5	2 hours	≧120 (140)	
3 hours	≧110 (130)	1			
Diabetes		≧2	Diabetes	any 2 values	Diabetes blood ≧ 500 plasma ≧ 600
Initial glucose load, 100 g			Initial glucose load, 1.75 g/kg		Initial glucose load, 30 g/m^2 body surface area

[a] U.S. Public Health Service.
[b] Blood.
[c] Plasma or serum.

diagnostic criteria for diabetes

sulfonylureas

drug interactions

cause either hypoglycemia or hyperglycemia, which may affect control of the condition.

Although insulin must be prescribed initially by a physician, pharmacists frequently are the health care professionals consulted concerning problems. Therefore pharmacists should be familiar with the various strengths and sources of insulin and with different onsets and durations of action.

Oral Hypoglycemic Agents

Even though this chapter deals with OTC products used in diabetes, pharmacist understanding of the proper use of sulfonylureas is necessary.

Sulfonylureas stimulate insulin secretion by the pancreas. The four products used in the United States are summarized in Table 5.

The most common side effect with the sulfonylureas is hypoglycemia. Frequent drug–drug interactions resulting in enhanced hypoglycemia occur with alcohol, anabolic steroids, chloramphenicol, dicumarol, monoamine oxidase inhibitors, phenylbutazone, propranolol, salicylates, sulfisoxazole, and theophylline (25). Drugs that may interfere with diabetes control by causing hyperglycemia include asparaginase, oral contraceptives, corticosteroids, thiazide diuretics, ethacrynic acid, furosemide, glucagon, phenytoin, dextrothyroxine, diazoxide, niacin (high doses), probenecid, and sympathomimetic amines (25).

Chlorpropamide is the most potent of the sulfonylureas in use in the United States. It can cause an increased sensitivity to circulating levels of antidiuretic hormone (ADH) which occur in approximately 4% of patients (32, 33). The chlorpropamide-induced inappropriate ADH activity is reversible. Improvement occurs within a week after the medication is discontinued. In insulinotardic and insulinoplethoric diabetics, diet is the main method of treatment, and sulfonylureas should be used only when diet fails. The physician should determine what constitutes dietary failure.

Conditions in which oral antidiabetic agents are contraindicated include acidosis or preacidotic states, severe infections accompanying diabetic onset, major surgery (during and after), sulfa sensitivity, and pregnancy.

Pharmacists dispensing sulfonylureas should explain to the patient that the medication is used to treat diabetes and that it is important to take the medication regularly, exactly as prescribed by the physician. If the patient develops a sore throat, fever, mouth sores, or dark-colored urine, the physician should be contacted. The pharmacist should caution the patient to avoid the use of alcoholic beverages and drugs containing salicylates and should stress the necessity of using the product in conjunction with the prescribed diet (34, 35). Pharmacists also should be aware that although initially 65–75% of insulinoplethoric and insulinotardic diabetic patients respond to sulfonylureas, there is a 5–30% failure in 6–12 months. Sulfonylureas also are possible teratogens; they should not be used early in pregnancy and are absolutely contraindicated late in gestation, since they may cause prolonged and severe hypoglycemia (35).

Insulin

Insulinopenic diabetics who have absolute insulin deficiency must be treated with exogenous insulin. Generally, persons who require insulin initially tend to be younger than 30, lean, prone to developing ketoacidosis, and markedly hyperglycemic, even in the fasting state (21). Insulin also is indicated for adult-onset diabetics with insulinopenia who do not respond to diet therapy, either alone or combined with oral hypoglycemic drugs (19). Insulin therapy is necessary in some stable diabetic patients who are subjected to stresses such as infections, pregnancy, and surgery. Occasionally in insulinoplethoric diabetics, doses of 10–20 units of intermediate-acting insulins are needed to bring hyperglycemia under control. Thus all classes of diabetics should be trained to inject themselves with insulin. Diabetic children should begin giving themselves their own shots at around age 8–9 (36), although parents should administer one or two injections per week to stay in practice and should inject in areas difficult for the child to reach (37). By combining the

Table 5. Basic Biopharmaceutics and Pharmacokinetics of the Oral Hypoglycemics

Drug	Recommended Dose, g	Maximum Dose, g	Half-Life, hours	Onset	Duration, hours	Metabolism and Excretion	Comments
Tolbutamide (Orinase)	0.5–3.0 divided doses	2–3	5.6	1 hour	6–12	totally metabolized to inactive form; inactive metabolite excreted in kidney	generally first drug of choice; most benign; least potent; short half-life; especially useful in kidney disease
Acetohexamide (Dymelor)	0.25–1.5 single or divided doses	1.5	5	1 hour	10–14	metabolite's activity equal to or greater than parent compound; metabolite excreted via kidney	essentially no advantage over tolbutamide, although few patients who fail on tolbutamide are controlled; significant uricosuric effects
Tolazamide (Tolinase)	0.1–1.0 single or divided doses	0.75–1.0	7	4–6 hours	10–14	absorbed slowly; metabolite active but less potent than parent compound; excreted via kidney	essentially no advantage over tolbutamide; said to be equipotent with less severe side effects
Chlorpropamide (Diabinese)	0.1–0.5 single dose	0.5	35	1 hour	72	previously thought not to be metabolized but recently found that metabolism may be quite extensive; activity of these unknown; significant percentage excreted unchanged	most potent in use; caution in elderly patients and those with kidney disease; disulfiramlike reactions may occur with alcohol
Phenformin (DBI, Meltrol)	0.05–0.2 single or divided doses	usually 0.2 (dose limited by GI effects)	3	3–4 days, then rapid	12 [a]	metabolized but activity of metabolite unknown; 90% excreted via kidney in 24 hours	FDA removed from market October 1977; was drug of choice for obese diabetics; used to treat secondary failures and to stabilize brittle juvenile diabetics

[a] For timed-release form.

characteristics of oral hypoglycemics

insulin use in ketoacidosis

appropriate modification of diet, exercise, and variable mixtures of short- and longer-acting insulins it has been possible to achieve acceptable control of blood glucose (19).

Use in Ketoacidosis

Regular insulin is the only insulin that should be used for the treatment of ketoacidosis. All regular insulin is now produced at a neutral pH.

Diabetic ketoacidosis constitutes an acute medical emergency, necessitating immediate diagnosis and therapy. It accounts for less than 1% of the deaths occurring in the diabetic population; however, the mortality rate associated with these acute episodes is 5–15%, indicating the need for strict attention to detail and management (38). The physician can diagnose diabetic ketoacidosis rapidly by examining urinary glucose and ketones, arterial blood pH and blood gas, and serum ketone laboratory values.

Shock and cerebral edema are among the complications encountered in diabetic ketoacidosis. Shock generally develops as a consequence of life-threatening stress such as sepsis, myocardial infarction, or acute pancreatitis (38). Treatment is directed at plasma volume expansion and correction of acidosis and hypotension. Low-dose insulin regimens are recommended to treat diabetic ketoacidosis and nonketotic hyperosmolar coma.

Insulin Preparations

The insulins are divided into three groups, according to their duration of action. Short-acting insulins include semilente and regular insulin. Intermediate-acting insulins include NPH, lente, and globin zinc insulin. The long-acting insulins include protamine zinc and ultralente insulin. Lente insulin is a combination of 70% ultralente and 30% semilente insulin. NPH insulin is a combination of two parts regular insulin and one part protamine zinc insulin.

It is expected that in the very near future the U-80 insulins will be taken off the market completely; such a proposal is now pending with the FDA. Some patients who use small insulin doses still prefer U-40 insulin, but manufacturers, the FDA, and the American Diabetes Association with the support of the American Pharmaceutical Association are attempting to convert all patients to U-100 insulins. Standardizing the strengths should help to eliminate errors resulting from the use of incorrectly calibrated syringes and reduce confusion in mixing insulins.

types of insulin preparations, their potency, duration of action, and identification

purity

sensitivity reactions

factors in absorption

Methods used to increase the duration of action of regular insulin have included the addition of zinc crystals, protein molecules, and acetate buffers. Globin, NPH, and protamine zinc are examples of intermediate- and long-acting insulins to which zinc and proteins have been added. The lente insulins result in longer- or shorter-acting types of insulin when the amounts of acetate buffer and zinc added to the insulin are varied.

All insulins except globin have a neutral pH; globin insulin has an acid pH. All regular insulins are at a normal pH of 7.4. All commercially available insulins are cloudy, except globin and regular insulins, which are clear. Vials and syringes are color coded to make for easier identification of the strengths of insulin. U-40 insulins (i.e., 40 units/ml) are color coded red; U-80 insulin, green; and U-100 insulin, orange with black lettering.

Factors Affecting Purity

The animal from which the insulin is derived can influence its effect on blood glucose control and insulin resistance and sensitivity (39). Most commercially available insulins are derived from beef and pork, and it is possible to obtain pure pork or pure beef insulin. High purification of pork NPH insulin is important in reducing insulin dose, lipoatrophy (subcutaneous concavities caused by a wasting of the lipid tissue), and insulin-binding capacity of serum. About 80% of patients with persistent local allergy to mixed beef–pork insulin improve if treated with pure pork insulin (10). Beef insulin has greater antigenicity because it is more unlike human insulin than pork insulin (10).

Another factor that has affected the use of insulin in diabetic patients is purity. Thanks to new analytical techniques using chromatography and electrophoresis to separate and isolate proteins, purer forms of insulin are now available. The average content of certain minor components of insulin, such as pro-insulin, desamido insulin, arginine insulin, esterified insulin, and glucagon, have been decreased, and this decrease has resulted in fewer insulin sensitivity reactions. The new forms of insulin are often referred to as "single-peak" insulins because the spectrophotometric curves of the insulin contents show lower amounts of noninsulin protein material and increased amounts of insulin. The purity of insulins has been improved from 92% to approximately 98% (21). It is possible to purify insulin to the "monocomponent" insulin (99% pure) level. The highly purified monocomponent insulins are available in some foreign countries but are not commercially available in the United States. One study has shown that the monocomponent type of insulin produces less antigenicity and, in the average patient, allows a 15% decrease in dose (40).

Diabetic patients who develop a sensitivity to insulin display a redness, usually at the site of injection. When a diabetic initially begins taking insulin, these reactions are quite common and may occur over a period of several weeks before subsiding gradually. If the reactions continue, however, they may be treated with an antihistamine such as diphenhydramine (25 mg).

Insulin resistance, a state requiring more than 200 units of insulin per day for more than 2 days in the absence of ketoacidosis or acute infection, occurs in only about 0.001% of diabetic patients. These patients almost invariably are found to have high titers of insulin-neutralizing antibodies. Glucocorticoids are indicated; usually, prednisone in a dose of 60–80 mg/day is indicated. Monocomponent pork insulin also is recommended.

Another factor that can affect the clinical use of insulin preparations is how they are administered parenterally (41). Insulin injection by the intramuscular route provides a faster absorption of insulin with a concomitant greater drop in plasma glucose than does injection by the subcutaneous route. Intravenous insulin produces the highest pharmacological level of insulin in the least amount of time.

Insulin absorption is affected by exercise. Leg exercise accelerates insulin absorption from the leg. Arm or abdominal injection avoids the acceleration during leg exercise and reduces exercise-induced hypoglycemia (42). Thus a diabetic whose day includes a hard game of tennis might do well to inject that day's insulin into the abdomen rather than into the arm or leg (43).

Another complication of insulin therapy is insulin lipodystrophy. Lipoatrophy is cosmetically difficult for the patient to accept. When single-peak insulin is injected into the affected areas, lipoatrophy improves in the majority of patients (44, 45). Lipohypertrophy is generally seen in patients who favor particular sites for insulin injection. This condition provides one of the main reasons for educating patients to rotate their injection sites. Besides being cosmetically unattractive, these areas of hypertrophy may decrease insulin absorption.

Mixing and Storage

Neutral regular insulin may be mixed with NPH or

lente insulin in any proportion desired, and the combination is stable for periods of up to 3 months before use. Regular insulin may be added to protamine zinc insulin, but because of the excess protamine in protamine zinc insulin, mixtures in a ratio of less than 1:1 have the same activity as protamine zinc insulin alone. As the proportion of regular to protamine zinc insulin nears 2:1, a time–activity curve approximating that of NPH insulin is obtained. When the ratio exceeds 2:1 (i.e., the amount of regular insulin is increased further), the time–activity of the mixture approaches that of a regular NPH combination.

Mixtures of regular and protamine zinc insulin may be prepared at any time. Semilente, ultralente, and lente insulins may be combined in any ratio desired at any time. Because of excess globin molecules in globin insulin, mixing with regular insulin produces globin insulin and therefore has no advantages. Regular insulin also may be mixed in any proportion with normal saline, but the combination should be used within 2–3 hours after mixing, since pH changes and dilution of buffer may affect stability. Regular insulin also may be mixed with Lilly's Insulin Diluting Fluid in any proportion and will be stable indefinitely.

Because insulin is a heat-labile protein, care must be exercised in storing all preparations so that potency and maximum stability will be maintained. With regular insulin, loss of potency begins after 18 months if the insulin is kept at room temperature. There is an increase in the loss of potency as the temperature increases with regular insulin. The lente forms of insulin retain their potency when stored at room temperature for 24 months, but signs of loss of potency do not occur until after 30 months. With NPH and protamine zinc insulin, loss of potency does not occur at room temperature for up to 36 months. Thus insulins are stable unrefrigerated for long periods. However, the pharmacist should advise patients to keep extra bottles of insulin in the refrigerator and keep the bottle being used at room temperature. Higher temperatures may cause the suspensions of insulin (NPH, protamine zinc, and lente) to clump. Potency is not necessarily lost, but there is a problem in drawing up the correct dose when clumping has occurred. Freezing also may cause clumping but does not necessarily affect potency (10). Injection of insulin stored at room temperature is recommended because refrigerated insulin produces more pain.

Adverse Reactions

The major complications of insulin therapy is hypoglycemia. Factors predisposing the patient to insulin reactions include insufficient food intake (skipping meals, vomiting, or diarrhea), excessive exercise, inaccurate measurement of insulin, concomitant intake of hypoglycemic drugs, and termination of diabetogenic conditions or drugs. Symptoms include a parasympathetic response (nausea, hunger, or eructation), diminished cerebral function (confusion, agitation, lethargy, or personality changes), a sympathetic response (tachycardia, sweating, or tremor), coma, and convulsions. Ataxia and blurred vision also are common (46). In elderly patients with decreased nerve function, diabetics with advanced neuropathy, or patients receiving propranolol the symptoms of hypoglycemia are lacking, and the reaction may go undetected and untreated. All manifestations of hypoglycemia are relieved rapidly by glucose administration.

Because of the potential danger of insulin reactions, the diabetic patient should always carry packets of table sugar or a candy roll for use at the onset of hypoglycemic symptoms. Patients also may swallow orange juice or any sugar-containing beverage or food. An ampule of glucagon (1 mg) should be provided to every diabetic receiving insulin therapy to be injected by family or friends in case of unconsciousness.

If a hypoglycemic person is mistakenly thought to be hyperglycemic and given insulin, severe brain damage may result. Thus when there is doubt whether a diabetic is in insulin shock or hyperglycemic, sugar should be given.

insulin mixing and storage conditions

complications of therapy

diabetic control and weight control

Nondrug Therapy

One of the objectives in maintaining diabetic control is maintaining normal weight. The pharmacist should stress the importance of proper exercise and diet.

Exercise

Although exercise is nearly always recommended by physicians as part of the treatment of diabetes, it is seldom prescribed. Physicians should prescribe an individualized daily exercise schedule for diabetic patients. Exercise allows glucose to penetrate the muscle cell to be metabolized without the assistance of insulin. Glucose may be utilized to varying degrees without insulin in all types of cells (17). Exercise also lowers blood sugar and increases circulation, enabling the blood vessels to perform more effectively. This function relieves the circulatory system and helps to withstand the abuse the diabetic condition imposes on it. Exercise also helps maintain normal body weight and aids breathing, digestion, and metabolism. An exercise log may help the patient maintain a regular daily schedule.

Diet

Diet is the most critical treatment method in insulinoplethoric and insulinotardic diabetics and, in combination with exercise and insulin, is a necessary treatment method for insulinopenic diabetics (47). However, diet therapy failure occurs often and creates feelings of frustration, pessimism, failure, and anger, which in turn result in poorly informed and inadequately motivated patients (48).

Factors in Dietary Control

Successful diet programs require behavior modification on the part of the patient. Patients should be encouraged to join groups such as Weight Watchers and to keep a diet log similar to the exercise log. They should write down (for a period of 4–10 days) each time they ate, how much they ate, and why they ate—whether food ingestion was due to social pressure, loneliness, depression, nervousness, or the time of day, or whether the patient truly needed nourishment. By having patients use smaller plates, take only one helping of food, and try to be conscious of why they eat, it is possible to change their dietary behavior (49). One reason for diet therapy failure in diabetics is that physicians or dieticians prescribe changes in diet without first adjusting the dose of insulin or oral agents. The first step in diet therapy should be to prescribe an exercise program, lower the medication dose, and put the patient on a diet containing fewer calories.

Insulin overtreatment is probably one of the most common causes of diabetic instability and weight gain (50). In one group of diabetic patients, 75% were found to need a reduction in insulin dose of at least 10%; 35% of the overtreated patients had large appetites, and 30% had hepatomegaly and headaches. A system should be developed in diabetic patients to detect whether or not they have involved themselves in a vicious cycle of taking too much insulin and then eating up to that level of insulin.

saccharin
sorbitol
other diet factors
use of alcoholic beverages

The pharmacist has a supportive role to play in diet therapy. Pharmacists need to encourage diabetic patients to follow the prescribed diet and should discourage prolonged fasting or using "fad" diets as a means of losing weight. Patients should obtain dietician or physician approval for any change in dietary habits. The pharmacist should caution diabetic patients that "dietetic" labeling of products does not mean "diabetic." Patients should be encouraged to read the labels of all foods marked "dietetic" because the foods may not be sugarless or even intended for diabetics. Some dietetic foods actually have more calories than regular foods.

Artificial Sweeteners

In general, there are two ways in which food may be adapted or prepared for the diabetic: by restricting the sugar content and by restricting both the sugar content and the caloric value (51). In preparing special foods, sucrose is omitted, and other sweetening agents may be substituted. The safety of some of these substitutes often has been in doubt. Saccharin, which is 400 times as sweet as sucrose, is the most common sucrose substitute in the United States. Because it has been implicated in causing cancerous tumors in rats, the FDA may ban saccharin. Currently, a cautionary statement on food and drugs containing saccharin is required. Cyclamates are used as a sugar substitute in other countries and eventually may be permitted back on U.S. markets, since little evidence of harm to humans has ever been documented (51).

Sorbitol is a glucose alcohol 60% as sweet as sugar. It is absorbed slowly from the gut with little effect on blood glucose levels. Sorbitol is without side effects unless large quantities are taken, when osmotic effects may cause diarrhea and abdominal discomfort. However, it is metabolized after conversion to glucose, and its energy value as calories must be counted for patients whose weight needs control. Sorbitol is one of the end products of the polyol pathway of glucose metabolism that results in some of the late complications of diabetes. Fructose is another sucrose substitute that is an end product of glucose metabolism by insulin-independent pathways and thus has a potential for adding to the late complications of diabetes (51).

Dietary Cautions

The aim of dietary treatment in diabetes is to control weight and blood glucose levels and to prevent the development and progression of vascular complications. Because about 75% of deaths among diabetics are due to cardiovascular disease, compared with 50% of deaths in the general population (52), diabetics should avoid dietary factors, e.g., animal fats, that have been shown to result in cardiovascular disease. The American Diabetes Association recently recommended a diet that contains 50% carbohydrates, 20% protein, and no more than 35% fat. Cholesterol also is restricted to less than 300 mg/day. Simple and refined sugars should be avoided in all diabetics because of the stress put on the patient (19).

Many diabetic patients believe that since diabetes results in increased blood glucose levels, carbohydrates in general should be avoided. One long-term clinical trial has shown that an increased proportion of dietary carbohydrate does not cause deterioration of diabetic control—especially when the carbohydrate source is in the form of bread, potatoes, or rice, and not simple sugars—as long as total calories are limited to maintain or achieve ideal body weight (19). Diabetic patients who follow their diet therapy can keep their serum triglyceride and serum cholesterol levels within a normal range (19). Restriction of saturated fats and avoidance of pie, sugar, syrups, candy, alcoholic beverages, sweetened soft drinks, and cake are advised for all diabetics.

Diabetic patients also should take a vitamin and mineral product. Patients taking vitamin supplements that contain high amounts of ascorbic acid should keep in mind that these vitamins may affect urine test values, and thus they should be sure to double-void (urinate, drink a glass of water, then urinate again) and use the second void when testing their urine.

A high-fiber diet is valuable in the diabetic patient. Adequate dietary roughage reduces intraluminal pressure in the bowel and decreases the absorption rate of saccharides (47). When guar and pectin, components of dietary fiber, were added to a carbohydrate meal, the postprandial rise of blood glucose was delayed significantly (53).

Fiber does not have miraculous weight-controlling properties. It simply makes it easier for a person to take in fewer calories without feeling hungry. Patients should be warned when changing to a high-fiber diet to do it gradually. A sudden large increase may cause temporary flatulence and bloating (54).

Alcohol

In general, alcohol use is discouraged in diabetic patients, but each individual diabetic should be assessed to see whether alcohol's advantages (e.g., reducing emotional tension, relieving anxiety, and stimulating appetite) outweigh its potential effect on blood glucose control (52).

Either hyperglycemia or hypoglycemia may develop in diabetics who ingest alcohol. Hypoglycemia is the most common effect. The hypoglycemic effect of alcohol is believed to be due either to increased early endogenous insulin response to glucose or to inhibition of hepatic gluconeogenesis. Relatively small quantities of alcohol (48 ml of 100 proof) may cause this effect. Thus if a diabetic patient is fasting and consumes alcohol, hypoglycemia may be severe. If a diabetic has adequate amounts of glucose in the blood, then alcohol has a less clinically significant effect.

The additive hypoglycemic effects of alcohol with insulin have produced severe hypoglycemia resulting in coma, brain damage, and even death. Diabetic patients who are well fed and drinking alcoholic beverages with a high level of carbohydrates eventually develop hyperglycemia.

Tolbutamide and chlorpropamide have been reported to interact with alcohol (55), resulting in an "Antabuse-like" reaction.

It has been recommended that diabetics avoid alcoholic beverages, if possible, including alcohol-containing drug products (56). However, avoidance is not always possible, and more realistic guidelines should be established. Diabetics who wish to drink should use small quantities of dry wines. Some diabetologists even recommend the use of small amounts of dry wine for their diabetic patients. Dry wine has been considered by many as part of the therapy in diabetes (57). Alcohol is one of the most readily oxidizable food substances known and, unlike sugar, can be metabolized readily without insulin participation. After the ingestion of wine, blood glucose levels may rise slightly.

Recent studies have shown that diabetics who are on a diabetic diet alone or taking insulin or a sulfonylurea can consume up to 2 ounces (60 ml) of dry wine without any significant alteration in the blood glucose values (57). The data available concerning diabetics taking strong forms of alcohol, such as in distilled liquors, are different. If strong alcohol is taken in excess, ketosis may arise, but there is little evidence to demonstrate concern over consumption of moderate amounts of hard liquor.

Alcohol has been shown to reduce cardiac output in diabetic patients with diseased hearts. A typical 4-ounce serving of dry table wine contains 90–100 calories with a sugar content generally averaging 0.4 g. Rosé wines tend to be sweeter; a 4-ounce serving contains about 1.3 g. Champagne contains about 1.4 g of sugar. The sweeter white wines may contain as much as 5 g of glucose per 4-ounce serving. The caloric intake for fortified wines is about twice as much as for an equal volume of dry wine, and the sugar content may be as high as 6 g for a 2-ounce serving of sweet sherries, ports, and muscatels. Thus, for example, 4 ounces of dry wine could be consumed with the evening meal without difficulty as long as calorie and carbohydrate adjustments were made for the wine (57).

Preventing Complications

The complications of diabetes include microangiopathy, macroangiopathy, dermopathy, retinopathy, neuropathy, and nephropathy, plus a decreased ability to overcome infections. The prevention of complications through good diabetic control is the treatment of choice. Diabetic patients must be careful in using products that can influence their diabetes. For example, the ingestion of large quantities of aspirin, or even ascorbic acid, may influence urine tests and affect diabetic control. Diabetic patients using products containing ascorbic acid or aspirin should be sure to double-void when using these products in testing their urine. Nasal sprays, asthma medications, decongestants, allergy medications, hay fever medications, cold preparations, and cough preparations that can contain sympathomimetic amines also should be used with caution in diabetic patients. Diabetics should avoid medications containing either sugar or alcohol. Antihistamines or other products that produce drowsiness may result in skipped insulin doses.

Specific measures to prevent problems that require special attention in diabetic patients include general hygiene, foot care (see Chapter 31), dental care (see Chapter 21), and prevention of hypoglycemic episodes.

alcohol use by diabetics

influence of other drugs on diabetic control

development of gangrene

General Hygiene

In general, diabetic patients are more susceptible to bacterial infection and particularly to monilial infection than the general population (58). The most easily infected part of the body is the skin. Infections in diabetic patients do not heal easily, and thus minor cuts and scratches should be thoroughly cleansed, and an antibiotic ointment applied. Diabetic patients should be encouraged to keep an OTC antibiotic ointment for use with minor cuts and scratches. It is recommended that these products be used no longer than 1 week. If any serious cut, burn, or puncture occurs, diabetic patients should see their physician immediately.

Monilial infection of the vagina or anus is a problem that is much more common in diabetic patients. The first order of treatment of monilial infections in diabetic patients is to bring the diabetes under control. A product found useful in treating pruritus ani contains three parts Amphogel, one part kaolin powder, and one part Unibase. Application of this product to the anal area reduces itching and irritation. Daily bathing with thorough drying also is recommended for diabetic patients. Diabetics should use mild soaps and avoid all harsh chemicals including caustic powders, iodine preparations, and any other product that may produce or exacerbate vascular or neurological complications.

Foot Care

Gangrene has been reported to be 50 times more frequent in diabetics over 40 than in nondiabetics of the same age (59). Before the advent of antibiotics, amputation of the leg was the operation performed on 9 of 10 diabetic patients undergoing surgery for gangrene of the foot. Even with the discovery of antibiotics, approximately 50% of major leg amputations are performed on diabetic patients (59). Because of vascular changes, as well as neuropathy in the lower extremities of diabetic patients, the ability to counteract infection is greatly decreased. Thus when foot tissue is exposed to minor trauma or infection, the thick-walled vessels become more easily obliterated, and gangrene may occur (59).

proper foot care

comparison of syringes

dead space volume

Control of diabetes is the first step in foot care. To prevent foot problems, diabetic patients must be educated to care properly for their feet. In addition to the procedures described in Chapter 31, these measures include:

- Rubbing dry feet thoroughly with either vegetable oil or lanolin to keep them soft and to prevent dryness (if feet become too soft and tender, they should be rubbed with alcohol once per week) (19);
- Avoiding bruises, cuts, and skin irritations, avoiding burning or freezing the skin of the feet, and not going barefooted;
- Cutting or filing toenails straight across, never shorter than the underlying soft tissue of the toe; and never cutting the corner of the nails;
- Never cutting corns or calluses;
- Preventing callus formation under the ball of the foot by exercise, finishing each step on the toes and not on the ball of the foot, and wearing shoes that are not too short and do not have excessively high heals;
- Avoiding corn medications, which all contain corrosive acid;
- Not sitting with crossed legs, since this posture constricts the circulation and promotes nerve pressure;
- Abstaining from the use of tobacco, which can cause vasoconstriction in the extremities;
- Selecting a podiatrist familiar with diabetic foot problems.

Circulation may be improved by the use of contrast baths. With the contrast bath, a patient will require a bath thermometer and two pails. One pail is filled with water at 105°F (use a thermometer), and the other with water at 50°F. The feet and legs are immersed alternately for 4 minutes in the warm water and 1 minute in the cold water, and this process is repeated 5 times.

Patients with any type of foot problem should see a physician or podiatrist immediately. All diabetic patients should examine their feet daily for cuts, scratches, and changes in color (24, 60).

Dental Care

Hidden abscesses of the teeth are common in brittle diabetics, and the diabetic patient should be advised to have teeth checked at least twice per year. Diabetic patients should brush and floss their teeth at least twice per day, and the gums should be massaged with a brush or fingers. At the first sign of abnormal condition of the gums, the patient should consult a dentist. Diabetic patients should inform their dentists that they are diabetic.

PRODUCT SELECTION GUIDELINES

Pharmacists should be able to advise the diabetic patient on purchasing the proper equipment. Injection aids are available for patients with handicaps such as impaired vision. Patients who travel should take special precautions. An identification tag should be worn.

Urine testing is important in controlling diabetes. The pharmacist should be able to explain the use of urine testing kits to diabetic patients, as well as the need to keep accurate records.

The pharmacist should be aware of any effects other OTC products may have on diabetic patients. Because these patients are more subject to certain types of infections (e.g., monilial infections), the pharmacist should recommend that appropriate products be kept handy and that strict hygiene measures be followed.

Syringes and Needles

Pharmacists have a responsibility to assure that the diabetic patient is purchasing the proper type of insulin and the proper insulin syringe that corresponds to the strength of insulin used. Problems with insulin dosage occur when patients use the wrong syringe with their insulin. Insulin is administered in units and not in milliliters, and therefore syringes are calibrated in units (23). The calibration of the syringe should correspond to the concentration of the insulin used.

There are two types of syringes available: glass (reusable) and plastic (disposable). Both short and long syringes are available; the long type resembles the tuberculin syringe and holds 1 ml of insulin. The long syringe is preferred most often. Automatic injectors are available but take only the short-type syringe. Although some centers recommend the automatic injector for use with children, many believe that children should be taught to inject themselves.

The advantages of the disposable syringes and needles include assured sterility, ease of penetration due to 25% less angle in the cut, side bevels, thinner metal, and silicone coating. However, they are more expensive than the glass syringes. Patients should be cautioned not to reuse disposable syringes, since they may cause infection. Some of the disposable syringes (Becton-Dickinson's Plastipak and Sherwood's Monoject) contain less "dead space," which can be an important factor in diabetes control. "Dead space" volume is defined as the volume of insulin contained in the hub of the syringe, the hub of the needle, and the shaft of the needle (61). This volume becomes a potential source of error when two different fluids are drawn, measured, and mixed in the same syringe.

The amount of dead space volume of various U-100 insulin syringes from various manufacturers was significant in all but the Becton-Dickinson Plastipak insulin syringe and needle (61). In another study, dead space in some commercially available disposable insulin syringes caused substantial differences in the actual mixed dose delivered (62). Errors of up to 60% in the amount of intermediate-acting insulin were found. New disposable syringes with a capacity of 0.5 ml may be used with U-100 insulin only. Patients who inject 50 units or less of U-100 insulin may use these syringes, with the advantage that the syringe is graduated in 1-unit increments which allow for more accurate measurement of the dose. Other syringes, both glass and disposable, are graduated in 2-unit increments. The least convenient type uses 5-unit increments.

Mixing Insulins

It is important that the patient understand how to mix insulin properly within the syringe. The technique generally recommended is as follows:

- Observing aseptic technique, inject a volume of air equal to the dose into the first vial of intermediate- or long-acting insulin. Withdraw the needle without withdrawing the dose.
- In the usual manner, take the second vial of regular or short-acting insulin; inject air and withdraw the proper dose of insulin.
- Invert the first vial of intermediate- or long-acting insulin several times. Withdraw the dose of that insulin into the syringe containing the regular insulin; remove the syringe from the vial.
- Holding the syringe with needle upright, draw an air bubble into the syringe, invert the syringe, and roll the bubble through to mix.
- Expel the air bubble and administer the insulin to the patient in the usual manner.
- Insulins also may be premixed in a bottle in the proper short, intermediate, and long-acting proportions.

Sterilization Methods

Glass syringes are sterilized by keeping the syringe and needle in alcohol or by boiling them in distilled water before each use. Even if the syringe is kept in alcohol, it should be boiled at least once per week. A new product available for sterilizing glass syringes, Ster-Inge, is portable, safe, and reusable every 90 minutes and provides the patient with a sterile syringe and needle for each injection. One-half cup of fresh distilled water should be used each time a syringe and needle are sterilized. If tap water is used for sterilization, the syringe may become caked on the inside with hard water deposits. These deposits can be removed by soaking the syringe in vinegar. Heavily chlorinated water or chemical solutions for the sterilization of syringes should be avoided.

When boiling is inconvenient, the syringe and the needle may be sterilized by immersion in 70% ethyl alcohol or 91% isopropyl alcohol for at least 5 minutes. No other kind of alcohol should be used. The syringe then must be dried thoroughly by pumping the plunger in and out several times. If large quantities of isopropyl alcohol are introduced into a vial of insulin, the preparation turns cloudy. In addition, introduction of alcohol under the skin, even in minimal amounts, may lead to considerable irritation. Isopropyl alcohol is preferred because there is less corrosion, it is not denatured, it does not counteract insulin, and there is less water that can cause hydrolysis of insulin (63).

Injection Technique

Pharmacists should make sure that their diabetic patients know the correct manner in which to withdraw insulin into a syringe. The following procedure is recommended:

- Wash the hands with soap and water.
- Make sure that the proper equipment is used—correct insulin in the correct strength from the animal source normally used, e.g., beef–pork mixture.
- Roll the insulin bottle between the hands, inverting to assure mixing. To avoid generating air bubbles in the insulin, do not shake the bottle.
- Wipe off the top of the bottle with a piece of cotton moistened with alcohol.
- Remove the clean syringe from storage. Touch only the handle of the plunger, the barrel of the syringe, and the hub of the needle.
- If necessary, remove any excess water or alcohol from the syringe by pushing the plunger back and forth a few times. If any liquid is left in the syringe, it will cause an error in measuring the insulin. For disposable syringes this step is unnecessary.
- Pull the plunger backward to the prescribed number of units on the barrel.
- Put the needle through the rubber cap on the bottle and force the air into the bottle by pushing the plunger down.
- Turn the bottle upside down and pull the plunger back slowly to the prescribed number of units. If air bubbles appear in the barrel, hold the bottle up straight and force the air back into the bottle by pushing the plunger. It may be necessary to rap the barrel of the syringe briskly with the fingers to remove some of the air bubbles.
- When the correct number of units of insulin, without air bubbles, has been measured, pull the bottle away from the needle.
- Lay the syringe on a flat surface such as a table or shelf with the needle over the edge to avoid contamination.
- Clean the injection site with a cotton ball moistened with alcohol, or use an alcohol swab.
- Check the record to see where insulin was injected the previous day.
- Pinch a fold of skin with one hand. With the other hand, hold the syringe like a pencil and push the needle quickly through the fold of skin at an angle of 45–90°, depending on the degree of obesity. Before injecting the insulin, draw back slightly on the plunger to be sure a blood vessel has not been hit (aspirate). If blood appears in the syringe barrel, withdraw the needle and repeat the injection in another spot.
- Inject the insulin by pressing the plunger in as far as it will go.
- Withdraw the needle quickly and press on the injection site with the cotton ball moistened with alcohol.
- Record the injection site.
- Discard the syringe and needle, if disposable, by breaking the needle off to prevent reuse.

steps for proper insulin mixing

glass syringe sterilization

correct injection technique

Patients should be taught that insulin is to be injected deep into subcutaneous tissue. Properly injected insulin leaves only the needle puncture dot to show the injection site. The technique for injection may need to be altered with each individual depending on the amount of subcutaneous tissue present. For many, the use of a 90° angle with the skin stretched will accomplish the deep subcutaneous injection needed. For a thin person a 45° angle with the skin pinched up may be the best to avoid penetrating the muscle. The purpose of pinching is to lift the fat off the muscle. Fibrosis and atrophy can be prevented by injection in the same site at no less than 14-day intervals.

The needle sizes recommended for diabetic patients for subcutaneous injection are in the 25–27 gauge, ½–⅝-inch range.

rotation of injection sites

problems during travel

proper urine testing

Pharmacists should stress to their diabetic patients the importance of rotating injection sites. Injection sites include the arms, thighs, hips, and abdomen. Rotation entails moving in a straight line, giving each injection approximately 1 inch (2.5 cm) apart. For example, the patient starts on the right arm and gives four injections, moving in a straight line, and then finishes the line by moving to the left arm; the patient proceeds to the right leg, then the left leg, left abdomen, right abdomen, right hip, and left hip. Then the patient returns to the beginning, dropping down approximately 1 inch below the original line.

If insulin leaks through the puncture in the skin, the needle should be inserted at a right angle to the skin, and a longer needle should be used. It should be stressed to patients that good rotation will help to avoid local irritation, tissue reaction, and lipodystrophy.

Injection aids are available for visually impaired diabetic patients. For blind persons, special aids may be used, or disposable syringes may be filled and stored by a sighted person.

Cautions in Traveling

Diabetic patients traveling abroad should take their own syringes with them, since there is no uniformity of syringes in foreign countries—for example, it may be difficult to find a U-100 syringe. They also should bring additional insulin along when traveling to ensure that they have insulin derived from the same protein source. Traveling diabetics should control their diets carefully and also carry candy or sugar to combat possible hypoglycemic attacks.

All diabetics, but especially traveling diabetics, should carry a card or wear an identification bracelet that shows that they are not intoxicated in the event that a hypoglycemic or hyperglycemic attack occurs. Diabetics changing time zones should plan their diet, exercise, and insulin adjustments carefully. It is wise for diabetic patients to carry some insulin and syringes with them rather than placing all of it in their luggage. Not only is this good practice in case luggage is lost (64), but also keeping insulin on the person avoids exposing it to extreme temperature changes.

The sale of syringes in various states differs. In some states there are no regulations governing the sale of insulin syringes. In others the sale of syringes must be made by a pharmacist. Certain states require a prescription for the purchase of syringes and needles. The patient should be aware that procedures may be different.

Urine Testing and Record Keeping

The pharmacist's role in emphasizing to the diabetic patient the importance of urine glucose testing and keeping records of urine sugars, medication dose, diet, and exercise is significant in improving the patient's diabetic control (65). The pharmacist should assist the patient in selecting and using urine equipment and should make available samples of urine testing products in the pharmacy's diabetic center so that patients may practice technique and demonstrate their ability to test their urine properly for glucose and ketones. Pharmacists also should encourage diabetic patients to bring in their urine testing, weight, and medication use records to check how well the patient's diabetes is being controlled. Record cheaters are easy to spot: their records are neat, clean, written with the same pen or pencil, and obviously filled out from memory.

Proper urine testing for glucose and acetone, as well as adequate records of daily control, is essential for diabetic patients. Pharmacists should monitor patients' drug therapy for drugs that interfere with either the copper reduction or glucose oxidase methods of testing for glucose in the urine.

Factors in Selection

Proper urine testing is especially important to the diabetic patient who is using insulin and must adjust the daily insulin dose according to test results (66). Several studies have shown that most diabetic patients do not perform urinary glucose tests properly (67–69), and therefore care should be used in adjusting insulin dose based on patient tests of urine glucose. Periodic plasma glucose measurements are recommended to confirm impressions obtained from urine tests (67). A recent study observed that the unpredictability of Clinitest in the critically ill is due not only to error, but also to a changing rate of renal glucose reabsorption (70). It was concluded that blood glucose values are essential to rational dosing of insulin in the critically ill patient. A diabetic patient's control may be vastly improved by home blood glucose determinations using Dextrostix and Eyetone. Home blood glucose determination by pregnant and unstable diabetics can greatly improve control and thus prognosis.

In ambulatory diabetic patients who have a relatively normal renal threshold for glucose (160–200 mg/100 ml) the testing of urine glucose is a valuable means of determining diabetic control. The renal glucose threshold varies dramatically from individual to individual. As a patient ages, the renal glucose threshold increases. Conditions other than diabetes that may cause renal glucosuria are pheochromocytoma, acute pancreatitis, ingestion of very large amounts of glucose, acromegaly, Cushing's syndrome, and other reducing sugars, e.g., fructose, lactose, and galactose. Other factors that may make urine glucose determinations unreliable include residual urine (prostate hypertrophy) and neurogenic bladder, which is a complication of diabetes that prevents the collecting of urine specimens at the correct time.

A number of factors need to be considered in selecting a product to test the urine of a diabetic patient.

Diabetic Category

Insulinoplethoric diabetics who are being treated with diet, or diet and sulfonylureas, need test their urine only once per day approximately 2 hours after the main meal. Insulinoplethoric diabetics also are not as concerned with the quantitative amount of glucose in their urine and therefore can use glucose oxidase tests such as TesTape or Clinistix. Labile insulinopenic diabetics receiving exogenous insulin should test their urine three to four times per day, using quantitative or semiquantitative methods such as Clinitest or Diastix.

Patient Ability and Motivation

Patients unable to perform the more complex tests should be tested with simple tests, even though they are not as quantitatively accurate. Willingness of the patient to learn and perform the more complicated test (the more complex drop method of Clinitest versus the strip method of TesTape or Clinistix) also should be taken into account.

Physical Handicaps

Patients with poor vision, which is common in diabetics, cannot see the Clinitest drops and therefore would have difficulty performing that test. Special kits are available for visually impaired diabetics. Patients with trembling hands cannot perform the Clinitest test correctly without special precautionary measures (65).

Patients who are ketosis prone should be educated not only to test their urine for glucose but also to test for ketones whenever their urine glucose is high for any period of time. All diabetic patients should test their urine periodically for protein as a warning of nephropathy. Protein in the urine can be tested easily by using Uristix, Labstix, or Combistix.

Urine Glucose Tests

glucose tests, copper reduction and glucose oxidase

There are two methods of testing for glucose in the urine: copper reduction tests and glucose oxidase tests. In the copper reduction tests, cupric sulfate (blue) in the presence of glucose yields cuprous oxide (green to orange). Copper reduction tests are not specific for glucose and may detect the presence of other reducing substances in the urine. Glucose in the urine in the presence of glucose oxidase yields gluconic acid plus peroxide (H_2O_2), which, in the presence of *o*-tolidine, results in a color change and is the basis of glucose oxidase tests (TesTape, Clinistix, and Diastix).

Pharmacists should be careful to explain to patients that various urine glucose tests can be interpreted in different manners, resulting in different degrees of glucose in the urine. It is therefore important that the patient understand which testing method the physician referred to when recommending a "sliding scale" for adjusting insulin dose. For example, a +1 with the Clinitest represents 0.005% glucose, whereas with Diastix it represents 0.0025% glucose, and with TesTape it represents 0.001% glucose. Table 6 shows comparative readings for various urine glucose tests (71).

Tests for Urinary Ketones

urinary ketone tests

Since the ketones in the blood overflow into the urine, urinary ketone levels can be tested as a means of detecting whether or not ketoacidosis is occurring. All diabetic patients should be counseled on the proper use of tests for ketones in the urine. The basis for the test is that sodium nitroprusside alkali in the presence of acetone or acetoacetic acid turns lavender.

Tests for Other Chemicals

A number of products are available that test for pH, protein, glucose, acetone, and other factors such as bilirubin, blood, and urobilinogen in the urine. These multiple tests are not often used by patients and are more commonly used in physicians' offices, but patients may be instructed to use one of these reagents to test for various chemicals in the urine that may indicate the degree of diabetic control. In all of the tests used, fresh urine is required. Urine may be refrigerated for a short time—up to 4 hours before testing—but the actual test must be run with the specimen at room temperature.

Identification Tags

No diabetic should be without an identification bracelet, necklace, tag, or card. This identification may be lifesaving if hypoglycemia or ketoacidosis occurs. If a diabetic patient does become unconscious through an accident or hypoglycemic or hyperglycemic coma, medications regularly taken by the patient may be missed. A hypoglycemic (insulin) reaction may be confused with drunkenness; there have been reports of diabetic patients being jailed rather than given medical care (58).

A tag that can be seen easily on any patient should indicate that the patient is diabetic and receiving medication. A diabetic identification card should include the patient's name, address, and telephone number, the amount and type of medication used, the patient's physician, and how the physician can be contacted.

Diabetic patients should be encouraged to inform friends, teachers, and others of the fact that they are diabetic. This is quite a challenge in diabetic patient education, since some patients are embarrassed that they have the condition and need special coaxing to overcome this problem. Diabetic patients also should carry a candy roll or quick energy source such as instant glucose.

OTC Products Affecting Diabetes

Reading the label on all food and drug products is essential to maintaining diabetic control. Patients should develop this habit early to avoid adverse effects.

Sugar-Containing Products

A list of sugar-free preparations (72) is useful to keep on hand in the pharmacy so that the pharmacist can suggest a suitable sugar-free product for diabetic patients. For example, cough preparations that contain simple syrup could have a clinically significant effect on a brittle insulinopenic diabetic. However, the amount of extra sugar ingested to relieve a cough would not be significant in most well-controlled diabetics. To put this into perspective, the difference between a large and a small orange could include more sugar than would be found in 2 tsp of most cough syrups. Although sugar-con-

Table 6. Comparative Readings for Various Urine Glucose Tests

Test	0	Trace	+	++	+++	++++	
Glucose oxidase tests							
TesTape	0%	—	0.1%	0.25%	0.5%	2%	
Diastix	0%	0.1%	0.25%	0.5%	1.0%	2%	
Clinistix	0%	—	0.25%	present	0.5%	—	
Copper reduction tests							
Clinitest	0%	0.25%	0.5%	0.75%	1.0%	2%	
Clinitest 2-Drop[a]	0%	Trace	0.5%	1.0%	2%	3%	5%

[a]The two-drop method has seven possible readings; other tests have six possible readings.

taining medicinals may affect control in some diabetics, those who are properly educated to monitor their condition should have no clinically significant problems.

effects of OTC products on diabetes control

monitoring and education—the keys to control

Sympathomimetic Amines

Ephedrine, pseudoephedrine, phenylpropanolamine, phenylephrine, and epinephrine increase blood glucose and cause increased blood pressure by vasoconstriction. These substances should be used cautiously in diabetic patients. The major problem would occur in brittle insulinopenic diabetics; the effect should not be significant in most insulinotardic and insulinoplethoric diabetics.

Salicylates

Aspirin products do not bear a warning statement for diabetic patients. However, aspirin in diabetics may cause hypoglycemia, possibly by stimulation of general cellular metabolism. In strictly controlled diabetics the degree of hypoglycemia resulting from aspirin could stimulate a hypoglycemic reaction (22). However, the clinical significance of aspirin is questionable if a diabetic patient is monitoring diabetes control. Aspirin also may give misleading results in urine tests for sugar.

DIABETIC PATIENT MONITORING

The therapeutic goal of diabetes therapy (insulin, diet, exercise, or drug) is to control the patient's blood sugar. Diabetic patients vary considerably in their responses to therapy and in their adherence to prescribed instructions. The pharmacist can play a key role in assisting the patient to adhere to the prescribed regimen.

A two-page diabetic patient monitoring checklist has been developed by the APhA Academy of Pharmacy Practice Section on Clinical Practice to help the pharmacist perform the monitoring function (Figure 3). The checklist is a patient profile, especially designed to record data necessary to effectively monitor the drug therapy of the diabetic patient. Use of the checklist enables the pharmacist to bring together pertinent information about the patient, e.g., blood and urine glucose test results and blood pressure readings; prescribed therapy, e.g., special diet and therapy for concurrent diseases; and the patient's drug therapy, including a special section for recording insulin type(s), dosage, and dosage changes. The checklist may be used as the sole patient profile, or it may be used in conjunction with existing profiles.

The checklist, available in pads of 50 from APhA, also includes an instruction booklet, which contains specific instructions and suggestions for use, a completed sample checklist, and a suggested transmittal form for obtaining blood sugar data from the patient's physician. The transmittal form, which can be reproduced easily on a 5″ × 8″ card, is given to the patient, who asks the physician to complete the form during a regular office visit and then returns it to the pharmacist.

PATIENT EDUCATION

Patient education is the key to success in controlling the diabetic patient. Some diabetologists insist that the patient know as much about diabetes from the practical management aspect as the physician (73). Diabetics live with their disease 24 hours a day, so it is essential that they know not only all the details but also when they are in trouble and when to call for help. Every diabetic patient should know:

- What diabetes is and why treatment is necessary;
- How to select the proper foods at each meal;
- How to test urine for sugar and acetone;
- How to administer insulin;
- The symptoms of uncontrolled diabetes and ketosis;
- The symptoms of hypoglycemia;
- The emergency treatment of hypoglycemia;
- When to return for follow-up;
- How to contact the attending physician or assistant;
- How to modify treatment for exercise or illness;
- How to care for the feet;
- The dosage and time of administration of oral agents, if appropriate.

A team approach to patient education is essential. The physician explains the disease and the treatment objectives to the patient. The dietician emphasizes the importance of reaching and maintaining an ideal body weight. The nurse trains the patient in using syringes and needles, mixing insulins, and injecting insulin subcutaneously; the nurse also gives advice on proper personal hygiene, foot care, urine testing techniques, and record keeping.

Diabetes checklist

This Diabetic Patient Drug Monitoring Checklist has been developed by the Academy of Pharmacy Practice, Section on Clinical Practice, American Pharmaceutical Association. ©Copyright APhA, 1979.

PATIENT'S NAME	Responsible Person	Insulin (Type)	Type of Diabetic: Diet: (calories)
Telephone	Telephone	Needle Size / Syringe Size	Age Onset: Diet Oral Insulin Hist: __ to __ to __ to __
Address	Relationship to Patient	Physician / Telephone	Physician / Telephone

Date of Birth	Ideal Weight	Family Members Diabetic: Have Children Been Tested Yes ☐ No ☐

KNOWN ALLERGIES/SENSITIVITIES: Name of Causative Agent	Description of Reaction	Date of Occurrence	Treatment	Outcome
1.				
2.				

CONCURRENT DISEASES:	Date Diagnosed	Treatment
1.		
2.		
3.		

Urine Tests: (List Type(s))	Normal Value	DATE ▶
1.		
2.		
Blood Sugar Code: (1) FBS (2) 2HPP		Code / Result

Insulin Therapy	
	Date ▶
(Type)	Units ▶
(Frequency)	Time ▶
	Date ▶
(Type)	Units ▶
(Frequency)	Time ▶

Examinations/Diagnostic Items:	Date
Code 1)—General 2)—Podiatry 3)—BUN 4)—Serum Creatinine 5)—Electrolytes 6)—Pulse (A-Apical; R-Radial) 7)—Blood Pressure 8)—Weight 9)—Diet	Code / Result; Code / Result; Code / Result

General Comments: (Record here comments regarding patient health status; courses of action you take; physician instructions; etc.)

This Checklist was prepared with the cooperation and support of Hoechst-Roussel Pharmaceuticals, Inc.

HOECHST-ROUSSEL PHARMACEUTICALS INCORPORATED SOMERVILLE, NEW JERSEY 08876

Figure 3. Diabetic patient drug monitoring checklist.

Pharmacists have a special role in patient education with reference to mixing, storing, and injecting insulin. They also should be able to answer questions concerning urine testing, record keeping, foot care, diet, treatment of cuts and scratches, the use of antihistamines and decongestants, products safe to use in weight control, and the alcohol and sugar content of both prescription and OTC drugs.

The pharmacist's role in patient education is significant. The challenge of understanding diabetic products and teaching patients how to use them properly brings many rewards. Diabetic patient education methods have been summarized in some excellent articles available from major manufacturers (38, 47, 74–81). Additional diabetes information sources for pharmacists and their patients are listed in the appendix. With the aid of this information, pharmacists should be prepared to discuss with patients any of the following topics:

- The relationship among diet, exercise, and insulin;
- The strength, dose, times of administration, and types of insulin;
- The correct use of insulin syringes, needles, and dead space;
- Diabetic diet and the prescribed caloric level;
- Injection sites and proper site rotation;
- Syringe preparation technique (insulin withdrawal and mixture);
- Oral hypoglycemic agents—dosage and times of administration;
- Urine testing methods and techniques;
- Urine testing times (insulinopenic versus insulinoplethoric diabetics);
- Proper interpretation of testing results and record keeping;
- Signs and symptoms of hypoglycemic versus hyperglycemic reactions;
- Appropriate treatment for hypoglycemic and hyperglycemic reactions;
- Proper identification, including diabetic information card and Medic Alert emblems;
- Skin and foot care.

Patient Education Techniques

pharmacist role in diabetes control and education

Pharmacists interested in giving special care to diabetic patients can use a number of educative techniques.

Diabetic Care Center

To emphasize to diabetic patients that the pharmacist is truly concerned and interested in serving their needs, a clearly identified section may be established in the pharmacy. The center should include a complete line of diabetic products: sugar-free food and drink products, OTC products safe for use by diabetics (e.g., sugar-free cough syrup), and diabetic services available. An area also may be set up in which patients can practice testing their urine and using syringes properly.

Diabetic Detection Programs

Free diabetes testing kits may be distributed to pharmacy patients. The American Diabetes Association may be helpful in providing information on how to set up a detection program. It is a good idea to establish 1–2 days each month when patients can be tested for diabetes in the pharmacy. Ames company representatives can also provide assistance.

Diabetic "Hotline"

Pharmacists who are knowledgeable about diabetes may advise patients with questions concerning diabetes and diabetic products to call them for information.

Communication

Team effort and coordination are vital in patient education, and communication must be part of that effort. Pharmacists concerned about diabetes control should become involved in their local diabetes association or local Juvenile Diabetes Foundation. In addition, they should become familiar with community internal medicine specialists who treat diabetes and should develop a working relationship with them.

A system for communicating with diabetic patients may be developed. Using a diabetic patient drug monitoring checklist or merely a series of questions allows the pharmacist to show concern for the patient and gather information helpful in monitoring the condition.

SUMMARY

Diabetes control requires team effort on the part of the physician, dietician, nurse, pharmacist, and patient. The pharmacist may play an important role by monitoring patient therapy and being informed about all aspects of the disease. Patient consultation should reinforce the patient's understanding of diabetes and should emphasize the importance of controlling blood glucose levels, urine testing, and accurate record keeping.

Concerned pharmacists may join their local diabetes association and consult recent literature to keep their knowledge up to date. Products for diabetics including both OTC medications and food and beverage preparations may be displayed in the pharmacy's diabetic center along with diabetic patient information.

The pharmacist should be able to explain insulins and sulfonylureas to the patient and know how to mix, store, and inject insulins properly. The necessity of regular scheduled exercise and a balanced, nutritious diet in combination with prescribed medication should be made clear to the patient. Only by educating patients about diabetes is it possible to bring the disease under control.

REFERENCES

(1) R. A. Kerr, *New Environ. Pharm.*, *3*(2), 9 (1976).
(2) A. R. Van Son, *Wellcome Trends Hosp. Pharm.*, *5*(3), 1 (1977).
(3) "1976 Fact Sheet," Juvenile Diabetes Foundation, New York, N.Y., 1976.
(4) "1977 Fact Sheet," Juvenile Diabetes Foundation, New York, N.Y., 1977.
(5) *American Druggist*, *176*(3), 54 (1977).
(6) M. Ellenberg, *Pharm. Times*, *40*(6), 56 (1974).
(7) M. A. Kimble, *J. Am. Pharm. Assoc.*, *NS14*, 80 (1974).
(8) P. G. Sesin, *Apothecary*, *89*(5), 22 (1977).
(9) E. Cerasi and R. Luft, "Pathophysiology of Diabetes Mellitus: Diagnosis and Treatment," Vol. 3, American Diabetes Association, New York, N.Y., 1971, p. 37.
(10) "Diabetes Mellitus," 7th ed., S. O. Waife, Ed., Lilly Research Laboratories, Indianapolis, Ind., 1976, p. 1.
(11) J. E. Gerich, *Am. Fam. Physician*, *16*, 85 (1977).
(12) K. E. Sussman, in "The Older Diabetic Patient," Upjohn, Kalamazoo, Mich., 1973, p. 20.
(13) W. B. Spaulding, W. O. Spitzer, and P. W. Truscott, *Can. Med. Assoc. J.*, *89*, 329 (1963).
(14) M. Fabrykant and B. I. Ashe, *J. Am. Geriatr. Soc.*, *11*, 68 (1963).
(15) G. J. Hamwi, S. S. Fajans, G. F. Cahill, Jr., W. V. Greenberg, R. C. Hardin, E. A. Haunz, D. M. Kipnis, R. H. Unger, and K. M. West, *Diabetes*, *16*, 540 (1967).
(16) N. Baumslag, R. E. Yodaiken, and J. C. Varady, *Diabetes*, *19*, 664 (1970).
(17) P. H. Forsham, in "Diabetes Rounds," Medcom, New York, N.Y., 1973, p. 8.
(18) J. Palmer, "Diabetes Update," Vol. 1, Diabetes Education Center, Deaconess Hospital, Spokane, Wash., 1977, p. 1.
(19) J. H. Karam, in "Current Medical Diagnosis and Treatment," M. A. Krupp and M. J. Chatton, Eds., Lange Medical, Los Altos, Calif., 1978, p. 738.
(20) K. D. Hepp, *Diabetologia*, *13*, 177 (1977).
(21) T. G. Skillman and M. Tzagournis, "Diabetes Mellitus," Upjohn, 1977, pp. 3, 14.
(22) T. A. Gossell and R. J. Wuest, "Diabetes Mellitus, Part 1," Chain Store Age Continuing Education Program, New York, N.Y., 1977, p. 93.
(23) "A Pharmacist's Guide to Diabetes Mellitus," School of Pharmacy, University of California, San Francisco, Calif., 1977, p. 52.
(24) O. C. Olson, "Instruction Book for Diabetic Patients," 9th ed., Diabetes Education Center, Deaconess Hospital, Spokane, Wash., 1977, pp. ii–iii.
(25) M. A. Kimble, in "Applied Therapeutics for Clinical Pharmacists," L. Y. Young and M. A. Kimble, Eds., Applied Therapeutics Inc., San Francisco, Calif., 1975, pp. 225–260.
(26) "Monograph: 2, Diabetes," J. C. Kelly, Ed., Pfizer Laboratories, New York, N.Y., 1974, p. 24.
(27) R. Engerman, J. Bloodsworth, and S. Nelson, *Diabetes*, *26*, 760 (1977).
(28) D. Job, E. Eschwege, C. Guyot-Argenton, J. P. Aubry, and E. Tchobroutsky, *Diabetes*, *25*, 463 (1976).
(29) P. H. Forsham, in "Diabetes Mellitus," M. Ellenberg and A. Rifkin, Eds., McGraw-Hill, New York, N.Y., 1971, p. 697.
(30) G. D. Molnar, *Mayo Clinic Proc.*, *47*, 709 (1972).
(31) B. I. Chazon, *Diabetologia*, *6*, 565 (1970).
(32) D. Fine and H. Shedrovilsky, *Ann. Intern. Med.*, *72*, 83 (1970).
(33) P. N. Weismann, L. Shenkman, and R. I. Gregerman, *N. Engl. J. Med.*, *284*, 65 (1971).
(34) D. L. Smith, "Medication Guide for Patient Counseling," Lea and Febiger, Philadelphia, Pa., 1977, p. 396.
(35) R. K. Maudlin and L. Y. Young, "Drug Consultation Guide," Drug Intelligence Publications, Inc., Hamilton, Ill., 1976.
(36) D. G. Eastman, R. A. Guthrie, J. W. Hare, A. Krosnick, J. J. Kristan, C. R. Shuman, and K. E. Sussman, *Patient Care*, *19*(9), 12 (1975).
(37) D. W. Guthrie, *Am. J. Nursing*, *77*(2), 48, 54 (1977).
(38) P. Felig, *Postgrad. Med.*, *59*, 109 (1976).
(39) T. Deckert, O. O. Anderson, and J. E. Poulsen, *Diabetologia*, *10*, 703 (1974).
(40) P. Daggett, B. E. Mustaffa, and J. Nabarro, *Practitioner*, *218*, 563 (1977).
(41) S. M. O. Guerra and A. E. Kitabchi, *J. Clin. Endocrinol. Metab.*, *42*, 868 (1976).
(42) V. Koivisto and P. Felig, *N. Engl. J. Med.*, *298*, 79 (1978).
(43) *Medical World News*, *18*(14), 15 (1977).
(44) B. M. Watson and J. S. Calder, *Diabetes*, *20*, 628 (1971).
(45) D. K. Yue and J. R. Turtle, *Diabetes*, *26*, 341 (1977).
(46) K. E. Sussman, J. R. Crout, and A. Marble, *Diabetes*, *12*, 38 (1963).
(47) A. Bloom, *Clin. Endocrinol. Metab.*, *6*, 499 (1977).
(48) J. K. Davidson, *Postgrad. Med.*, *59*, 114 (1976).
(49) L. Howard, *Am. Fam. Physician*, *12*, 152 (1975).
(50) *Diabetes Outlook*, *11*(6), 2 (1976).
(51) J. M. Court, *Med. J. Aust.*, *1*, 841 (1976).
(52) "Diabetes and Cardiovascular Disease," Publication No. (NIH)77-1212, Department of Health, Education, and Welfare, 1977, p. 8.
(53) D. J. A. Jenkins, D. V. Goff, A. R. Leeds, K. G. M. M. Alberti, T. M. S. Wolever, M. A. Gassull, and T. D. R. Hockaday, *Lancet*, *2*, 172 (1976).
(54) H. R. Murdock, *Geriatrics*, *27*(7), 93 (1972).
(55) "Evaluations of Drug Interactions," 2nd ed., APhA, Washington, D.C., 1976, p. 240.
(56) G. E. Dukes, J. G. Kuhn, and R. P. Evens, *Am. Fam. Physician*, *16*(3), 97 (1977).
(57) S. Dippe, in "Important Data on Diabetes," Northern California Diabetes Association and Geigy Pharmaceuticals, San Francisco, Calif., 1970, p. 23.
(58) P. P. Lamy and M. E. Kittler, *J. Am. Pharm. Assoc.*, *NS10*, 610 (1970).
(59) M. C. Robson and L. E. Edstrom, *Surg. Clin. North Am.*, *57*, 1089 (1977).
(60) M. Kahan and Y. J. Chafiian, *Hosp. Med.*, *8*(2), 15 (1972).
(61) M. Kochwar and L. K. Fry, *Drug Intell. Clin. Pharm.*, *8*, 33 (1974).
(62) M. Rosoff, *Acad. Gen. Pract.*, *10*(7), 3 (1975).
(63) J. C. Scheller and M. D. Ormsby, *Hosp. Pharm.*, *6*(7), 7 (1971).
(64) O. Aagenes and H. K. Akerblom, *Acta Paediatr. Belg.*, *30*, 126 (1977).
(65) C. J. Nelson, *Drug Intell. Clin. Pharm.*, *8*, 422 (1974).
(66) S. R. Abel and R. W. Bennett, *Apothecary*, *89*(3), 12 (1977).
(67) J. M. Feldman and F. L. Leborwitz, *Diabetes*, *22*, 115 (1977).
(68) G. M. Shenfield and J. M. Steel, *Practitioner*, *218*, 147 (1977).
(69) J. I. Malone, A. L. Rosenbloom, A. Grgic, and F. T. Weber, *Am. J. Dis. Child.*, *130*, 1324 (1976).
(70) D. Smith and D. Angaran, "Urine Glucose Estimation of Blood Glucose in the Critically Ill," paper presented at the American Society of Hospital Pharmacists Midyear Meeting, Atlanta, Ga., Dec. 1977.
(71) P. A. Lawrence, *Am. Diabetes Assoc. Forecast*, *25*(2), 1, 12 (1972).
(72) *American Druggist*, *173*, 82 (May 1976).
(73) M. Ellenberg, *N.Y. State J. Med.*, *77*, 62 (1977).
(74) C. A. Sczupak and W. F. Conrad, *Am. J. Hosp. Pharm.*, *34*, 1238 (1977).
(75) K. W. Schilling, *Am. J. Hosp. Pharm.*, *34*, 1242 (1977).
(76) R. D. Scalley, K. Fiegen, and E. Kearney, *Am. J. Hosp. Pharm.*, *34*, 1245 (1977).
(77) E. W. Buruchien, *Drug Topics*, *120*(21), 31 (1976).
(78) L. A. Gieselman, "The Development and Evaluation of an Individualized Diabetic Education Program," 2nd Annual University of Nebraska Hospital Pharmacy Resident Seminar, 1975, p. 1.
(79) D. W. Guthrie, *Am. J. Nurs.*, *77*(2), 48 (1977).
(80) A. H. Dube, *N.Y. State J. Med.*, *69*, 1169 (1969).
(81) B. J. Dye, C. A. Blainey, P. L. Byre, and J. P. Palmer, *J. Fam. Pract.*, *5*, 341 (1977).

APPENDIX: DIABETES INFORMATION SOURCES

Information for Pharmacists

- Becton, Dickinson and Company
Rutherford, NJ 07070
"Notes on Syringes and Needles."

- California Syllabus
1494 MacArthur
Oakland, CA 94602
"A Pharmacist's Guide to Diabetes Mellitus," University of California at San Francisco School of Pharmacy, 1977.

- Eli Lilly and Company
Lilly Research Laboratories
Indianapolis, IN 46206
"Diabetes Mellitus," 7th ed., 3rd rev., S. O. Waife, Ed., 1976.

- Pfizer Laboratories
Division of Pfizer Incorporated
235 E. 42nd Street
New York, NY 10017
"Diabetes Rounds," P. H. Forsham, 1973.
"Diabetes Outlook—Newest Developments in Diagnosis and Management," published 10 times yearly for Pfizer Laboratories by Science and Medicine Publishing Company, 515 Madison Ave., New York, NY 10022.

- Smith Kline & French Laboratories
Philadelphia, PA 19101
"Low-Dose Insulin Therapy in Diabetic Ketoacidosis," in *Therapeutics Drug Monographs for the Pharmacist*, Biomedical Information Corporation, 919 Third Avenue, New York, NY 10022, 1977.

- The Upjohn Company
Kalamazoo, MI 49001
"The Child With Diabetes Mellitus," R. L. Jackson and R. A. Guthrie, Sept. 1975.
"On Spontaneous Hypoglycemia," J. W. Conn and S. Pek, 1970.
"Diabetes Mellitus," T. G. Skillman and M. Tzagournis, 1977.
"The Older Diabetic Patient," M. Ellenberg et al., 1973.
"Diagnosis and Management of Diabetic Nephropathy," H. H. Goldstein, 1974.
"Diagnosis and Management of Neuropathies," M. Ellenberg, 1973.
"Diagnosis and Management of Peripheral Vascular Disease," J. F. Fairbairn II, 1973.
"A Monograph on Diabetes Mellitus," A. G. Macloud, 1969.

Information for Patients

- American Diabetes Association, Inc.
One West 48th Street (600 Fifth Avenue)
New York, NY 10020
"What You Need to Know About Diabetes," 1976, plus numerous publications on subjects relevant to diabetes.

- Ames Company
Division of Miles Laboratories, Inc.
Elkhart, IN 46514
"Care of the Child With Diabetes: A Guidebook for Parents and Teachers of Diabetics," 1977.
"Home Urine Testing for the Diabetic," P. Sylbert, 1976.
"Straight Talk About Diabetes: A Guidebook for the Teenager and Young Adult Diabetic," 1977.
"Toward Good Control: Guidebook for Diabetics," 1977.
"Shopping List for Diabetic Patients," 1978.

- Baptist Hospitals Foundation of Birmingham, Inc.
3201 Fourth Avenue S.
Birmingham, AL 35222
"Body Map for Diabetics—To Record the Systematic Rotation of Insulin Injection Sites," 1974.

- Becton, Dickinson and Company
Rutherford, NJ 07070
"The Importance of Proper Dosage Accuracy for the Diabetic," 1977.
"An Illustrated Guide to Proper Diet Control for the Diabetic," 1977.
- California Canners & Growers Cookbook Department
3100 Ferry Building
San Francisco, CA 94106
"Diet Delight Cookbook for Diabetic Children," 3rd ed., J. Jones.

- Geigy Pharmaceuticals
Division of Ciba-Geigy Corporation
Ardsley, NY 10502
"Living With Diabetes," 1972.
"Urine Test Record," 1972.
"Daily Foot Care Checklist," 1972.

- The Juvenile Diabetes Foundation
23 E. 26th Street
New York, NY 10010
"What You Should Know About Juvenile Diabetes," plus numerous other brochures on subjects relevant to insulinopenic diabetes.

- Eli Lilly and Company
Lilly Research Laboratories
Indianapolis, IN 46206
"What Is Diabetes?" 1976.
"A Guide for the Diabetic," 1975.
"Basic Facts About Diabetes," 1972.
"Recent Advances in the Purification of Iletin," 1975.
"The Progress of Insulin," 1977.
"Iletin (Insulin, Lilly): The First Landmark in Control of Diabetes," 1975.

"Directions for Changing from U-40 or U-80 to U-100 Iletin," 1976.

"Tes-Tape For Fast, Accurate Determination of Glucose in Urine," 1975.

"How to Use Tes-Tape," 1971.

- Monoject, Division of Sherwood Medical
  Dept. T.I., 1831 Olive Street
  St. Louis, MO 63103
  "How to Take Insulin."

- Pfizer Laboratories
  Division of Pfizer Inc.
  235 E. 42nd Street
  New York, NY 10017

"Cooking With Style: Diabetic Recipes With a Difference," 1972.

"Take Good Care of Yourself," 1972.

"The Foods You Eat," 1971.

- E. R. Squibb and Sons, Inc.
  Princeton, NJ 08540

"Don't Be Afraid of Diabetes: A Handbook for Diabetics," 1977.

"An Instructional Aid on Juvenile Diabetes Mellitus," L. B. Travis, 1969.

- The Upjohn Company
  Kalamazoo, MI 49001
  "You and Diabetes," Jan. 1977.
  "Urine Test Record," July 1971.

"Illustrated Instructions for the Diabetes Patient," 1972.

Miscellaneous

The pharmacist should contact the local diabetes association for brochures to provide to diabetics.

- "Juvenile Diabetes—Adjustment and Emotional Problems," New Jersey State Department of Health, Diabetic Control Program, P.O. Box 1540, Trenton, NJ 08625. Single copies free.

- "How to Live With Diabetes," H. Dolger, Upjohn (available only through bookstores).

New information is constantly being published to help the diabetic patient maintain control. Pharmacists should ask the representatives of major pharmaceutical companies about what information is available for them and their diabetic patients.

Product[a] (Manufacturer)	Species[b] Source	Onset[c], hours	Peak[c], hours	Duration[c], hours	pH	Buffer	Preservative	Description	Stability at Room Temperature, months	Zinc Content, mg/100 U	Protein, mg/100 U
Rapid-Acting											
Beef Regular Iletin (Lilly)	B	1	3–5	5–8	7.4	none	phenol	round	10–18	0.01–0.04	none
Pork Regular Iletin (Lilly)	P	1	3–5	5–8	7.4	none	phenol	round	10–18	0.01–0.04	none
Regular Iletin (Lilly)	B,P	1	3–5	5–8	7.4	none	phenol	round	10–18	0.01–0.04	none
Regular Insulin (Squibb)	B,P	1	3–5	5–8	7.4	none	phenol	round	10–18	0.01–0.04	none
Semilente Iletin (Lilly)	B,P	1	4–6	12–14	7.0	acetate	methylparaben	U-40 + U-80 semilente in hexagon	24	0.2–0.25	none
Semilente Insulin (Squibb)	B	1	4–6	12–14	7.0	acetate	methylparaben	U-100 round	24	0.2–0.25	none
Sterile Diluting Fluid for Neutral Regular Insulin Injection (Lilly)	—	—	—	—	neutral	10% hydrochloric acid and/or 10% sodium hydroxide	phenol	—	10–18	—	—
Intermediate											
Beef Lente Iletin[e] (Lilly)	B	2–4	8–12	24–28	7.0	acetate	methylparaben	round	24–30	0.016–0.4	none
Beef NPH Iletin[c] (Lilly)	B	2–4	8–12	24–28	7.2	phosphate	phenol, *m*-cresol	round	36	0.25–0.35	protamine, 0.5
Globin Zinc[g] (Squibb)	B,P	1–3	6–10	16–22	3.6	none	phenol	round	18–20	0.2–0.25	globin
Lente Iletin[e] (Lilly)	B,P	2–4	8–12	24–28	7.0	acetate	methylparaben	U-40 + U-80 lente in hexagon	24–30	0.016–0.4	none
Lente Insulin[e] (Squibb)	B	2–4	8–12	24–28	7.0	acetate	methylparaben	round	24–30	0.016–0.4	none
NPH Iletin[f] (Lilly)	B,P	2–4	8–12	24–28	7.2	phosphate	phenol + *m*-cresol	round	36	0.25–0.35	protamine, 0.5
NPH (Isophane) Insulin (Squibb)	B,P	2–4	8–12	24–28	7.2	phosphate	phenol + *m*-cresol	round	36	0.25–0.35	protamine[g], 0.5
Pork Lente Iletin[e] (Lilly)	P	2–4	8–12	24–48	7.0	acetate	methylparaben	round	24–30	0.016–0.4	none
Pork NPL Iletin (Lilly)	P	2–4	8–12	24–28	7.2	phosphate	phenol + *m*-cresol	round	36	0.25–0.35	protamine, 0.5
Sterile Diluting Fluid for Dilution of NPH Iletin (Lilly)	—	—	—	—	neutral	10% hydrochloric acid and/or 10% sodium hydroxide	phenol + *m*-cresol	—	36	—	—
Long-Acting											
Beef Protamine Zinc Insulin (Lilly)	B	2–4	14–20	24–36	7.2	phosphate	phenol	round	36	0.2–0.25	protamine[h], 1.25

Insulin Preparations

Product[a] (Manufacturer)	Species[b] Source	Onset[c], hours	Peak[c], hours	Duration[c], hours	pH	Buffer	Preservative	Description	Stability at Room Temperature, months	Zinc Content, mg/100 U	Protein, mg/100 U
Pork Protamine Zinc Insulin (Lilly)	P	2–4	14–20	24–36	7.2	phosphate	phenol	round	36	0.2–0.25	protamine, 1.25
Protamine Zinc and Iletin (Lilly)	B,P	2–4	14–20	24–36	7.2	phosphate	phenol	round	36	0.2–0.25	protamine, 1.25
Protamine Zinc Insulin (Squibb)	B,P	2–4	14–20	24–36	7.2	phosphate	phenol	round	36	0.2–0.25	protamine, 1.25
Ultralente Iletin (Lilly)	B,P	3–6	16–18	30–36	7.0	acetate	methylparaben	U-40 + U-80 hexagon	24–30	0.2–0.25	none
Ultralente Insulin (Squibb)	B	3–6	16–18	30–36	7.0	acetate	methylparaben	round	24–30	0.2–0.25	none

Miscellaneous	
Glucagon for Injection (Lilly)	Used parenterally (subcutaneously, intramuscularly, or intravenously) for treatment of hypoglycemia. Stable in solution up to 3 months. Stimulates the conversion of liver glycogen to glucose. Intravenous glucose is drug of choice in hypoglycemia if available. To use, lyophilized glucagon is dissolved using accompanying solution and then injected.
Glutose (Reactose)	(C.R. Canfield and Co., 2744-46 Lyndale Ave. South, Minneapolis, MN 55408) Oral glucose solution used to treat insulin reaction (hypoglycemia) before unconsciousness occurs.
Instant Glucose	Available from Diabetes Association of Cleveland, 2022 Lee Road, Cleveland, OH 44118.
Insulin Allergy Desensitization Kits (Lilly)	Contain "single peak" pork insulin, "single peak" beef insulin, or "single-component" pork insulin with 0.1% human serum albumin, plus directions for use.
Monocomponent Insulin (various)	Highly purified (99% pure insulin) by diethylaminoethylcellulose chromatography. Not commercially available in United States but can be obtained from manufacturers on special request.

[a] Available in U-40 (coded red), U-80 (coded green), and U-100 (coded orange). Lilly also manufactures a regular (concentrated) Iletin (prescription only) containing 500 units of pork insulin/ml; used in patients with marked insulin resistance. Pure pork and pure beef insulin available only in U-100 strength.
[b] Insulins with a combination of beef and pork contain 70% beef and 30% pork; B = beef and P = pork.
[c] Biological response varies greatly in different individuals, so times are approximate.
[d] Mix regular with NPH or lente in any proportion; stable for 2–3 months. With protamine zinc insulin, use at least twice as much regular. Intermix lentes in any proportion. Stable for long periods. Lente plus regular stable for 2–3 months.
[e] Lente can be mixed with regular or semilente or ultralente in any proportion and is stable for 2–3 months.
[f] NPH plus regular. Mix in any proportion; stable for 2–3 months.
[g] No need to mix regular and globin—yields more globin.
[h] One part protamine zinc insulin to two parts regular equals NPH. Ultralente 70% plus semilente 30% yields lente. Lentes mix in any proportion—stable for 2–3 months.

Insulin Syringes and Related Products

Product (Manufacturer or Supplier)	Sizes Available or Description	Comments
Syringes		
Busher Auto Injector (Becton-Dickinson)	Connects to short-type reusable insulin syringe or with adaptor to long type. Provides quick automatic insertion of the needle at proper depth and angle.	Used in past to help patients overcome needle fear. Patients should be trained to overcome emotional factors and therefore not recommended.
Eisele Glass Tip Insulin Syringe (Eisele)	For U-100 insulin, 35 unit and 50 unit.	Can use with disposable or reusable needles. Useful for patients who take less than 35 or 50 units of U-100 insulin. Dead space a problem.

Product (Manufacturer or Supplier)	Sizes Available or Description	Comments
Syringes		
Eisele Hard Pak-Syrg Insulin Syringes (Eisele)	1 cc short type U-40, U-80, U-100, U-40/80. In 7 pack, 10 pack, 30 pack, and 100 pack with 26 G ½″ or 25 G ⅝″ needles attached.	Dead space is a problem.
Injector-Aid (Support Systems)	Model BD-1 for Becton-Dickinson disposable syringes, and MJ-1 for Monoject disposable syringes.	Injection helper. Useful for handicapped or sightless patients.
Insulin Syringe, Single Use Plastipak Lo-Dose (Becton-Dickinson)	0.5 cc with 26 G ½″ needle. 30/package.	Can't change needle size. Used for patients taking less than 50 units of U-100 insulin. Larger print of calibrations allows more accurate dosing. Should be available soon in 27 g.
Jelco U-100 Reduced Air Insulin Syringe (Jelco)	1-cc U-100 with 26 G½″ nonremovable needle.	Reduced dead space and air bubbling. Bold printed scale. Good product but not carried by all pharmacies.
Med-E-Jet Inoculator (Med-E-Jet)	Jet injector powered by carbon dioxide cartridges.	Provides a subcutaneous injection of insulin with less trauma. Can be used by sightless patients. Expensive, complicated to use, dosage adjustments in 5-unit increments. Not recommended.
Monoject Insulin Syringe (Sherwood)	1 cc with self-contained 27 G ½″ needle. U-40, U-80, and U-100. 30 pack or 120's. 27 G ⅝″ available in U-100. 0.5 cc for patients using 50 units or less of U-100 insulin	Bold numbers, preferred needle gauge, reduced dead space, sterile. 27 G less painful. Difficult to open, more storage space required. Recommended.
Plastipak Self Contained Insulin Syringe (Becton-Dickinson)	1 cc with 26 G ½″ in U-40, U-80, and U-100 1 cc with 25 G ⅝″ in U-40, U-80, and U-100 1 cc with 27 G ½″ and microfine needle in U-100	No dead space. Excellent for travel. More expensive than reusable but sterile and convenient. Needs to be manufactured in 27 G ⅝″. No dead space. Less pain with 27 G. Recommended.
Single Use, Long Type (Becton-Dickinson)	2 cc U-100 30 pack detachable needles	2 cc useful for patients taking large doses. Detachable needles produce clinically significant dead space if insulin mixing is needed.
Stylex Insulin Syringe (Pharmaseal)	1 cc U-40, U-80, and U-100 syringes with 25 G ⅝″ or 26 G ½″ needles	Needles pop off. Significant dead space. Lettering rubs off easily. Not carried by all pharmacies. Not recommended.
Syrijet (Mizzy Inc.)	High-quality jet injector. Up to 35 units/injection.	Easy to use but requires education program and physician monitoring. Can be used up to 4 times/day to improve control. Should be used with home blood glucose monitoring. Dosage adjustments in 2-unit increments. Comparatively inexpensive. Recommended.

Product (Manufacturer or Supplier)	Sizes Available or Description	Comments
Syringes		
Yale Glass Insulin Reusable Short Type Luer Tip Syringe (Becton-Dickinson)	1 cc U-40 1 cc U-80 1 cc U-40-80 dual scale 2 cc U-40	Can use with reusable or disposable needles. Preferred over Luer-Lok. Less expensive. Dual scale yields dose errors Switch to U-100.
Yale Insulin Reusable Hypodermic Short Type Luer-Lok Tip Syringe (Becton-Dickinson)	1 cc U-40 1 cc U-80 1 cc U-40-80 dual scale	Can use with 26 G ½″, 25 G ⅝″, or 27 G ½″ reusable or disposable needles. More expensive than Luer tip. Dual scale confusing and can cause dosing errors. Try to convince diabetics to switch to U-100.
Yale Insulin Reusable Long Type Luer Tip Syringe (Becton-Dickinson)	1 cc U-40 1 cc U-80 green plunger or blue plunger 1 cc U-40/80 dual scale, blue plunger or reg. plunger	More expensive than short type. Can use with 26 G ½″, 25 G ⅝″, or 27 G ½″ reusable or disposable needle. Dual scale confusing.
Yale 0.35 cc Special Insulin Syringe (Becton-Dickinson)	0.35 cc, calibrated up to 35 units	Available for patients using small doses of U-100 insulin
Aids for Visually Impaired		
Cornwall, Becton-Dickinson Adjustable Positive Stop (American Foundation for the Blind)	Metal, complicated device that covers most of syringe. Dose set with plunger springs.	Large and bulky. Use only with U-80 and U-100 glass syringe. Accurate but expensive.
Dos-Aid (American Foundation for the Blind)	Plastic tray that adjusts to hold syringe and insulin bottle. Plunger is pulled back to a plunger stop.	Uses all types of disposable syringes. Simple to teach; accurate. Can't mix insulins.
Eisele Truset Syringe (Eisele)	Thin, metal spring and stop catch that fits over glass syringe.	Inaccurate, easily broken, but inexpensive.
Hill Accurate Dosage Insulin Syringe (American Foundation for the Blind)	U-80 glass syringe with a metal plunger rod containing adjustable lock rings that are set by a sighted person.	Inaccurate by up to 4 units but simple to teach. Not used with U-40 or U-100.
IDM (Andros Inc.)	Plastic scale that attaches to plunger. Can be cut to proper length so when end reaches barrel of syringe correct dose is measured.	Inexpensive and simple to use. Can use only with U-100. Not as accurate as Insulgage.
Insulgage (Meditec Inc.)	Small plastic gauge that attaches to B-D long or Jelco disposable syringes. Gauge and plunger are pulled back until gauge drops into place between plunger end and barrel.	Accurate, simple to teach, can be used with mixed insulins. Available for U-100 disposable syringes and inexpensive. Highly recommended.

Product (Manufacturer or Supplier)	Sizes Available or Description	Comments
Aids for Visually Impaired		
Insulin Syringe MES 260 (American Foundation for the Blind)	Precision device consisting of a glass barrel inside a 3½″ metal casing. Units drawn up determined by an audible click.	Used only with U-40 and U-80 syringes. Expensive but accurate.
Syringe Magnifier (Cemco)	Unbreakable magnifier made of stainless steel.	Easy to snap on and off. Magnifies bubbles and calibrations on syringe. Not for totally blind.
Syringe Magnifier (Char-Mag Co.)	Magnifier made of optical quality plastic. Plastic can become scratched.	Easy to snap on and off. Magnifies bubbles and calibrations on syringe. Not for totally blind.
Miscellaneous		
Alcohol Swabs and Alcohol Wipes Spongettes (Becton-Dickinson, Sherwood Medical)	70% isopropyl alcohol for single use.	The unit dose of alcohol swabs. More expensive but great for travel.
Insulin-Aid (Seabee Enterprises)	Device made of Plexiglas that magnetically attaches to a metal surface and holds any insulin bottle inverted to make it easier to withdraw insulin into syringe.	Useful if one needs an extra hand to withdraw insulin into syringe.
91% Isopropyl Alcohol (Lilly and various manufacturers)	Used for sterilizing needles and syringes and for cleansing skin before injections. Preferred to rubbing alcohol due to less water and not denatured; therefore safer with insulin.	Lilly product is in plastic, nonbreakable bottles. Generic less expensive.
Needle Sharpener (Aloxite Safety Blade Hone) (Carborundum Co. and others)	Used to sharpen reusable needles.	Patients should be encouraged to use disposable needles.
Ster-Inge (Ster-Inge)	Device to sterilize glass syringes and disposable or reusable needles.	Simple to operate. Recommended for patients who do not use disposable syringes.
Syringe and Needle Destroyers (B-D's Destruclip) (Becton-Dickinson, Jelco)	Device to destroy disposable needles after use. Cuts off needle and cuts syringe into parts.	Useful in hospitals and nursing homes where large numbers of syringes are used.

Urine and Blood Glucose Tests

Product (Manufacturer)	Product Formulation and Sizes	Active Ingredients	Indication of Product Deterioration	Time Required to Evaluate	Drug Interference	Comments[a]
Clinistix (Ames)	Strip: 50's	glucose oxidase peroxidase *o*-tolidine	tan or dark test area	10 seconds	no false(+) some false(−) (levodopa, ascorbic acid, aspirin)	inexpensive, convenient use for insulinoplethoric; not quantitative

Urine and Blood Glucose Tests

Product (Manufacturer)	Product Formulation and Sizes	Active Ingredients	Indication of Product Deterioration	Time Required to Evaluate	Drug Interference	Comments
Clinitest (Ames) 5-drop method 2-drop method	Tablets: 36's, 100's, 250's, 1000's Foilwrap: 24's and 500's Tablets: 36's	copper reduction	deep blue tablet	15 seconds, then shake gently	false(+) in presence of reducing agents no false(−)	2-drop most reliable at high glucose levels; use for "sliding scale"; use for insulinopenic; inexpensive but inconvenient (requires water, dropper, test tube); not specific for glucose; only difference in 2-drop and 5-drop method is the amount of urine used
Dextrostix (Ames)	Strip: 25's 100's	glucose oxidase peroxidase *o*-tolidine	test area does not resemble "O" on color chart	60 seconds (test for blood glucose)	no false(+) some false(−)	useful in screening; accurate if read by analyzer; can use to correlate blood and urine glucose levels; home use improves control
Diastix (Ames)	Strip: 50's 100's	glucose oxidase peroxidase potassium iodide chromogen	variation from light blue or "neg" on color chart	30 seconds, dip, remove excess urine, and read	no false(+) some complete false(−) (see Clinistix)	easy to read; relatively expensive; more accurate than TesTape but less than Clinitest; underreading possible at high glucose levels; for use by both insulinopenic and insulinoplethoric
Mega-Diastix (with control tablets) (Ames)	Strip: 50's 100's	glucose oxidase peroxidase potassium iodide chromogen	variation from light blue or "neg" on color chart	30 seconds, dip, remove excess urine, and read	no false(+) some complete false(−) (see Clinistix)	extra large strips for visually impaired diabetic; control tablets used to test to see if patient can read accurately
TesTape (Eli Lilly & Co.)	Strip: 100 tests/ dispenser	glucose oxidase peroxidase *o*-tolidine yellow dye	brown color or doesn't resemble "O" on test with distilled water	1 minute	no false(+) some partial false(−) (see Clinistix)	most inexpensive test; convenient for home and travel; accuracy adequate if all 3+ read as 4+; not as quantitative as Diastix or Clinitest

[a] Protect all products from heat, light, and moisture.

Combination Urine Tests

Product (Manufacturer)	Product Formulation and Sizes	Active Ingredients	Indication of Product Deterioration	Time Required to Evaluate	Drug Interference	Comments
Chemstrip 8 (Biodynamics)	Strip: 50's	glucose oxidase peroxidase *o*-tolidine sodium nitroferricyanide others	discoloration of test area	0– 60 seconds (dip and read)	no false (+) (glucose)	Tests for glucose, protein, pH, blood, ketones, bilirubin, urobilinogen, and nitrite. Error potential is great. Specific individual tests recommended.

Product (Manufacturer)	Product Formulation and Sizes	Active Ingredients	Indication of Product Deterioration	Time Required to Evaluate	Drug Interference	Comments
Combistix (Ames)	Strip: 100's	glucose oxidase others	discoloration of test area	30–60 seconds (dip and read)	no false (+) (glucose) some false (−)	Test for glucose, protein, and pH. Not needed by diabetic.
Ketodiastix (Ames)	Strip: 50's 100's	glucose oxidase nitroprusside	glucose area green ketone area darkened	15–30 seconds (dip and read)	no false (+) (glucose) some false (−)	Useful combination product for glucose and ketones. No need to use this test often, only when passing 4+ glucose often.
Labstix (Ames)	Strip: 100's	glucose oxidase nitroprusside others	discoloration of test area	30–60 seconds (dip and read)	no false (+) (glucose) some false (−)	Test for blood, pH, glucose, acetone, and protein. Amount of use does not warrant expense for individual patient.
Multistix (Ames)	Strip: 100's	glucose oxidase peroxidase *o*-tolidine sodium nitroferricyanide others	discoloration of test area	0–60 seconds (dip and read)	no false (+) (glucose)	Same as N-Mulstix but does not test for nitrite.
N-Mulstix (Ames)	Strip: 100's	glucose oxidase peroxidase *o*-tolidine sodium nitroferricyanide others	discoloration of test area	0–60 seconds (dip and read)	no false (+) (glucose)	Tests for glucose, protein, pH, blood, ketones, bilirubin, urobilinogen, and nitrite. Error potential is great. Specific individual tests recommended.
Uristix (Ames)	Strip: 100's	glucose oxidase others	discoloration of test area	30–60 seconds (dip and read)	no false (+) (glucose) some false (−)	Test for glucose and protein. Useful to determine if protein in urine (diabetic nephropathy).

Urine Ketone Tests

Product (Manufacturer)	Product Formulation and Sizes	Active Ingredient	Indication of Product Deterioration	Time Required to Evaluate	Drug Interference	Comments
Acetest (Ames)	Tablets: 100's 250's	nitroprusside	darkened brown tablet	30 seconds (urine) 2 minutes (plasma) 10 minutes (whole blood)	false (+) possible but rare (levodopa)	Test for acetone and acetoacetic acid. Useful in determining whether or not a diabetic is developing ketoacidosis. Patient with 2% or more glucose should test for ketones.
Ketostix (Ames)	Strip: 50's 100's	nitroprusside	tan or brown	15 seconds	false (+) possible but rare (levodopa)	Test for acetone and acetoacetic acid. Useful in determining whether or not a diabetic is developing ketoacidosis. Patient with 2% or more glucose should test for ketones.

Product (Manufacturer)	Description
Clinilog (Ames)	A diary for diabetics to record date, urine sugars, urine acetone, and remarks plus a glossary of terms for diabetic patients, plus diet information. Patient should keep track of weight, changes in medication, exercise, diet, infections, or emotional stress.
Diabetic ID Tags	Bracelets and necklaces that indicate that the patient is diabetic. Available from Medic Alert Foundation (P.O. Box 1009, Turlock, CA 95380) and Health Enterprises, Inc. (P.O. Box 684, North Attleboro, MA 02751).
Eyetone Reflector Colorimeter (Ames)	A meter used with Dextrostix that provides accurate blood glucose determinations. Can be used by pregnant, brittle, or unstable diabetics to improve control by home blood glucose monitoring. Also useful for screening for diabetes.
Glucola (Ames)	100 g of glucose in 7-oz. disposable bottle. Requires 0.5 hour to evaluate. Caffeine-free carbonated cola-flavored prep. For use as a carbohydrate challenge in glucose tolerance testing.
Urine Specimen Jars	Pharmacist should keep available for diabetic patients and encourage patients to take urine specimens when seeing their physicians.

Infant Formula Products

Michael W. McKenzie, Kenneth J. Bender, and A. Jeanece Seals

Chapter 12

Questions to Ask the Patient

What are the child's age and weight?

Is the child under a physician's care?

Has your pediatrician recommended a formula?

Is the child allergic to milk? Are there other dietary restrictions?

Is diarrhea a problem? If so, what is the frequency?

Does the child have fever, dry skin, or loss of appetite?

Do you understand the directions for mixing the formula? Repeat them in your own words.

The popularity of infant formula products is reflected in the fact that commercially prepared milk-based or milk-free formulas account for approximately 75% of the milk and formula fed to infants (1). Most of these products are purchased as concentrated liquids requiring addition of water to supply the appropriate concentration of calories per fluid ounce. The more expensive ready-to-feed formulas which require no mixing or diluting also constitute a substantial proportion, while powdered formulas are used less frequently. Pharmacies and groceries are the major distributors of infant formulas, although about 6% are distributed by nutrition and infant care centers.

Results of market research by various infant formula manufacturers give fairly accurate data on milk and formula use. It is estimated that Similac, Enfamil, and SMA are used to feed 96% of all infants receiving commercially prepared milk-based formulas (1). Isomil, ProSobee, Neo-Mull-Soy, and Soyalac are used for an estimated 92% of all infants receiving commercially prepared milk-free formulas (1).

Milk, alone or in a mixture, is an infant's most important food. Early commercial formulas did not provide an adequate substitute for breast milk. They were high in carbohydrates and often were linked with bacterial infections because of poor sanitation. However, in the last 30 years there has been a considerable increase in formula feeding of infants. The main factors responsible for this increase are technical advances in producing sanitary formulas and the change in women's attitudes toward breast-feeding. The proportion of breast-feeding during the newborn period decreased from about 65% in the 1940's to 25% in 1958 (2). Although there appears to be a growing trend to breast-feed among mothers of middle and upper socioeconomic groups, the proportion of infants who are breast-fed at the age of 1 month remains constant—about 20% (3).

The composition of commercial infant formulas is in accordance with guidelines generated from extensive assessment of infant nutritional needs. Formula variation provides the opportunity to select a product that is acceptable to a particular infant and satisfies special nutritional requirements. These variations, however, have produced differences in palatability, digestibility, and convenience of administration. The pharmacist should be able to evaluate indications and advise on the selection and preparation of infant formulas.

NUTRITIONAL REQUIREMENTS

The growth rate of infants is faster from birth to 1 year than at any other time. Infants are expected to double their birth weight at 6 months and to triple it at 1 year. Because of this rapid growth rate the nutritional adequacy of an infant's diet is very important.

Three basic nutritional principles should be considered in evaluating an infant formula: it should contain adequate, but not excessive, amounts of all essential nutrients; it should be readily digestible; and it should have a reasonable distribution of calories derived from protein, fat, and carbohydrate. Metabolic studies suggest that 7–16% of the calories should be derived from protein, 30–55% from fat, and 35–65% from carbohydrate (4). Human milk provides 7, 55, and 38% of its calories from protein, fat, and carbohydrate, respectively; corresponding figures for whole cow's milk are 20, 50, and 30%.

Nutritional requirements are best expressed as the amounts needed per 100 kcal of total food intake, rather than amounts per kilogram of body weight (Table 1). This system provides a convenient way to reflect the interaction of one nutrient with another, e.g., vitamin A and unsaturated fatty acids, and it can be applied to formulas of different calorie concentrations (5).

Caloric Allowance

The metabolic calorie [large calorie or kilocalorie (kcal)] is the amount of heat required to raise the temperature of 1000 g of water from 15 to 16°C. The Recommended Daily Dietary Allowance (RDA), as established by the National Academy of Sciences/National Research

Council, is 117 cal/kg/day for infants from birth to 6 months and 108 cal/kg/day from 6 months to 1 year. A full-term, full-weight infant should have no difficulty in consuming enough of a standard diluted formula (20–30 cal/oz. or 20 cal/30 ml) to meet these needs. A premature or low birth weight infant has a higher caloric need and may require as much as 130 cal/kg/day (6). An infant recovering from illness or malnutrition also requires more calories (5).

Protein Allowance

nutritional guidelines for infants

protein RDA's for infants

essential amino acids

The RDA for protein is 2.2 g/kg from birth to 6 months and 2.0 g/kg from 6 months to 1 year. Low birth weight infants may have a higher protein requirement, although too much protein may overwhelm the ability of the infant kidney to excrete the necessary nitrogen (>4.5 g/100 kcal) (5). The Committee on Nutrition of the American Academy of Pediatrics recommends a minimum of 1.8 g/100 kcal of protein having a PER (protein efficiency ratio derived from the weight gain per gram of protein fed) at least 100% that of casein. This recommendation applies primarily to formulas; human milk contains 1.5 g/ 100 kcal and is adequate for the full-term infant.

It is important that the protein source contain the eight essential amino acids: isoleucine, leucine, lysine, methionine, phenylalanine, threonine, tryptophan, and valine. There is evidence that histidine also is essential for the newborn (7). Both human and cow's milk contain histidine in quantities exceeding estimated infant re-

Table 1. Infant Nutritional Recommendations per 100 kcal

Nutrient	Minimum	Maximum
Protein, g	1.8	4.5
Fat, g	3.3 (30.0% cal)	6.0 54.0
Essential fatty acids (linoleate), g	3.0 (300.0% cal)	—
Vitamins		
A, IU	250.0 (75 μg)[a]	750.0 (225 μg)[a]
D, IU	40.0	100.0
K, μg	4.0	—
E, IU[b]	3.0	—
C (ascorbic acid), mg	8.0	—
B_1 (thiamine), μg	40.0	—
B_2 (riboflavin), μg	60.0	—
B_6 (pyridoxine), μg[c]	35.0	—
B_{12} (cyanocobalamin), μg	0.15	—
Niacin, mg[d]	250.0 (800.0 mg equivalent)	—
Folic acid, μg	4.0	—
Pantothenic acid, μg	300.0	—
Biotin, μg	1.5	—
Choline, mg	7.0	—
Inositol, mg	4.0	—
Minerals		
Calcium, mg	50.0[e]	—
Phosphorus, mg	25.0[e]	—
Magnesium, mg	6.0	—
Iron, mg	0.15	—
Iodine, μg	5.0	—
Zinc, mg	0.5	—
Copper, μg	60.0	—
Manganese	5.0	—
Sodium	20.0 (6 mEq)[f]	60.0 (17 mEq)[f]
Potassium	80.0 (14 mEq)[f]	200.0 (34 mEq)[f]
Chloride	55.0 (11 mEq)[f]	150.0 (29 mEq)[f]

Excerpted from the report of the Committee on Nutrition of the American Academy of Pediatrics, *Pediatrics*, *57*, 278 (1976).
[a] Retinol equivalents.
[b] With 0.7 IU/g linoleic acid.
[c] With 15 μg/g of protein in formula.
[d] Although expressed as niacin, it is recognized that on the average, 1 mg of niacin is derived from each 60 mg of dietary tryptophan.
[e] Calcium-to-phosphorus ratio must be no less than 1.1 and no more than 2.0.
[f] Milliequivalent for 670 kcal/liter of formula.

quirements of 26 mg/100 kcal and may be fed to newborns until the body begins to synthesize histidine (2–3 months after birth). Tyrosine and cystine, as well as histidine, may be essential initially for the premature infant (7, 8).

Carbohydrate Allowance

Although there is no RDA for carbohydrates, a human infant efficiently uses 35–65% of the total calories from a carbohydrate source (4). Most carbohydrate sources used in infant formulas are monosaccharides or disaccharides, which are digested and absorbed more readily by the infant than polysaccharides (starch). Lactose, the "milk sugar" disaccharide, is the most common carbohydrate in an infant's diet. It is hydrolyzed by acids and the enzyme lactase to glucose and galactose. Disaccharide hydrolysis in a newborn may be incomplete, and because lactase activity develops late in fetal life, a premature infant is especially prone to lactose intolerance (manifested by diarrhea, abdominal distention, and cramping) during the first weeks after birth (9).

Fat Allowance

The Committee on Nutrition recommends a minimum of 3.3 g/100 kcal and a maximum of 6.0 g/100 kcal of fat (9). A normal caloric distribution in an infant's diet derives 30–55% of the calories from dietary fat. Diets that supply more calories from fat may cause ketosis because ketone bodies are formed from excess free fatty acids (4). Fat is an efficient calorie source because of its high caloric density. It contains 9 cal/g compared with 4 cal/g for protein and carbohydrate. Fat in a diet increases palatability and enhances the absorption of lipid-soluble vitamins.

Fat also supplies the essential fatty acids not synthesized in the human body. The American Academy of Pediatrics recommends linoleic acid intakes of 300 mg/100 kcal or 30% of total calories (10). Linoleic and arachidonic acids enable optimum caloric intake use and proper skin composition; four other fatty acids also are essential (11). Because these fatty acids are precursors of the prostaglandins, the manifestations of their deficiency may result from impaired prostaglandin synthesis. The actions of the prostaglandins appear to be related to cyclic adenosine monophosphate (cAMP) and range from mediating inflammatory response and hormone control to transporting water and electrolytes.

The digestibility of the fat source is important. Medium-chain fatty acids (8–10 carbons) that are unsaturated are most easily absorbed. Monounsaturated fatty acids have one double bond; polyunsaturated fatty acids are dienoic, trienoic, or tetraenoic, depending on the number of double bonds. Linoleic acid represents the bulk of polyunsaturated fatty acids in infant formulas.

Vitamin and Mineral Allowances

Although certain infants may need vitamin supplementation in their diets, indiscriminate vitamin supplementation, especially with lipid-soluble vitamins A and D, is potentially hazardous. (See Chapter 10 for a complete discussion of vitamins.) The use of vitamin supplements should be limited to infants with known problems in fat absorption and those receiving restricted diets because of allergies or metabolic disease (5).

Premature infants on restricted diets may need vitamin E supplementation. Hemolytic anemia has been reported in premature infants who have received formulas with high levels of polyunsaturated fatty acids without vitamin E supplementation (13).

Iron deficiency anemia is the most prevalent nutritional deficiency in infants. As a result, the American Academy of Pediatrics Committee on Nutrition recommends the use of iron-fortified formula in the first year of life (12). The RDA for iron is 10 mg; 32 oz (960 ml) of iron-fortified commercial formula provides adequate daily iron. Present recommendations for iron of 0.15 mg/100 kcal are based on the amount in human milk.

High iron intake levels (8 mg/kg or more) also contribute to hemolytic anemia in premature infants, possibly by interfering with the intestinal absorption of vitamin E in the infant (14). For this reason the premature infant should not receive iron in excess of the levels recommended by the Committee on Nutrition.

sugars, starch, and fats

vitamin supplementation in infants

composition of human milk

The fluoride concentration in human and cow's milk is 0.1–0.2 mg/liter (5). Foods provide the recommended intake of 0.5 mg/day for children under 3 in areas having a low fluoride concentration in the drinking water (<0.5 mg/liter). Fluoride supplementation of 0.5 mg/day (irrespective of the infant's milk or formula) increases tooth resistance to dental caries when the quantity of fluoride in the water supply is less than 1.0 mg/liter (15). However, the relationship of fluoride intake in the first 6 months of life to dental caries is unclear, and no recommendations concerning fluoride supplements in exclusively breast-fed infants can be made (5). Fluoride intake in excess of ~0.5 mg/day by the infant is unnecessary, and excessive intake will result in fluorosis and mottled tooth enamel.

CONTENT OF MILK AND FORMULAS

The initial comparison to be considered is that between the "standard" of human milk and cow's milk, which is used as the protein base for most commercial preparations.

Human Milk: Standard of Comparison

Human milk is the standard against which all formulas may be compared. Obviously, it is more effective than cow's milk in meeting the nutritional requirements of the human infant. The differences in composition reflect the needs of both the human infant and the calf. Although certain conditions in the infant may necessitate therapeutic formulas, human milk is the most appropriate diet for most infants.

Cow's milk has about three times the ash and protein normally found in human milk (Figure 1). This difference reflects the calf's larger growth rate and proportionate demand for protein and minerals. The urea formed from protein nitrogen combines with the mineral residue (ash) to create a higher renal solute load for the infant ingesting cow's milk. Although cow's milk usually is diluted with water and carbohydrates, the solute load requiring renal excretion generally remains greater than the load from human milk.

Not only does cow's milk contain a higher percentage of protein than human milk, but the protein differs in composition. The difference in protein composition alters digestibility and may create a milk "sensitivity" where the infant has difficulty in digesting a milk-based formula. Compared with human milk, cow's milk has a high proportion of casein protein (crude protein mixture of α-, β-, γ-, and κ-caseins) to lactalbumin protein (primarily α-lactoglobulin but includes α-lactalbumin). Casein is relatively insoluble and occurs in milk as a "tough" curd; lactalbumin is highly soluble and occurs in milk as whey. The large amount of curd in cow's milk slows the gastric emptying rate and may cause GI distress. Heating cow's milk reduces the curd tension. Milk sensitivity differs from milk allergy in that sensitivity may be relieved by altering the casein-to-lactalbumin ratio, but an allergic reaction requires that all animal milk protein be eliminated. Although heating cow's milk may increase digestibility by reducing curd tension, it will not alter its antigen activity in allergic infants.

composition differences between human and cow's milk

curd tension

fatty acids

carbohydrate percentage

The fat in cow's milk differs from that in human milk in two ways. The triglycerides in cow's milk contain primarily short- and long-chain fatty acids (e.g., butyric and caproic). Human milk fat includes medium-chain fatty acids (e.g., capric and lauric) but not the short-chain group. In addition, human milk contains a majority of monounsaturated fatty acids, and cow's milk butterfat primarily consists of saturated fatty acids. Commercial milk-based formulas incorporate the highly digestible, unsaturated, medium-chain triglycerides by replacing butterfat with vegetable oil and special medium-chain triglyceride oils.

The carbohydrate percentage in cow's milk is smaller than that in human milk, and carbohydrate supplementation is often necessary. Honey and other unrefined foods are probably poor choices for carbohydrate supplementation, since they may contain botulism spores that are possible contributors to crib death in susceptible infants (16). Lactose, the carbohydrate source in both cow's milk and human milk, is absorbed into the brush border of the small intestine and cleaved by the disaccharidase into galactose and glucose which then are absorbed actively against concentration gradients.

Cow's milk and human milk differ in absolute and proportionate amounts of calcium and phosphorus. The effect of this difference on calcium absorption is not clear because of the interrelation of additional factors such as vitamin D, fat absorption, and active transport. For the premature infant a low phosphorus intake is required to minimize renal solute load.

Evaporated Milk

Evaporated milk is standardized with respect to concentrations of protein, fat, carbohydrate, and major minerals. Cow's milk evaporated to one-half its original volume is preferred over the natural product because it is sterile and convenient and because the curd formed

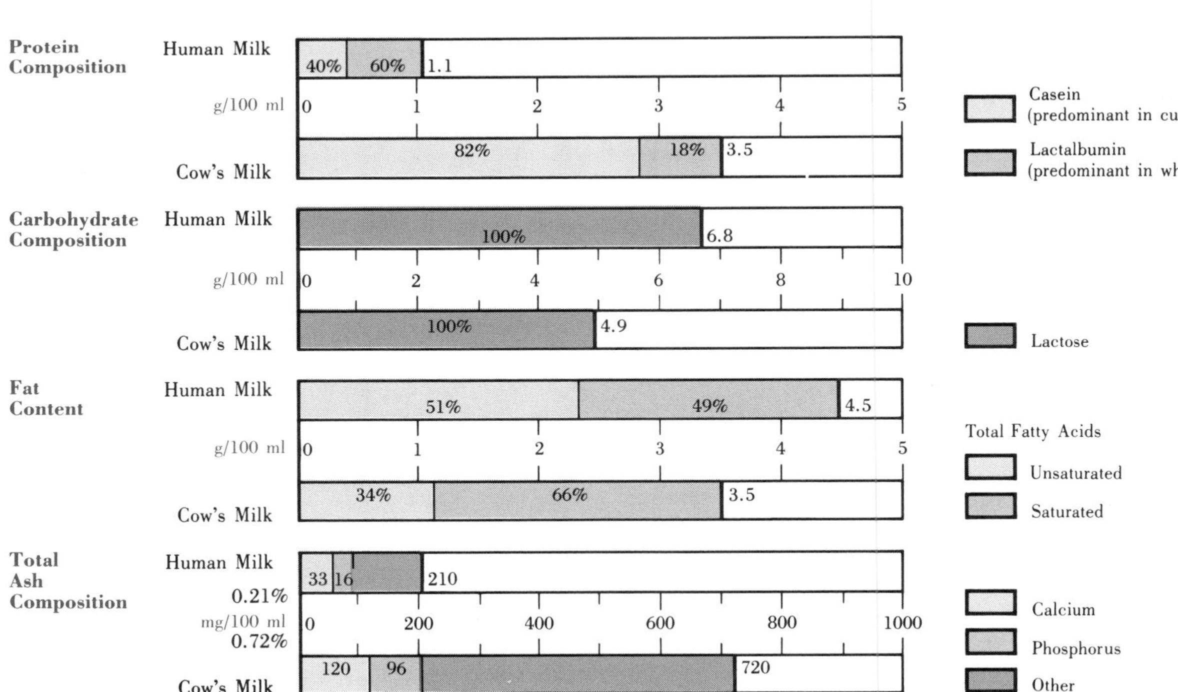

Figure 1. Comparison of human and cow's milk.

after coagulation by gastric secretions is smaller and softer. Formulas made with evaporated milk, water, and sucrose must take into account that evaporated milk has one-half the fluid content of whole milk and its caloric content is twice as great. For a 3000-g infant a formula with 150 ml of evaporated milk, 300 ml of water, and 45 g of sucrose supplies enough fluid (450 ml) and calories (380 cal) to meet the RDA (17), although evaporated milk formulas and unmodified cow's milk fail to meet current recommendations for ascorbic acid, vitamin E, and essential fatty acids (5, 10).

other kinds of milk

Skim Milk

Skim milk, from which fat has been removed by centrifugation, generally contains 0.1% fat. Skim milk may be fed to infants, beginning at 4–6 months of age, to help treat or prevent obesity and perhaps to aid in preventing atherosclerosis. Infants fed skim milk gain somewhat less in weight and slightly, but not significantly, more in length than infants fed whole milk (18). Although this result may seem desirable, considerations of energy balance offer cause for concern.

Infants fed skim milk utilize more of their stores of body fat. Over an extended period, once fat stores have been depleted, the infant's ability to respond adequately to a major illness may be compromised (19). In addition, infants receiving a major percentage of caloric intake from skim milk may receive exceedingly high protein intake and low fat intake and an inadequate intake of essential fatty acids.

Goat's Milk

Goat's milk is not widely used, but it is generally accepted as being nutritionally adequate. It contains primarily medium- and short-chain fatty acids and may be digested more readily than cow's milk. Because goat's milk is deficient in folates, supplementation of about 50 μg/day of folate (as folic acid) should be given to prevent megaloblastic anemia in infants fed only with goat's milk.

benefits of breast-feeding

Breast-Feeding Considerations

Human milk provides certain advantages over cow's and goat's milk. Because of its cleanness (lack of opportunity for contamination) and its abundance of "host resistant factors" (including bifidus factor, lactoferrin, lymphocytes, lysozyme, macrophages, and secretory IgA), infectious agents such as *Escherichia coli* and poliomyelitis virus that affect or enter the body through the GI tract have less chance of causing an infection (20–24). These anti-infective properties of human milk may be lifesaving with poor home hygiene and also provide protective effects in well-sanitized homes (25). *E. coli* and *Klebsiella* organisms, which may be etiological in some cases of necrotizing enterocolitis, are very uncommon in the intestine of the breast-fed infant (26, 27).

The most common food allergen in infancy is β-lactoglobulin, a cow's milk protein. Secretory IgA in human milk helps prevent absorption of food allergens. The best prophylaxis against food allergy in infancy is breast-feeding and avoiding semisolid food (until 4–6 months of age) (28).

Breast-feeding, when other food is withheld and suckling occurs throughout the day, also contributes to child spacing, owing to endocrinological effects of prolactin secreted from the anterior pituitary in response to suckling (29). Limited daytime breast-feeding, however, does not effectively produce this "lactation amenorrhea."

The closer contact between mother and infant during breast-feeding with resultant increase in maternal hormone secretion and neonatal somatosensory, olfactory, and auditory stimulation may increase maternal–neonate bonding (30). This intense attachment formed via breast-feeding may be helpful in preventing later psychosocial emotional disturbances, including "disorder of mothering" with subsequent child abuse (31–33).

Breast-feeding also prevents the infant from being exposed to emulsifiers, additives such as carrageenan, lecithin, and sodium citrate, thickening agents, antioxidants, and pH adjusters found in commercial formulas. Although these agents generally are not associated with ill effects and are approved by the *Codex Alimentarius* of the Food and Agricultural Organization of the United Nations (30), they are not found in human milk.

Study results demonstrate a greater gain in weight and length of bottle-fed than breast-fed infants (34). Bottle-fed infants generally gain more weight for a specified gain in length than breast-fed infants. This condition could reflect an overfeeding of bottle-fed infants. Overfeeding may contribute to subsequent obesity because an abnormally large population of adipocytes develops or because a habit of overeating is established. However, a correlation between obesity in infancy and obesity in the adolescent or adult has not been conclusively demonstrated.

Often, human milk is not chosen because the mother prefers not to breast-feed. Past experience of the mother or her family and friends is important in deciding whether to begin and continue breast-feeding (35). Educational programs, technical information, and support are needed for women who breast-feed to avoid early cessation. Breast-feeding is estimated to decrease from 20% during the first month of life to 5% in the fifth month (36).

One minor problem associated with human milk is created by a substance secreted by some women, 3α,-20β-pregnanediol, which seems to increase the incidence and severity of hyperbilirubinemia in infants by inhibiting glucuronide formation. This substance does not pose a significant drawback to breast-feeding, and an interruption of breast milk for 1–2 days is usually enough to reverse the infant's raised bilirubin.

drug use and breast-feeding

Another potential problem in using human milk arises when the mother is taking medication. Drugs excreted in human milk may have undesirable effects on the infant and also may alter breast milk composition (37–39). For example, changes were reported in milk protein, fat, and calcium content in women taking combination-type oral contraceptives (40). Although these contraceptive agents are not specifically contraindicated for nursing mothers, the infant should be observed for adverse effects. Also, lactation is diminished by progesterone–estrogen combinations taken before adequate milk secretion is established, i.e., 3–4 weeks postpartum (41).

Many drugs taken by the lactating woman may be found in her milk (38). The degree of drug distribution across the membrane between plasma and milk is influenced by its solubility in lipid and water, by its pKa′ or degree of ionization, and by selective transport mechanisms. The pH of milk is less than that of plasma; consequently, milk may act as an "ion trap" for basic compounds. Conversely, acidic drugs tend to be inhibited from entering milk.

The following drugs are not recommended for nursing women: anticoagulants, antimetabolites, atropine, most cathartics, dihydrotachysterol, ergot, thiouracil, iodides, metronidazole, radioactive drugs, and tetracycline. In addition, oral contraceptives, lithium carbonate, sulfonamides, reserpine, steroids, diazepam, diuretics, nalidixic acid, barbiturates, phenytoin, and cough medicines with codeine should be used only under supervision (39).

drugs that may affect breast-fed infants

composition considerations for formulas

milk allergy

electrolyte replacement

Standard Formula

A formulation may be altered by the manufacturer in response to changes in availability of ingredients or modifications in recommended allowances. For example, the carbohydrate source for Lofenalac was changed from a combination of maltose, sucrose, dextrins, and arrowroot starch to corn syrup and tapioca starch when arrowroot starch became unavailable. The fat source of Similac was modified by adding soy oil to the combination of corn and coconut oils in response to the decreased availability and rising cost of corn oil. Accurate listing of current ingredients and quantities then may be obtained only by direct communication to the manufacturer. Texts rapidly become outdated, and even product labels may reflect old formulations until their supply is depleted and new labels are printed.

Calories

In normal dilution, most formulas provide 20 cal/oz., approximating the caloric content of human and cow's milk. The caloric recommendations are based traditionally on comparison studies of varied concentrations fed ad libitum to normal infants. These studies show that although infants in the first 41 days do not consume enough dilute formula to obtain their required calories, they exceed the acceptable caloric intake when given formulas of higher caloric concentration (42). Advantages and disadvantages of high caloric intake in infancy are debatable because the increased weight gain may be proportionate to the gain in body length. Most nutritionists agree, however, that the incidence of overfed and overweight infants is higher than that of underfed infants.

Protein

Evaporated cow's milk supplies two-thirds the calories of most standard formulas; about 15% of these calories are derived from casein. This protein source may be altered to produce a lactalbumin-to-casein ratio resembling that of human milk. Through electrodialysis or ion exchange processes the protein components then may be demineralized, and additions made to produce the average concentrations found in human milk.

Variations in protein source have been developed because of milk allergy. Soy is the most frequently used alternative protein source; others include beef heart and hydrolysates of casein. The hydrolysates are enzymatic breakdown products with reduced antigenicity. As measured by weight gain in rats, beef heart is about 80% as efficient as casein, soy about 70%, and casein hydrolysates about 100% (43). Serum albumin levels obtained from infants are used as a more direct measurement of satisfactory protein nutritional status (44).

Fat

To obtain an easily digestible fat source, most commercial formulas have replaced butterfat with vegetable oil. Vegetable oil digestibility is increased with a high proportion of unsaturated fatty acids and decreased with a large amount of long-chain fatty acids. Corn and soy oils are easier to digest than coconut oil, which has a relatively high number of long-chain saturated fatty acids. Commercial formulas have been produced from which about 85% of the fat is absorbed—the absorption rate of fat in human milk (45).

Carbohydrates

Carbohydrates supply 40% of the calories of most standard formulas. If more than 50% of the calories are derived from carbohydrates, an infant's ability to hydrolyze disaccharides may be compromised. The increased passage of disaccharides in the feces creates an osmotic gradient in the colon which results in loose, characteristically acidic, watery stools. The excess lactose in the ileocecal region is fermented by bacteria to produce carbon dioxide and lactic acid. This process irritates the colon and may cause diarrhea, resulting in dehydration and electrolyte imbalance.

Formulas that contain sucrose and corn syrup as carbohydrate sources have a sweeter taste than those that contain lactose. Although there are differences in response to the sweeter formulas (female infants are more responsive than males, and newborns who weigh more than 3540 g at birth are more responsive than those who have a lower birth weight), the consequences of long-term use of the sweeter formulas and the criteria with which to select an optimum carbohydrate source are unknown (46).

Electrolytes and Minerals

The amount of sodium, potassium, and chloride in standard formulas is calculated on the basis of the infant's relatively high obligatory losses and the smaller amount required for growth. If fluid retention is a concern, a product with a low sodium content, e.g., Lonalac, should be considered. Commercial therapeutic formulas with no nutritional value, such as Pedialyte and Lytren, have been developed to replace electrolytes and are used in cases of diarrhea or vomiting. Because of the critical nature of electrolyte imbalance and dehydration associated with infant diarrhea and vomiting, oral electrolyte replacements should be used cautiously as temporary treatment for conditions that may require intravenous therapy and inpatient monitoring. In certain cases the initial step in correcting infant diarrhea is to withhold the feeding temporarily.

The amount of calcium and phosphorus needed to replace an infant's obligatory loss is less than that required for growth. In milk and milk-based formulas, much of the available phosphorus is released from the slowly digested casein and may not be available during calcium absorption (45). This "bound" phosphorus alters the calcium-to-phosphorus ratio and enhances calcium absorption. When a formula combines this effect with a well-absorbed fat mixture and an adequate supply of vitamin D, optimum calcium absorption is achieved. The ratio of calcium to phosphorus in a formula should be between 1.1 and 2.0 (5).

Iron and Vitamins

Supplementation of certain infant diets may be required, even when the diet is breast milk. Supplementation may be particularly important in breast-fed infants of mothers whose own diet is not well balanced (47). Supplementary iron and vitamin D are required by infants receiving human milk or unfortified cow's milk. Most commercially prepared infant formulas, with the exception of Similac and Enfamil without iron (both are available with or without iron), provide 8–12 mg of iron per quart (36). Approximately 60% of all infants fed commercially prepared formulas receive 8–12 mg of iron per quart of formula (36). Precooked infant cereals are fortified with finely divided electrolytic iron that is absorbed as well as the iron in prepared formulas (48). Iron availability may be less in formulas with higher protein concentration; iron deficiency is more common in infants fed 2.4% protein (3.6 g/100 kcal) than in those fed 1.5% (2.3 g/100 kcal) in a milk formula (49).

Ascorbic acid supplementation is necessary with cow's milk but may be unnecessary with human milk from a well-nourished woman. Supplementing ascorbic acid with commercially prepared strained foods often is difficult because of losses of the vitamin during processing. Strained fruits are inadequate as ascorbic acid sources except those whose juices are fortified with ascorbic acid or strained bananas, to which ascorbic acid is added to prevent color change.

Cyanocobalamin supplementation is necessary in breast-fed infants of vegetarian women (47, 50). Many young people consuming largely or exclusively vegetarian diets are not aware of the absence of cyanocobalamin in plant foods. Severe deficiency may develop in the infant in the absence of signs in the mother (47).

Contaminants in Milk

DDT and lead in milk

The residue limit for total DDT in cow's milk is 0.05 ppm (approximately 50 μg/liter) (51). DDT concentrations in cow's milk generally have been maintained within limits specified by the World Health Organization. Human milk contains more DDT than cow's milk, since pesticides tend to become more concentrated and stored in meat eaters than in herbivores (52). DDT concentrations in human milk generally have averaged 450 μg/liter in a studied black population and 75 μg/liter in whites, but no documentation of adverse effects in infants has been reported (38). Levels appear to be decreasing in urban areas since the DDT ban.

Results of studies suggest that lead concentrations in human milk and whole cow's milk may be quite low, but greater concentrations are present in evaporated milk and infant formulas (53). The medical significance of lead in milks and of the lead content of other foods consumed by infants and preschool children is difficult to evaluate. In view of the uncertainty regarding permissible lead intakes and the additive effects of dietary and nondietary lead intakes, it is not known whether the lead content of current diets of infants and children in the United States is regularly within the safety limits (54–56).

THERAPEUTIC FORMULA USE

Milk Allergy

products for milk allergy

Most therapeutic formulas provide a protein substitute for milk proteins. Food allergy may occur in infants because the immature digestive and metabolic processes may not be completely effective in converting dietary proteins into nonantigenic amino acids. Estimates that 1% of the infant population is allergic to cow's milk (as measured by symptoms such as rash and wheezing) may be conservative because syndromes such as failure to thrive, anemia, and recurrent infections have been linked to serum antigen–antibody reactions to milk protein.

The formulas that include water-soluble soy isolates (Isomil, Neo-Mull-Soy, ProSobee, and Nursoy) are whiter and more palatable than soy-based formulas that derive their protein from soy flour (Mull-Soy). Some "hypoallergenic" formulas incorporate enzymatic hydrolysates of casein (Nutramigen, Pregestimil). Meat Base Formula derives its substitute for milk protein from beef heart and may require carbohydrate supplementation.

Fat Restriction

Fat and protein composition may be altered to achieve a more easily digested "humanized" formula. The fat in these formulas is made up of triglycerides of mainly medium-chain fatty acids. The digestibility of medium-chain triglyceride oil closely approximates that of human milkfat. Medium-chain triglyceride oil ensures acceptance by infants who will not tolerate long- or short-chain fatty acids. In combination with a fat source, such as corn oil, it provides lecithin phospholipids.

Conditions that may necessitate a low or moderate fat intake include cystic fibrosis and celiac disease. The latter is characterized by an intolerance to the gluten protein of wheat and rye and by the transient inability to absorb fat and starch. Formulas with a moderate amount of medium-chain triglyceride oil are helpful in these conditions because their fat is more easily assimilated than butterfat (Pregestimil, 2.8 g/100 ml; Portagen, 3.1 g/100 ml). Soy-based formulas are not recommended for patients with cystic fibrosis because of the reported hypoproteinemic edema resulting from their use by individuals with this disease (57).

Caloric/Carbohydrate Considerations

Low birth weight infants (less than 2 kg at 3 weeks) or premature infants (born before 37 weeks from the first day of the last menstrual period) need a higher caloric content for growth than full-term infants because of an increased caloric need and decreased ability to consume an adequate volume of formula. Examples of commercial preparations that provide the required higher caloric concentrations and are used in the hospital setting for these infants are Premature Formula and specifically concentrated SMA-Improved and Similac PM 60/40 (80 cal/100 ml).

Disaccharidase deficiency may occur as a congenital defect or secondary to cystic fibrosis or celiac disease. The absence of disaccharidase leads to malabsorption and acidic diarrhea. In these cases the formula CHO-Free, which has no carbohydrates, may be given temporarily. Formulas without the suspect disaccharide then may be tried to re-establish the infant's diet.

other conditions requiring formula modifications

In cases of galactosemia, a relatively rare disorder resulting from a deficiency of either galactose 1-phosphate uridyl transferase or galactokinase, it is necessary to eliminate dietary lactose, so that the body may convert glucose only to the amount of galactose it requires. Dietary lactose may be essentially eliminated by using soy isolates or Nutramigen, which contains only 16 mg/67 cal of lactose (equivalent to 8 mg galactose) as a contaminant of its casein protein, or Meat Base Formula, which has only trace amounts of galactose from the heart muscle protein.

Galactosemia from an inborn enzyme deficiency is characterized in untreated infants by failure to thrive, liver disease, cataracts, and mental retardation.

Congenital Heart Disease

Infants with congenital heart disease often require a formula with an increased caloric concentration because they may tire in feeding before a volume with sufficient nutrients has been consumed. In addition, an excessive renal load must be avoided.

Lonalac, a sodium-free formula, may be used to limit sodium intake, but only for a short time before sodium must be supplemented. This formula presents a renal solute load slightly less than that of whole cow's milk, and caution is required in view of the limited liquid volume intake characteristic of the seriously ill heart patient.

Phenylketonuria

Phenylketonuria results from the failure of phenylalanine to be converted to tyrosine in the body. Phenylalanine accumulation alters brain development and leads to mental retardation. Phenylalanine restriction is the only indication for Lofenalac, which may be used to eliminate dietary phenylalanine. Because it is an essential amino acid, phenylalanine then must be supplied in monitored quantities. For this purpose, formulas are used that have a predominance of whey protein, which has less phenylalanine than casein.

Excessive phenylalanine restriction bringing blood levels below 2 mg/100 ml has resulted in retarded bone growth, vacuolization of bone marrow cells, megaloblastic anemia, hypoglycemia, and death (58). Lofenalac, like other therapeutic formulas, should be used only as directed and indicated. Using therapeutic formulas indiscriminately or interchanging them arbitrarily with standard formulas must be avoided.

FORMULA/BOTTLE PREPARATION

preparing formulas and bottles

Infant formula preparation requires careful technique, and the pharmacist should explain the directions adequately to parents to ensure satisfactory nutrition for their infant. There are three forms of infant formulas—ready-to-feed, concentrated liquid, and concentrated powder. The latter two require the addition of water or, to add calories, a water–carbohydrate solution such as water–dextrose. Failure to dilute a concentrated formula properly could result in a hypertonic solution, precipitating diarrhea and dehydration. In an extreme case, overconcentrated formula produced renal failure, disseminated intravascular coagulation, gangrene of the legs, and coma (59).

Equal amounts of water and concentrated liquid formula provide the necessary 20 cal/30 ml. The powdered formula requires one packed level measure of powder (1 tbsp) to 60 ml of water. For special dilutions of therapeutic formulas and other modified formulas the directions on the product should be followed.

terminal heating

Infants are highly susceptible to infections because of insufficient antibody formation and decreasing maternal antibody titer. Until an infant can produce adequate antibodies, it is especially important to sterilize all equipment used in formula preparation. Bottles, nipples, can opener, funnel, caps, and other equipment should be washed with hot soapy water and rinsed thoroughly with hot running water (water should be squeezed through the holes in the nipples) (Table 2).

Formula may be prepared for individual feedings or for a 24-hour supply, the latter procedure being more advantageous and efficient for milk, water, and carbohydrate mixtures. Formula may be prepared to prevent bacterial contamination by terminal heating or aseptic technique (60). The American Academy of Pediatrics Committee on Fetus and Newborn does not recommend the use of washed equipment and hot tap water to prepare formula. The Committee recommends that some method of sterilization (preferably the terminal heating method) with emphasis on the need for 25 minutes of active boiling and the necessity for clean equipment be used before feeding milk mixtures to infants (61).

Although the terminal heating method has been recommended as being the most effective, there are some special formulas, e.g., CHO-Free liquid and Meat Base Formula, which should not be heated terminally because the procedure may cause the ingredients to separate and make feeding difficult. The terminal heating method is more convenient than aseptic technique for preparing a day's supply.

The commercially sterilized liquid formulas and bacteriologically safe powdered formulas may be prepared more conveniently in single bottles. A day's supply of bottles may be sterilized in advance, and the formula added at feeding time. This practice eliminates the need for refrigeration of bottled formula and prefeeding warming.

The terminal heating method may allow bacterial growth during storage if instructions are not followed or bottles are not cleaned thoroughly of milk film (62). However, evaporated milk formula carefully prepared just prior to feeding in bottles cleaned with hot tap water is bacteriologically safe (63). Milk formulas mixed at feeding time in "unsterilized" but clean bottles showed a definite bacteriological advantage over the stored formula in homes where sanitary conditions were poor and instructions for terminal heating and formula storage were not followed properly (64).

steps in three methods of formula/bottle preparation

Table 2. Formula Preparation

Terminal Heating [a]	Aseptic [a]	Single-Bottle [b]
1. Rinse the bottle and nipple with cool water immediately after the feeding. Wash the day's supply of bottles, nipples, and caps with hot, soapy water, and rinse well.	1. Rinse the bottle and nipple with cool water immediately after the feeding. Wash the day's supply of bottles, nipples, and caps with hot, soapy water and rinse well.	1. Rinse the bottle and nipple with cool water immediately after the feeding. Wash the day's supply of bottles, nipples, and caps with hot, soapy water and rinse well.
2. Rinse the outside of the formula can and shake the contents well. Open the can with a clean can opener, mix the formula with water, or water–carbohydrate solution if prescribed, and pour the solution into bottles, Attach the nipples and cover them loosely with caps.	2. Boil the bottles, nipples, caps, can opener, and mixing utensils for 5 minutes in a deep cooking utensil with enough water to cover each item. Remove the items with tongs, and place the bottles on a clean towel or rack.	2. For formulas that require water, pour into each bottle the amount of water needed to prepare the feeding. Attach the nipples and cover them loosely with caps. Place the bottles on a rack in a deep cooking utensil containing ~5–8 cm of water. Bring water to a boil, cover, and allow it to boil gently for 25 minutes. Remove the cooking utensil from the stove, allow it to cool, and tighten the caps and bottles. The bottles may be left inside the cooking utensil until they are needed.
3. Place the bottles on a rack in a deep cooking utensil containing ~5–8 cm of water. Heat water to boiling, and allow it to boil gently for 25 minutes while covered before removing from the stove.	3. While the equipment is being cleaned, boil some water in a covered saucepan or tea kettle for 5 minutes (slightly more water than the prescribed amount should be used to allow for evaporation).	3. For formulas that need no water, boil the bottles, nipples, caps, and can opener for 5 minutes. Put the nipples and caps on the bottles with aseptic care.
4. After the sides of the cooking utensil have cooled enough to be touched comfortably, remove the lid and the formula bottles. (Leaving the utensil closed for this period is recommended to prevent formation of milk film on bottles and clogging of nipples.) [c]	4. Remove the boiled water from the stove, allow it to cool, and measure the required amount.	4. At feeding time, remove the cap and nipple aseptically. Add the appropriate amount of formula and replace the nipple. With the powdered formula, also replace the cap, and shake the bottle vigorously to mix.
5. Warm the bottle of formula to the desired temperature before feeding.	5. Rinse, shake the can well, and add the commercially processed formula or evaporated milk and carbohydrate mixture to the boiled water and stir with a clean spoon. (If bottled milk or other unsterilized milk is used, it should be boiled with the water. Evaporated milk, carbohydrate modifiers, and commercially processed formulas usually are not boiled.)	5. Feed the infant while formula is at room temperature.
	6. Pour the formula into bottles, and attach the nipples and caps with aseptic care. Store them in the refrigerator. Formula should be used within 24 hours.	
	7. Warm the bottle of formula to the desired temperature before feeding.	

[a] *Handbook of Infant Formulas*, 6th ed., J. B. Roerig, Division of Pfizer, New York, N.Y., 1969, p. 86.
[b] For supplementing the diet of breast-fed infant or when traveling; from *Handbook of Infant Formulas*, 6th ed., J. B. Roerig, Division of Pfizer, New York, N.Y., 1969, p. 88.
[c] H. K. Silver, *Pediatrics*, *20*, 997 (1957).

Common Problems

Infants are particularly susceptible to dehydration because of their high metabolic rate and ratio of surface area to weight and height. Fluid volume depletion by diarrhea may quickly (within 24 hours) produce severe dehydration with fluid electrolyte imbalance, shock, and possibly death. A common etiology of diarrhea in infants is improper dilution of concentrated liquid or powder formula, and therefore care must be taken to ensure proper formula preparation.

If diarrhea is a problem, the pharmacist should ascertain the severity, frequency of stools, duration, and method of preparing the infant formula. If the diarrhea is serious (many more stools per day than the normal range of one to five) or has continued for 48 hours, or if the infant is clinically sick (fever, lethargy, anorexia, irritability, or dry skin), the infant should be referred to a physician for appropriate care.

diarrhea—a serious problem in the infant

feeding schedules and amounts

Medical care should be directed at identifying the cause of the diarrhea as well as correcting the physiological imbalances. Reducing fat intake, using medium-chain triglyceride sources, or temporarily eliminating lactose may be helpful in determining whether the diarrhea is diet related.

Mild diarrhea of short duration may resolve without medical measures, but the infant should be observed closely. Because improper digestion of the infant's formula may initiate diarrhea and because continuation of a formula while diarrhea persists may yield only marginal nutrient absorption, a temporary (24 hours) discontinuation of usual foods may be helpful. Lytren or Pedialyte may be used cautiously for short-term management of electrolyte loss. However, it is important to re-emphasize that these solutions should not be used when parenteral rehydration is required, nor should they be used to provide nutritional value. Parents should be reminded that a solution such as Pedialyte is not a new infant formula for the baby after diarrhea has ceased and that resumption of a nutritionally adequate formula should begin under a physician's direction.

Feeding the Infant

The newborn infant may want to be fed at intervals of 2–3 hours. This schedule is permissible, but it does not allow the mother very much rest, and the infant may consume only small amounts (e.g., 15 ml) of formula at a time. The baby should be encouraged to lengthen the interval to 4 hours as soon as possible. Most infants readily adopt a 4-hour schedule by the time they are 3–4 weeks old, but some prefer a shorter interval for several months (18).

Babies vary considerably in the amount of formula desired. It is customary for no formula to be given until 12–24 hours of age, and then at 15 ml per feeding (18). An increase of 15 ml at each feeding is offered up to satiety. Further increments may be added as hunger symptoms appear. The amount given should be consistent with the RDA for caloric intake (Table 1). Some pediatricians prescribe more formula than babies probably will accept, relying on each baby's own appetite to limit intake. This method works well if the mother does not urge or force the infant to take more than is desired at any one feeding. If an infant finishes a bottle and still seems hungry, another bottle should be offered.

Complaints about an infant's rejection of a formula may be resolved in some cases by examining the specific feeding problem. "Spitting up" is often caused by improper burping, feeding a large amount too quickly, laying the infant face down too soon after feeding, or having excess mucus in the nasopharynx. During feeding, the infant should be held in a well-supported position at a 45° angle, preferably with the head nestled in the curve of the arm. Infants should not be given a bottle in the crib while lying flat. They should be burped after every 30–45 ml of formula by gently patting or rubbing the back interchangeably. After feeding, the infant should be positioned on the abdomen (on the right side) to prevent regurgitation and aspiration of formula. Many infants are chronic "spitters" of formula; if they are growing and gaining weight, there is no reason to be greatly concerned.

Larger nipple holes may be required to aid feeding. The nipple hole may be enlarged with a hot needle, or a cross-cut nipple may be used.

Indiscriminate vitamin supplementation may lead to hypervitaminosis. An infant should not receive vitamin supplementation if an iron-fortified standard formula is used unless it has been prescribed to correct a deficiency.

PRODUCT SELECTION GUIDELINES

In recommending the type of infant formula and its method of preparation, the pharmacist should take into consideration the parents' ability to follow directions, their attitudes and preferences, and the sanitary conditions and refrigeration facilities available. Instruction in cleaning techniques may include a step-by-step emphasis on the importance of sanitary conditions. For example, the top of the infant formula container should be cleaned thoroughly before opening, either by rinsing the top with hot tap water or by dipping it in boiling water for about 15 seconds before it is opened. Partially used formula cans should be kept covered, placed in the refrigerator, and stored no longer than 48 hours.

For many parents, cost may be a critical factor in the selection of an infant formula. The concentrated formula preparations are less expensive than the ready-to-feed products; powdered preparations range between the two. Convenience is also a consideration. The powder and concentrated liquid formulas require more manipulative functions in preparation and more attention to aseptic technique. A formula that is well tolerated by the infant, convenient to prepare for the parents, and within the family budget should be used.

SUMMARY

Infant formulas should supply the basic nutritional elements necessary to a baby's healthy development. Whether it comes in concentrated liquid, powder, or ready-to-feed form, the product should be easily digestible and contain reasonable distributions of protein, fat, and carbohydrate.

Commercial formulas have become more popular in the last 30 years because of technological advances in manufacturing coupled with a decline in breast-feeding of newborn infants—down to about 20% for 1-month-old babies.

The pharmacist should make sure that parents purchasing commercial infant formula understand completely the directions for preparing the product and the importance of storage in clean containers. If any serious problems, e.g., severe diarrhea, develop in spite of these precautions, the parents should be referred to a physician.

REFERENCES

(1) S. J. Fomon, *Pediatrics, 56,* 350 (1975).
(2) S. J. Fomon, "Infant Nutrition," 2nd ed., Saunders, Philadelphia, Pa., 1974, p. 7.
(3) P. S. Berman, "Report of Market Research Data," Ross Laboratories, Columbus, Ohio, Jan. 1974.
(4) "Infant Nutrition," Medcom, New York, N.Y., 1972, p. 31.
(5) C. W. Woodruff, *J. Am. Med. Assoc., 240,* 657 (1978).
(6) "Infant Nutrition," Medcom, New York, N.Y., 1972, p. 29.
(7) *Ibid.*, p. 121.
(8) G. Gaull, J. A. Sturman, and N. C. Räihä, *Pediatr. Res., 6,* 538 (1972).
(9) "Infant Nutrition," Medcom, New York, N.Y., 1972, p. 194.
(10) Committee on Nutrition, American Academy of Pediatrics, *Pediatrics, 57,* 278 (1976).
(11) H. Schlenk, *Fed. Proc., 31,* 1430 (1972).
(12) Committee Statement, Committee on Nutrition, American Academy of Pediatrics, "Iron-Fortified Formulas," Newsletter Supplement (Dec. 15, 1970).
(13) S. A. Hashim and R. H. Asfour, *Am. J. Clin. Nutr., 21,* 7 (1968).
(14) "Infant Nutrition," Medcom, New York, N.Y., 1972, p. 28.
(15) "Infant Nutrition," 2nd ed., Saunders, Philadelphia, Pa., 1974, p. 351.
(16) S. S. Arnon, T. F. Midura, D. Damus, R. M. Wood, and J. Chinn, *Lancet, 1,* 1273 (1978).
(17) H. M. Seidel, in "Pediatrics," 2nd ed., M. Ziai, Ed., Little, Brown, Boston, Mass., 1975, p. 209.
(18) S. J. Fomon, "Infant Nutrition," 2nd ed., Saunders, Philadelphia, Pa., 1974, p. 80.
(19) *Ibid.*, p. 81.
(20) A. S. Goldman and C. W. Smith, *J. Pediatr., 82,* 1082 (1973).
(21) J. Winberg and L. Gothefors, *J. Trop. Pediatr., 21,* 260 (1976).
(22) *British Medical Journal, 1,* 1167 (1976).
(23) M. Behar, *Bull. Pan Am. Health Organ., 9,* 1 (1975).
(24) O. A. Stoliar, E. Kaniecki-Green, R. P. Pelley, M. H. Klaus, and C. C. J. Carpenter, *Lancet, 1,* 1258 (1976).
(25) A. S. Cunningham, *J. Pediatr., 90,* 726 (1977).
(26) L. Gothefors, S. Olling, and J. Winberg, *Acta Paediatr. Scand., 65,* 225 (1976).
(27) L. J. Mata and J. J. Urrulia, *Ann. N.Y. Acad. Sci., 176,* 93 (1971).
(28) D. J. Matthew, A. P. Norman, B. Taylor, M. W. Turner, and J. F. Soothill, *Lancet, 1,* 321 (1977).
(29) R. C. Kolodny, L. S. Jacobs, and W. H. Daughaday, *Nature, 238,* 284 (1972).
(30) D. B. Jelliffe and E. F. P. Jelliffe, *N. Engl. J. Med., 297,* 912 (1977).
(31) M. H. Klaus, J. H. Kennell, N. Plumb, and S. Zuehlke, *Pediatrics, 46,* 187 (1970).
(32) M. H. Klaus and J. H. Kennell, "Mother-Infant Bonding: The Impact of Early Separation or Loss on Family Development," Mosby, St. Louis, Mo., 1976, p. 43.
(33) M. A. Lynch, *Lancet, 2,* 317 (1975).
(34) S. J. Fomon, "Infant Nutrition," 2nd ed., Saunders, Philadelphia, Pa., 1974, p. 79.
(35) E. Eastham, D. Smith, D. Poole, and G. Neligan, *Br. Med. J., 1,* 305 (1976).
(36) S. J. Fomon, *Pediatrics, 56,* 352 (1975).
(37) *Medical Letter on Drugs and Therapeutics, 16,* 25 (1974).
(38) P. O. Anderson, *Drug Intell. Clin. Pharm., 11,* 208 (1977).
(39) C. S. Catz and G. P. Giacoia, in "Dietary Lipids and Postnatal Development," C. Galli, G. Jacini, and A. Pecile, Eds., Raven Press, New York, N.Y., 1972, p. 247.
(40) V. M. Barsivala and K. D. Virka, *Contraception, 7,* 307 (1973).
(41) C. S. Catz and G. P. Giacoia, *Pediatr. Clin. North Am., 19,* 151 (1972).
(42) "Infant Nutrition," Medcom, New York, N.Y., 1972, p. 27.
(43) S. J. Fomon, "Infant Nutrition," 2nd ed., Saunders, Philadelphia, Pa., 1974, p. 59.
(44) *Ibid.*, p. 128.
(45) "First After Mother's Milk," Wyeth Laboratories, Philadelphia, Pa., 1971, p. 6.
(46) R. E. Nisbelt and S. B. Gurwitz, *J. Comp. Physiol. Psychol., 73,* 215 (1970).
(47) M. Higginbottom, L. Sweetman, and W. L. Nyhan, *N. Engl. J. Med., 299,* 317 (1978).
(48) E. Rios, R. E. Hunter, J. D. Cook, N. J. Smith, and C. A. Clement, *Pediatrics, 55,* 686 (1975).
(49) P. R. Dallman, *J. Pediatr., 85,* 742 (1974).
(50) B. C. Lamphin and E. F. Saunders, *J. Pediatr., 75,* 1053 (1969).
(51) S. J. Fomon, "Infant Nutrition," 2nd ed., Saunders, Philadelphia, Pa., 1974, p. 374.
(52) G. M. Woodwell, *Sci. Am., 216,* 24 (1967).
(53) J. F. Rosen and S. H. Lamm, *Pediatrics, 53,* 143 (1974).
(54) D. G. Mitchell, *Pediatrics, 53,* 142 (1974).
(55) J. S. Lin-Fir, *N. Engl. J. Med., 289,* 1229 (1973).
(56) S. Lamm, B. Cole, K. Glynn, and W. Ullmann, *N. Engl. J. Med., 289,* 574 (1973).
(57) P. A. di Sant'Agnese, in "Current Pediatric Therapy," S. S. Gellis and B. M. Kagan, Eds., Saunders, Philadelphia, Pa., 1973, p. 234.
(58) "Amino Acid Metabolism and Genetic Variation," W. L. Nyhan, Ed., McGraw-Hill, New York, N.Y., 1967, pp. 6–63.
(59) C. A. L. Abrams, L. L. Phillips, C. Berkowitz, P. R. Blackett, and C. J. Priebe, Jr., *J. Am. Med. Assoc., 232,* 1136 (1975).
(60) H. K. Silver, *Pediatrics, 20,* 998 (1957).
(61) Committee on Fetus and Newborn, American Academy of Pediatrics, *Pediatrics, 28,* 674 (1961).
(62) H. K. Silver, *Pediatrics, 20,* 997 (1957).
(63) C. C. Fischer and M. A. Whiteman, *J. Pediatr., 55,* 118 (1959).
(64) V. C. Vaughn III, R. B. Dienst, C. R. Sheffield, and R. W. Roberts, *J. Pediatr., 61,* 547 (1962).

Product[a] (Manufacturer)	Calories per 30 ml	Calories per 100 ml	Protein, g/100 ml	Fat, g/100 ml	Carbo-hydrate, g/100 ml	Sodium, mEq/100 ml	Potas-sium, mEq/100 ml	Chloride, mEq/100 ml	Calcium, mg/100 ml	Phos-phorus, mg/100 ml
Standard Formulas										
Advance (Ross)	16	54	2.0	2.7	5.5	1.3	2.2	1.6	51.0	39.0
Breast Milk	22	75	1.1	4.5	6.8	0.7	1.3	1.1	33.6	16.0
Cow's Milk, whole, fortified	21	69	3.5	3.5	4.9	2.5	3.6	2.7	120.0	96.0
Evaporated Milk, diluted 1:1, fortified	21	69	3.5	4.0	4.9	2.8	3.9	3.2	134.6	102.5
Goat's Milk, fresh	21	69	3.6	4.0	4.6	1.4	4.6	4.5	128.0	104.9
Enfamil (Mead Johnson)	20	66	1.5	3.7	7.0	1.2	1.8	1.5	55.0	46.0
Enfamil with Iron (Mead Johnson)	20	66	1.5	3.7	7.0	1.2	1.8	1.5	55.0	46.0
Similac (Ross)	20	68	1.55	3.6	7.23	1.1	2.0	1.5	51.0	39.0
Similac with Iron (Ross)	20	68	1.55	3.6	7.23	1.1	2.0	1.5	51.0	39.0
SMA Improved (Wyeth)	20	68	1.5	3.6	6.9	6.5	1.4	1.0	44.0	33.0
Therapeutic Formulas										
Milk Allergy										
Isomil (Ross)	20	68	2.0	3.6	6.80	1.3	1.8	1.5	70.0	50.0
i-Soyalac (Loma Linda)	20	66	2.1	3.75	6.65	1.8	1.9	2.6	63.4	52.8
Meat Base Formula (1:1 dilution) (Gerber)	20	65	2.8	3.3	6.2	0.8	1.0	0.6	98	65.0
Mull-Soy (Syntex)	20	66	3.1	3.6	5.2	1.6	4.0	1.6	120.0	78.2
Neo-Mull-Soy (Syntex)	20	66	1.8	3.5	6.4	1.7	2.5	0.6	84.0	41.0
Nursoy (Wyeth)	20	67.6	2.3	3.6	6.8	0.87	1.9	1.0	63	44
Nutramigen (Mead Johnson)	20	66	2.2	2.6	8.8	1.4	1.7	1.3	63	47
Pro-Sobee (Mead Johnson)	20	66	2.5	3.4	6.8	1.8	1.9	1.2	79	53
Soyalac (Loma Linda)	20	66	2.1	3.8	6.65	—	2.0	1.3	63.4	52.8
Electroylte Imbalance										
Lytren (Mead Johnson)	9	30	none	none	7.6	3.0	2.5	2.5	7.9	8.6
Pedialyte (Ross)	6	20	none	none	5.0	3.0	2.0	3.0	8.0	none
Medium Chain Triglyceride Requirement										
Portagen (Mead Johnson)	20	66	2.4	3.2	7.8	1.4	3.2	1.6	63.0	47
Carbohydrate and/or Fat Restriction										
CHO-Free Formula Base (Syntex)	12	40	1.8	3.5	0.02	1.6	2.2	0.6	87.0	66.9
Pregestimil (Mead Johnson)	20	66	2.2	2.8	8.8	1.4	1.7	1.3	63	47
Skim milk, fortified, market average	11	36	3.6	trace	5.3	2.3	3.6	3.0	122.7	98.0
High Protein and/or Caloric Requirement										
Premature Formula (Mead Johnson)	24	81	2.2	4.1	9.2	1.4	2.3	1.9	127	63
Probana (Mead Johnson)	20	66	4.2	2.2	7.9	2.7	3.1	2.1	116	89
Similac PM 60/40 (Ross)	20	68	1.58	3.5	68.8	0.7	1.5	0.7	40.0	20.0
Sodium Restriction										
Lonalac (Mead Johnson)	20	66	2.2	2.7	8.8	1.4	1.7	1.3	63	47
Phenylketonuria										
Lofenalac (Mead Johnson) (℞)	20	66	3.4	3.5	4.8	0.1	2.6	1.7	113.2	103.3

[a] Values are based on ready-to-use strength and were obtained with cooperation of the Dietary Service, Shands Hospital, Gainesville, Florida, and manufacturers.

Iron, mg/ 100 ml	Type of Carbohydrate	Source of Protein	Type of Fat	Vit. A, IU/ liter	Vit. D, IU/ liter	Thiamine, mg/liter	Niacin[b] (Equivalent), mg/liter	Ascorbic Acid, mg/liter
1.2	corn syrup, lactose	cow's milk, soy protein	soy, corn oils	2,400	400	0.75	10.0	50
0.15	lactose	human milk	human milk fat	2,400	5	0.16	3.5	8
0.05	lactose	cow's milk	butterfat	1,850	400	0.29	1.0	10
0.05	lactose	cow's milk	butterfat	1,850	400	0.20	1.0	7
0.1	lactose	goat's milk	goat's milk fat	2,074	24	0.40	1.9	15
trace	lactose	cow's milk	soy, coconut oils	1,690	420	0.5	8.0	54
1.2	lactose	cow's milk	soy, coconut oils	1,690	420	0.5	8.0	54
trace	lactose	cow's milk	soy, coconut oils	2,500	400	0.65	7.0	55
1.2	lactose	cow's milk	soy, coconut oils	2,500	400	0.65	7.0	55
1.3	lactose	demineralized whey	safflower oil (blend), soy, coconut oils	2,640	423	0.71	10.1	58
1.2	sucrose, corn syrup	soy protein	soy, coconut oils	2,500	400	0.40	9.0	55
1.6	sucrose	soy	soy oil	2,113	423	0.53	8.5	63
1.37	sucrose, modified tapioca starch	beef heart	sesame, beef fat	1,740	460	0.60	7.2	59
0.5	sucrose, inverted sucrose	soy	soy oil	2,000	400	0.53	9.5	42
0.8	sucrose	soy isolate	soy oil	2,000	400	0.50	7.0	50
1.3	sucrose, corn syrup	soy isolate	safflower oil (blend)	2,640	420	7.1	10.0	58
1.2	sucrose, arrowroot starch	hydrolyzed casein	corn oil	1,690	420	0.5	8.0	54
1.2	sucrose, corn syrup solids	soy isolate	soy oil	1,690	420	0.5	8.0	54
1.6	sucrose, dextrose, maltose, dextrins	soy	soy oil	2,113	423	0.53	8.5	63
none	corn syrup solids, glucose	none	none	none	none	none	none	none
none	dextrose	none	none	none	none	none	none	none
1.2	corn syrup solids, sucrose	casein	corn, MCT[c] oils	5,285	528	1.1	13.7	54
0.8	none	soy	soy oil	2,000	400	0.50	7.0	52
1.2	glucose, tapioca starch	hydrolyzed casein	corn, MCT[c] oils	2,000	400	0.60	8.0	52
trace	lactose	cow's milk	none	4,167	400	0.40	trace	19
trace	lactose, sucrose	cow's milk	MCT[c], coconut, corn oils	2,029	507	0.6	10.1	65
trace	dextrose, lactose	cow's milk, casein hydrolysate	butterfat, corn oil	5,285	1,057	0.60	8.0	54
0.26	lactose	demineralized whey, casein	corn, coconut oils	2,500	400	0.65	7.3	55
trace	lactose	casein	coconut oil	960	none	0.42	0.8	none
1.2	corn syrup, tapioca starch	hydrolyzed casein	corn oil	2,000	400	0.60	8.0	52

[b] See Table 1 for explanation of niacin equivalent.
[c] MCT = medium-chain triglycerides.

Weight Control Products

Glenn D. Appelt

Chapter 13

Questions to Ask the Patient

What are your age, height, and weight?

How long have you had a weight problem?

Is there a family history of obesity?

Do you tend to eat excessively when you are anxious or nervous?

Have you consulted a physician about the problem?

Are you following a diet?

What diet preparations have you used previously? Were they effective?

What attempts at behavioral modification have you made in an effort to lose weight? Do you belong to a self-help group, such as Weight Watchers?

Do you have a regular exercise program?

Are you being treated for any chronic disease, such as hypertension or diabetes?

What medication(s) are you currently taking?

Obesity is the pathological accumulation of fat in excess of that needed for normal body functioning (1). From a practical viewpoint, obesity may be defined as the physical state where body weight in relation to height is more than 20% above the ideal (Table 1) (2), caused by caloric intake exceeding caloric expenditure. Although "obesity" often is associated with "overweight," the terms are not interchangeable. Athletes, for example, may be overweight but not obese. Daily caloric allowances for persons with moderate physical activity vary with age and sex (3). Values for males (weight, 70 kg; height, 1.78 m) in a temperate climate range from 3200 cal at age 25 to 2550 cal at age 65. Corresponding figures for females (weight, 58 kg; height, 1.63 m) are 2300 and 1800 cal. The values for women increase slightly (300 cal) during pregnancy and significantly (1000 cal) during lactation.

It takes 3500 excess calories to result in 0.454 kg (1 lb.) of fat. Most obesity cases involve overeating, particularly of carbohydrates or fats. The calories ingested beyond those necessary for normal energy requirements usually are deposited and stored as fat. Because the lack of food is rarely a problem in the United States, Americans must decide how much and what type of food to consume. Apparently, many make unwise choices, since obesity is a chronic American affliction. Some researchers estimate that 35% of Americans are overweight by accepted standards (4).

CLINICAL CONSIDERATIONS

Obesity in individuals is a subject of intense study. Many factors enter into the concept of metabolic equilibrium. Appetite control is only part of the answer. Since overeating leading to obesity may result from psychological components, often self-therapy groups help in treating the cause, while pharmacological agents tend to treat only the symptoms.

Etiology of Obesity

The question of why individuals ingest more calories than they expend is complex. The answer may be related to physiological, genetic, environmental, or psychological factors. A possible physiological factor, endocrine disorders, apparently is rarely involved in obesity. Obesity may result from an anatomical or biochemical lesion in the brain's feeding centers, although this hypothesis is not proven in humans (5). Another theory suggests that in the obese person there is a deficiency of an enzyme responsible for α-glycerophosphate oxidation, resulting in increased availability of this substrate for triglyceride synthesis (6). A recent hypothesis holds that prostaglandins are involved in the development of obesity through an effect on lipogenesis (7). Prostaglandin overproduction in the adipose cells may result in increased fat tissue.

Some researchers believe that thin and obese people differ in the degree of thermogenesis after food ingestion (8). Overeating in nonobese subjects causes increased heat production, which tends to dissipate the excess calories. In obese subjects, thermal energy dissipation is less pronounced, resulting in fat storage. The thermogenesis theory has been expanded to include a specialized form of fat tissue (brown fat) which functions in thermogenesis. The role of brown fat is unclear, but it appears to favor increased triglyceride hydrolysis (9).

Another hypothesis relates infantile obesity to excess fat cells during infancy that predispose the individual to obesity later in life (10). Obese patients have not only

Table 1. Desirable Weights for Adults

Height (in Shoes)[a]	Weight (in Indoor Clothing), lbs Small Frame	Medium Frame	Large Frame
Men			
5 ft 2 in	112–120	118–129	126–141
5 ft 3 in	115–123	121–133	129–144
5 ft 4 in	118–126	124–136	132–148
5 ft 5 in	121–129	127–139	135–152
5 ft 6 in	124–133	130–143	138–156
5 ft 7 in	128–137	134–147	142–161
5 ft 8 in	132–141	138–152	147–166
5 ft 9 in	136–145	142–156	151–170
5 ft 10 in	140–150	146–160	155–174
5 ft 11 in	144–154	150–165	159–179
6 ft 0 in	148–158	154–170	164–184
6 ft 1 in	152–162	158–175	168–189
6 ft 2 in	156–167	162–180	173–194
6 ft 3 in	160–171	167–185	177–199
6 ft 4 in	164–175	172–190	182–204
Women			
4 ft 10 in	92–98	96–107	104–119
4 ft 11 in	94–101	98–110	106–122
5 ft 0 in	96–104	101–113	109–124
5 ft 1 in	99–107	104–116	112–128
5 ft 2 in	102–110	107–119	115–131
5 ft 3 in	105–113	110–122	118–134
5 ft 4 in	108–116	113–126	121–138
5 ft 5 in	111–119	116–130	125–142
5 ft 6 in	114–123	120–135	129–146
5 ft 7 in	118–127	124–139	133–150
5 ft 8 in	122–131	128–143	137–154
5 ft 9 in	126–135	132–147	141–158
5 ft 10 in	130–140	136–151	145–163
5 ft 11 in	134–144	140–155	149–168
6 ft 0 in	138–148	144–159	153–174

For adults 25 years and older; prepared by the Metropolitan Life Insurance Company, derived primarily from data of the Build and Blood Pressure Study, 1959.
[a] Based on 1-inch heels for men and 2-inch heels for women.

ideal weights

causes of obesity

environmental and psychogenic factors

role of hypothalamus

larger than normal fat cells but also an increased number of these cells. Apparently, as people lose weight on a low-calorie diet, the size of each fat cell decreases, but the total number of fat cells remains the same; when people return to increased weight levels, the fat cells regain their original size. Obesity in children may result from new fat cells, whereas "adult onset obesity" may represent an expansion of fat cells already present (11). Some experiments suggest that the earlier the onset of obesity, the greater the number of fat cells (12). After the age of 20, obesity is caused almost exclusively by the expansion of existent cells. Accordingly, an overweight child or adolescent may be more susceptible to obesity as an adult.

A child who has one obese parent has a 40% chance of being obese; if both parents are obese, there is an 80% possibility (13). These data suggest a direct genetic component, and although it has not been proven in human obesity, animal studies indicate this relationship (14). In experimental animals, genetic transmission of obesity is associated with modified organ size and composition (15, 16). Human data suggest fundamental relationships between body build and obesity (17, 18). These studies reveal that obese women differ from nonobese women in a morphological characteristic other than the degree of adiposity. Obese women were more endomorphic than nonobese women; i.e., abdomen mass overshadowed thoracic bulk; all regions were notable for their softness and roundness; and the hands and the feet were relatively small.

Obesity may result from environmental influence, such as the widespread advertising of food products. Occupational, economic, and sociocultural concepts also may be considered in the broad environmental sense. It now appears that socioeconomic status and related social factors are important in obesity's development. Obesity is seven times more common among women of low socioeconomic groups than among those of high-level groups (19). The mental health indexes of the obese subjects in the low socioeconomic group reflected "immaturity," "rigidity," and "suspiciousness" in comparison with those of average weight individuals in the same group. A defect in impulse control might be suspected by the high "immaturity" rating. Obesity was more prevalent in young females of lower socioeconomic status than in those of upper socioeconomic status (20). Another study confirmed the greater incidence of obesity among women of low socioeconomic status and found a similar but less marked trend in men. In addition, suggestive relationships between ethnic and religious factors and obesity were found for both sexes (21).

Obesity has a psychogenic component in 90% of the cases (22). Although the psychological aspect of caloric excess usually is exemplified by compulsive overeating replacing other gratifications, other factors are involved. Obesity may be related to physical activity and emotions (23). Decreased physical activity may play a role in the development and maintenance of obesity. This theory involves the aspect of caloric expenditure rather than caloric ingestion and stresses the function of caloric disequilibrium in obesity. Mental depression may not be a purely incidental occurrence in obese people but rather one of the main reasons for the obesity (23). Another psychological aberration in obese patients is the disturbance in body image, where the body is viewed as "grotesque and loathsome" (24).

Appetite Control

The hypothalamus apparently contains centers that are intimately involved in the food ingestion process. Studies in rats show a "satiety center" and an "appetite center" located in the hypothalamic region (25). Destroying the satiety center leads to marked overeating with subsequent obesity; conversely, obliterating the appetite center results in emaciation. These results indicate that there may be a feedback inhibition of the appetite center by impulses from the satiety center after food is ingested. The glucostatic hypothesis of appetite regulation states that hunger is related to the degree that glucose is used by cells called "glucostats" (26). When glucose utilization by glucostats in the satiety center is low, the inhibitory effect on the appetite center is reduced, favoring eating behavior. Conversely, when glucose utilization is high, the appetite center is inhibited, and the desire for food intake is reduced.

The hypothalamus contains high concentrations of noradrenergic terminals (27). A discrete fiber system that supplies the hypothalamus with most of its norepinephrine-secreting terminals is called the "ventral noradrenergic bundle." Destroying the noradrenergic terminals in the hypothalamus or damaging the ventral noradrenergic bundle results in obesity in animals (28). It is suggested that this noradrenergic bundle normally mediates satiety and that it may serve as a substrate for amphetamine-induced appetite loss (29).

The interpretation of visual and chemical food-related stimuli occurs in the cerebral cortex, and acceptance or rejection of the sight, aroma, or taste of foods involves this area of the CNS. An obese person may respond differently from people of normal weight to the appearance, taste, and sight of food (30). Research involving the trigeminal nerve, a pathway relaying sensory input from the oral cavity to the hypothalamus, indicates this system's possible role in food intake. The trigeminal circuit is a system of oral touch, and the excessive nibbling common to obese individuals may be due to their greater sensitivity to this stimulus (31).

Role of Obesity in Other Conditions

Studies show a significant association between early mortality and obesity. Cardiovascular diseases account for many early deaths (32). There is evidence that sustained hypertension is more common in overweight people, although the correlation between blood pressure and adiposity is weak (33). However, there appears to be a definite relationship between obesity and hypertension, and it seems reasonable to suggest that high-risk people (e.g., those with a positive family history of youthful obesity) should reduce salt intake (34). If a patient cannot control obesity by any reasonable means, the pharmacist may recommend salt intake reduction. Weight reduction due to water loss by reduced sodium intake may be of psychological benefit; however, it should be stressed that this weight loss is not relevant to effects on adipocytes. Vascular change and cerebrovascular disease have been associated with obesity (35, 36).

The relationship between obesity and diabetes mellitus is clear-cut (32). An early study revealed that 85% of those over 40 who developed diabetes mellitus were overweight (37). Glucose intolerance commonly occurs with obesity, and relative insulin resistance is noted in obese subjects (38, 39). The hyperinsulinemia that occurs in obesity is related to increased body fat (see Chapter 11) (40). Weight reduction results in improved glucose tolerance in the obese diabetic and reduced hyperinsulinemia in both nondiabetic and diabetic obese persons (41, 42). The severity of diabetes mellitus and the need for medication often may be decreased by weight reduction.

In addition to the correlations of obesity with these disease states, obesity results in higher death rates in nephritis, pneumonia, cirrhosis, biliary disease, appendicitis, postoperative complications, and accidents (43). Obesity also may be related to cholesterol gallstone formation, since the level of this compound is characteristically elevated in obesity (44).

Hyperostosis of the spine (formation of bony bridges between the vertebrae) has been associated with hyperglycemia and obesity, although these factors are at least partly independent of each other (45). Excess obesity may contribute to respiratory stress. Obesity alters pulmonary function resulting in plethora, reduced lung volume, hypercapnia, and pulmonary hypertension (46). The description by Charles Dickens of Joe (the fat boy) in *The Pickwick Papers* reveals a person with marked obesity and somnolence. This description may be the first account of this condition in the literature; the "Pickwickian syndrome" describes a person who is obese, exhibits narcoleptic behavior, and has an excessive appetite (47).

Although obesity generally denotes overeating, it may not always denote overnourishment. Obesity may mask malnutrition due to overusing carbohydrate at the expense of deleting essential factors such as protein, vitamins, and minerals (48).

glucostatic hypothesis

relation to cardiovascular disease and diabetes

therapy

Signs and Symptoms of Obesity

Common patient complaints regarding obesity are often cosmetic, involving a desire to "look slim." Remarks such as "I can't tie my shoes without getting out of breath" indicate actual physical discomfort. The obese patient may complain of persistent backache and varicose veins.

Because obesity may be caused by the inactivity resulting from mental depression, patients who remain obese after prolonged self-medication with OTC obesity control products should be referred to a physician (20). A psychogenic component involving inactivity due to depression or a compulsive anxiety reaction related to repeated "snacking" may be involved in such cases. The pharmacist should emphasize that weight loss will not occur unless caloric disequilibrium is corrected. Chronic use of OTC drugs to correct obesity may indicate a more severe underlying problem.

TREATMENT

Drug treatment of obesity is of limited value (49). Amphetamines have been prescribed for obesity. Amphetamine and related drugs are thought to suppress appetite by an effect on the appetite centers in the hypothalamus (50). Unfortunately, tolerance develops to amphetamine's appetite-suppressant activity, making long-term use undesirable. Because overeating seems to be controlled primarily by psychological behavioral factors, overeating will occur as soon as the anorexigenic effects disappear. Amphetamine and related drugs have the potential for abuse and dependence, and their value is limited to short-term use in obesity control as an adjunct to a controlled diet.

Human chorionic gonadotropin has been used by some clinicians in treating obesity. However, its effectiveness has not been established (38).

Dietary management through proper guidance and patient motivation are essential to any weight reduction program. The first few months of a weight reduction program seem to be the most successful, possibly because patients are willing to subject themselves to self-discipline.

Ingredients in OTC Products

OTC obesity control products are represented by phenylpropanolamine (a drug that may act similarly to amphetamine), bulk producers such as methylcellulose, and benzocaine (a local anesthetic). It is reasonable to expect weight loss in an individual taking OTC weight reduction drugs or other substances such as carbohydrate dietary aids, if the overall calorie intake is reduced so that caloric expenditure is greater. Whether the agent is pharmacologically active or a placebo, if it assists the patient in accomplishing this goal, weight will be lost.

components of weight control products, their mechanisms, side effects, and interactions

cellulose derivatives

Phenylpropanolamine

Phenylpropanolamine is a sympathomimetic agent related chemically and pharmacologically to ephedrine and amphetamine. It acts as an indirect sympathomimetic, exerting more prominent peripheral adrenergic effects compared to weak central stimulant actions (51). In the past, controversy has existed as to phenylpropanolamine's effectiveness as an anorexigenic agent (52). Early animal studies indicated its usefulness in diminishing food intake in animals (53, 54). Later clinical studies indicated a possible appetite-suppressant activity. Results from one double-blind experiment indicated that phenylpropanolamine (25 mg), taken 30 minutes before lunch, reduced intake of a liquid diet (55). In another double-blind study, subjects taking the same dosage reported a significant reduction in the size of supper and the number of snacks (56). A double-blind clinical evaluation of a phenylpropanolamine/caffeine/vitamin combination compared to a placebo and diet showed a significantly greater weight loss by patients on a 1200-cal diet over a 4-week period (57).

All authorities, however, do not agree on the effectiveness of phenylpropanolamine as an anorexigenic agent. The *AMA Drug Evaluations* states (58), "This agent is probably ineffective in the dose provided (25 mg)." A basic pharmacology textbook states that the drug is ineffective as an appetite suppressant (59). In addition, no mention of its use in obesity is made in a standard pharmacy reference (51). However, in recent deliberations an FDA advisory panel approved phenylpropanolamine as safe and effective when used for up to about 12 weeks as an adjunct in weight reduction. This action reverses previous opinions voiced by this agency (60).

Potential Side Effects

Amphetamine and related prescription drugs apparently depress appetite by stimulating the satiety center in the hypothalamic ventromedial nucleus. This process may occur indirectly on the frontal lobes of the cortex (61). Although phenylpropanolamine's effects on the cardiovascular system and CNS are not as strong as those of amphetamine, side effects may occur, particularly if the recommended dosage is exceeded. Nervousness, restlessness, insomnia, headache, nausea, and excessive rise in blood pressure are some of phenylpropanolamine's adverse effects (51). Recent evidence suggests that phenylpropanolamine may reduce vitamin A levels in experimental animals (63). Various adverse reactions of the cardiovascular system have been reported, and the label on products containing phenylpropanolamine warns against exceeding 25 mg three times per day (62, 64–67).

Although the FDA OTC Panel on Cold, Cough, Allergy, Bronchodilator, and Antiasthmatic Products was not reviewing anorectics as such (68), it concluded that nervousness, insomnia, motor restlessness, and nausea may occur with phenylpropanolamine doses of 50 mg every 3 hours. However, these side effects occur almost as often with a placebo. A dose of 25–30 mg every 4 hours, not to exceed 150 mg in 24 hours, is considered safe.

Because phenylpropanolamine is an adrenergic substance, it may elevate blood glucose levels and produce cardiac stimulation. For these reasons the labels on products containing this drug warn that individuals with diabetes mellitus, heart disease, hypertension, or thyroid disease should seek medical advice before taking the drug.

Drug Interactions

Many drug interactions with adrenergic agents are theoretically possible, but clinically, phenylpropanolamine has been implicated only in interactions with monoamine oxidase inhibitors (69–71). Severe hypertensive episodes may be more likely when preparations containing phenylpropanolamine in a free form, rather than in a slow-release form, are ingested by patients taking monoamine oxidase inhibitors concurrently (70, 71). There is one report of a positive phentolamine pheochromocytoma test in hypertension induced by phenylpropanolamine (72). Reserpine and guanethidine may interfere with actions of phenylpropanolamine (51). Some OTC products contain caffeine and phenylpropanolamine; the possibility of an additive effect with these two cardiac stimulants should be considered (65).

Bulk Producers

Typical examples of bulk producers are methylcellulose, carboxymethylcellulose, psyllium hydrophilic mucilloid, agar, and karaya gum. It has been suggested that the bulk-producing activity produces a sense of fullness, reducing the desire to eat. The usefulness of the bulk-forming agents as appetite suppressants in controlling obesity has not been established (73). A radiographic study shows that a methylcellulose mass is almost entirely gone from the stomach in 30 minutes. In addition, intestinal peristalsis is increased following the rapid gastric emptying (74). Neither bulk production by methylcellulose nor gastric transport rate increase offers a mechanism to produce satiety. No experimental evidence exists to support an appetite-suppressant claim. Bulk-producing substances have been approved for dietary use by the FDA (75).

It is assumed that the benefit of bulk producers in obesity control is related to caloric intake reduction, irrespective of the ingestion of the bulk producer. Bulk producers probably are no more effective than a low-calorie, high-residue diet in a weight reduction program. Moreover, their laxative effect may not always be desirable. There is some danger of esophageal obstruction with methylcellulose wafers, and it is recommended that generous amounts of water accompany the ingestion of the bulk producers to minimize this danger (73). Drugs with anticholinergic properties reduce bowel motility, and using these drugs concurrently with bulk producers may be hazardous because they may produce blockage.

Benzocaine

Benzocaine was first incorporated into a weight control preparation in 1958 (76). A preparation containing benzocaine and methylcellulose in chewing gum wafers was tried for 10 weeks in 50 patients who were 5.5–46 kg overweight. The patients were instructed to chew one or two wafers, then to drink a glass of water, just before meals. They also were placed on low-calorie diets and were directed to chew the gum every 4 hours if there was a strong desire to eat. Results showed that 90% of the subjects lost weight. However, the study was not placebo controlled, and the weight loss could have been caused by the benzocaine, the methylcellulose, or the diet itself. The benzocaine dose used was small, and any marked degree of numbness in the oral cavity was questionable. It is conceivable that subtle effects on taste sensitivity or taste modification occur and that perceived analgesia or numbness is not necessary for possible appetite-suppressant activity. Obese persons may be more sensitive to taste stimuli (31).

Constant "snacking" is characteristic of the "oral syndrome" in many obese persons. A nontraditional appetite control plan using benzocaine, glucose, caffeine, and vitamins in a hard candy form was tried (76). The subjects ingested the candies when they wanted a snack and before and after meals. The purpose of this approach was to keep the patients orally active and at the same time elevate their blood glucose levels. Benzocaine's influence was considered to be a requisite for "meaningful losses" in this study.

side effects of bulk producers

anesthetics

Capsules or tablets containing benzocaine are designed to be swallowed, and hence the drug does not come into contact with the oral cavity. Any appetite suppression would depend on an effect on the GI mucosa. There are no conclusive clinical data to support such an activity.

Although they are rare, cyanotic reactions have been reported following benzocaine administration (77). Methemoglobinemia in infants also has been reported (78–81). These reactions refer mainly to infants and therefore are

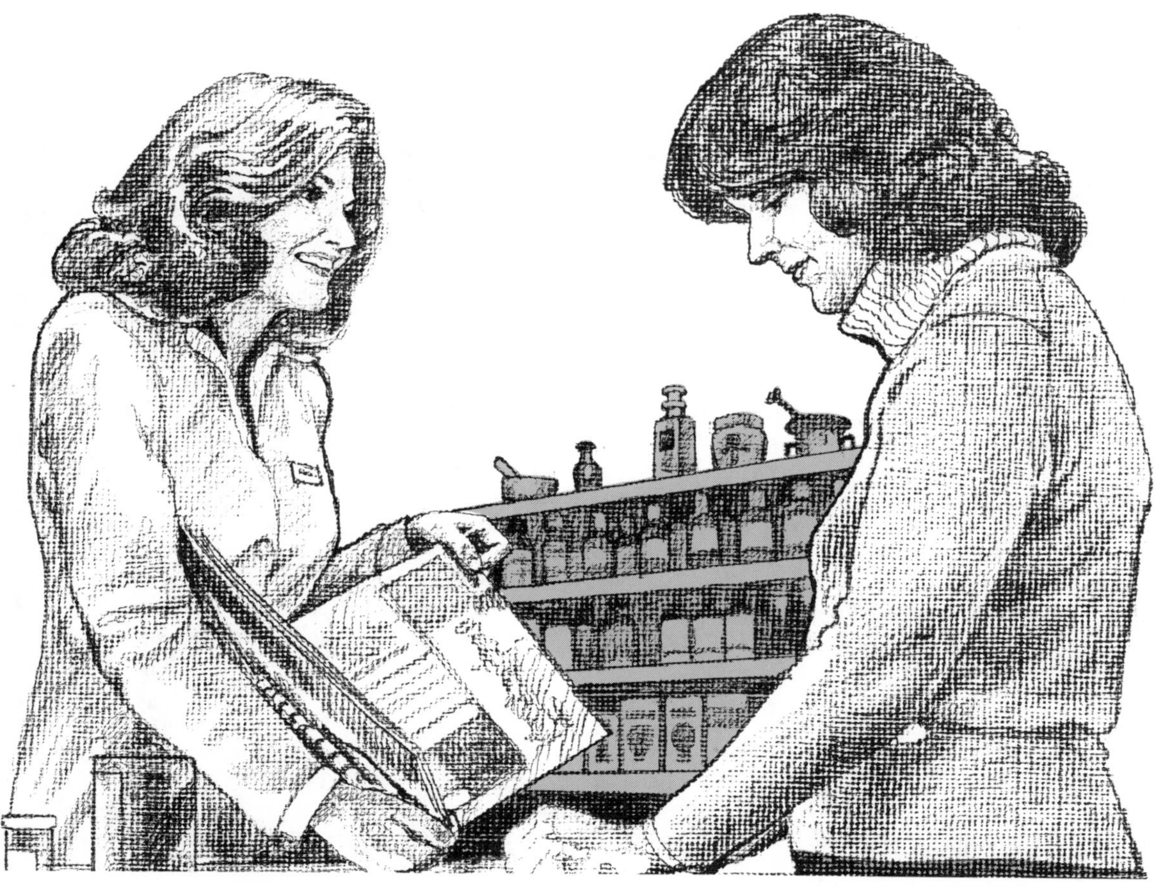

not specifically relevant to the drug's use in the noninfant obese population. It is important, however, to be aware of potential benzocaine toxicity. A fatal anaphylactic reaction occurred in an adult a few minutes after the ingestion of a throat lozenge containing benzocaine (82). Obese persons taking preparations containing benzocaine over long periods may expose themselves to the consequences of drug-induced sensitivity. Also, there are no conclusive data to support benzocaine's appetite-suppressant effect.

Other Products

Dietary aids such as carbohydrate "candy" type foods and low-calorie nutritionally balanced liquids are not considered drugs but are available as adjuncts in a weight reduction program. In addition, synthetic sweeteners such as saccharin may be valuable in reducing excess sugar consumption and thus lowering caloric intake.

dietary aids
canned diets
saccharin
xylitol
aspartame

Glucose

Preparations containing glucose and vitamins are claimed to elevate blood glucose levels when taken before meals or at snack time, so that the satiety center exerts an inhibitory influence on the appetite center. This assertion, however, is questionable. A clinical study reported that a glucose load (50 g) taken 20 minutes before lunch depressed caloric intake relative to control load at lunch ($p < 0.01$) (83). Reactions to a glucose load's oral qualities may constitute the principal factor in the first 20 minutes rather than GI or postabsorptive effects on satiety. However, the efficacy of glucose in long-term weight control programs has not been established.

Low-Calorie Balanced Foods

The "canned diet" products are considered substitutes for the usual diet. One product typical of this group supplies 70 g of protein per day, an amount the manufacturer states "is the recommended daily dietary allowance of protein for normal adults." It also contains 20 g of fat and 110 g of carbohydrate in a daily ration. Powder, granule, and liquid forms are available, and these products are also formulated as cookies and soups.

These dietary foods are low in sodium. Weight loss in the first 2 weeks is probably caused, in part, by water loss from the tissues. Whether a weight loss over a short period is significant with regard to the effective long-term treatment of obesity is somewhat questionable.

The pharmacist should be aware that products that substitute 900 cal/day for the usual diet are usually effective in reducing weight. Moreover, it appears that any diet of 900 cal that supplies adequate protein and lower carbohydrate and fat intake should enable an obese patient to lose weight.

Artificial Sweeteners

Sucrose overuse is common. A sucrose substitute, saccharin, provides no calories and may allow significant calorie reduction in certain patients. Saccharin is about 400 times more potent than sucrose as a sweetener. It produces a bitter taste in some individuals, and it is not heat stable; nevertheless, it is the most popular artificial sweetener, especially since the prohibition of nonregulated use of cyclamates. Saccharin may have considerable importance in reducing caloric intake for some persons. For instance, if saccharin is used to sweeten a cup of coffee instead of 1 tsp of sugar, 33 cal are removed from the diet. In 1972, bladder tumors were discovered in rats fed saccharin in utero and throughout life. The FDA then removed saccharin from the list of food additives generally recognized as safe. Saccharin is presently permitted in products labeled specifically as diet foods or beverages. It may accumulate in fetal tissues and should not be used during pregnancy (84). As of June 1, 1978, pharmacies carrying saccharin-containing OTC products are required to display posters containing the following warning statement (85):

> SACCHARIN NOTICE. This store sells food including diet beverages and dietetic foods that contain saccharin. You will find saccharin listed in the ingredient statement on most foods which contain it. All foods which contain saccharin will soon bear the following warning: Use of this product may be hazardous to your health. This product contains saccharin, which has been determined to cause cancer in laboratory animals. This store is required by law to display this notice prominently.

In November 1977 an 18-month moratorium was imposed on any regulatory action by the FDA against the use of saccharin in foods. Several studies, including one by the National Cancer Institute and one by the National Academy of Sciences, are currently in progress to determine whether or not there is a relationship between human bladder cancer and saccharin.

As alternatives to saccharin, two sugar alcohols are being tested to determine their suitability as sucrose substitutes. Sorbitol is about 60% as sweet as sucrose, whereas xylitol (birch sugar) is about 100% as sweet as sucrose. Certain advantages tend to accrue, since apparently neither of these products causes tooth decay and some xylitol products have a more pleasing taste (86). However, some evidence implicates xylitol in the development of bladder tumors in mice. Further tests are under way to evaluate this possibility. As a result, xylitol use is declining. Ingesting sufficient amounts of dietetic candies containing sorbitol may result in an osmotic catharsis in small children (87).

Aspartame is a synthetic dipeptide about 180 times as sweet as sugar. The manufacturer suspended testing this compound after a metabolite of aspartame was reported to produce uterine polyps in rats.

Dosage Forms

OTC products for obesity control are available as liquids, powders, granules, tablets, capsules, sustained-release capsules, wafers, cookies, soups, chewing gum, and candy preparations. If candy cubes, wafers, or chewing gum are substituted for high-calorie desserts or "snacks," the confectionogenic nature of the dosage form may offer patients a psychological aid that is not found when a standard tablet or capsule is used. Ingesting large quantities of diet candy would, of course, contribute significantly to caloric intake.

Adjunctive Therapy

Some cases of obesity may be treated by dieting. The pharmacist should make sure that any diet is being followed under a physician's supervision. Patients having difficulty losing weight may find reinforcement in self-help groups and behavior modification.

Diet

Diets in the 800 to 1000-cal/day range are used frequently in weight reduction programs. Total fasting or semistarvation sometimes is proposed as a means of weight reduction in grossly obese persons (88, 89). Starvation, either total or partial, depletes the body of lean tissue and essential electrolytes in addition to fat (90). The ketosis and ketoacidosis of a fasting state reflect a metabolic alteration. If total fasting is employed as a means of treating obesity, hospitalization is recommended so as to deal effectively with mood changes or alteration of physiological functions such as cardiac arrhythmias (91). "Crash" diets involving 500 cal/day for 4–8 weeks have been implicated in scalp hair loss (92). This effect apparently reflects the trauma of semistarvation.

The extent of injuries and deaths due to the use of extremely low calorie protein diets is unclear. However, it is apparent that studies oriented toward geographical incidence, concurrent pathology, age, and other factors need careful scrutiny. The complaints reported to the FDA frequently include nausea, vomiting, diarrhea (liquid preparations), constipation (dry preparations), faintness, muscle cramps, weakness or fatigue, irritability, cold intolerance, decreased libido, amenorrhea, hair loss, skin dryness, cardiac arrhythmias, gout recurrence, dehydration, and hypokalemia (93). The Commissioner of Food and Drugs has proposed that the following warning labeling be attached to protein supplements (94):

> Warning: Very low calorie protein diets may cause serious illness or death. DO NOT USE FOR WEIGHT REDUCTION OR MAINTENANCE WITHOUT MEDICAL SUPERVISION. Do not use for any purpose without medical advice if you are taking medication. Not for use by infants, children, or pregnant or nursing women.

It is also pertinent to point out the possibility of drug–"food" interactions with low-calorie protein diets. Patients taking prescription drugs such as diuretics, antihypertensive drugs, hypoglycemic agents, insulin, adrenergic medications, high doses of corticosteroids, thyroid preparations other than those used in replacement therapy, and lithium therapy should not use the liquid protein diet.

The pharmacist should warn the patient not to undertake this type of diet approach without medical supervision. The patient's age also should be taken into consideration, since elderly obese persons may be more susceptible to cardiovascular stress and gout, usually prevalent in this age group.

Group Therapy

Group therapy and behavior modification sometimes are effective in treating obesity. Groups such as TOPS (Take Off Pounds Sensibly) and Weight Watchers have been successful in the treatment of obesity (95). The group pressure resulting from praise or criticism apparently is an effective deterrent to overeating for many persons. Behavior modification involving eating considered as a "pure" activity, as well as eating more slowly, may be beneficial. In addition, keeping a "diet diary" and using a "unit dose" concept of foods may prove helpful in a weight reduction program. Psychotherapeutic approaches also show promise in helping control obesity (96).

Other (Surgical Intervention)

In refractory cases of gross obesity, intestinal bypass operations have been performed (97). This type of procedure is probably the most hazardous measure used to treat extreme obesity.

PRODUCT SELECTION GUIDELINES

nondrug approaches
protein diets

In recommending an OTC product for weight control, the pharmacist should stress the importance of a diet plan or program. Weight cannot be lost without a concerted effort to change one's eating and exercise life style and maintain it. In light of the pharmacist's role in total health care, emphasis should be placed on alternative means of obesity control. The pharmacist should inquire about previous diet control regimens the patient has attempted so that other OTC diet management programs may be recommended. The pharmacist also may wish to monitor the patient's weight reduction efforts.

As a health care professional, the pharmacist also should emphasize the importance of a rational, low-calorie, balanced diet and proper exercise to correct caloric imbalance, as well as the importance of individual effort in maintaining a diet management program. The patient may be referred to a reinforcing group.

The patient should appreciate the caloric value of various food types. An OTC obesity control product should be considered only as an adjunct to a planned weight reduction program. Vitamins sometimes are added to such products on the assumption that dieting individuals may not have an adequate vitamin intake. This practice may be justified in individual cases but cannot be applied to all patients. Caffeine is included in some preparations, probably in an effort to allay fatigue, a contributing factor that may lead to an impulsive desire to eat.

SUMMARY

The effectiveness of a weight reduction program depends largely on the patient's education and acceptance of the regimen necessary to achieve long-term weight control. A patient should recognize the many facets of a successful weight reduction program, including motivation, physical activity, reduced caloric intake, and possibly a pharmacological "crutch" such as an OTC drug. The role of the pharmacist as a qualified health professional is to supply pertinent and accurate information regarding these matters.

REFERENCES

(1) R. S. Goodhart and M. E. Shils, "Modern Nutrition in Health and Disease," Lea and Febiger, Philadelphia, Pa., 1973, p. 625.
(2) *Metropolitan Life Insurance Company Statistical Bulletin, 47,* 1 (1966).
(3) M. G. Wohl, "Modern Nutrition in Health and Disease," Lea and Febiger, Philadelphia, Pa., 1960, p. 532.
(4) M. G. Wagner, *J. Am. Diet. Assoc., 57,* 311 (1970).
(5) J. Mayer, *Annu. Rev. Med., 14,* 111 (1963).
(6) D. J. Galton, *Br. Med. J., 2,* 1498 (1966).
(7) P. B. Curtis-Prior, *Lancet, 1,* 897 (1975).
(8) D. S. Miller, P. Mumford, and M. J. Stock, *Am. J. Clin. Nutr., 20,* 1223 (1967).
(9) R. E. Smith and B. A. Horowitz, *Physiol. Rev., 49,* 330 (1969).
(10) J. Hirsch and J. L. Knittle, *Fed. Proc., 29,* 1516 (1970).
(11) A. Angel, *Can. Med. Assoc. J., 110,* 540 (1974).
(12) L. B. Salans, S. W. Cushman, and R. E. Weismann, *J. Clin. Invest., 52,* 929 (1973).
(13) S. R. Williams, "Nutrition and Diet Therapy," Mosby, St. Louis, Mo., 1967, p. 477.
(14) J. Mayer, *Bull. N.Y. Acad. Med., 36,* 323 (1960).
(15) K. J. Carpenter and J. Mayer, *Am. J. Physiol., 193,* 449 (1958).
(16) N. B. Marshall, S. B. Andrus, and J. Mayer, *Am. J. Physiol., 189,* 342 (1957).
(17) C. C. Seltzer and J. Mayer, *J. Am. Med. Assoc., 189,* 677 (1964).
(18) C. C. Seltzer and J. Mayer, *J. Am. Diet. Assoc., 55,* 454 (1969).
(19) M. E. Moore, A. Stunkard, and L. Srole, *J. Am. Med. Assoc., 181,* 962 (1962).
(20) A. Stunkard, E. d'Aquili, S. Fox, and R. D. L. Filion, *J. Am. Med. Assoc., 221,* 579 (1972).
(21) P. B. Goldblatt, M. E. Moore, and A. J. Stunkard, *J. Am. Med. Assoc., 192,* 1039 (1965).
(22) "Drugs of Choice 1972–1973," W. Modell, Ed., Mosby, St. Louis, Mo., 1972, p. 285.
(23) A. Stunkard, *Psychosom. Med., 20,* 366 (1958).
(24) A. Stunkard and M. Mendelson, *J. Am. Diet. Assoc., 38,* 328 (1961).
(25) A. W. Hetherington and S. W. Ransom, *Am. J. Physiol., 136,* 609 (1942).
(26) J. Mayer, *Ann. N.Y. Acad. Sci., 63,* 15 (1955).
(27) V. Vngorstedt, *Acta Physiol. Scand. Suppl., 365,* 1 (1971).
(28) J. E. Ahlskog and B. G. Hoebel, *Science, 182,* 166 (1973).
(29) R. M. Gold, *Science, 182,* 488 (1973).
(30) B. G. Hoebel, *Annu. Rev. Physiol., 33,* 533 (1971).
(31) H. P. Ziegler, *Psychology Today,* Aug. 1975, p. 62.
(32) H. H. Marks, *Metabolism, 6,* 417 (1957).
(33) G. V. Mann, *N. Engl. J. Med., 291,* 178 (1974).
(34) J. Stamler, "The Hypertension Handbook," Merck Sharp & Dohme, West Point, Pa., 1974, p. 15.
(35) S. L. Wilens, *Arch. Intern. Med., 79,* 120 (1947).
(36) S. Heyden, C. G. Hames, A. Bartel, J. C. Cassal, H. A. Tyroler, and J. C. Cornoni, *Arch. Intern. Med., 128,* 956 (1971).
(37) G. F. Baker, "Clinic and Metropolitan Life Insurance Co.: Diabetes in the 1940's," New York Metropolitan Life Insurance Co. Press, 1940.
(38) G. V. Mann, *N. Engl. J. Med., 291,* 226 (1974).
(39) S. M. Genuth, *Ann. Intern. Med., 79,* 812 (1973).
(40) A. Z. El-Khodary, M. F. Ball, I. M. Oweiss, and J. J. Canary, *Metabolism, 21,* 641 (1972).
(41) J. H. Karam, G. M. Grodsky, F. C. Pavlatos, and P. H. Forsham, *Lancet, 1,* 286 (1965).
(42) R. S. Yalow et al., *Ann. N.Y. Acad. Sci., 131,* 357 (1965).
(43) "The Merck Manual," 9th ed., Merck and Co., Inc., Rahway, N.J., 1956, p. 324.
(44) "Muir's Textbook of Pathology," 9th ed., D. F. Cappell and J. R. Anderson, Eds., Edward Arnold Ltd., London, England, 1971, p. 587.
(45) H. Julkunen, O. P. Heinonen, and K. Pyörälä, *Ann. Rheum. Dis., 30,* 605 (1971).
(46) R. H. L. Wilson and N. L. Wilson, *J. Am. Diet. Assoc., 55,* 465 (1969).
(47) C. S. Burwell, E. D. Robin, R. D. Whaley, and A. G. Bickelmann, *Am. J. Med., 21,* 811 (1956).
(48) J. Woodsworth, "Diet Revolution," St. Martins Press, New York, N.Y., 1977, p. 66.
(49) *FDA Drug Bulletin* (Dec. 1972).
(50) S. Cole, *Psychol. Bull., 79,* 13 (1973).
(51) "Remington's Pharmaceutical Sciences," 15th ed., A. Osol et al., Eds., Mack, Easton, Pa., 1975, p. 820.
(52) H. I. Silverman, *Am. J. Pharm., 135,* 45 (1963).
(53) M. L. Tainter, *J. Nutr., 27,* 89 (1944).
(54) A. Epstein, *Comp. Physiol. Psychol., 52,* 37 (1959).
(55) B. G. Hoebel, J. Cooper, M. Kamin, and D. Willard, *Obesity Bariatric Med., 4,* 192 (1975).
(56) B. G. Hoebel, J. Krauss, J. Cooper, and D. Willard, *Obesity Bariatric Med., 4,* 200 (1975).
(57) S. I. Griboff, R. Berman, and H. I. Silverman, *Curr. Ther. Res., 17,* 535 (1975).
(58) "AMA Drug Evaluations," 3rd ed., Publishing Sciences Group, Littleton, Mass., 1977, p. 488.
(59) A. Goth, "Medical Pharmacology," 7th ed., Mosby, St. Louis, Mo., 1974, p. 110.
(60) *American Druggist, 178*(3), 3 (1978).
(61) W. C. Bowman, M. J. Rand, and G. B. West, "Textbook of Pharmacology," Blackwell, Oxford, England, 1968, p. 332.
(62) P. R. Salmon, *Br. Med. J., 1,* 193 (1965).
(63) P. B. Acosta and P. J. Garry, *Fed. Proc., 37,* 485 (1978).
(64) S. R. Shapiro, *N. Engl. J. Med., 280,* 1363 (1969).
(65) R. B. Peterson and L. A. Vasquez, *J. Am. Med. Assoc., 223,* 324 (1973).
(66) S. Ostern and W. H. Dodson, *J. Am. Med. Assoc., 194,* 472 (1965).
(67) P. H. Livingston, *J. Am. Med. Assoc., 196,* 1159 (1966).
(68) Summary Minutes of the FDA OTC Panel on Cold, Cough, Allergy, Bronchodilator, and Antiasthmatic Products, Washington, D.C., June 19–20, 1973.
(69) C. M. Tonks and A. T. Lloyd, *Br. Med. J., 1,* 589 (1965).
(70) A. M. S. Mason and R. M. Buckle, *Br. Med. J., 1,* 875 (1969).
(71) M. F. Cuthbert, M. P. Greenberg, and S. W. Morley, *Br. Med. J., 1,* 404 (1969).
(72) F. C. Duvernoy, *N. Engl. J. Med., 280,* 877 (1969).
(73) "The Pharmacological Basis of Therapeutics," 5th ed., L. S. Goodman and A. Gilman, Eds., Macmillan, New York, N.Y., 1975, p. 979.
(74) E. J. Drenick, *J. Am. Med. Assoc., 234,* 271 (1975).
(75) D. C. Fletcher, *J. Am. Med. Assoc., 230,* 901 (1974).
(76) C. W. McLure and C. A. Brusch, *J. Am. Med. Women's Assoc., 28,* 239 (1973).
(77) B. M. Bernstein, *Rev. Gastroenterol., 17,* 123 (1950).
(78) H. de C. Peterson, *N. Engl. J. Med., 263,* 454 (1960).
(79) N. Goluboff and D. J. MacFadyen, *J. Pediatr., 47,* 22 (1955).
(80) J. A. Wolff, *Pediatrics, 20,* 915 (1957).
(81) N. Goluboff, *Pediatrics, 21,* 340 (1958).
(82) D. J. Hesch, *J. Am. Med. Assoc., 172,* 62 (1960).
(83) D. A. Booth, A. T. Campbell, and A. Chase, *Nature, 228,* 1104 (1970).
(84) *The Medical Letter, 17,* 61 (1975).
(85) *Federal Register, 43,* 8793 (1978).
(86) *Pharmacy Times,* p. 25 (Jan. 1977).
(87) J. R. Gryboski, *N. Engl. J. Med., 275,* 718 (1966).
(88) W. L. Bloom, *Metabolism, 8,* 214 (1959).
(89) S. M. Genuth, J. H. Castro, and V. Vertes, *J. Am. Med. Assoc., 230,* 987 (1974).
(90) R. E. Bolinger, B. P. Lukert, R. W. Brown, L. Guevara, and R. Steinberg, *Arch. Intern. Med., 118,* 3 (1966).
(91) I. C. Gilliand, *Postgrad. Med. J., 44,* 58 (1968).
(92) R. B. Odum and D. K. Goette, *J. Am. Med. Assoc., 235,* 476 (1976).
(93) *FDA Drug Bulletin* (Jan.–Feb. 1978).
(94) *Federal Register, 42,* 232 (1977).
(95) A. Stunkard, H. Levine, and S. Fox, *Arch. Intern. Med., 125,* 1067 (1970).
(96) A. Stunkard, *Arch. Gen. Psychiatry, 26,* 391 (1972).
(97) H. F. Conn, "Current Therapy," Saunders, Philadelphia, Pa., 1975, p. 406.

Product (Manufacturer)	Phenylpropanolamine Hydrochloride	Bulk Producer	Other
Anorexin Capsules (Thompson)	25 mg	carboxymethylcellulose sodium, 50 mg	caffeine, 100 mg; vitamin A, 1667 IU; vitamin D, 133 IU; thiamine, 1 mg; riboflavin, 1 mg; pyridoxine hydrochloride, 0.33 mg; cyanocobalamin, 0.33 μg; ascorbic acid, 20 mg; niacinamide, 7 mg; calcium pantothenate, 0.33 mg
Appedrine Tablets (Thompson)	25 mg	carboxymethylcellulose sodium, 50 mg	caffeine, 100 mg; vitamin A, 1667 IU; vitamin D, 133 IU; thiamine, 1 mg; riboflavin, 1 mg; pyridoxine hydrochloride, 0.33 mg; cyanocobalamin, 0.33 μg; ascorbic acid, 20 mg; niacinamide, 7 mg; calcium pantothenate, 0.33 mg
Appress (North American)	25 mg	—	caffeine, 100 mg
Ayds Weight Suppressant Droplets (Purex)	25 mg	—	—
Coffee Break Cubes Weight Reduction Plan (O'Connor)	37.5 mg	—	—
Coffee, Tea & A New Me (Thompson)	25 mg	—	—
Dex-A-Diet II (O'Connor)	75 mg	—	caffeine, 200 mg
Dexatrim Capsules (Thompson)	50 mg	—	caffeine, 200 mg
Diadax Capsules (O'Connor)	50 mg	—	—
Diadax Tablets (O'Connor)	25 mg	—	—
Diet-Trim Tablets (Pharmex)	NS [a]	carboxymethylcellulose	benzocaine
Grapefruit Diet Plan with Diadax Tablets (O'Connor)	10 mg	—	natural grapefruit extract, 16.6 mg; ascorbic acid, 10 mg; vitamin E, 3.6 mg
Grapefruit Diet Plan with Diadax Vitamin Fortified Continuous Action Capsules (O'Connor)	30 mg	—	natural grapefruit extract, 50 mg; ascorbic acid, 30 mg; vitamin E, 11 mg
Grapefruit Diet Plan with Diadax Chewable Tablets Extra Strength (O'Connor)	25 mg	—	natural grapefruit extract, 33 mg; ascorbic acid, 20 mg; vitamin E, 10 IU
Grapefruit Diet Plan with Diadax Extra Strength Vitamin Fortified Continuous Action Capsules (O'Connor)	75 mg	—	natural grapefruit extract, 100 mg; ascorbic acid, 60 mg; vitamin E, 30 IU
Odrinex Tablets (Fox)	25 mg	methylcellulose, 50 mg	caffeine, 50 mg
Pro Dax 21 (O'Connor)	75 mg	—	—
Prolamine Capsules (Thompson)	35 mg	—	caffeine, 140 mg
Slim Line Candy (O'Connor)	—	methylcellulose, 45 mg	benzocaine, 5 mg; corn glucose syrup; natural and artificial flavoring
Slim Line Gum (O'Connor)	—	—	benzocaine, 6 mg
Spantrol Capsules (North American)	75 mg	carboxymethylcellulose sodium, 135 mg	caffeine (anhydrous), 150 mg; benzocaine, 9 mg; ascorbic acid, 30 mg; thiamine hydrochloride, 1 mg; riboflavin, 1.2 mg; niacinamide, 10 mg; pyridoxine hydrochloride, 1 mg; iron, 10 mg

Appetite Suppressant Products

Product (Manufacturer)	Phenylpropanolamine Hydrochloride	Bulk Producer	Other
Vita-Slim Capsules (Thompson)	50 mg	—	vitamin A, 2500 IU; vitamin E, 15 IU; ascorbic acid, 30 mg; folic acid, 0.2 mg; thiamine, 0.75 mg; riboflavin, 0.85 mg; niacinamide, 10 mg; pyridoxine hydrochloride, 10 mg; cyanocobalamin, 3 μg; calcium pantothenate, 5 mg; iron, 9 mg; iodine, 75 mg

[a] Quantity not specified.

Weight Control Products

Product (Manufacturer)	Dosage Form	Calories Supplied	Essential Composition
Bulk Producers			
Diet-Aid (Rexall)	tablet	not stated	alginic acid, 200 mg; carboxymethylcellulose sodium, 100 mg; sodium bicarbonate, 70 mg
Instant Mix Metamucil (Searle)	powder in single-dose packets	3/packet	psyllium mucilloid, 3.7 g; citric acid; sodium bicarbonate (equiv. to 250 mg sodium)
Melozets (Calgon)	wafer	30	methylcellulose, flour, sugar
Metamucil (Searle)	powder	14/tsp	psyllium mucilloid, 50%; dextrose, 50%
Reducets (Columbia Medical)	capsule	0	benzocaine, 5 mg; methylcellulose, 100 mg; multivitamins; minerals
Artificial Sweeteners			
Ril-Sweet (Plough)	liquid	0	saccharin sodium, 3.3%
Sucaryl Sodium (Abbott)	tablet liquid	0	saccharin sodium, 16 mg/tablet 1.21% (liquid)
Sweeta (Squibb)	tablet liquid	0	saccharin, 15 mg/tablet, 7 mg/drop
Low-Calorie Foods			
Dietene (Doyle)	powder	353/100 g powder	nonfat dry milk, cocoa, carrageenan, artificial flavor, lecithin, polysorbate 80, malt, vitamins, sucrose, calcium caseinate, minerals
Metrecal (Drackett)	cookie	25	flour, sugars, milk protein concentrate, vegetable shortening, yeast, vitamins, minerals
Slender (Carnation)	liquid powder to be mixed with milk bar	225/can 170 mixed with 6 oz. skim milk 225 mixed with 6 oz. whole milk 275/2 bar serving	nonfat dry milk, sucrose, vegetable oil, artificial flavors, vitamins, minerals
Low-Calorie Candy			
Ayds (Purex)	candy cube	25/cube	corn syrup, vegetable oils, sweetened condensed skim milk, vitamins, minerals

Sleep Aid, Sedative, and Stimulant Products

James P. Caro and Charles A. Walker

Chapter 14

Questions to Ask the Patient

Sleep Aid and Sedative Products

How long has insomnia been a problem? Do you have difficulty sleeping every night or only occasionally?

Is the problem related to falling or staying asleep?

Can you relate the insomnia to a cause such as a change in work shifts, anxiety, or pain?

Are you using tranquilizers, sleeping tablets, or other medication?

Do you drink coffee, tea, cola, or alcohol?

Do you have any chronic diseases?

Are you under a physician's care?

Stimulant Products

How long do you intend to use a stimulant product?

Are you a regular drinker of coffee and other caffeinated beverages?

Have you ever experienced unpleasant reactions to coffee?

Which stimulant products have you used before? How well did they work?

Are you now being treated for a condition that requires the use of other drugs?

Almost nothing is as restful as a good night's sleep, but almost half the American population fails to achieve this relatively simple goal. Some people have trouble falling asleep, and others awaken in the middle of the night, from psychological or physiological problems.

At the opposite end of the spectrum are individuals who need stimulants to stay awake. Boredom and fatigue have a soporific effect, and the tedium of extended periods of activity such as highway driving may induce sleepiness.

Nonprescription drugs are available to combat both these disorders. Pharmacists should counsel patients on correct use of sedatives and stimulants. Most of the time a restful sleep pattern may be established without drugs; for example, taking a walk before bedtime may relax the body enough to facilitate falling asleep. Excessive use of caffeine as a stimulant is unwise under any circumstances and may have untoward effects, such as nervousness and irritability.

SLEEP AID/SEDATIVE PRODUCTS

Although many nonprescription preparations are promoted as providing "safe and restful sleep" or relief from "simple nervous tension," claims for the safety and efficacy of these products are unsubstantiated. Many contain drugs found in prescription medications (e.g., antihistamines and scopolamine) but in much lower doses, and it is assumed that these lower doses minimize the untoward effects of these agents. Unfortunately, the sedative effects also are minimal because in most cases, sedation is only a secondary (or side) effect rather than the drug's primary pharmacological effect. In addition, the sedative effect of these agents is subject to considerable personal variation; some individuals may even experience a paradoxical state of excitement. The low efficacy of these preparations may pose an additional hazard because individuals who do not experience sedation at normal doses may exceed the recommended dose and suffer toxic effects.

Considering the widespread use of OTC sedatives without medical supervision, the need to ensure that they are used appropriately and safely is essential. The FDA OTC Panel on Sleep Aid Drug Products questions the safety and efficacy of many products on the market (1).

Physiology of Sleep

The sites and mechanisms of action of sleep-inducing drugs are largely unknown. Neurophysiological investigations have yielded many theories concerning the influence of brain structures on consciousness and have provided some insight into the complex feedback systems that control consciousness. It is now known that the brain stem coordinates the activity of these systems.

The brain stem contains the reticular activating system (RAS), which monitors and selectively limits all sensory input to the brain. Although the reticular activating system responds to stimuli by arousing the brain, the cerebral cortex discriminates between stimuli even during sleep. For this reason, only selected stimuli will produce arousal from sleep (2).

stages of sleep
REM sleep
insomnia

Sleep is characterized by a diminution of activity in the ascending and descending reticular activating system pathways. This reticular deactivation occurs by passive limitation of sensory input (e.g., sleeping in a dark, quiet room) and by active influence from the cerebral cortex, medulla, and possibly other structures (3).

Sleep is classified into rapid eye movement (REM) and non-rapid eye movement (non-REM) stages (Figure 1). Non-REM sleep is subdivided into Stages I–IV, according to increasing depth of sleep. In young adults, REM sleep constitutes about 25% of a night's sleep. During REM sleep the body is generally physiologically more active than it is in non-REM stages. In young adults there is an initial awake period (sleep latency) followed by a rapid progression through Stages I–IV of non-REM. This sequence is then reversed, followed by the first REM period. This initial sequence of non-REM sleep (REM latency) lasts about 70 minutes. The first REM period is very short and is followed by another cycle. In each successive cycle, less time is spent in Stage IV, and more time is spent in the other stages, including REM. In the elderly, both sleep latency and REM latency are increased, Stage IV may be decreased or absent, and awakenings are more frequent (4).

Etiology of Insomnia

The occasional inability to attain restful sleep is a common problem. It is estimated that about 50% of the population experiences insomnia at some time, and 33% voices it as an ongoing complaint (5). Although insomnia is usually transient and self-limiting, it may be of sufficient duration or severity to interfere with an individual's

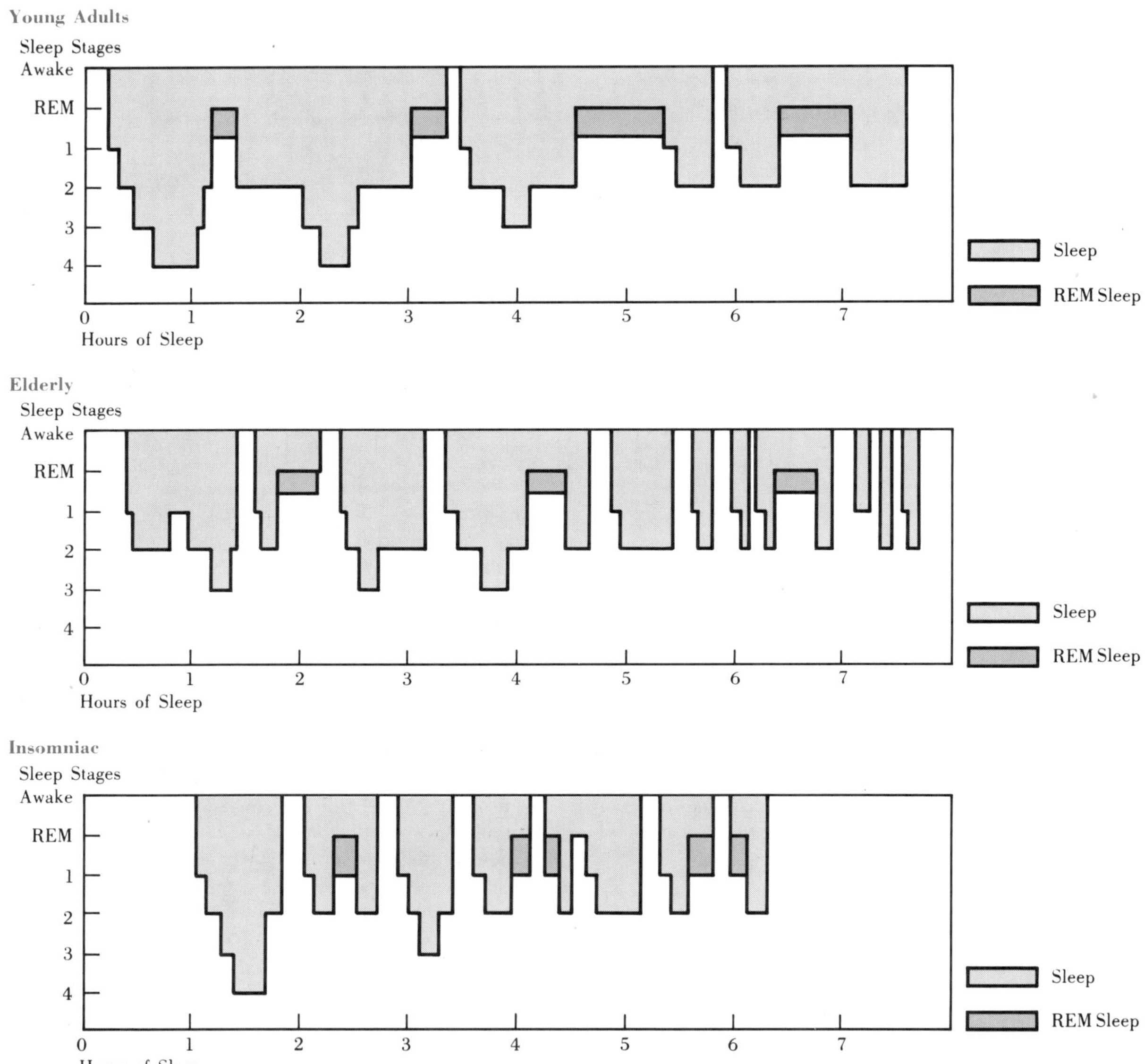

Figure 1. Hours of sleep and sleep stages in young adults, the elderly, and insomniacs. Adapted from *Patient Care*, *X*(3), 113 (1976).

functioning during the waking hours. Severe or chronic insomnia may be a symptom of serious psychological or physical illness.

Insomnia may be classified as either difficulty in falling aleep, difficulty in remaining asleep, or too early final wakening (6). Many factors may be involved.

Situational Stress and Anxiety

These conditions cause difficulty in falling asleep. Usually acute and transient, they include anything that may cause worry or excitement. Situational stress and anxiety are probably the most frequent causes of insomnia in young people.

Pain or Physical Discomfort

Pain such as headache and dental pain frequently prevents falling asleep.

Change in Daily Rhythm

A change in work shift and "jet lag" are typical occurrences that may precipitate insomnia.

Age

Elderly individuals are prone to early or frequent awakening because sleep cycles change with age.

Depression

Some types of depression are associated with awakenings during the night or early morning. If anxiety occurs with depression, the patient may complain of difficulty in falling and remaining asleep.

Conditions With Nocturnal Exacerbation

Autonomic nervous system bursts during REM sleep precipitate angina attacks, vascular headaches, and duodenal ulcer distress that disturb sleep. Asthma, epilepsy, and lumbosacral and cervical disc disease also have been implicated in sleep disturbances.

Endocrine Abnormalities

Hypothyroidism and hyperthyroidism as well as other endocrine disorders disturb sleep patterns, but the mechanism is unknown.

Sleep Apnea

This sleep disturbance, which is most common in men over 40, is manifested by loud, irregular snoring. In this syndrome, respiration actually stops for periods of 20–90 seconds many times during the night, resulting in partial awakening and sleep disruption. The patient may be unaware of irregular respiration and may complain only of feeling tired during the day. Researchers believe that sleep apnea is caused by a defect in CNS respiratory control which, in some cases, is complicated by an anatomical upper airway obstruction.

Nocturnal Myoclonus

This syndrome consists of recurrent, rhythmic movement of one or both legs. The patient may not awaken fully and so may be unaware of what has been happening.

Drug Use

Drugs may cause sleep disturbances. Certain anorexic preparations (prescription and OTC) containing CNS stimulants, caffeine, and aminophylline may cause nervousness and prevent sleep in some individuals. Alcohol, amphetamines, barbiturates, diphenhydramine, ethchlorvynol, glutethimide, methyprylon, narcotics, scopolamine, and tricyclic antidepressants are drugs that cause sleep disturbances by suppressing REM (7). Amphetamines, barbiturates, benzodiazepines, chloral hydrate, glutethimide, and reserpine decrease Stage IV sleep. Abrupt withdrawal of a REM suppressant after chronic use precipitates a compensatory rebound of REM sleep. This rebound is associated with disturbances in sleep patterns and accompanying nightmares. REM rebound also may occur as a patient develops tolerance to a REM-suppressing hypnotic. Deprivation of Stage IV sleep results in symptoms that suggest a depressive and hypochondriacal reaction (7).

factors involved in insomnia

effects of other drugs on sleep

agents used in sleep aid products

Ingredients in OTC Products

Drugs used to treat insomnia include antihistamines, salicylates and salicylamide, and scopolamine (an anticholinergic). None has proven satisfactorily safe and effective, and patients using sedative products containing these agents, particularly pregnant women, should be warned of possible adverse effects. The pharmacist should urge patients to try adjunctive nondrug measures to help them sleep.

Antihistamines

Antihistamines can induce symptoms of both CNS stimulation and depression. Although drowsiness usually results from therapeutic doses, excitation is a symptom of intoxication. The mechanisms by which antihistamines exert their CNS effects are unclear, but similarities between the actions of antihistamines and scopolamine suggest that acetylcholine antagonism in the CNS is common to both (8). The CNS depressant action of antihistamines is unpredictable because individuals vary in sensitivity to this effect and tolerance develops with continued use.

Antihistamines' efficacy as sleep aids is questionable. The results of one study indicate that 50 mg of methapyrilene is no more effective than placebo (9). The FDA Panel on Sleep Aid Drug Products has recommended an additional testing period of 3 years because data on the safety and efficacy of these products are lacking (1).

Side effects of antihistamines include dizziness, tinnitus (ringing in the ears), blurred vision, GI disturbances, and dryness of the mouth and throat. Antihistamines may also cause CNS stimulation, resulting in nervousness and insomnia. However, this effect is uncommon, occurring primarily in children.

Although the antihistamines have a wide margin of safety, potential poisoning with these agents should not be discounted if an acute overdose is taken, especially in combination with alcohol. The symptoms observed with intoxication result from the CNS effects—the pupils become fixed and dilated, fever may be present, and excitement, hallucinations, and convulsions occur. In severe cases these symptoms are followed by coma and cardiorespiratory collapse. Treatment consists of preventing the drug's absorption, emesis, and supportive measures such as assisting ventilation and controlling convulsions.

The antihistamines commonly used in OTC sleep aid products are methapyrilene and pyrilamine maleate, alone or in combination. The dosage range is 10–50 mg/dose.

Antihistamines have produced teratogenic effects in animals and therefore should be avoided by pregnant women. High doses may precipitate convulsions and should be used with caution in persons with epilepsy. The CNS depressant effect of antihistamines is enhanced by alcohol and other CNS depressant drugs.

Salicylates and Salicylamide

Salicylates are included in sleep aid products primarily to relieve minor pain which may hinder sleep. Salicylamide is not metabolized to salicylate in the body.

methapyrilene

pyrilamine maleate

drug interactions with salicylates

anticholinergics

Although salicylamide also has sedative properties, the doses contained in OTC preparations (200–400 mg) probably are insufficient to produce sedation (10). In addition, the results of one study indicate that salicylamide's bioavailability is poor because the drug is relatively insoluble and rapidly inactivated in the GI tract and liver (11).

The side effects most commonly associated with salicylates are those involving the GI tract. (See the discussion in Chapter 9 on side effects and toxicities of salicylates.)

Salicylates are present in OTC sleep aid products as various salts, in doses of 80–200 mg. Salicylamide is included in doses of 200–400 mg.

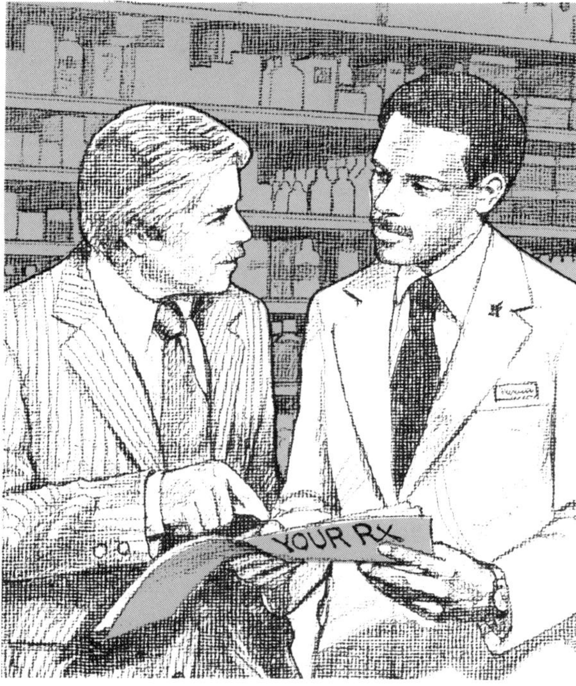

Salicylates should not be used by patients with GI ulcers or allergy to salicylates. Salicylates potentiate the action of oral anticoagulants and methotrexate, and concurrent use of these drugs may result in serious toxic effects. Salicylates antagonize the uricosuric effect of sulfinpyrazone and probenecid and cause additive ulcerogenic effects on the gastric mucosa when used concurrently with alcohol or with corticosteroids (12).

Scopolamine

Scopolamine is a belladonna alkaloid anticholinergic agent that differs from atropine in that it lacks a CNS stimulant effect. Scopolamine acts as a hypnotic by depressing the cerebral cortex, especially the motor areas (13). It suppresses spontaneous electrical activity as well as the arousal response to photostimulation (14). In animals, scopolamine antagonizes the electroencephalogram (EEG) response produced by stimulation of the reticular formation and hypothalamus (15). These findings indicate that scopolamine suppresses the brain structures responsible for maintaining consciousness.

Scopolamine is absorbed readily from the GI tract. Therapeutic doses (0.6 mg orally or parenterally) produce drowsiness, euphoria, fatigue, and dreamless sleep (16). In some individuals, therapeutic doses cause an idiosyncratic reaction manifested by excitement, restlessness, and delirium; this reaction occurs most commonly when severe pain is present.

Scopolamine may disrupt the sleep cycle by decreasing REM time. When scopolamine is discontinued after several days of use, a rebound in REM occurs. This effect may result in nightmares, insomnia, and a feeling of having slept badly (3). Although the scopolamine dose in OTC preparations probably is insufficient to produce "REM rebound," patients who use these preparations chronically or who exceed the recommended dosage may experience this effect.

Scopolamine has been used as a preanesthetic medication for its sedative action. In obstetrics it was combined with narcotics to produce a state of amnesia and partial analgesia ("twilight sleep"). Although scopolamine is effective in preventing motion sickness, it has been replaced by newer agents (e.g., dimenhydrinate) with fewer side effects.

The most common side effect of scopolamine is dryness of the mouth and throat. Other effects such as blurred vision, photophobia, and urinary retention are uncommon at the dosage provided in OTC preparations.

Infants and young children are particularly susceptible to the toxic effects of belladonna alkaloids. The fatal scopolamine dose in children may be as low as 10 mg (17). The symptoms of poisoning are delirium, tachycardia, fever, and hot, dry, flushed skin. In severe cases, respiratory depression and coma may result.

Treatment of oral scopolamine poisoning consists of delaying and preventing the drug's absorption by administering milk or activated charcoal, inducing emesis, and counteracting its central peripheral effects with physostigmine. In addition, general measures such as reducing fever, controlling convulsions, and maintaining urinary output are used.

Scopolamine is available for nonprescription use as the aminoxide hydrobromide salt. Theoretically, the use of this salt minimizes toxic effects and provides sustained action because the aminoxide hydrobromide is slowly metabolized to the parent base. The advantages of this compound over others have not been proved conclusively (1). The amount of scopolamine in OTC products may be 0.1–0.5 mg/dose. Scopolamine alone is ineffective as a sleep aid at these doses. However, it may enhance sedation produced by other components of OTC products.

Scopolamine should not be used in children under 12 or in patients with narrow-angle glaucoma, coronary insufficiency, or prostatic hypertrophy. This agent should be used cautiously with other drugs possessing anticholinergic activity (e.g., other belladonna alkaloids, phenothiazines, tricyclic antidepressants, and antihistamines) and CNS depressants because concurrent use may enhance the anticholinergic action or the CNS depression.

scopolamine dosage considerations

Adjunctive Measures

recommended nondrug measures

Before advising patients on the proper use of OTC sleep aid preparations, the pharmacist should recommend the following nondrug measures appropriate to help relieve insomnia:

- Abstaining from beverages containing caffeine;
- Avoiding heavy meals several hours before bedtime;
- Avoiding naps during the day;
- Performing light exercise before bedtime;
- Designating a specific time for sleep;
- Relaxing by engaging in positive activities such as reading in bed, watching television, or listening to relaxing music;
- Minimizing external stimuli that might disturb sleep, e.g., by using dark shades over the windows to keep out light and ear plugs to keep out noise.

STIMULANT PRODUCTS

caffeine

OTC stimulant products used today contain caffeine (1,3,7-trimethylxanthine) as the active component and are classified as "stay-awake aids." The related dimethylxanthines, theophylline and theobromine (Figure 2), are not used therapeutically as stimulants. The caffeine content of nonalcoholic beverages is:

- Brewed coffee, 100–150 mg per cup;
- Cola drinks, 40–60 mg per glass;
- Decaffeinated coffee, 2–4 mg per cup;
- Instant coffee, 86–99 mg per cup;
- Tea, 60–75 mg per cup.

More than 25 OTC analgesic products contain as much as 64 mg of caffeine per dose. Caffeine is considered a relatively safe substance administered orally in doses of less than 200 mg (18).

Approximately 7 million kilograms of caffeine are consumed yearly in the United States. Caffeine is used most commonly to induce wakefulness and to relieve the sense of boredom and fatigue associated with performing tedious work for extended periods. For example, it is used to prevent "highway hypnosis" encountered during long periods of continuous driving. Caffeine is also used inappropriately to combat hangover symptoms and to antagonize the depressant properties of alcohol and other sedatives.

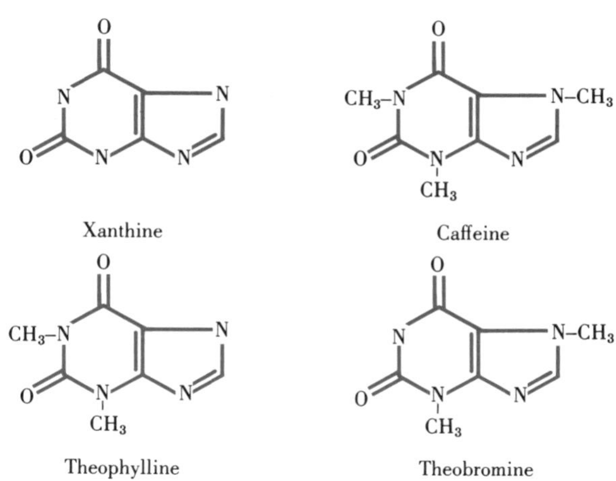

Figure 2. Structure of methylated xanthines.

Caffeine Effects on Nervous System

nervous system effects

Indications for stimulant use are drowsiness and fatigue. In a study on driver performance it was found that caffeine improves alertness, but contradictory evidence exists on caffeine's sobering effect. Mental activity was improved by caffeine in tests that involved simple arithmetic, typing, and decoding, especially in long sessions, when fatigue and boredom are possible factors (18).

Improvement of skeletal muscle tone is a fundamental property of caffeine useful in combating fatigue (19). At typical therapeutic doses this effect is produced mainly by CNS stimulation and in part by the direct action on the voluntary musculature. It is difficult to separate the central from the peripheral influences, but the central effects probably are more important and pronounced.

In humans the physiological consequences of various caffeine doses have been studied. Small doses (50–200 mg) stimulate cerebrocortical areas associated with conscious mental processes (Figure 3)—ideas become clearer, thoughts flow more easily and rapidly, and fatigue and drowsiness decrease (19). Doses larger than 250 mg often cause insomnia, restlessness, irritability, nervousness, tremor, headaches, and, in rare cases, a mild form of delirium manifested as perceived noises and flashes of light. In investigations of caffeine's objective and subjective effects a study evaluating the effects of placebo versus caffeine (150–300 mg) on objective performance and mood showed that although caffeine produces a subjective feeling of increased alertness and physical activity, objective performance requiring alertness and psychomotor coordination is not improved (20).

Injected doses of caffeine larger than 250 mg stimulate vagal respiratory and vasomotor areas of the medulla oblongata (21). Caffeine is therapeutically effective in

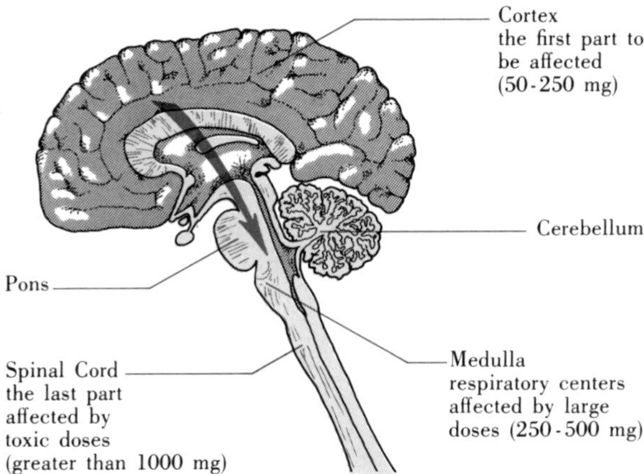

Figure 3. The site of action of caffeine in the central nervous system. (The arrow indicates the progression of the effect.)

effects on cardiovascular system

vasoconstriction

caffeinism

treating drug-induced depression of the medullary respiratory center. Doses of more than 10 g ingested orally are required to induce convulsions (19). In cases of oral overdosage the stomach should be emptied by inducing emesis or by using gastric lavage. Depressants, such as barbiturates, have been used to control caffeine-induced convulsions.

Effects on Cardiovascular System

Xanthines may stimulate the myocardium directly, promoting an increase in cardiac force, rate, and output (22). These cardiac effects may be masked, however, because xanthines, especially caffeine in large doses, also stimulate the medullary vagal nuclei and tend to produce a reflex decrease in heart rate. Large doses (more than 250 mg) may induce cardiac irregularities attributed to caffeine's direct effects on the myocardium (19). Experimentally, caffeine has been shown to stimulate norepinephrine synthesis and release in the brain and epinephrine release from the adrenal medulla (19). However, the evidence does not implicate these amines in human cardiovascular problems (due to caffeine intake).

In humans, caffeine does not cause a consistent decrease in systemic mean blood pressure despite a decrease in peripheral resistance. Generally, with moderate caffeine doses, blood pressure is maintained by increased cardiac output. However, large intravenous doses of caffeine have been shown to cause a transient fall in blood pressure due to medullary vagal nuclei stimulation, which also may result in bradycardia and a slight decrease in cardiac output (19).

Xanthine compounds have been shown to cause marked vasoconstriction of cerebral blood vessels. The property has been reported to be a mechanism of action in relieving hypertensive headache with caffeine (21).

In an investigation regarding the effect of 140 mg of caffeine in tea on hemodynamic measures in patients with cardiac disease, there was a significant rise in the cardiac index, stroke index, oxygen consumption, and minute ventilation (23). A small but significant increase in brachial arterial pressure and ventricular filling pressure also occurred. No arrhythmias were seen in any of the patients as a result of drinking tea.

There have been conflicting reports of positive correlation between coronary artery disease and coffee consumption. One study compared the histories of 700 heart attack patients with the histories of 13,000 other patients (24). Patients who drank as many as five cups of coffee per day had a 50% greater risk of heart attack than those who abstained; patients who drank six or more cups per day had a 100% greater risk of heart attack than abstainers. These results have been disputed by other studies that failed to show a correlation among coffee consumption, serum lipids, serum cholesterol, and coronary disease (25, 26).

Other Caffeine Effects

"Caffeinism" is the syndrome associated with excessive caffeine intake. Ingesting more than 1000 mg/day of caffeine (about 10 cups of coffee) may produce symptoms similar to those of anxiety neurosis. The CNS symptoms related to excessive stimulation include nervousness, irritability, agitation, headache, tachypnea, tremulousness, and muscle twitches. Sensory disturbances such as hyperesthesia, tinnitus, and visual hallucinations may occur. Insomnia characterized by a delay in sleep onset or by frequent awakenings may be a consequence of caffeinism.

The effects of regular coffee, decaffeinated coffee, and caffeine on gastric acid secretion and lower esophageal sphincter pressure have been investigated in healthy subjects (27). The results of this study suggest that regular and decaffeinated coffee are more potent stimulants of gastric acid secretion than caffeine, that decaffeination diminishes coffee's acid secretory potency only minimally, and that regular and decaffeinated coffee increase lower esophageal sphincter pressure, whereas caffeine alone has only a minimal effect. Clinical recommendations based on the known GI effect of caffeine thus may bear little relation to the actual observed action of regular or decaffeinated coffee (27). Moreover, the effects of caffeine alone may not be similar to the effects of beverages in which caffeine is present. However, decaffeination does not necessarily completely remove undesirable effects of caffeinated beverages.

Caffeine's value in mixtures for relief of headache and other pain is questionable except in the treatment of vascular headache. In one study, caffeine in combination with aspirin was no more effective than aspirin alone for headache (28). Caffeine generally is believed to play a minor role in the toxic effects from excessive analgesic use (29, 30). Caffeine taken with analgesics may, by its stimulant properties, act as a mood enhancer when pain is accompanied by minor depression.

Because caffeine has a hyperglycemic effect, it may elevate blood glucose levels and produce high readings for serum uric acid when the Bittner (1963) assay is used (31). Caffeine or its metabolites interfere in vanillylmandelic acid [4-hydroxy-3-methoxymandelic acid (VMA)]

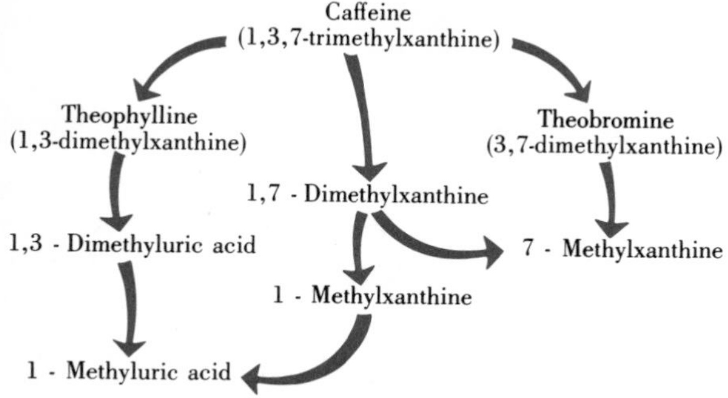

Figure 4. Caffeine metabolism in humans.

determination. The test is used to detect elevated adrenal or sympathetic catecholamine levels as seen in pheochromocytoma or neuroblastoma. An increase in catecholamine urine levels may be detected following caffeine ingestion (31).

Figure 4 shows the human metabolism of caffeine, after which approximately two-thirds of the drug is excreted in the urine as monomethylxanthine or dimethyluric acid. Although coffee and preparations containing caffeine often are prohibited in individuals suffering from gout, this prohibition may not be justified (19). Uric acid is not formed following caffeine ingestion, and the methylxanthines and methyluric acids that do appear as metabolites do not provoke attacks of gout. Therefore it is doubtful that therapeutic doses of caffeine aggravate the disease.

In a study of caffeine use in hyperkinetic children it was concluded that caffeine may have a place in the therapeutic management of children with minimal brain dysfunction syndrome and consequent hyperkinetic impulse syndrome (32).

A mild degree of tolerance and physical dependence occurs with caffeine ingestion. Irritability, nervousness, and headache were reported in habitual coffee users (five or more cups per day) following withdrawal from the beverage (33). Although these symptoms do not prove actual caffeine physical dependence, they may indicate psychological dependence. Another study conducted to determine tolerance to caffeine in healthy subjects provided some information on physiological changes associated with chronic caffeine administration (34). It was established that 150 mg of caffeine taken at bedtime reduces pulse rate significantly in non-coffee-drinkers but not in those who habitually consume caffeinated beverages. The study also indicated that caffeine administration (150 mg) to non-coffee-drinkers delays the onset of sleep patterns. On the other hand, chronic coffee drinkers show no symptoms of bradycardia or insomnia (34). Although results indicate possible physical changes in coffee drinkers, it is the general opinion that caffeine tolerance in chronic users occurs because of increased metabolism.

Chronic caffeine use may produce a degree of tolerance to insomnia and a decrease in the mental alertness produced by caffeine, i.e., a decrease in caffeine's ability to act as a stimulant (35).

Caffeine Toxicity

Fatal caffeine poisoning is extremely rare. Death has been reported in only a few cases following intravenous injection or oral administration. In adults the lethal intravenous dose of caffeine was reported to be 3.2 g; the reported oral lethal dose range is 18–50 g (36). The administration route influences the severity of toxic manifestations. Peak blood levels occur within 2 hours after oral administration (37). The average half-life is 3–3.5 hours (38). Children are very susceptible to caffeine toxicity; caffeine-containing drugs should be kept out of their reach.

The following treatment for caffeine overdosage is suggested:

- Ingestion of aluminum hydroxide gel as an antacid and protective agent against GI irritation;
- Oxygen inhalation;
- Short-acting barbiturates injected cautiously to control neuromuscular irritability and convulsions;
- Intravenous fluids to combat dehydration;
- Antibiotics for complicating infections;
- Evacuation.

caffeine metabolism and toxicity

overdose treatment

FDA Panel recommendations

diphenhydramine

Renal irritation and nephrotoxicity may occur following chronic abuse of caffeine-containing analgesic drug mixtures. One study reported a significant number of renal tubular cells and red blood cells in the urine of 10 healthy volunteers following the ingestion of 1.2 g/day of caffeine for 5 days (32).

SUMMARY

Insomnia usually is a transient, self-limiting condition caused by stress or change of location or schedule. Patients who request OTC sleep aid or sedative products should be informed that these products are only for occasional use at recommended dosages. Scopolamine preparations should not be recommended because they are ineffective at recommended doses and higher doses may precipitate toxicity. The antihistamines are the most satisfactory ingredients of OTC sleep aid and sedative products. The FDA OTC Panel on Sleep Aid Drug Products has recommended additional testing of these agents at doses greater than those presently used and is considering the introduction of diphenhydramine as an OTC sleep aid.

The use of an antihistamine product along with nondrug measures is probably the most rational advice a pharmacist can give a patient suffering from insomnia. Patients using any OTC sleep aid or sedative product should be cautioned that their ability to drive or operate hazardous machinery may be impaired and that concurrent use of these products with alcohol or other CNS depressants will intensify the CNS depression.

The pharmacist should advise caffeine product users of the possible side effects and dangers of overconsumption of these compounds. Because of caffeine's possible interactions with other drugs, caffeine intake should be reduced during the treatment of specific diseases, especially cardiovascular, psychological, or renal problems.

The use of analgesic combinations that contain caffeine is not advisable for patients with rheumatoid arthritis or other conditions that require large doses (10–30 tablets per day) of medication because in these amounts there is danger of caffeine toxicity. Caffeine consumption should be avoided prior to blood or urine analysis.

The pharmacist should caution against caffeine overuse. Habitual overuse may lead to sleep deprivation. CNS stimulants may facilitate the ability to ignore the sensation of tiredness, but they do not replenish depleted energy. Continuous use of coffee or caffeine tablets does not allay emotional fatigue. Neither coffee nor caffeine tablets taken after alcohol consumption induce sobriety, but the degree of CNS depression is lessened, and somnolence is diminished or eliminated. In other words, a person may still be inebriated without feeling sleepy.

REFERENCES

(1) *Federal Register*, 57297 (1975).
(2) "The Anatomy of Sleep," Roche Laboratories, Nutley, N.J., 1966, pp. 39–59.
(3) "The Nature of Sleep," G. E. W. Wolstenholme and M. O'Connor, Eds., Little, Brown, Boston, Mass., 1961, pp. 86–102.
(4) K. L. Melmon and H. F. Morrelli, "Clinical Pharmacology—Basic Principles in Therapeutics," 1st ed., Macmillan, New York, N.Y., 1972, pp. 482–490.
(5) J. Moriarity, *Dis. Nerv. Syst.*, *36*, 279 (1975).
(6) C. C. Brown, E. L. Hartmann, G. L. Usdin, E. D. Weitzman, D. J. Greenblatt, and L. E. Hollister, *Patient Care*, *10*, 98 (1976).
(7) G. Fass, *Am. J. Nurs.*, *71*, 2316 (1971).
(8) R. H. Dreisbach, "Handbook of Poisoning," 8th ed., Lange Medical, Los Altos, Calif., 1974, pp. 606–608.
(9) G. Teutsch, D. L. Mahler, C. R. Brown, W. H. Forrest, Jr., K. E. James, and B. W. Brown, *Clin. Pharmacol. Ther.*, *17*, 195 (1975).
(10) "The Pharmacological Basis of Therapeutics," 5th ed., L. S. Goodman and A. Gilman, Eds., Macmillan, New York, N.Y., 1975, p. 348.
(11) L. Fleckenstein, G. R. Mundy, R. A. Horovitz, and J. M. Mazzullo, *Clin. Pharmacol. Ther.*, *19*, 451 (1976).
(12) "Evaluations of Drug Interactions," 2nd ed., APhA, Washington, D.C., 1976.
(13) "Martindale: The Extra Pharmacopoeia," 26th ed., N. W. Blacow, Ed., Pharmaceutical Press, London, England, 1972, p. 295.
(14) A. M. Ostfeld and A. Arugete, *J. Pharmacol. Exp. Ther.*, *137*, 133 (1962).
(15) K. A. Exley, M. C. Fleming, and A. D. Espdlien, *Br. J. Pharmacol.*, *13*, 485 (1958).
(16) "The Pharmacological Basis of Therapeutics," 5th ed., L. S. Goodman and A. Gilman, Eds., Macmillan, New York, N.Y., 1975, p. 517.
(17) R. H. Dreisbach, "Handbook of Poisoning," 8th ed., Lange Medical, Los Altos, Calif., 1974, p. 305.
(18) "Drill's Pharmacology in Medicine," 4th ed., J. R. DiPalma, Ed., McGraw-Hill, New York, N.Y., 1971, p. 537.
(19) "The Pharmacological Basis of Therapeutics," 5th ed., L. S. Goodman and A. Gilman, Eds., Macmillan, New York, N.Y., 1975, p. 368.
(20) A. Goldstein, S. Kaizer, and R. Warren, *J. Pharmacol. Exp. Ther.*, *150*, 146 (1965).
(21) "The Pharmacological Principles of Medical Practice," 7th ed., J. C. Krantz and C. J. Carr, Eds., Williams and Wilkins, Baltimore, Md., 1969, pp. 256–260.
(22) I. Starr, C. J. Gamble, A. Margolies, J. S. Donal, Jr., N. Joseph, and E. Eagle, *J. Clin. Invest.*, *16*, 799 (1937).
(23) L. Gould, M. K. Gofwami, C. V. Reddy, and R. F. Gomprecht, *J. Clin. Pharmacol.*, *13*, 469 (1973).
(24) Boston Collaborative Drug Surveillance Program, *Lancet*, *2*, 1278 (1972).
(25) S. Heyden, *Z. Ernaehrung*, *9*, 388 (1969).
(26) J. A. Little, H. M. Shanoff, A. Csima, and R. Yano, *Lancet*, *1*, 732 (1966).
(27) S. Cohen and G. H. Booth, *N. Engl. J. Med.*, *293*, 897 (1975).
(28) C. G. Moertel, D. L. Ahmann, W. F. Tyler, and N. Schwartau, *J. Am. Med. Assoc.*, *229*, 55 (1974).
(29) L. J. Cass and W. S. Fredrik, *Curr. Ther. Res. Clin. Exp.*, *4*, 583 (1962).
(30) M. Grotto, S. Dikstein, and F. G. Sulman, *Arch. Intern. Pharmacodyn.*, *155*, 365 (1965).
(31) F. H. Meyers, E. Jawetz, and A. Goldfein, "Review of Medical Pharmacology," 4th ed., Lange Medical, Los Altos, Calif., 1974, p. 678.
(32) R. C. Schnackenber, *Am. J. Psychiatry*, *130*, 796 (1973).
(33) R. H. Dreisbach and C. Pfeiffer, *J. Lab. Clin. Med.*, *28*, 1212 (1942).
(34) T. Colton, R. E. Gosselin, and R. P. Smith, *Clin. Pharmacol. Ther.*, *9*, 31 (1968).
(35) K. H. Pieper, *Arzneim. Forsch.*, *13*, 585 (1963).
(36) R. H. Cheney, *J. Pharmacol. Exp. Ther.*, *53*, 304 (1935).
(37) J. Axelrod and J. Reichenthal, *J. Pharmacol. Exp. Ther.*, *107*, 519 (1953).
(38) C. Landis, in "Problems of Addiction and Habituation," Vol. 13, P. H. Hoch and J. Zubin, Eds., Grune and Stratton, New York, N.Y., pp. 37–48.

stimulant products

Stimulant Products

Product (Manufacturer)	Caffeine	Other
Amostat Tablets (North American)	100 mg	—
Caffedrine Capsules (Thompson)	200 mg	—
Double-E Alertness Capsules (Keystone)	200 mg	—
Nodoz Tablets (Bristol-Myers)	100 mg	—
Quick-Pep Tablets (Thompson)	150 mg	—
Summit (Pfeiffer)	100 mg	acetaminophen, 325 mg
Tirend Tablets (Norcliff Thayer)	100 mg	—
Verb T.D. Capsules (Amer. Pharm.)	200 mg	—
Vivarin Tablets (J.B. Williams)	200 mg	dextrose, 150 mg
Wakoz (Jeffrey Martin)	200 mg	—

Product (Manufacturer)	Scopolamine	Antihistamine	Analgesic
Compoz Tablets (Jeffrey Martin)	—	methapyrilene hydrochloride, 15 mg pyrilamine maleate, 10 mg	—
Dormin Capsules (Dormin)	—	methapyrilene hydrochloride, 25 mg	—
Nervine Capsule-Shaped Tablets (Miles)	—	methapyrilene hydrochloride, 25 mg	—
Nervine Effervescent Tablets (Miles)	—	methapyrilene fumarate, equivalent to 25 mg of hydrochloride	—
Nervine Liquid (Miles)	—	methapyrilene fumarate, equivalent to 5 mg of hydrochloride/ml	—
Nite Rest Capsules (Amer. Pharm.)	aminoxide hydrobromide, 0.25 mg	methapyrilene hydrochloride, 50 mg	—
Nytol Capsules and Tablets (Block)	—	methapyrilene hydrochloride, 50 mg/capsule 25 mg/tablet	—
Quiet World Tablets (Whitehall)	—	pyrilamine maleate, 25 mg	aspirin, 227.5 mg acetaminophen, 162.5 mg
Relax-U-Caps (Columbia Medical)	—	methapyrilene hydrochloride, 25 mg	—
Sedacaps (Vitarine)	—	methapyrilene hydrochloride, 25 mg	—
Seedate Capsules (Amer. Pharm.)	aminoxide hydrobromide, 0.125 mg	methapyrilene hydrochloride, 25 mg	—
Sleep-Eze Tablets (Whitehall)	—	pyrilamine maleate, 25 mg	—
Sleepinal Capsules (Thompson)	—	methapyrilene hydrochloride, 50 mg	—
Sominex Tablets and Capsules (J. B. Williams)	aminoxide hydrobromide, 0.25 mg/tablet 0.5 mg/capsule	methapyrilene hydrochloride, 25 mg/tablet 50 mg/capsule	salicylamide, 200 mg/tablet or capsule
Somnicaps (Amer. Pharm.)	—	methapyrilene hydrochloride, 25 mg	—
Tranqium Capsules (Thompson)	—	methapyrilene hydrochloride, 50 mg	—
Tranquil Capsules (North American)	—	methapyrilene fumarate, 25 mg	sodium salicylate, 25 mg acetaminophen, 25 mg
Twilight Capsules (Pfeiffer)	—	methapyrilene hydrochloride, 25 mg	salicylamide, 300 mg

Menstrual Products

Laurel E. Ashworth

Chapter 15

Questions to Ask the Patient

When was your last period?

What contraceptive measures (if any) do you use?

How do the present symptoms vary from those of your normal cycle (flow, duration, intensity)?

Are you under the care of a physician?

Do you have discharge between your periods? Is the discharge accompanied by pain, itching, pus, or foul odor?

Have you had these symptoms before? What treatment was used? Was it helpful?

The biological phenomenon of menstruation is a fact of life for women during their childbearing years. Many symptoms have been associated with various phases of the menstrual cycle including headaches, fluid accumulation, backaches, breast tenderness, irritability, abdominal cramping, anxiety, and depression.

The range and severity of symptoms experienced vary considerably from individual to individual. Pharmacists should be familiar with the relatively few pharmacological agents comprising the host of OTC preparations marketed to alleviate premenstrual and menstrual discomfort.

MENSTRUAL CYCLE

Approximately every 28 days an ovum (egg) passes down one of the fallopian tubes toward the uterus, where it impacts on the uterine endometrium. If the egg is not fertilized, it is discarded along with the endometrial lining in the menstrual flow which passes through the cervix, down the vaginal canal, and out of the body. This process is referred to as menstruation (1). A more succinct definition of the menstrual process is a periodic cyclic bleeding from the uterus, accompanied by desquamation of the endometrium (2).

Menarche, or the appearance of the first menstrual period, occurs near the end of puberty and generally is preceded by a growth spurt and the development of secondary sex characteristics. The age at which the first period occurs may be as low as 10 or as high as 16 years, but the average age for menarche in North American girls is 12.5 years (3).

The typical menstrual cycle, i.e., the interval between the first day of menstruation and (up to and including) the day prior to the onset of the next period, is 28 days. This interval varies widely among different women and from month to month even in the same individual. A range of 25–32 days is generally acceptable. The cycle is most irregular in puberty and near menopause and is interrupted by pregnancy.

The beginning of the cycle (day 1) is designated arbitrarily as the first day of menstruation because for most women the initial appearance of blood is the most accurately determined event of the cycle. Menstrual bleeding usually persists for 3–5 days. In any one woman the duration and pattern of flow are usually standard from one cycle to the next.

The amount of blood lost during a normal menstrual cycle is difficult to quantitate but sufficient to cause a slight lowering of the hemoglobin value in a healthy woman receiving adequate dietary intake. In a study involving 476 women a mean loss of 33.2 ± 1.6 ml of blood per cycle was reported; in this study, blood losses in excess of 80 ml were considered pathological (4). The total body fluid loss during menstruation may be 60–200 ml (5). This monthly blood loss may be significant in women who have poor dietary habits or underlying anemia attributable to nonmenstrual factors.

The menstrual discharge has a characteristic dark-reddish color. The offensive odor of the menstruum is attributable to decomposed blood elements and to the admixture of vulvar sebaceous gland secretions. In addition to the blood elements, the flow contains cervical mucus, vaginal mucosa, numerous bacteria, and degenerated endometrial particles.

PHYSIOLOGY

The menstrual cycle may be considered as consisting of three interrelated phases. Phase I (menstruation, menses) has an average duration of 5 days. During this time a portion of the endometrium degenerates and is lost along with blood from the ruptured endometrial vessels to form the menstrual discharge.

Phase II (follicular, estrogenic, or proliferative stage) persists from about day 5 to the time of ovulation, around day 14. The uterus hypertrophies and becomes hyperplastic under the influence of rising estrogen titers. Together, phases I and II constitute the preovulatory phase.

phases of the menstrual cycle

hormonal levels and changes

physiological effects

Phase III (progestational, or secretory stage) extends from the time of ovulation (around day 15) to the beginning of menstruation, approximately 14 days or half the cycle. During this phase the uterus shows changes characteristic of progesterone stimulation and is ideally prepared to facilitate implantation. Phase III is called the postovulatory phase.

In the preovulatory phase the anterior pituitary gland secretes follicle-stimulating hormone (FSH) which initiates the development in the ovary of an ovum-containing follicle. During follicular maturation, estrogen is secreted in increasing quantities due to the biochemical activity of the follicular apparatus.

In addition to promoting the development of secondary sex characteristics in the maturing female, estrogen supports oogenesis (production of eggs) and stimulates the endometrium to exhibit active proliferative changes in its vascular system, glandular tissue, and stroma. A high blood level of estrogen diminishes further pituitary secretion of follicle-stimulating hormone and appears to trigger the sudden release of luteinizing hormone (LH), which is responsible for ovulation.

The fluid pressure building inside the follicle eventually causes the follicle to burst, thereby ejecting the ovum into the fimbria of the nearby oviduct. Subsequent events are determined by whether or not the ovum is fertilized. In this chapter it is assumed that fertilization does not occur.

During the postovulatory phase, estrogen influence gradually subsides as luteinizing hormone transforms the pre-existing follicle cells into the corpus luteum, a structure that functions as an endocrine gland in that it secretes progesterone.

Progesterone's primary role is the continued development of the uterine endometrium. Under progesterone's influence the endometrium more than doubles in thickness. Its glands become increasingly convoluted, and the surrounding stroma is characterized by cellular hypertrophy and edema. Abundant quantities of a thick mucoid secretion rich in glycogen are produced.

Maintenance of the corpus luteum and its secretory activity is conventionally claimed to depend on a continuing hormone supply from the pituitary. The importance of this relationship has been questioned (6). The corpus luteum synthesizes and secretes estrogen and progesterone for 12–14 days, then gradually degenerates and becomes a scar tissue known as the corpus albicans. The resultant drop in the hormone levels initiates a sloughing of the uterine endometrium, and menstruation occurs. The low circulating progesterone level in turn triggers the pituitary to secrete follicle-stimulating hormone once more, and the next month's cycle begins. This sequence of events is depicted in Figure 1.

Most symptoms of menstrual or premenstrual discomfort may be attributed to elevated circulating estrogen levels (Table 1) (6). Two estrogen peaks, the maximal at ovulation (near day 14) and a lesser one at the midluteal stage (days 24–25), correlate well with the appearance

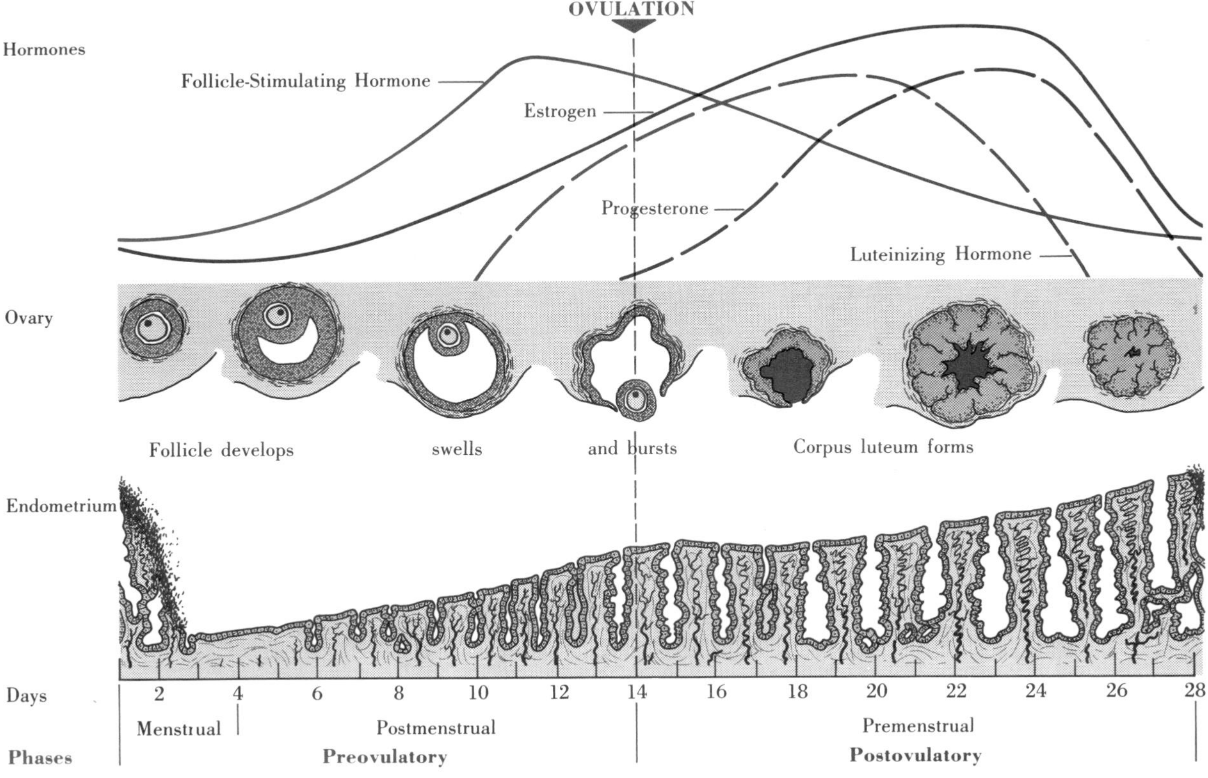

Figure 1. Menstrual cycle. Adapted with permission from C.W. Young, G.L. Stebbins, and F.G. Brooks, *Introduction to Biological Sciences,* Harper & Row, New York, N.Y., 1956.

Table 1. Estrogen Levels in Women of Childbearing Age

	Menses	Ovulation	Midluteal
Serum estrogen, IU/liter	20	60	55
Urinary estrogen excretion, μg/24 hours	13	56	43

Data taken from *Medical Physiology*, 12th ed., V. B. Mountcastle, Ed., Mosby, St. Louis, Mo., p. 1003.

of typical premenstrual and menstrual complaints: breast fullness and tenderness, fluid retention and weight gain, premenstrual tension, and menstrual cramping.

Studies in human subjects revealed that estrogen administration results in sodium and chloride retention, decreased urinary volume, increased extracellular fluid and blood volumes, and increased body weight (8). The mechanism involved appears to be increased sodium reabsorption from the urinary tubules, which is independent of the adrenals or ovaries but may involve the neurohypophysis.

MENSTRUAL ABNORMALITIES

Menstrual function should not entail such great discomfort as to restrict one's daily activities. A general feeling of "puffiness" (with or without breast tenderness) at ovulation and for several days prior to menstruation is normal for many women. These symptoms usually regress with the onset of menstruation. The pharmacist should question complaints of unusually severe and/or unprecedented premenstrual and menstrual symptoms, since referral to a gynecologist may be indicated.

Dysmenorrhea

Dysmenorrhea is a term used to describe painful menstruation. The discomfort may range from minor abdominal cramping to intense pain that may be accompanied by diarrhea, nausea, and vomiting.

Primary dysmenorrhea is encountered in the absence of any significant pelvic lesion and is normally attributed to intrinsic uterine factors. The pain, which may be colicky or aching, characteristically begins with the onset of menstruation and persists for several hours. On occasion it may continue for several days. The discomfort associated with primary dysmenorrhea may be severe enough for some women to necessitate 1 day or more of bed rest each month.

The causes of primary dysmenorrhea may be constitutional, endocrine, or psychogenic. The sensations of pelvic heaviness, breast fullness, and occasional cramping are within normal limits for the usual menstrual period. However, the demarcation between normal discomfort and frank dysmenorrhea is a very subjective distinction which the patient herself draws on the basis of the degree of incapacity she feels her monthly cycle produces.

Family attitudes—in particular, the ways in which a girl's mother regards the menstrual process—greatly influence the daughter's accommodation to menstruation as a part of her daily activities. An excellent article discusses the importance of folk beliefs about the normal body and its functions in health behavior (8). Clearly, a patient's understanding of menstruation or the lack of such knowledge has a direct bearing on her ability to cope with the inconveniences the process places on her daily routine.

On the basis of clinical impressions, the cramping of primary dysmenorrhea generally is attributed to exaggerated uterine contractility. Estrogenic hormones have long been regarded as stimulants of uterine contractility, whereas progesterone is considered an inhibitor of this contractility. Over the last 15 years or so the role of prostaglandins in menstrual cramping has been advanced.

fluctuations in estrogen levels

cramps

role of prostaglandins

absence of menstruation

mittelschmerz

It was first suggested almost 20 years ago that under the influence of progesterone, prostaglandin $F_{2\alpha}$, a neurohormone that causes smooth muscle contraction, is synthesized by the secretory endometrium (9). Prostaglandin $F_{2\alpha}$ is released as the endometrium breaks down at menstruation, and its action on uterine muscle and vasculature provokes contraction and pain. When excessive amounts of the substance are released into the circulation, the systemic characteristics associated with dysmenorrhea such as diarrhea, nausea, and vomiting result.

Secondary dysmenorrhea occurs with diseases or abnormal conditions of the uterus and surrounding pelvic structures. The sudden or gradual onset of difficult menstruation in a patient who has had years of menstrual bleeding with absent or minimal discomfort should be investigated. Pelvic pathology such as endometriosis, intrauterine polyps or myomas, or assorted obstructions of the reproductive tract may be present.

Amenorrhea

Amenorrhea, the absence of menstruation, is a symptom of some underlying problem. Primary amenorrhea refers to the failure of menses to occur before a given age, normally the eighteenth birthday. Patients exhibiting primary amenorrhea have a relatively high incidence of chromosomal disorders. Secondary amenorrhea is the cessation of menses for at least 3 months. Irregular menses over a period of months or unusual patterns are often diagnosed and treated as secondary amenorrhea. This symptom usually results from emotional or psychogenic causes and functional disorders. Secondary amenorrhea also may occur in women who have stopped taking oral contraceptives.

Intermenstrual Pain and Bleeding

Both of these conditions occur at or near the midinterval of the menstrual period, and their occurrence is associated with ovulation. Intermenstrual pain, or "mittelschmerz," may be slight or as severe as the more intense forms of dysmenorrhea. Most commonly, the discomfort lasts only a few hours; rarely does it persist longer than 2–3 days. Midcycle bleeding may range from

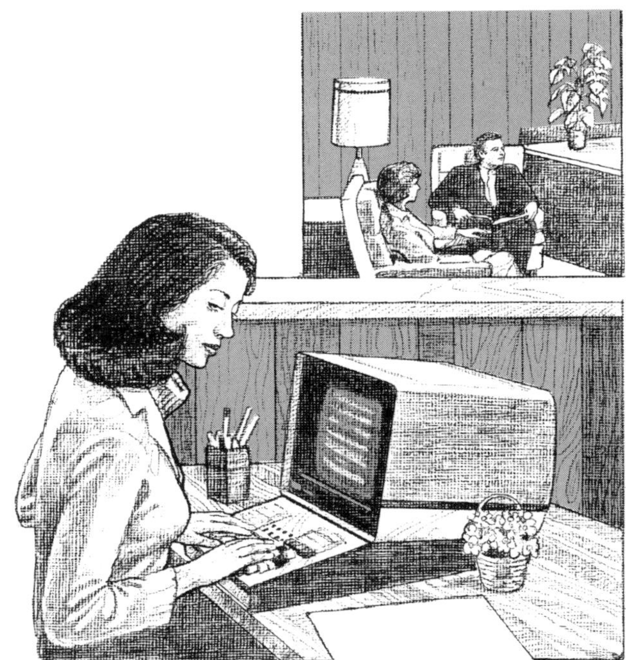

premenstrual effects

phenacetin, acetaminophen, aspirin, and salicylamide

a scant brownish discharge to a significant flow termed "kleine Regel," or little period.

Premenstrual Tension and Edema

Minor tension 2–3 days before menstruation is relatively common. This disorder is associated most characteristically with headache and less so with nervousness and depression.

Premenstrual edema may be experienced by menstruating females of any age but occurs most commonly in women in the late 30's to mid-40's. It is normal for most women to experience a slight weight gain prior to menses. In one study, 30% of a group of normal women exhibited a weight gain of 1.3 kg or more that could be attributed to premenstrual fluid retention (10).

The edema characteristically appears a few days before menstrual onset and provokes complaints of swollen feet and/or ankles and a "puffy" face. Once menstruation has begun, there is a noticeable polyuria and a rapid disappearance of edema.

EVALUATION

Most women who purchase OTC menstrual products are healthy females who are experiencing midcycle or premenstrual edema, headache, and/or cramping secondary to the normal hormone elevations that occur at these points in the cycle. Before recommending any product for a patient, the pharmacist should establish that the symptoms are indeed normal functional menstrual discomforts, in keeping with previous cycles, or whether they are unusually severe for her typical menstrual pattern. Any irregularities concerning the frequency, volume, or character of the menstrual discharge and any complaints of unusually pronounced pain and/or fluid retention indicate the need for immediate referral to a gynecologist. Pharmacist/patient consultation must be carried out in a private atmosphere. Confidentiality of the discussion is important. The pharmacist should strive to empathize with the patient in seeking to assist her with her problems.

If the evaluation seems to indicate that the patient's discomfort is simply that of a normal menstrual cycle, the pharmacist should inquire about products taken previously for relief of monthly symptoms so as to avoid recommending any product that has failed to give relief and to ascertain whether the dosage taken was sufficient to effect relief. The presence or absence of salicylate allergy always should be established, and menstrual products selected accordingly. Recommendation of any OTC product always should be accompanied by appropriate patient counseling regarding its proper use and dosage considerations.

TREATMENT

The pharmacist should avoid recommending any combination OTC menstrual products that contain subtherapeutic doses of analgesics, ineffective amounts of antiquated diuretics, and obscure natural products which are assumed to be innocuous. The pharmacist should be familiar with effective doses of agents that are rational ingredients for the relief of particular symptoms.

Ingredients in OTC Products

Analgesics

Phenacetin and acetaminophen appear in many menstrual products. Acetaminophen is the major active metabolite of both acetanilid and phenacetin and is traditionally reported to have less overall toxicity than its parent compounds (11). The analgesic effects of acetaminophen are similar to those of aspirin and are generally adequate to relieve the moderately intense pain commonly associated with menstrual headaches and dysmenorrhea. Acetaminophen has minimal if indeed any anti-inflammatory properties.

The relatively low incidence of minimal side effects hitherto associated with acetaminophen has led to its increased use by the American public to treat minor aches and pains. The sense of safety that all too many people associate with acetaminophen use is a false one. Patients using this product should be instructed to adhere strictly to the recommended adult dosage of 325–650 mg taken orally every 4–6 hours, not to exceed 2.6 g in 24 hours (12).

Until recently, the potential danger of fatal hepatic necrosis resulting from acetaminophen overdose was not appreciated fully in the United States. More than 100 fatal cases have been documented in England, where the annual incidence of overdoses averages 7000 with ~1% fatality rate (13). Because of the increased advertising of the agent's more potent forms throughout the United States the misuse and overuse of acetaminophen preparations are expected to increase. Many excellent articles address this problem and its treatment (13–15).

The salicylates (aspirin and salicylamide) constitute the second major group of analgesic compounds found in OTC menstrual products. Salicylamide possesses anti-inflammatory, antipyretic, and analgesic effects similar to those of aspirin even though it is not metabolized to aspirin per se in the body. It also possesses mild sedative properties.

Salicylamide generally is considered less effective than aspirin in relieving pain of slight to moderate intensity such as the pain of premenstrual and menstrual discomfort. One explanation offered for this clinical observation is that salicylamide is rapidly inactivated during absorption and during its initial pass through the liver (16). Salicylamide is no longer an official drug, primarily because its effects in humans are unreliable and hence other salicylate preparations are preferable. The conventional analgesic salicylamide dose is 650 mg orally four times per day. Thus the doses of 225–250 mg in most menstrual products that do contain salicylamide are probably ineffective.

Many potential adversities associated with aspirin use are not experienced by women who only occasionally use aspirin-containing menstrual products several days of each month. Aspirin-induced gastric ulceration and other salicylate-associated effects are seen with the chronic high-dose aspirin therapy used in the collagen diseases, but these complications are seldom of concern for the patient who now and then consumes the 325- to 650-mg aspirin dose every 4–6 hours recommended for menstrual discomfort. See Chapter 9 for a more complete discussion of adverse effects associated with aspirin ingestion.

In selecting a nonprescription menstrual product for any given patient, the pharmacist should routinely establish the presence or absence of salicylate sensitivity. The pharmacist also should inquire about disease states and/or other medications the patient is taking that would preclude her use of an aspirin-containing product.

Antihistamines

Antihistamines are used for their sedative side effects, which possibly help relieve the nervousness and irritability associated with premenstrual tension. Their usefulness is questionable, however, because the amounts of antihistamines contained in menstrual products are one-eighth to one-half the usual recommended dose for this effect (11, 17). The antihistamine used most frequently in menstrual products is pyrilamine maleate. Methapyrilene fumarate and phenindamine tartrate also are used. Even in the low dosages contained in menstrual products the antihistamines cause drowsiness in some women. The pharmacist also should determine whether the patient is taking any other antihistamine-containing OTC or prescription drug products.

Diuretics

Menstrual products commonly contain subtherapeutic doses of minimally effective diuretic agents. Pamabrom, caffeine, and ammonium chloride frequently are employed.

Pamabrom

Pamabrom used in conjunction with an analgesic and an antihistamine is marketed for the relief of premenstrual tension and related discomforts. Depending on the individual manufacturer, the recommendation is made that the combination product be taken for 4–7 days before menstrual onset to effect relief. The daily dose of pamabrom should not exceed 200 mg (18). While pamabrom has received positive reviews in the past, present-day clinical evaluations are lacking, and its use therefore is not strongly advocated (19).

Caffeine

With respect to diuretic properties, caffeine is the least potent member of the xanthine family. In doses approaching or exceeding 100 mg, caffeine may augment gastric secretions and thereby provoke gastric irritation. At these doses, caffeine behaves as a CNS stimulant. However, in the usual 30-mg doses employed in OTC products, caffeine increases the sodium and chloride excretion rate by acting directly on the renal tubule to effect a slight diuresis (20).

Ammonium Chloride

Ammonium chloride is one of the acid-forming salts with limited value (1–2 days' duration) in promoting diuresis. Therapeutic doses of 8–12 g/day are associated with gastric irritation, nausea, and vomiting even when administered in divided doses after meals. Therapeutic doses are contraindicated in the presence of markedly impaired renal function because uncompensated acidosis may develop. The effectiveness of the 325- to 500-mg ammonium chloride doses present in various OTC preparations is questionable.

Alternative Therapy

Having read the preceding material, the pharmacist may be wondering how a competent, concerned health professional acting in clear conscience and good faith can recommend some of the available OTC menstrual products to patients. A more rational and professional approach to treating premenstrual and menstrual discomfort using the available nonprescription agents involves patient counseling as to proper use of a single analgesic agent (acetaminophen or a salicylate) and dietary modification (e.g., salt restriction on days of the cycle known to be troublesome with respect to edema formation). Patients in whom premenstrual edema is a problem should be instructed to avoid salt-rich foods, such as pickles, snack chips, and fried potatoes, and to avoid salting their regular food for 3–4 days before menstruation. A reduced sodium intake should minimize or alleviate their edema.

For a patient troubled regularly with menstrual edema the pharmacist may wish to consider asking her physician to prescribe a small quantity of a diuretic to be used judiciously as needed for menstrual edema. Such professional involvement is preferable to merchandising an OTC product of questionable value.

Related Menstrual Products

The pharmacist should be familiar with feminine protection products and should know what to recommend under the particular circumstances. If possible, the pharmacist should discourage frequent douching (more than

other ingredients in OTC menstrual products

other measures

feminine protection products

twice weekly) in favor of regular bathing (see Chapter 17).

Feminine Napkins and Tampons

Feminine napkins are available in a wide assortment of sizes and absorbancies. Some require a belt to hold them in place over the perineum so that they will absorb the menstruum effectively, while newer styles are held in position with an adhesive strip on the underside of the pad, which affixes to the crotch of the patient's undergarment.

Feminine napkins are composed of absorbent cotton layers covered with a lightweight paper gauze. A layer of cellulose or thin plastic is incorporated into the side of the pad worn away from the perineum to discourage leakage and soiled undergarments.

related products

Most women experience their heaviest menstrual flow on day 2 of the menstrual cycle. "Super" napkins or "maxi" pads may be used at this time by women who do not use tampons. The napkins should be changed frequently to minimize the development of unpleasant odors arising from the breakdown of the menstrual products collected on the napkin. Frequent changing of sanitary napkins also helps to reduce the degree of irritation and chafing of the upper inner thigh associated with napkin use. Dusting the area with a talcum or medicated powder is beneficial in alleviating chafing. During periods of heavy flow (day 2), napkins may need to be changed every 2 hours, while changing every 4–6 hours is adequate for days of moderate flow.

"Mini" or "light" pads and "junior" or "teen" napkins accommodate nicely to the smaller anatomy and lighter flow of the adolescent female. Many mature women prefer the light pads to the more cumbersome belted napkins for the first and last days of their cycle. These shields also may be used to protect undergarments from being stained by the vaginal leakage of vaginal creams and suppositories.

Tampons are attractive to many women from the standpoint that they are worn intravaginally and hence do not pose the problems of bulkiness, chafing, and irritation associated with feminine napkin use. Some women use both a tampon and a napkin on days of heavy menstrual flow or on days when they know their schedule will not permit frequent changing. Deodorant tampons containing polysorbate 20 and assorted fragrances are available in addition to the conventional nonscented cotton tampons. The possibility that these additives may act as sensitizers in some women must not be overlooked.

Many misconceptions still exist regarding limitations in one's daily activities during menstruation. One of the most common misconceptions is that women should not bathe or wash themselves during this time. Good hygiene that includes routine showering or bathing during these days is one of the most effective ways of reducing menstrual odors.

Cleansing Products

Various feminine products including towelettes, sprays, and douches are marketed to assist the menstruating female in her personal hygiene. Inasmuch as perspiration and menstrual discharge have minimal odor until they are allowed to remain on the skin surface, regular showering or bathing is the most effective and economical way to ensure a body that is odor free during menstruation.

The practice of vaginal douching is coming under increasing disfavor from the medical community. A relationship between frequent, vigorous vaginal douching and salpingitis or pelvic inflammatory disease has been established. Douching is being associated with the upward spread (ascending infection) of whatever pathogens happen to be present in the vagina, including gonococcus (21). A more detailed presentation on feminine hygiene products appears in Chapter 17.

SUMMARY

Premenstrual and menstrual discomfort is a component of the lives of millions of American women, and, while it is inconvenient, the functional discomfort is rarely so severe as to prevent a woman from carrying out her daily activities. The rational and judicious use of nonprescription menstrual products can provide relief of discomfort and enable the patient to go more easily about her daily activities. The pharmacist has an important role in recommending safe and effective procedures and/or drug products to accomplish these goals.

REFERENCES

(1) P. D. Anderson, "Clinical Anatomy and Physiology for Allied Health Sciences," Saunders, Philadelphia, Pa., 1976, p. 423.

(2) R. F. Vollmann, "The Menstrual Cycle," Vol. 7 in *Major Problems in Obstetrics and Gynecology*, E. A. Friedman, Ed., Saunders, Philadelphia, Pa., 1977.

(3) E. R. Novak, G. S. Jones, and H. W. Jones, "Novak's Textbook of Gynecology," 9th ed., Williams and Wilkins, Baltimore, Md., 1975, p. 91.

(4) L. Hallberg, A. M. Hogdahl, L. Nilsson, and G. Rybo, *Acta Obstet. Gynecol. Scand.*, *45*, 320 (1966).

(5) "Harrison's Principles of Internal Medicine," 8th ed., G. W. Thorn, R. D. Adams, E. Braunwald, K. J. Isselbacher, and R. G. Petersdorf, Eds., McGraw-Hill, New York, N.Y., 1977, pp. 241–245.

(6) "Medical Physiology," 12th ed., V. B. Mountcastle, Ed., Mosby, St. Louis, Mo., 1968, p. 1003.

(7) *Ibid.*, p. 1008.

(8) L. F. Snow and S. M. Johnson, *J. Am. Med. Assoc.*, *237*, 2736 (1977).

(9) H. J. Clitheroe and V. R. Pickles, *J. Physiol. (London)*, *156*, 225 (1961).

(10) E. R. Novak, G. S. Jones, and H. W. Jones, "Novak's Textbook of Gynecology," 9th ed., Williams and Wilkins, Baltimore, Md., 1975, p. 726.

(11) "The Pharmacological Basis of Therapeutics," 5th ed., L. S. Goodman and A. Gilman, Eds., Macmillan, New York, N.Y., 1975, p. 343.

(12) "Product Information," McNeil Laboratories, Fort Washington, Pa.

(13) G. J. Merritt and P. U. Joyner, *Drug Intell, Clin. Pharm.*, *11*, 458 (1977).

(14) J. Ambre and M. Alexander, *J. Am. Med. Assoc.*, *238*, 500 (1977).

(15) R. G. Peterson and B. H. Rumack, *J. Am. Med. Assoc.*, *237*, 2406 (1977).

(16) "Facts and Comparisons," E. K. Kastrup and J. R. Boyd, Eds., Facts and Comparisons, Inc., St. Louis, Mo., 1977, p. 249-c.

(17) "AMA Drug Evaluations," 3rd ed., Publishing Sciences Group, Littleton, Mass., 1977, p. 675.

(18) "Martindale's Extra Pharmacopoeia," 27th ed., Pharmaceutical Press, London, England, 1977, p. 1792.

(19) R. B. Greenblatt, *Group Pract.*, *11*, 66 (1955).

(20) "The Pharmacological Basis of Therapeutics," 5th ed., L. S. Goodman and A. Gilman, Eds., Macmillan, New York, N.Y., 1975, p. 840.

(21) H. H. Neumann and A. DeCherney, *N. Engl. J. Med.*, *295*, 789 (1976).

Product[a] (Manufacturer)	Analgesic	Diuretic	Antihistamine	Caffeine	Other
Aqua-Ban (Thompson Medical)	—	ammonium chloride, 325 mg	—	100 mg	—
Cardui (Chattem)	acetaminophen, 325 mg	pamabrom, 25 mg	pyrilamine maleate, 12.5 mg	—	—
Femcaps Capsules (Buffington)	acetaminophen[b]	—	—	citrate[b]	ephedrine sulfate, 8 mg atropine sulfate, 0.03 mg
Flowaway Water 100's (DeWitt)	—	uva ursi extract, 98 mg buchu leaves extract, 24 mg	—	20 mg	potassium nitrate, 171 mg
Fluidex (O'Connor)	—	buchu powdered extract, 65 mg couch grass powdered extract, 65 mg corn silk powdered extract, 32.5 mg hydrangea powdered extract, 32.5 mg	—	—	—
Fluidex-Plus with Diadax (O'Connor)	—	buchu powdered extract, 65 mg couch grass powdered extract, 65 mg corn silk powdered extract, 32.5 mg hydrangea powdered extract, 32.5 mg	—	—	phenylpropanolamine hydrochloride, 25 mg
Humphrey's No. 11 (Humphrey's Pharmacal)	—	—	—	—	cimicifuga, 3X pulsatilla, 3X sepia, 3X
Lydia Pinkham (Smith, Miller & Patch)	—	—	—	—	extract of Jamaica dogwood, pleurisy root, and licorice[b] ferrous sulfate[b]
Lydia Pinkham Vegetable Compound Liquid (Smith, Miller & Patch)	—	—	—	—	extract of Jamaica dogwood, pleurisy root, and licorice[b] alcohol[b]
Midol (Glenbrook)	aspirin, 454 mg	—	—	32.4 mg	cinnamedrine, 14.9 mg
Odrinil (Fox)	—	buchu powdered extract, 34.4 mg uva ursi powdered extract, 34.4 mg corn silk powdered extract, 34.4 mg juniper powdered extract, 16.2 mg	—	extract, 16.2 mg	—
Pamprin (Chattem)	acetaminophen, 325 mg	pamabrom, 25 mg	pyrilamine maleate, 12.5 mg	—	—
Pre-Mens Forte (Blair)	—	ammonium chloride, 500 mg	—	100 mg	—
Sunril (Emko)	acetaminophen, 300 mg	pamabrom, 50 mg	pyrilamine maleate, 25 mg	—	—
Trendar (Whitehall)	acetaminophen, 325 mg	pamabrom, 25 mg	—	—	—
Tri-Aqua (Pfeiffer)	—	extracts of buchu, uva ursi, triticum, zea	—	100 mg	—

[a] Tablet unless specified otherwise.
[b] Quantity not specified.

Contraceptive Methods and Products

James Huff and Luis Hernandez

Chapter 16

Questions to Ask the Patient

Are you currently using a contraceptive method or product? If so, what do you use?

Have you consulted a physician or family planning service?

Do you understand the principles of contraception?

Do you have any problems possibly related to your method/product of contraception, such as irritation, inconvenience, or unusual symptoms?

Do you think you might have VD?

Are you pregnant?

Recent trends to smaller families and the increase in venereal disease suggest that the pharmacist and other health care practitioners must be able to supply accurate, unbiased, and definitive information on methods of contraception and venereal disease prevention. In addition, with the therapeutic safety controversy that surrounds oral contraceptive therapy, OTC contraceptive items represent a viable alternative for many persons.

Pharmacists, who are frequently the first health professionals consulted, should be knowledgeable about the various methods of contraception and should assist their patients in determining which methods or products best suit the patients' needs.

CONCEPTION

Conception (impregnation) is the union of an ovum (egg) from the female and a spermatozoon (sperm) from the male; contraception is the voluntary prevention of conception. Anything that blocks any part of the fertilization process in the male or female or anything that prevents or even delays the union of a sperm with the egg can prevent conception and is called a contraceptive agent, device, or method.

After ovulation, the egg remains fertilizable for about 6–24 hours, possibly as long as 48 hours. (See Chapter 15 for a discussion of the female reproductive cycle.) After ejaculation, sperm retain their ability to fertilize an egg for about 24–48 hours, although normal sperm life may be 72 hours in the presence of cervical mucus and as long as 5 or more days under "optimum conditions." In general, to result in conception, sexual intercourse must take place within the 4-day period including 2 days before the egg's release, the day of ovulation, and 1 day afterward.

The survival time of sperm in a condition in which they can fertilize the egg is a major consideration in preventing conception. Although the sperm may remain active (maximum duration of motility is 48–60 hours), they may be beyond the point where they can fertilize an egg (1–4). Sperm remain viable in the vagina for 2.5 hours, in the cervix for perhaps 48 hours, in the cavum uteri for 48 hours, and in the fallopian tube, where they can fertilize an egg, for a maximum of 48 hours (1). The time periods are not additive.

The ejaculated sperm of mammals with scrotal testicles eventually lose their fertility because of the temperature in the female genitalia and because of the alkaline secretion of the accessory male sex glands with which sperm are mixed during ejaculation (5).

CONTRACEPTION

Contraception is accomplished by preventing the semen containing sperm from entering the vagina or the cervical canal, by preventing follicular development, by preventing attachment of a mature egg to the endometrium, by limiting intercourse to times when a mature egg is not available for fertilization, or by immobilizing sperm that have entered the vaginal canal. The ideal method should be effective, safe, simple, easy to use, inexpensive, reversible, and acceptable. Several methods approach this ideal, but none has achieved it.

By 1973, 18.6 million of the 26.6 million married couples in the United States were using some type of contraception (6). Choosing the most acceptable method of contraception is an important issue. Selection of a contraceptive method is extremely personal and should be individualized. The key to success of any one method is motivation: if a couple strongly wishes to prevent conception, nearly any properly used contraceptive method will be reasonably successful (7).

Contrary to popular belief, many persons in the United States do not understand the basic principles of reproduction and conception (8, 9). Family planning services generally are lacking or unused at colleges and universities, and although many elementary and secondary schools attempt to provide sex education and birth control programs, they are frequently inadequate, underfunded, or instituted after sex patterns have been established (10–15). Fortunately, these inadequacies are being overcome as more and more people become positively concerned and involved.

Illegitimacy and unwanted pregnancies are frequent occurrences (16, 17). Recent statistics (18) indicate that 14.2% of all births are to unmarried women; 11,000 babies are born each year to mothers under 15. The report conservatively places the number of legal abortions at 643,000/year. Because pregnancy among teenagers remains a major public health problem, a recent survey was taken in 153 cities to catalogue the services available to pregnant teenagers (19).

In 1977 the incidence of venereal disease in the United States, which had been increasing at an annual rate of 10% during the previous 10 years, decreased. Nonetheless, VD is still considered to hover at epidemic levels; an estimated 360,000 cases of syphilis and 2.7 million cases of gonorrhea occur each year (20). In the United States, 3 million adolescents and young adults are infected at any given time (20). Each year, 1 million new cases are reported, three times the number of all other reportable infectious diseases. Even this statistic does not represent a true picture of the disease's epidemic proportions, since apparently only one case in eight is reported. A marked reversal has occurred in the national trend of reported cases of early syphilis. After decreasing for four consecutive 6-month periods, reported cases for January–June 1978 increased 1.0% over cases reported for January–June 1977 (21). VD stays rampant (22), and several factors explain its prevalence. First, gonorrhea infection confers little or no immunity against subsequent infections. In addition, many affected persons are not inconvenienced by the signs and symptoms and do not seek treatment. Finally, nearly 50% have no noticeable symptoms and thus are unsuspecting carriers.

venereal disease

contraceptive methods and OTC products

reasons for condom failure

METHODS OF CONTRACEPTION

Methods of contraception that do not require a prescription order include abstinence, coitus interruptus (withdrawal), coitus reservatus, condoms, creams and jellies, douching, foaming tablets, foam, rhythm, sponges, and vaginal suppositories. The pharmacist should suggest that the patient consult a physician or a family planning service before selecting a birth control method.

OTC Contraceptive Products

Contraceptive agents are available without prescription for both men and women. The pharmacist should be familiar with the various types of condoms, jellies, creams, tablets, and vaginal suppositories. The pharmacist also should encourage the patient to seek medical consultation before recommending a particular product.

Condoms

Contraceptive methods used by males are receiving increased attention (23–25). The most common methods throughout the world are coitus interruptus and the use of condoms. Both require control and forethought.

Condoms (bags, balloons, French letters, prophylactics, protectives, rubbers, safes, scum bags, sheaths, or skins) are among the most widely used, most effective, and most practical OTC contraceptives. They are simple to use, harmless, inexpensive, and easy to buy and do not require a physical examination or physician's advice. They are the only relatively effective, easily obtained contraceptive used by males, and their purpose and function are easy to understand: sperm are deposited in the condom and not the vagina.

Offering dual protection against pregnancy and VD (it is the only contraceptive method that prevents VD), the condom today is a carefully produced, rigorously tested, and highly effective contraceptive product readily available through nonclinical channels (26–28). In the United States, more than 300 million condoms are purchased each year at a cost to consumers of about $160 million. Nearly 50% of the purchases are made in pharmacies (29).

Condoms are made of rubber (or latex) and collagenous tissue (frequently obtained from lamb cecum). These materials are elastic, strong, and thin. The skin condom, the first type developed, generally is considered a luxury, and rubber condoms are used more frequently.

The psychological and physiological needs of the potential condom user are met by a wide choice of styles (opaque, transparent, colored, plain-ended, reservoir-ended, rippled or pagoda shaped, strictured or contoured, flocked with a rough rubber surface, dry, or lubricated with a water-soluble substance or silicone) and several different sizes (26). Condom thickness appears better correlated with durability (and therefore effectiveness) than with other features. Condoms usually are thicker toward the closed end.

Although condoms provide a high degree of protection against conception, accidents may happen, even when condoms are used correctly. Failure resulting from tearing or rupture of the condom is the major cause of fertilization; fortunately, it is infrequent (30).

Two techniques help prevent the condom from bursting: if it is plain ended, it should be unrolled on the erect penis with about 1.75 cm of space left at the end to accommodate the ejaculate; if the natural moisture in the woman's genital tract is scant, the outside of the condom should be lubricated with a contraceptive cream or jelly to prevent tearing on insertion (31). A water-soluble jelly is preferable owing to ease of cleansing. Petroleum jelly, liquid petrolatum, and other oils should not be used as lubricants because they may cause the rubber to deteriorate.

An often overlooked reason for inadvertent impregnation is improper use of the condom, probably due to lack of knowledge. First, prior to ejaculation, sperm in the urethral secretions may cause conception. Second, because of loss of erection following ejaculation, semen may leak out the open end of the condom, or the condom may slip off while the penis is still in the vagina or while it is being withdrawn. For best contraceptive effectiveness the condom must be put on before the penis comes into contact with the vagina and must be worn throughout coitus. Following ejaculation the penis should be withdrawn immediately. Accidents may be avoided if the ring (or open end) at the top of the condom is held securely

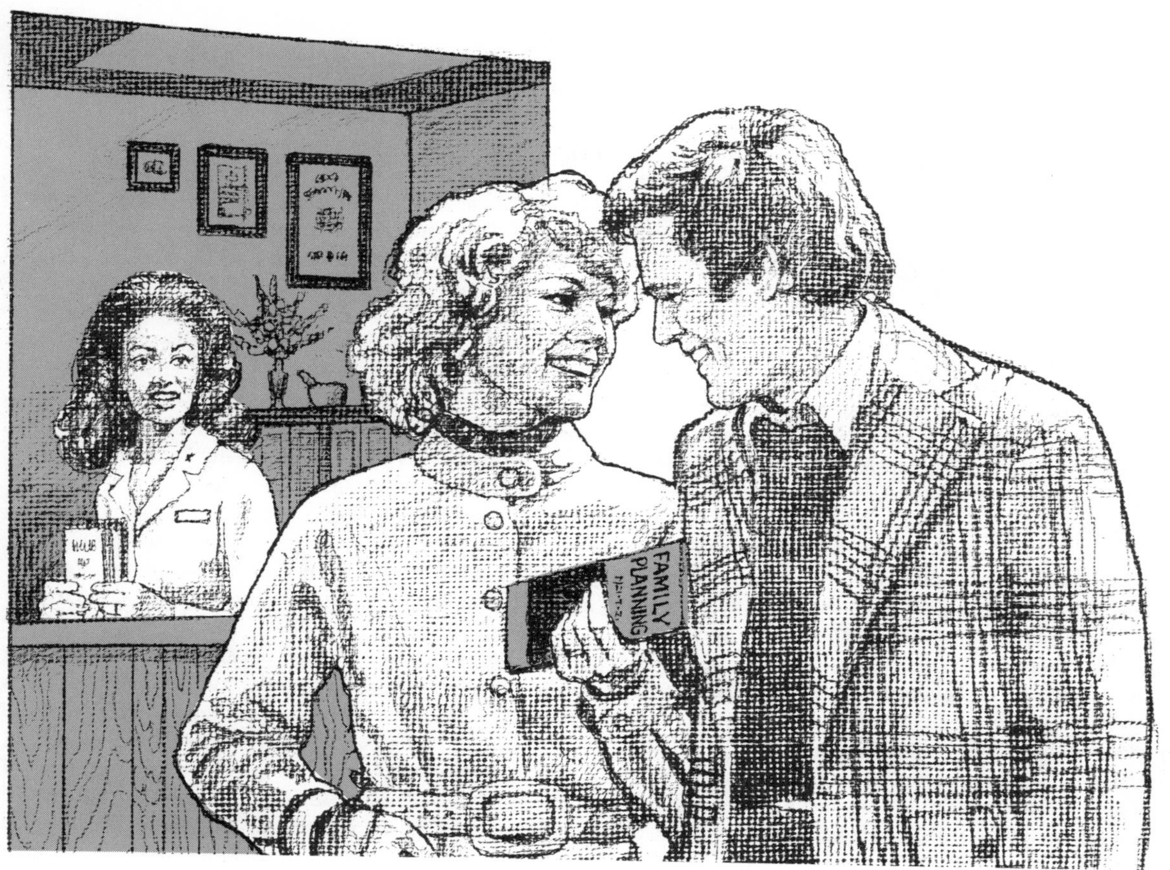

recommended condom type

role of condom in VD prevention

spermicides

to prevent spillage during withdrawal. As an added protection, the condom may be coated with a vaginal contraceptive (foam, cream, or jelly) in conjunction with the use of a vaginal contraceptive prior to intercourse. This method provides lubrication and a secondary defense against spilled semen.

The reservoir-ended condom is less likely to burst because there is ample space to hold the ejaculated semen; the lubricated kind allows easier insertion. The lubricated, reservoir-ended condom is the recommended type; however, the user may prefer another type.

As the only contraceptive that prevents both the contact and the infection, the condom substantially reduces the risk of transmitting gonorrhea and syphilis (32, 33). Its use should be encouraged, especially among younger people. Improvement of the product, its packaging, design, and promotion has resulted in its wider use and a decrease in unwanted pregnancies and VD (34).

In 1975, fewer than 6 in 10 pharmacies displayed condoms (29). Major reasons were fear of community disapproval or pharmacists' personal disapproval. Most pharmacists are not reluctant, however, to show female contraceptive products, although a significant number in 1972 would not sell contraceptives to unmarried minors (35). Such practices are detrimental to the pharmacist's role as an active member of the health team, especially in the area of preventive medicine. Today, more pharmacists are overcoming their reluctances as they recognize societal needs and as they assume a more active position on the health care team.

Vaginal Contraceptives

Four basic dosage form types of chemical contraceptives are used vaginally: creams, jellies, and pastes, usually squeezed from a tube; suppositories; gels; and foams, either in tablet form or in pressurized containers (36). Research is being directed toward identifying vaginal preparations with both contraceptive and prophylactic properties.

Vaginal Spermicides

The combination of a diaphragm and chemical spermicide has been used for years as an effective method of contraception. Also available are vaginal spermicidal preparations designed to be used without either a diaphragm or other contraceptive devices. Both types contain two components: a spermicidal chemical that actively immobilizes and kills sperm and an inert base that mechanically guards the cervical os (opening of the uterus). The base is formulated to provide for spreading over the os. Spermicides are relatively inexpensive, dermatologically harmless, and generally accepted as imparting an effective contraceptive action. The nonreactive bases may be formulated in dosage forms such as creams, foams, gels, jellies, vaginal suppositories, and vaginal tablets.

Choice depends on individual preference. The cream provides greater lubrication during intercourse. The jelly affords easier removal and dissipation because it is completely water soluble. Foams, on the other hand, do not contribute any appreciable lubrication but have the advantage of being almost totally undetectable during use.

The vaginal spermicidal preparations are not the same as preparations intended for use with a diaphragm. The former generally are more potent and have a different consistency from that of the agents used with other contraceptive devices. This distinction should be considered carefully in dispensing these products. The most commonly used spermicidal chemicals are the polyoxyethylated alkylphenols (nonionic surfactants). The number of polyoxyethylene groups in the side chain determines spermicidal activity. Some products are formulated to create a distinctly acid pH in the vaginal tract. A pH below 3.5 is considered spermicidal, with increasing effectiveness as the pH decreases. Boric acid, phenylmercuric acid, and ricinoleic acid are used in vaginal spermicidal products for this purpose.

polyoxyethylated alkylphenols as spermicides

mechanism of vaginal spermicides

diaphragm–spermicide combination

formulations

The method of use is fairly simple. A special applicator deposits the required amount of vaginal spermicide near the cervix, and coital movements distribute the agent throughout the vagina and over the cervix. The spermicide should be inserted not more than 1 hour, preferably 10–30 minutes, before intercourse. One applicatorful of spermicide is enough for only one intercourse; if intercourse is repeated, another dose of the contraceptive must be inserted. Douching (see Chapter 17) should not be attempted for 6–8 hours after intercourse, since it dilutes and/or removes the spermicidal agent, without necessarily removing the remaining viable sperm.

The vaginal spermicide alone is less effective in preventing pregnancy than the use of a diaphragm and cream, which together provide a better mechanical barrier. However, the foam, cream, or jelly alone is simpler to use and avoids a medical examination and prescription.

Used properly, the diaphragm–spermicide combination is among the most effective methods of contraception. In a study of 2168 women conscientiously using the diaphragm and jelly, accidental pregnancies in the first 12 months of use ranged from 1.9/100 for women under 18 to 3.0/100 for women 30–34 years old (37). These rates compared favorably with those for prescription oral contraceptive agents and the intrauterine device (IUD).

Allergic reactions to spermicides are uncommon. However, if either partner experiences an allergic response, the pharmacist should instruct the person to discontinue use immediately, change products, and contact a physician. Another method of contraception should be recommended for use until the patient sees the physician. In some cases a chemical contraceptive may cause local irritation or soreness. In general, switching to another brand of contraceptive (being sure the ingredients are different) is sufficient to ameliorate any signs and symptoms. If the person prefers not to see a physician, the pharmacist should recommend an alternative product with a different formula.

Aerosol Foams

This method of contraception involves the use of an aerosol dispenser to load a vaginal applicator by which the spermicidal foam is inserted before coitus. Basically, the foam is a spermicidal cream, packaged as an aerosol, that foams when it is released. The user attaches the applicator to the aerosol container of foam, fills the applicator (prefilled ones also are available), inserts it well into the vagina, and depresses the plunger to deposit the foam at the cervical os. Good adherence to the vaginal walls and tenacious covering of the cervical os make the foams one of the best vaginal contraceptives, and they are considered by many women to be more esthetically pleasing than vaginal jellies or tablets. The foams leak very little during or after intercourse. The newer, prefilled applicators may be prepared for use as many as 7 days prior to insertion. With either type, foam must be inserted and applied less than 1 hour before sexual intercourse and should remain in the vaginal tract for 8 hours after intercourse. Before each subsequent intercourse, an additional applicatorful should be inserted.

As with all topically applied chemical contraceptives, irritation of the vagina and penis may occur, although rarely, and in these cases the foams should be discontinued immediately and another type of contraceptive used.

Used correctly, vaginal foam is one of the most effective contraceptive methods. (Of course, use of a diaphragm together with foam increases effectiveness.) In one study, foam was used by nearly 3000 women for approximately 28,000 cycles with a pregnancy rate of 3.98/100 woman-years (38). The rate is relatively low for a vaginal contraceptive; effectiveness was attributed to patient instruction and motivation as well as frequent contact between patient and clinic staff. The only side effect that caused patients to stop using the foam was irritation—107 women, 17 men.

Suppositories and Tablets

Suppositories contain spermicides, usually mercurial compounds or nonoxynol-9, incorporated into a cocoa butter or polyethylene glycol base that melts or dissolves at body temperature. After insertion the user should wait at least 20 minutes before intercourse to allow for melting and distribution over the cervical os. This waiting period can be a disadvantage and, along with variations in melting time, contributes to lower effectiveness. Another suppository contains nonoxynol-9 in a water-soluble base that effervesces to aid dispersion, and the manufacturer claims that after a waiting period of only 10 minutes, protection is provided for up to 2 hours with this product.

Foaming tablets disintegrate and release carbon dioxide on contact with vaginal moisture, covering the uterine entrance with foam to block the sperm. A tablet should be inserted into the vagina near the cervix a few minutes to 1 hour before intercourse. To determine the tablet's freshness, it should be moistened with a drop of water. Then when the bubbling begins, the tablet should be inserted immediately. Foaming tablets should be stored in a dry, cool place and should be used within 6 months of purchase. Successful use depends on the presence of adequate fluid in the vagina to produce complete disintegration prior to intercourse. As with the aerosol foam, a new tablet should be inserted before each intercourse.

Suppositories and foaming tablets probably are less

protective than the foams, creams, or jellies. However, if they are used regularly, they provide a higher degree of protection than other methods used irregularly.

Sponges

A circular sponge, commercial or homemade, has been used as a barrier-type contraceptive agent. Sponges generally are 1.2–1.9 cm thick and 5–7.5 cm in diameter, generally with a retrieval string attached. For greater protection, both sides should be coated with a contraceptive agent prior to insertion deep into the vagina. Alone, the sponge is better than nothing.

Douching

Flooding and flushing out the vagina mechanically (with water alone or with a spermicidal agent) immediately after coitus to remove the semen is an age-old means of attempting to avoid pregnancy. Unfortunately, this after-the-fact method is totally unreliable for conception control. Douching is the least effective of the methods in use and should be discouraged.

The idea behind the practice is that a quick and thorough douching washes the semen from the vagina before the sperm can enter the uterus, thus preventing conception. However, if no other means of contraception is used, douching cannot, even theoretically, be effective because direct cervical insemination occurs prior to douching. Sperm may reach the cervix within 90 seconds of ejaculation. Immediate postcoital tests revealed active spermatozoa in the endocervix within 1.5–3 minutes after coitus, and spermatozoa have been recovered from the fallopian tubes 30 minutes after insemination (39). It is highly improbable that douching can be initiated quickly or thoroughly enough to remove all traces of semen, and therefore all sperm, from the vagina.

The method is mentioned only because douching apparently is practiced widely and a number of commercial douche products are available. No convincing evidence shows that douching with or without added chemicals is an effective contraceptive.

If any nonprescription contraceptive is used following unprotected coitus, a vaginal contraceptive foam or cream probably is best, not only because these agents are effective but because less time is needed to load and discharge an applicatorful than to douche.

The FDA Obstetrics and Gynecology Advisory Committee has been studying vaginal douches to determine whether they exert any contraceptive effect (40). Advertising for most of these products stresses their use for hygienic purposes, not for contraception.

Toxicity Potential

The active ingredients in many spermicidal preparations are potentially toxic if they are ingested in pure form, but the toxic agents are present only in small percentages (41). Signs and symptoms of toxicity vary depending on the ingredient ingested. The possibility remains remote that a child or adult would ingest enough of the toxic agent to cause overt signs and symptoms of acute toxicity; nevertheless, contraceptive preparations should be kept out of the reach of children.

Nonpharmaceutical Methods

Rhythm

The rhythm method is abstinence from sexual relations during the fertile period of the female cycle. Rhythm is one of the least effective methods, although some couples, especially if the woman has a regular menstrual cycle, find it satisfactory.

The major, relatively simple techniques for establishing the time of ovulation are the calendar method (Ogino-Knaus), the thermal or temperature method (basal body temperature, or BBT), and the cervical mucus method (ovulation method) (42). The calendar method predicts ovulation on the basis of probabilities calculated from a woman's menstrual history; the thermal method detects, whereas the cervical mucus method predicts, ovulation on the basis of specific physiological changes that occur during the menstrual cycle.

nondrug techniques

establishing ovulation in rhythm method

If ovulation could be determined accurately, rhythm undoubtedly would become a more acceptable method of contraception. Theoretically, if intercourse were avoided for 2 days prior to ovulation, the day of ovulation, and 1 day after ovulation, conception would not occur. These 4 days constitute the fertile (unsafe) phase of the menstrual cycle; the intermenstrual days before and after are the infertile (safe) phase. The alternation of the fertile phase with the preceding and succeeding infertile phases is called the rhythm (43). Unfortunately, the widely differing lengths of most women's menstrual cycles make it nearly impossible to determine precisely when ovulation takes place (44).

When ovulation begins, a woman's basal body temperature drops slightly, followed by a rise of about 0.5°F (0.28°C) over 24–72 hours. After 2 days of elevated temperature the safe period begins. The temperature fluctuation and a meticulous graphical record of at least 1 year's menstrual cycles form the basis for predicting ovulation and using the rhythm method. For added safety, intercourse should be avoided a few days before and after the unsafe period.

A thermometer (basal thermometer) specifically designed to check basal body temperature records 96–100°F (35.6–37.8°C) with 0.1°F intervals, allowing detection of small changes in body temperature. Better accuracy is achieved from a rectal recording of 5 minutes taken immediately on awakening, before getting out of bed (45). The thermometer should be shaken down the night before and placed at the bedside (to prevent physical exertion on awakening, which causes a rise in temperature). Charts for recording the basal body temperature during the menstrual cycle are available.

For Catholic patients, pharmacists should be aware that the methods of contraception approved by the Catholic Church are abstinence and rhythm (42). The patient should be fully informed of the risks and difficulties inherent in practicing rhythm.

Coitus Interruptus or Withdrawal

coitus interruptus and reservatus

Coitus interruptus involves the removal of the stimulated penis from the vagina and the area of external genitalia before ejaculation. Coitus reservatus differs from coitus interruptus in that penetration takes place in the normal way, but ejaculation is avoided, and the penis remains in the vagina until it becomes flaccid. The problem with both methods is that sperm in the urethral secretions released prior to ejaculation may fertilize the egg.

CONTRACEPTIVE EFFECTIVENESS

A contraceptive method's reliability is in direct proportion to the user's motivation—the most frequent cause of contraceptive failure is simply failure to use the contraceptive. Any contraceptive method works better than none at all, but even the most effective method must be used consistently. Effectiveness depends on acceptability and suitability to a couple's needs at a particular time.

reliability of various methods

reasons for contraceptive failure

pregnancy rate by contraceptive method

immunoassay in pregnancy testing

Contraceptive failure often is caused by ambivalent feelings about pregnancy (46). A study of the main psychological reasons behind undesired pregnancies caused by the misuse or rejection of contraception (47) concluded that from "the large number of illegitimate births, legally and illegally induced abortions, and legitimate but undesired pregnancies in this country and abroad," it is obvious "that contraceptive measures are commonly ignored or actively rejected by a substantial proportion of coitally active human beings who consciously deny procreative intent."

Contraceptive failure may be due to lack of proper education about birth control. A report involving 562 women who had applied for or had obtained abortions stated that the main reasons for unplanned pregnancies were misinformation about the menstrual cycle, the risk of pregnancy, improper use of contraceptives, fear of side effects, and actual method failure (48). In one group studied, deficiencies in medical management were emphasized—most women were given inadequate information or poor advice from their physicians. Types or methods of contraception used in the other group were rhythm, withdrawal, foam, condom, diaphragm, IUD, and oral contraceptives. Lack of understanding of conception and contraception were important factors. Results from both groups indicated that better sex education is needed to reduce the number of unplanned pregnancies ending in abortion. Better education among health care professionals is also needed not only to increase knowledge, but also to reduce their inhibitions and to correct their misconceptions.

Theoretical contraceptive effectiveness relies on the assumption that the method is used according to instructions. Actual effectiveness is reduced by inconsistent or incorrect use (49). Effectiveness in use depends on factors other than biological efficiency, e.g., personal preference, the mores of the social group, availability, cost (initial and long-range), storage, use (ease, frequency, and propensity), timing in relation to intercourse, interference with intercourse, requirements for medical consultation, and side effects. The overall usefulness of a contraceptive method is determined essentially by its ability to reduce the probability of conception—by consistency of use and continuation of use (50).

Among women who use no method of contraception, 80% may expect to become pregnant within 1 year. Table 1 shows the pregnancy rates of various contraceptive methods as determined from current use–effectiveness data. The 1970 National Fertility Study in the United States (51) reported failure rates of 31% with contraceptive foams and 39% with douching. The study also found that one-third of married couples using a contraceptive method fail within 5 years to prevent an unplanned pregnancy. Although these figures are outdated, they remain historically instructive.

Table 1. Pregnancy Rates of Various Contraceptive Methods

Method Used	Percentage
Hysterectomy	0.001
Tubal ligation	0.04
Vasectomy	0.15
Combined oral contraceptive pills	4–10
Low-dose oral progestogen	5–10
Intrauterine device	5
Condom	10
Diaphragm with spermicide	17
Coitus interruptus	20–25
Rhythm (calendar)	21

Data show approximate number of pregnancies per 100 women during first year of use. From R.A. Hatcher et al., *Contraceptive Technology 1976–1977*, 8th rev. ed., Irvington, New York, N.Y., 1976, 144 pp.

PREGNANCY TESTING

The first laboratory test for the detection of pregnancy, a bioassay developed by Ascheim and Zondek in 1928, was based on the observation that urine from a pregnant woman, which contained high levels of human chorionic gonadotropin (HCG), when injected into mice or rats would cause corpus luteum formation with accompanying swelling and hemorrhaging. The test required 5 days for results, and a year later, Friedman developed a similar test which used a rabbit as the test animal and required only 48 hours. Other bioassays for pregnancy that have been used include production of ovarian hyperemia in the rat, extrusion of eggs in the frog, and extrusion of sperm in the toad following injection of HCG-containing urine from pregnant females.

Currently, immunoassay is the most widely used method for pregnancy testing. Two techniques are utilized. One involves inhibition of hemagglutination in a test tube, and the other, inhibition of latex particle agglutination on a slide. The slide test is fast, requiring only a few minutes to perform, but requires experienced personnel to obtain reliable results. The hemagglutination inhibition test performed in a test tube requires about 2 hours to perform and is the method used for the "do-it-yourself" early pregnancy test now being marketed in the United States[1].

[1] e.p.t. In-Home Early Pregnancy Test (Warner-Chilcott, Division of Warner-Lambert Company, Morris Plains, NJ 07950).

The early pregnancy test kit includes a test tube containing dried sheep red blood cells on which HCG has been absorbed and sufficient HCG antiserum to prevent agglutination of these cells when suspended in the water provided in the kit. If the urine being tested contains HCG, it will react with the available HCG antiserum and permit visible agglutination of the sheep red cells. In performing the test, exactly three drops of first morning urine are added carefully to the tube containing the HCG red blood cells and the HCG antiserum; then the premeasured water is added, and the tube is stoppered and shaken for at least 10 seconds. The tube must then be placed in the holder provided and left undisturbed for 2 hours. It is important to avoid any vibration during this time as well as direct sunlight. After 2 hours a positive test produces a dark doughnut-shaped brownish ring (agglutination), and a negative test an evenly dispersed brownish deposit (no agglutination).

The accuracy of this test when performed at home by the consumer was observed to be about 97% for positive readings and 80% for negative readings (52).

The test is intended to be sensitive to HCG urine levels at 23 days or more after ovulation in pregnant females (9 days after the missed menstrual period). If a negative result is obtained with the first test and menses does not occur in 7 days, the manufacturer recommends that the test be repeated. The accuracy of the negative test results increases to 91% on these second tests. If the second test is negative, a physician should be consulted.

It is felt that the lower accuracy rate with negative test readings results primarily from a miscalculation of the time when menses should have occurred and therefore an insufficient HCG level in the urine. Disturbance of the test tube during the 2-hour waiting period also can result in false negative readings.

False positive readings can result from detergent residue in the urine collection container as well as blood or high protein concentrations in the urine sample.

All pregnancy tests that are based on the detection of HCG will be positive in the presence of hydatiform mole, while ectopic pregnancies will most likely produce negative rest results.

FAMILY PLANNING/CONTRACEPTION

Much information is available on contraception and family planning techniques, methods, and practices. The 1970 *Manual of Family Planning and Contraceptive Practice* (53) details the methods of population control recommended in hospitals, public health services, and offices of private physicians. A bibliography of international family planning programs (54) and an account of family planning personnel (55) are examples of current efforts in the search for better methodology and implementation. Other organizations (see the appendix) are excellent sources of educational material and should assist the pharmacist in becoming an expert information outlet on family planning and birth control. In dispensing a birth control agent the pharmacist should discuss the available literature on the particular method and should be able to answer individual questions.

Manufacturers of contraceptive products should make available displays of all forms of contraceptive devices, products, and literature. This approach will promote increased knowledge and use. Condoms, especially, should be displayed.

Table 2 documents the lack of rapport between pharmacists and patients in the area of family planning and contraception (11). The results should motivate pharmacists to re-evaluate their present policies. According to this 1970 report, 65–93% of patients purchasing a contraceptive rarely or never ask for advice. The pharmacist must take a more active role as a qualified consultant in the area of contraception information.

home pregnancy testing

pharmacists as advisors on contraception

In another study, low-income women in Hawaii indicated that they needed and wanted to learn more about contraceptives (56). More than one-third of the women preferred to go to a private doctor for contraceptive supplies, 26% to clinics, 16% to pharmacies, and 6% to hospitals; 11% did not know where to go. Again, these results point out the need for accurate information on where contraceptives can be prescribed, which ones are prescription-only or nonprescription, and where they are available.

At the end of 1969, despite a 42% growth in family planning services in the United States over the previous 18 months, only one in five women estimated to be in need of subsidized family planning help was receiving it. The first national family planning service resource list identifies about 4500 facilities in the United States and three territories that provide these services: 90% offer oral contraceptives, IUDs, and foam, 75% the condom, and 67% the diaphragm and jelly (57).

Pharmacists should become more familiar with family planning programs and should be able to supply the appropriate information. They should not refuse to offer advice on birth control and contraception to anyone, regardless of the circumstances. To dictate that sex without marriage is wrong not only endangers pharmacist/patient rapport but also damages the pharmacist's reputation as a reliable, unbiased source of birth control information.

Table 2. Persons Seeking Advice on Contraception From the Pharmacist

Frequency	From Male Pharmacists, %	From Female Pharmacists, %
Male		
Often	21	3
Rarely	68	73
Never	11	20
Female		
Often	19	35
Rarely	71	52
Never	10	13

Two opposite viewpoints have been expressed concerning the pharmacist's role in advising on birth control and contraception. One advocates a more active role for the pharmacist as a birth control consultant (58); the other insists that the pharmacist is a poor choice for this very special liaison and ultimately disrupts the necessary intimacy and rapport between the physician and the patient (59).

pharmacist role in birth control and VD prevention

Pharmacists profess to take their consultant role seriously when it comes to birth control. Four of five responding pharmacists in one survey believed that providing contraceptive advice and information should be part of their professional duties (58). Unfortunately, only 1% displayed condoms on self-service counters; 85% required a prescription, and 13% did not carry condoms. A significant 58% placed vaginal foams, creams, and jellies on self-service counters, 20% sold them on request, 9% required a prescription, and 7% did not stock them. The report suggests that because pharmacies are distributed widely and "already respond to many consumer needs insofar as services and hours are concerned, a more formal, coordinated effort to enlist the professional involvement of the pharmacist seems in order." Whether or not the pharmacist makes this effort is a moot point; "not to make the attempt, however, will certainly help perpetuate those dismal statistics on unwanted births, illegitimacy, and deadened lives" (45).

SUMMARY

The pharmacist's role as a health consultant in the area of conception control is important. The practicing pharmacist can and should be integrally involved in supplying information on all methods of contraception. The specific concerns of the pharmacist center on those agents that do not require the services of a physician. Moreover, because the pharmacist dispenses prescription-only contraceptives, a knowledge of them and of IUD's and surgical techniques also is essential.

The personal nature of contraception should be considered and dealt with in a professional way. The more objectively the conception control methods are presented, the easier it is for the informed patient to make a choice.

Pharmacists should be on the alert for side effects experienced by patients taking oral contraceptives or using vaginal spermicides and should advise immediate physician referral in these cases. The pharmacist also should contact the patient's physician to discuss the untoward reactions.

REFERENCES

(1) W. J. Dignam, in "Birth Control: A Continuing Controversy," Charles C Thomas, Springfield, Ill., 1967, pp. 142–151.
(2) G. Pincus, "The Control of Fertility," Academic, New York, N.Y., 1965, p. 96.
(3) B. J. Duffy and M. J. Wallace, "Biological and Medical Aspects of Contraception," University of Notre Dame Press, Notre Dame, Ind., 1969, pp. 83–85.
(4) T. Mann, "The Biochemistry of Semen and of the Male Reproductive Tract," Wiley, New York, N.Y., 1954, pp. 29–30.
(5) H. Knaus, "Periodic Fertility and Sterility in Woman: A Natural Method of Birth Control," Chicago Medical Book, Chicago, Ill., 1934, p. 32.
(6) C. F. Westoff, *Fam. Plann. Perspect.*, *8*, 54 (1976).
(7) R. W. Kistner, *J. Am. Med. Assoc.*, *215*, 1162 (1971).
(8) T. Crist, *Obstet. Gynecol. News*, *5*, 16 (Dec. 15, 1970).
(9) E. M. Nash and L. M. Louden, *J. Am. Med. Assoc.*, *210*, 2365 (1969).
(10) G. Hollis and K. Lashman, *Fam. Plann. Perspect.*, *6*, 173 (1974).
(11) N. N. Wagner, P. R. Millard, and R. J. Pion, *J. Am. Pharm. Assoc.*, *NS10*, 258 (1970).
(12) B. N. Fujita, N. N. Wagner, and R. J. Pion, *Am. J. Obstet. Gynecol.*, *109*, 787 (1971).
(13) N. N. Wagner, N. Perthou, B. Fujita, and R. J. Pion, *Postgrad. Med.*, *46*, 68 (Oct. 1969).
(14) S. O. Gustavus and C. A. Huether, *Fam. Plann. Perspect.*, *7*, 203 (1975).
(15) M. L. Finkel and D. J. Finkel, *Fam. Plann. Perspect.*, *7*, 256 (1975).
(16) M. Zelnik and J. F. Kanter, *Fam. Plann. Perspect.*, *6*, 74 (1974).
(17) J. Sklar and B. Berkov, *Fam. Plann. Perspect.*, *6*, 80 (1974).
(18) "Statistical Abstract of the United States," 98th ed., U.S. Government Printing Office, Washington, D.C., 1977, 1048 pp.
(19) H. Goldstein and H. M. Wallace, *Public Health Rep.*, *93*, 46 (1978).
(20) *American Druggist*, *175*, 45 (1977).
(21) *Morbidity Mortality Weekly Report*, *26*, 296 (1978).
(22) P. O. Roberts, *Am. J. Public Health*, *68*, 13 (1978).
(23) "Control of Male Fertility," J. J. Sciarra, Ed., Harper and Row, Hagerstown, Md., 1975, 337 pp.
(24) "Schering Workshop on Contraception: The Masculine Gender," G. Raspe and S. Bernhard, Eds., Pergamon, New York, N.Y., 1973, 332 pp.
(25) P. E. Pothier, National Library of Medicine, Literature Search No. 75-24, 1-11, 142 citations, Jan. 1973–Nov. 1975.
(26) I. A. Dalsimer, P.T. Piotrow, and J. J. Dumm, *Popul. Rep.*, *H*, H/1 (1973).
(27) J. J. Dumm, P. T. Piotrow, and I. A. Dalsimer, *Popul. Rep.*, *H*, H/21 (1974).
(28) "The Condom: Increasing Utilization in the United States," M. H. Redford, G. W. Duncan, and D. J. Prager, Eds., San Francisco Press, San Francisco, Calif., 1974, 320 pp.
(29) P. Schwartz, *Am. Drug.*, *177*, 23 (March 1978).
(30) C. Tietze, "Family-Planning Programs: An International Survey," Basic Books, New York, N.Y., 1969, pp. 183–191.
(31) A. F. Guttmacher, W. Best, and F. S. Jaffe, "Planning Your Family," Macmillan, New York, N.Y., 1964, pp. 41–42.
(32) *Medical Letter on Drugs and Therapeutics*, *13*, 85 (1971).
(33) *Medical Letter on Drugs and Therapeutics*, *13*, 108 (1971).
(34) P. D. Harvey, *Fam. Plann. Perspect.*, *4*, 27 (1972).
(35) *Fam. Plann. Digest*, *1*, 1 (1972).
(36) R. Belsky, *Popul. Rep.*, *H*, H/37 (1975).
(37) M. E. Lane, R. Arceo, and A. J. Sobrero, *Fam. Plann. Perspect.*, *8*, 81 (1976).
(38) G. S. Bernstein, *Contraception*, *3*, 37 (1971).
(39) C. C. Marcus and S. L. Marcus, in "Progress in Infertility," Little, Brown, Boston, Mass., 1968, pp. 21–62.
(40) W. Rinehart, *Popul. Rep.*, *J*, J/41 (1976).
(41) R. E. Gosselin, H. C. Hodge, R. P. Smith, and M. N. Gleason, "Clinical Toxicology of Commercial Products: Acute Poisoning," 4th ed., Williams and Wilkins, Baltimore, Md., 1976, Sec. II, pp. 1–273; Sec. V, pp. 1–799.
(42) C. Ross and P. T. Piotrow, *Popul. Rep.*, *I*, I/1 (1974).
(43) J. Rock, in "Manual of Family Planning and Contraceptive Practice," 2nd ed., M. S. Calderone, Ed., Williams and Wilkins, Baltimore, Md., 1970.
(44) L. Mastroianni, Jr., *Fam. Plann. Perspect.*, *6*, 209 (1974).
(45) B. J. Pisani, in "Manual of Family Planning and Contraceptive Practice," 2nd ed., M. S. Calderone, Ed., Williams and Wilkins, Baltimore, Md., 1970.
(46) H. Lehfeldt, *Mod. Aspects Hum. Sexual.*, *5*, 68 (1971).
(47) E. C. Sandberg and R. I. Jacobs, *Am. J. Obstet. Gynecol.*, *110*, 227 (1971).
(48) *Fam. Plann. Perspect.*, *8*, 72, 75 (1976).
(49) C. Tietze, in "Manual of Family Planning and Contraceptive Practice," 2nd ed., M. S. Calderone, Ed., Williams and Wilkins, Baltimore, Md., 1970, pp. 268–269.
(50) C. Tietze and S. Lewit, *Fertil. Steril.*, *22*, 508 (1971).
(51) N. B. Ryder, *Fam. Plann. Perspect.*, *5*, 133 (1973).
(52) Warner Chilcott, Studies 2C0814 and 2C0815, Morris Plains, N.J.
(53) "Manual of Family Planning and Contraceptive Practice," 2nd ed., M. S. Calderone, Ed., Williams and Wilkins, Baltimore, Md., 1970.
(54) K. C. Lyle and S. J. Segal, "International Family Planning Programs, 1966–1975: A Bibliography," University of Alabama Press, University, Ala., 1977, 207 pp.
(55) W. L. Barton, in "Health Manpower Planning: Principles, Methods, Issues," T. L. Hall and A. Mejia, Eds., World Health Organization, Geneva, Switzerland, 1978, pp. 223–232.
(56) R. J. Wolff and B. Z. Bell, *Stud. Fam. Plann.*, *56* (Aug. 1970).
(57) *Family Planning Perspectives*, *8*, 130 (1976).
(58) M. J. Rumel, L. C. Stringfellow, and R. J. Pion, *Fam. Plann. Perspect.*, *3*, 80 (1971).
(59) P. Cutright, *Fam. Plann. Perspect.*, *3*, 25 (1971).

APPENDIX: FAMILY PLANNING INFORMATION

- Planned Parenthood Federation of America, Inc.
  810 Seventh Avenue
  New York, NY 10019

Offers family planning services, infertility therapy, pregnancy counseling, abortion and sterilization services or referral for such services, education for marriage and sex education, prenatal care, and a variety of special programs. Patient-level pamphlets cover all methods or individual ones (some in Spanish). Teaching aids, posters, and subscription periodicals are offered.

- The Population Council
  Publications and Information Office
  One Dag Hammarskjold Plaza
  New York, NY 10017

Publishes the monthly *Studies in Family Planning* and *Population and Development Review*, as well as books and monographs. The Council endeavors to advance knowledge in the broad field of population by fostering research, training, and technical consultation and assistance in the social and biomedical sciences.

- Zero Population Growth
  1346 Connecticut Avenue, N.W.
  Washington, DC 20036

Activities aimed at population education and political action to remove laws that inhibit or restrict individual freedom of choice of medically approved contraception techniques. Advocates an end to population growth in the United States through its population policy.

- The Alan Guttmacher Institute
  515 Madison Avenue
  New York, NY 10022

Publishes *Family Planning Perspectives* (bimonthly), *International Family Planning Perspectives and Digest* (quarterly), *Family Planning/Population Reporter*, and *Planned Parenthood Washington Memo*; the Institute has prepared a detailed two-volume manual, *Developing Statewide Family Planning Programs: A Planning Handbook* (available for $50), to assist administrators and program officials in developing a statewide approach to family planning programs that will meet federal and state requirements. The Institute also has published *Contraceptive Services for Adolescents: Each State and County, 1975*, a nationwide study (available for $5.00).

- Population Information Program
  The Johns Hopkins University
  624 N. Broadway
  Baltimore, MD 21205

Publishes *Population Reports*, an excellent series that provides an accurate and authoritative overview of important developments in the population field.

- The Population Program
  The Rockefeller Foundation
  1133 Avenue of the Americas
  New York, NY 10036

Strives toward the goal of population stabilization through support of research, training, and experimental programs in a broad range of fields related to population.

- Special Programme of Research, Development
  and Research Training in Human Reproduction
  World Health Organization
  Avenue Appia
  1211 Geneva 27, Switzerland

The objectives are geared to meet the expressed needs of Member States for technology for family planning and infertility that is safer, more effective, better adapted to the needs of their populations, and to focus on the development of new methods and service approaches that emphasize ease of provision through primary health care, simplicity of use, and low cost.

Product (Manufacturer)	Dosage Form	Spermicide	Other
Vaginal Spermicides Used Without a Diaphragm			
Anvita (A. O. Schmidt)	suppositories	phenylmercuric borate, 1:2000	boric acid, aluminum potassium sulfate, thymol, chlorothymol, aromatics, cocoa butter
Because (Emko)	foam	nonoxynol 9, 8%	benzethonium chloride, 0.2%
Conceptrol (Ortho)	cream	nonoxynol 9, 5%	—
Dalkon (Robins)	foam	nonoxynol 9, 8%	benzethonium chloride
Delfen (Ortho)	foam cream	nonoxynol 9, 12.5% nonoxynol 9, 5%	—
Emko (Emko)	foam	nonoxynol 9, 8%	benzethonium chloride, 0.2%; stearic acid; triethanolamine; glyceryl monostearate; poloxamer 188; polyethylene glycol 600; substituted adamantane; dichlorodifluoromethane; dichlorotetrafluoroethane
Encare Oval (Eaton)	suppository	nonoxynol 9, 2.27%	effervescent, water-soluble base
Koromex (Holland-Rantos)	foam	nonoxynol 9, 12.5%	propylene glycol, isopropyl alcohol, laureth 4, cetyl alcohol, polyethylene glycol stearate, fragrance, dichlorodifluoromethane, dichlorotetrafluoroethane
Koromex II Cream (Holland-Rantos)	cream	octoxynol, 3.0%	propylene glycol, stearic acid, sorbitan stearate, polysorbate 60, boric acid, fragrance
Koromex II and II-A Jelly (Holland-Rantos)	gel	octoxynol, 1% (II) nonoxynol 9, 2% (II-A)	propylene glycol, cellulose gum, boric acid, sorbitol, starch, simethicone, fragrance
Lanteen (Lambda)	jelly	—	chlorothymol, 0.0077% ricinoleic acid, 0.5% hexylresorcinol, 0.1%
Ramses 10 Hour (Schmid)	jelly	dodecaethylene glycol monolaurate, 5%	—
Semicid (Gynechemie)	suppository	nonoxynol 9, 5%	—
S'Positive (Jordan-Simner)	suppository	nonoxynol 9, 10%	vegetable oil base benzethonium chloride
Vaginal Spermicides Used With a Diaphragm			
Koromex II (Holland-Rantos)	jelly cream	octoxynol, 1% octoxynol, 3%	— —
Ortho-Creme (Ortho)	cream	nonoxynol 9, 2%	—
Ortho-Gynol (Ortho)	jelly	*p*-diisobutylphenoxy-polyethoxyethanol, 1%	—

Brand Name (Supplier)	Type
Conceptrol Shields, Lubricated (Ortho Pharmaceutical)	rubber shaped and/or ribbed, packaged with lubricant
Conceptrol Shields, Non-lubricated (Ortho Pharmaceutical)	rubber shaped and/or ribbed, packaged dry
Conture (Akwell)	rubber-shaped and/or ribbed, packaged with lubricant
Excita Sensitol (Schmid)	rubber-shaped and/or ribbed, packaged with lubricant
Fetherlite (Schmid)	rubber-plain end, packaged dry rubber-plain end, packaged with lubricant
Fiesta Sensi-Color (Schmid)	rubber-reservoir end, packaged with lubricant
Fourex (Schmid)	lamb cecum-regular end, packaged with lubricant
Guardian (Youngs)	rubber-reservoir end, packaged with lubricant
Naturalamb (Youngs)	lamb cecum-regular end, packaged with lubricant
Nuda (Akwell)	rubber-reservoir end, packaged with lubricant
Nuform Sensi-Shape, Lubricated (Schmid)	rubber-shaped and/or ribbed, packaged with lubricant
Nuform Sensi-Shape, Non-lubricated (Schmid)	rubber-shaped and/or ribbed, packaged dry
Prime (Akwell)	rubber-reservoir end, packaged with lubricant
Prime, Non-Lubricated (Akwell)	rubber-reservoir end, packaged dry
Ramses (Schmid)	rubber-plain end, packaged dry
Ramses Sensitol (Schmid)	rubber-plain end, packaged with lubricant
Sheik Plain End (Schmid)	rubber-plain end, packaged dry
Sheik Reservoir End, Lubricated (Schmid)	rubber-reservoir end, packaged with lubricant
Sheik Reservoir End, Non-lubricated (Schmid)	rubber-reservoir end, packaged dry
Stimula (Akwell)	rubber-shaped and/or ribbed, packaged with lubricant
Tahiti (Akwell)	rubber-reservoir end, packaged with lubricant
Trojan-Enz, Lubricated (Youngs)	rubber-reservoir end, packaged with lubricant
Trojan-Enz, Non-lubricated (Youngs)	rubber-reservoir end, packaged dry
Trojans (Youngs)	rubber-plain end, packaged dry
Trojans Plus (Youngs)	rubber-shaped and/or ribbed, packaged with lubricant
Trojans Ribbed (Youngs)	rubber-shaped and/or ribbed, packaged with lubricant

Feminine Cleansing and Deodorant Products

Stephen G. Hoag

Chapter 17

Questions to Ask the Patient

Have you noted a discharge?

Have you experienced pain or itching?

Are there any sores in the genital area?

How long has the condition been present?

Do you douche? How frequently? What method do you use?

Have you ever had a reaction to ointments or sprays?

What drugs, either prescription or nonprescription, are you currently using?

To your knowledge, are you pregnant?

Do you have diabetes?

American society today is probably unsurpassed in history in its concern for cleanliness, personal hygiene, and elimination of body odors. The many products promoted are intended to keep us clean and odor free from head to toe. Included in this group of personal toiletry and cosmetic products are douches and feminine deodorant products. Vaginal douches are not new. Feminine deodorant sprays, on the other hand, are relative newcomers to the field, having been introduced in the mid-1960's.

Feminine toiletry and cosmetic products are used (appropriately or not) for general cleansing of the vaginal or perineal areas, for deodorizing, for relief of itching, burning, erythema, and edema, for removing secretions or discharge, and for psychological reasons, such as producing a soothing and refreshing feeling. Some of these feminine products, such as douches, may be prescribed by physicians for altering vaginal pH to affect microscopic flora.

Many gynecologists believe that the healthy vagina cleanses itself and that the perineal area may be cleaned adequately with soap and water. Others seem to feel that douching, done properly, promotes healthy vaginal tissues. The value of feminine deodorant sprays is also controversial. Their efficacy as deodorants is often questioned, and possible adverse effects, such as irritation of vaginal mucous membranes, have come to light since the sprays first appeared.

In this chapter the word "hygiene" is not used in connection with these products because most of the products do not possess medicinal properties, especially the deodorant sprays. Their action and benefit are cosmetic. Furthermore, the few douche preparations that do have therapeutic properties should not be purchased for self-medication in the presence of disease; their use may delay the user from seeking medical attention. Nonprescription vaginal cleansing and deodorant products always should be used as cosmetics and toiletries unless a physician or pharmacist is supervising their use for therapeutic purposes.

PHYSIOLOGY OF VAGINAL TRACT

The important physiological considerations concerning feminine cleansing and deodorant product use include vaginal epithelial thickness and glycogen content, normal bacterial flora, vaginal pH, production of secretions and discharge, and production of objectionable odor (see Chapter 15). Vaginal surfaces are lined with squamous epithelium, and estrogens are mainly responsible for controlling the thickness of this lining. Epithelial cell height increases at menarche and decreases at menopause. Before menarche and after menopause the vaginal epithelium is apparently less resistant to infection. Glycogen content of vaginal epithelium is increased during the childbearing years.

Vaginal health depends on pH, normal bacterial flora, epithelial cellular height, and epithelial glycogen content. The normal vaginal bacterial flora include Döderlein's bacillus, diphtheroids, staphylococci, and anaerobic streptococci. Döderlein's bacillus (a strain of lactobacillus) metabolizes epithelial glycogen to lactic acid. Vaginal pH is normally alkaline before menarche and after menopause but is normally acid during the childbearing years as a result of this metabolic production of lactic acid by bacteria. The vaginal pH ranges from 3.0 to 6.1; the average range is usually 3.5–4.2 (1–3). The acidic vaginal pH and the presence of normal flora usually preclude pathogen growth, but a pH shift toward alkalinity may render the area more susceptible to infection.

Vaginal mucous secretion is composed in part of the endocervical mucus as well as bacteria and desquamated vaginal epithelium. This discharge is a natural cleansing mechanism, but in the absence of personal cleanliness the discharge or secretion may accumulate on external genital surfaces and produce an odor. The vulvoperineal area contains sebaceous, apocrine, and exocrine glands, each producing minimal secretions, as well as Bartholin's glands, which secrete a very small amount of mucus during sexual stimulation. In addition, there is a clear, alkaline transudate in the vagina during sexual excitement. Vaginal discharge may increase noticeably during periods of emotional stress and ovulation.

The mucous, sebaceous, and apocrine perineal secretions and the vaginal discharge are subject to bacterial decomposition if left on the skin for long periods. This bacterial decomposition of normal secretions is the main cause of objectionable odor.

VAGINITIS

Etiology and Classification

origins and types of vaginitis

predisposing factors

leukorrhea and pruritus

Besides cosmetic and deodorant considerations, the most common reasons for using douches and other feminine cleansing products are probably vulvar pruritus (and/or a burning sensation) and excessive vaginal discharge (leukorrhea). One of the most frequent causes of these symptoms is vaginitis, an inflammation of vulvar and vaginal epithelium usually caused by disturbances of the normal flora or by pathogenic microorganisms. In most instances, vaginitis causes more discomfort than danger to the patient (4–6). A classification of vaginitis is given in Table 1, but most cases may be placed in one of four categories: *Trichomonas vaginalis* vaginitis, *Candida albicans* (monilial) vaginitis, nonspecific vaginitis, or atrophic vaginitis. Because there are no nerve endings in the vagina to perceive pain and pruritis, the patient has no symptoms until the external genitalia become involved in the infection.

Trichomonal and monilial vaginitis are the most common types in women of childbearing age. Prolonged tetracycline use, steroid therapy (including oral contraceptives), cancer, pregnancy, and diabetes are among the factors possibly predisposing to the overgrowth of monilial organisms (*C. albicans*) (7). Atrophic vaginitis occurs after menopause when vaginal epithelium thins. *Proteus* may be implicated in a significant number of chronic cases of atrophic vaginitis. Although childhood vulvovaginitis is relatively uncommon, it usually has the same cause and manifestations as atrophic vaginitis. Monilial and trichomonal infections may occur simultaneously, and both organisms may be present in the normal, healthy vagina (8, 9). *Trichomonas* and *Hemophilus* vaginitis frequently are transmitted by sexual contact.

Symptoms

The symptoms of vaginitis, leukorrhea and pruritus, may cause a woman to seek medical attention or to self-medicate. Offensive odor may be caused by discharge associated with trichomonal or *Hemophilus* organisms. The description of a purulent vaginal discharge should alert the pharmacist to the possibility of vaginitis and the need for a specific diagnosis and prescribed therapy. In postmenopausal women a thin, watery discharge accompanied by pruritus indicates possible atrophic vaginitis or malignancy. The pharmacist should determine whether vaginitis symptoms are present, how long they have persisted, and whether predisposing factors exist. The patient also should be asked whether any previous attempts at self-treatment have been made, because symptoms may be an adverse reaction to an OTC product.

Depending on the specific diagnosis of vaginitis, antitrichomonal, antimonilial, or antibacterial therapy may be prescribed by the physician. In atrophic vaginitis, however, systemic or local estrogenic hormone therapy may be prescribed because estrogen stimulates vaginal epithelium, increasing its thickness and resistance to infection. Nonprescription feminine cleansing and deo-

Table 1. Classification of Vaginitis

Type	Organism	Age Group Affected
Infectious		
Atrophic (senile)	coliforms, staphylococci, streptococci	postmenopausal (prepubertal, rarely)
Gonorrhea	*Neisseria gonorrhoeae*	adult
Herpes II	herpes II	all
Monilial	*Candida albicans*	adult (especially if pregnant or diabetic)
Mycoplasma	mycoplasma	all
Nonspecific	*Hemophilus vaginalis*[a], coliforms, staphylococci, streptococci	all
Preadolescent (childhood vulvovaginitis)	helminths, coliforms, staphylococci, streptococci	prepubertal
Trichomonal	*Trichomonas vaginalis*	adult (prepubertal, rarely)
Tuberculous	*Mycobacterium tuberculosis*	all
Noninfectious		
Allergic and chemical	—	all (when foreign chemicals are instilled vaginally)
Postirradiation	—	all (when irradiation is used for treatment of cervical carcinoma)
Traumatic	—	all

[a] *Hemophilus* vaginitis is frequently considered by itself because *H. vaginalis* is the most frequent pathogen in nonspecific bacterial vaginitis.

dorant products should be used in cases of vaginitis only on a pharmacist's or physician's advice.

Pruritus with or without a malodorous discharge may occur in conditions other than vaginitis such as cystitis, urethritis, chemical irritation, venereal disease, and carcinoma of the cervix, endometrium, and vagina. Regardless of the cause, these symptoms are an indication for diagnostic evaluation by a physician, especially if they are persistent, severe, or recurrent.

VAGINAL DOUCHES

Douches may exert cleansing effects by lowering surface tension, mucolytic action, and proteolytic action, although standards for evaluating these effects have not been established (10). Douche products are available in disposable or nondisposable form as liquids, liquid concentrates to be diluted in water, powders to be dissolved in water, and powders to be instilled as powders. The term "douche" is not limited to a stream of water.

Ingredients

ingredients in douches recommended concentrations

Recommended concentrations for many ingredients in feminine cleansing and deodorant products are listed in Table 2, but many manufacturers do not list concentrations.

Antimicrobial Agents

Most antimicrobial agents in douche products are present in concentrations that provide preservative properties to the product per se, not therapeutic activity. They include benzethonium and benzalkonium chlorides, chlorothymol, hexachlorophene, and parabens. Other compounds, such as boric acid, cetylpyridinium chloride, eucalyptol, menthol, oxyquinoline, phenol, sodium perborate, and thymol, may be included for purported antiseptic or germicidal activity. However, the value of these ingredients as antimicrobials is questionable, depending in some cases on the concentration used. Because many manufacturers do not list concentrations of ingredients if the products are considered cosmetics, it is impossible to assess their efficacy. Boric acid (5%) under physician supervision is an effective antimicrobial for treating monilial vaginitis, and povidone-iodine is an effective antimicrobial agent for adjunctive therapy in monilial and trichomonal vaginitis (11, 12), although questions of safety have arisen (13). The possibility of local irritation or sensitization exists with many antimicrobial agents found in douches, and if these effects are encountered, the patient should be instructed to discontinue use of the product and to consult a physician.

Local Anesthetics/Antipruritics

Compounds such as eucalyptol, menthol, and phenol are included in douches for local anesthetic or antipruritic effects. Possible antipruritic effects are not substantiated. Eucalyptol, because of its fragrance, also may provide some deodorant effect.

Counterirritants

Many douche products contain substances such as menthol, methyl salicylate, and thymol for counterirritant

Table 2. Recommended Concentrations for Components of Feminine Cleansing and Deodorant Products

Agent	Recommended Concentration
Alum	0.5–5.0% [a]
Benzalkonium chloride	1:5,000–1:2,000 vaginally 0.02–0.2% externally
Benzethonium chloride	1:750 [a]
Benzocaine	1.0–2.0% [a]
Boric acid [b]	1.0–4.0% [a]
Cetylpyridinium chloride	1:10,000–1:2,000 on mucous membranes 1:1,000–1:100 externally
Hexachlorophene	0.2% [c]
Menthol	0.1–2.0% [a]
Methylbenzethonium chloride	1:10,000–1:100 [a]
Methyl salicylate	10–25% [a]
Oxyquinoline	1:1,000 vaginally or externally
Parabens (total)	0.05–0.3% [a]
Phenol	0.5–1.0% [a]
Phenylmercuric acetate	0.02% on mucous membranes, 0.2% externally, 0.002–0.125% as a preservative
Povidone-iodine [d]	10% (0.5–3.0% of available iodine) [a]
Resorcinol	2.0–20% [a]
Salicylic acid	2.0–20% [a]
Thymol	1.0% [a]
Zinc oxide	15–25% [a]
Zinc sulfate	0.25–4.0% [a]

From *Remington's Pharmaceutical Sciences*, 14th ed., A. Osol and J. E. Hoover, Eds., Mack, Easton, Pa., 1970.
[a] Recommendation does not specify difference in concentration between external skin and mucous membranes and should be viewed cautiously because mucous membranes may be more sensitive.
[b] From T. E. Swate and J. C. Weed, *Obstet. Gynecol.*, *43*, 893 (1974).
[c] Present legal FDA maximum allowable concentration in OTC products (From FDA Minutes of the OTC Panel on Contraceptives and Other Vaginal Drug Products.)
[d] From J. J. Ratzan, *Calif. Med.*, *110*, 24 (1969).

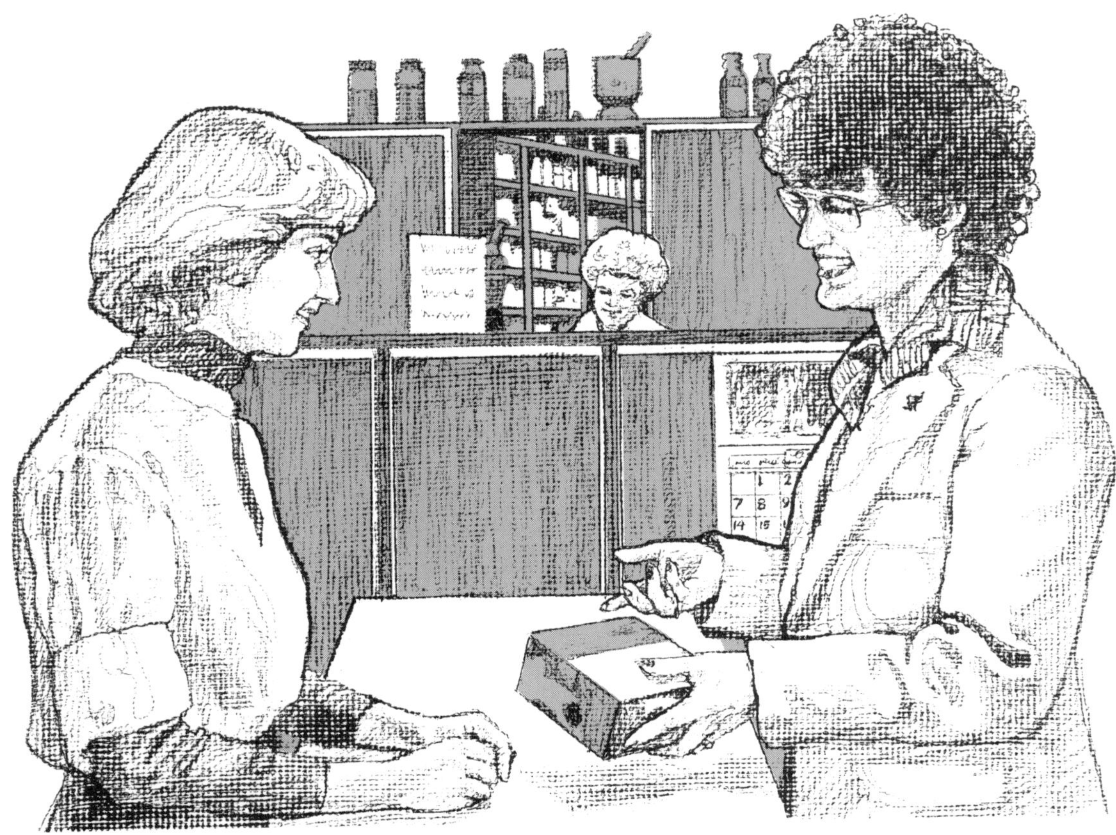

ingredients in douches

syringes and their use

effects, although their value has not been substantiated. Offensive odor may be masked by the fragrance of methyl salicylate.

Astringents

Astringent substances such as ammonium and potassium alums and zinc sulfate are included in some douches to reduce local edema, inflammation, and exudation. Micronized aluminum powder also has been used as an astringent douche (2). The astringent concentration is important because many astringents are irritants in moderate or high concentrations (14).

Proteolytics

At least one proteolytic agent, papain, is used in a douche product to remove excess vaginal discharge. Papain may elicit allergic reactions.

Surfactants

Dioctyl sodium sulfosuccinate, nonoxynol 4, and sodium lauryl sulfate are used to facilitate the douche's spreading over vaginal mucosa and penetrating the mucosal folds and rugae (1). Cetylpyridinium chloride also has surface-active properties.

Substances Affecting pH

Many vaginal douche products are buffered or contain substances that purposely render them either acidic or alkaline. For example, sodium perborate and sodium bicarbonate provide alkalinity, and lactic acid and citric acid provide acidity. The significance of pH and buffering is discussed in the section on advisability of douching.

Miscellaneous Ingredients

Other ingredients occasionally found in douches are emollients, emulsifiers, keratolytics, and substances intended to raise the preparation's osmolarity. Liquid vehicles are alcohol, propylene glycol, water, or combinations of these substances. Talc is used as a vehicle for douche powders intended to be instilled as powders (insufflations). Lactose may be added as a bacterial nutrient, but the reason for its inclusion is unclear. Aromatic agents (chlorothymol, eucalyptol, menthol, thymol, or methyl salicylate) may be added for the general effect of producing a soothing and refreshing feeling. Many urologists feel that a simple douche consisting of small amounts of white vinegar and tap water (2 tbsp of vinegar per quart of water) is as good as commercially available products.

Types of Syringes

Several types of syringes are used for douching. The combination water bottle–syringe (fountain syringe) and the folding feminine syringe are held above hip level while the douche liquid is instilled into the vagina via gravity. These syringes are supplied with the necessary tubing and tips for use with douches or with enemas. Patients should be advised of the difference between douche and enema tips. The main advantage to the combination (fountain) and folding feminine syringes is that fluids are instilled with gentle gravity force only, thereby minimizing the chance of excessive fluid force.

Bulb-type feminine syringes also may be used with douche liquids via gentle squeezing of the bulb. The main advantage of bulb-type feminine syringes is ease of handling, since it is not necessary to use tubing or to hold the syringe at an elevated level. Care must be exercised, however, to avoid excessive squeezing and excessive fluid force on instillation of the douche. Excessive force may introduce fluid into the cervix which may cause an inflammatory response, depending on the degree of uterine involvement.

Techniques of Douching

recommended procedures for safe instillation

To avoid the possible dangers of improper douching, several investigators recommended procedures to ensure safe instillation (7, 15–17):

- Douches should never be instilled with excess pressure. The force of gravity is sufficient if a bag, tube, and nozzle are used. The douche bag should not be more than 60 cm above the hips. If a syringe is used, minimum pressure should be applied.
- Most douches should be instilled while the patient is lying down, the knees drawn up and the hips raised.
- Water used to dilute powder or douche solutions should be lukewarm, not hot.
- Douching equipment should be cleaned thoroughly before and after use. Sterilization by boiling is also recommended. (The use of disposable douche products eliminates this inconvenience.)
- Douches should not be used during pregnancy.
- Douches should not be used when practicing the cervical mucus method of birth control (see Chapter 16).

Recommendations concerning the frequency of douching vary widely. One study found that 175 women douching daily had higher vaginal epithelial glycogen concentrations than 199 women douching less often than daily, implying that the group douching more frequently experienced a beneficial effect (18). Water and a medicinal powder douche were used, but the ingredients and nature of the medicinal powder were not stated.

Some studies recommend avoiding routine douching altogether (13, 16, 19). A common recommendation, however, is that a woman who prefers routine douching should not do so more than twice per week unless otherwise advised by the physician or pharmacist. The potential for harm from frequent douching depends in part on formulation and technique of instillation, both of which may be incorrect. Properly prepared and properly instilled, a douche used twice per week should cause no harm, but it has not been proven that twice-weekly or even less frequent douching is necessary at all.

An alternative self-bathing method for vaginal and perineal areas has been studied for benefits and possible adverse effects in more than 500 women, including 180 with symptoms or diagnosis of vaginitis (20). The technique involves gentle washing with the fingers of the vulvar, perineal, and anal regions and the vagina, using only lukewarm water and a mild soap. (See Chapter 26 for a discussion of antimicrobial soaps.) The technique was effective as a cleansing practice and was 94% effective in clearing the symptoms of vaginitis, whose recurrence rate was slightly more than 5%.

Advisability of Douching

pros and cons of douching

Evaluating whether or not a woman should use a douche for routine vaginal cleansing is quite difficult; both sides of the conflict are well represented in the literature. The current FDA position regarding safety and efficacy of vaginal douching is that there are no standards for evaluating or substantiating claims (10).

Adverse effects of douches on vaginal pH, flora, and cytology have been cited as potential hazards of routine douching. However, the effects of acid, alkaline, and vinegar douches on vaginal pH and vaginal mucosal cytology are not significant (3, 21). An alkaline douche is said to be more effective than an acid douche for removing vaginal discharge and relieving pruritis, and it is effective as adjunctive therapy in vaginitis (21–23).

Other reports also support douching as a safe, effective cleansing mechanism that does not alter vaginal pH significantly if the douche preparation is unbuffered (1, 2, 24); acidic rather than alkaline douches are advised, however, because shifts toward alkalinity may inhibit normal flora and promote pathogen growth (1, 2). Of course, care should be taken that the douche is not excessively acidic, causing irritation or injury.

In one study, douching caused no significant alterations in normal vaginal flora (18). Moreover, significant increases in vaginal epithelial glycogen content were observed in women who douched, and it was concluded that douching was not only harmless but even beneficial to vaginal and cervical epithelium. Others (25, 26) also have attested to the safety of routine douching carried out according to physician instructions. No evidence was found that douche ingredients may be absorbed systemically in significant quantities. Boric acid and phenylmercuric acetate may be absorbed but not in toxic amounts (11, 13).

A significant number of case reports described adverse effects, suggesting that douching may be unwise without specific indication. Five cases were studied in which salpingitis, endometritis, or pelvic inflammatory disease was associated with douching (17). Instillation pressure of the douche fluid was implicated in each case. In another study, 90% of 101 patients with pelvic inflammatory disease were reported as being "vigorous" douchers (27). Other conditions linked to douching are infection, hemorrhage, trauma, embolism, and chemical peritonitis (15, 16, 20, 28).

Perhaps the most frequent adverse effects of douches are direct, primary mucosal/dermal irritation or allergic contact sensitivity from specific ingredients. No well-controlled clinical studies of these effects on vaginal mucosa after douching could be found, but many ingredients of douche preparations have been implicated in these dermal effects. Dermal irritants or sensitizers may affect the vaginal epithelium similarly. Compounds incorporated into douche products which cause direct chemical effects, especially allergic contact sensitivity, include benzalkonium and benzethonium chlorides, benzocaine, chlorhexidine hydrochloride, chloroxylenol, parabens, phenol, propylene glycol monostearate, and triethanolamine (29–34).

Potential hazards must be weighed against the questionable value of routine douching in the absence of symptoms. According to one position (17), in spite of reported adverse effects, we must "recognize that a douche properly prepared and administered is harmless." The key words in this statement are "properly prepared and administered." This is where the pharmacist can help by proper counseling.

Douche products should not be considered contraceptive agents. Douches of normal volume, properly instilled, are ineffective in removing seminal fluid (19). Precoital douches also are ineffective as contraceptives (17). Postcoital douching is preferred by some women, but the benefits are probably psychological or placebo because the superiority of douching over cleansing with soap and water has not been demonstrated conclusively. Douching should be done no sooner than 6–8 hours after the use of a spermicide because spermidical agents may be removed in the douching process.

components of vaginal sprays

benefits and hazards of sprays

FEMININE DEODORANT SPRAYS

Feminine deodorant sprays are aerosol products intended for use on the external genital area to reduce or mask objectionable odor. They are available in mist or powder form. A typical formula includes an antimicrobial agent, an emollient carrier, a perfume, and a propellant. Talc is added to spray powders. The FDA considers these products cosmetics and prohibits references to "hygiene" by manufacturers (35). The sprays do not possess therapeutic or medicinal properties. They may be used as deodorants or simply for placebo or psychological benefits as toiletries.

Ingredients

Some concentrations of feminine deodorant spray ingredients may be safe for external skin but not necessarily for vaginal mucosa.

Perfumes

The main ingredients of feminine deodorant sprays, fragrances, or perfumes are responsible for deodorant activity. They should be selected with care because some may be irritating to perineal and vaginal mucosa (36). Fragrances are characterized as mild or strong, short- or long-lasting, sweet, medicinal, and floral, among other categories (37). Some products contain encapsulated perfumes that are released slowly on contact with moisture.

Antimicrobials

Antimicrobial compounds in sprays include benzalkonium and benzethonium chlorides, chloroxylenol, and hexachlorophene. These and similar compounds are preservative rather than therapeutic. Although a deodorant action may be achieved by inhibiting or eradicating vulvoperineal bacteria, the sprays do not deodorize by this mechanism. Properly used, they do not alter normal vulvovaginal flora, but if they are used improperly, they may do so (38). Holding the spray too close to the body may result in an excessively high surface concentration of the antimicrobial agent or may cause the agent to enter into the vagina, where the concentration also may be excessive.

Emollients

A number of emollient substances are included in these formulations as vehicles and for their soothing effect on the skin. The most commonly used are fatty esters such as fatty alcohols, isopropyl myristate, and polyoxyethylene derivatives of fatty esters. Unfortunately, some of these substances also may be sensitizers (30, 32, 36).

Propellants

The fluorinated hydrocarbon propellants that have been used in feminine deodorant sprays also may be responsible for some adverse reactions. If the spray is held too close to the body and the propellant reaches the skin, the chilling effect when the spray evaporates may cause irritation and edema (36, 39, 40). With proper application, propellants are not likely to be irritants.

Advisability of Sprays

As with douche products, the advisability and benefits of using feminine deodorant sprays are controversial. Their efficacy even as deodorants has been questioned, and adverse effects have been reported (41). When the sprays are used as directed, however, manufacturers report that extensive testing fails to demonstrate adverse effects.

A feminine deodorant spray was evaluated in 1400 women after more than 200,000 test applications by direct application and patch testing (42). However, the results of the study are difficult to judge because many details were not provided. The authors felt that their study supported the position that the sprays were nonirritating and nonsensitizing. It was also reported that, in one group of 300 women, 8% of the control group experienced erythema from soap and water, but only 3% of those using the spray experienced this effect. The authors offered other explanations for consumer complaints of vulvar irritation after the use of these sprays. It was possible, they said, that close-fitting and/or nonabsorbent undergarments caused vulvar irritation even if no spray was applied; that the symptoms might appear if sprays are used immediately after intercourse; or that the sprays were held too close to the body when applied.

In another study, only one case of erythema and one of irritation were reported, and it was concluded that the preparation was suitable for use (43). Other authors also have attested to the safety of feminine deodorant sprays (39, 44).

Despite reports that these aerosol products are not hazardous when evaluated in controlled studies and when properly used, there is evidence that hazards do exist.

Physicians in private practice reported vulvar irritation in some of their female patients (45–47), and feminine deodorant sprays were strongly suspected as being the cause. The FDA receives many reports of adverse local reactions, all locally severe and all attributed to the use of these products (48). In most of these cases, systemic steroid treatment was required even when the sprays were discontinued. The specific ingredients responsible for adverse effects, however, were not identified. Four positive patch-test reactions to specific ingredients were reported after 30 women and 2 men were tested with the individual ingredients in 12 different sprays (36). The ingredients eliciting positive responses were benzethonium chloride, chlorhexidine, isopropyl myristate, and perfume. Ingredients in douches that cause either direct primary irritation or allergic contact sensitization also are found frequently in feminine deodorant sprays. Women who use sprays immediately before sexual intercourse also may exhibit local reactions (36).

Most evidence criticizing feminine deodorant spray use is from case reports or complaints received by manufacturers, physicians, and the FDA; most evidence in defense of these products is cited by the authors as the findings of controlled studies. However, in controlled studies, subjects are given instructions on proper application. The use of sprays throughout the population is uncontrolled, and it is especially difficult to assess the incidence of improper application. It seems that feminine deodorant sprays are harmless to most users, but reports of adverse effects are too frequent to be ignored, and the significant potential hazards must be considered. Furthermore, the superiority of these sprays over soap and water has been questioned (49, 50). In the absence of conclusive demonstrations of prominent adverse effects, they continue to be marketed.

Proper Application of Sprays

Most manufacturers recommend that sprays be held at least 20 cm from the body when applying. By following this indication, premarketing evaluations of sprays consistently demonstrate safety. The most frequent adverse effect resulting from applying a spray held too closely is irritation as a result of evaporation and "chilling" from propellants inappropriately reaching the skin, excessive concentrations of ingredients on cutaneous surfaces, or accidental penetration of ingredients into the vagina from the force of the spray (ingredients are intended only for external use).

The relationship between frequency of use and the incidence of adverse effects has not been described well in the literature. It is reasonable to assume, however, that frequent application, perhaps several times per day, elicits more frequent local reactions than less frequent use. If women are fully informed of the possibility and nature of side effects, they can, with the help of the pharmacist, determine a desirable frequency of application for themselves.

MISCELLANEOUS PRODUCTS

Although their uses and ingredients are similar to the douche or spray formulations, some OTC vaginal products are available as suppositories, premoistened towelettes, and local anesthetic cream.

The antimicrobial agents used in vaginal antiseptic suppositories are chloramine-T and phenylmercuric acetate, each contained in a greaseless, water-dispersible suppository base. Both compounds are effective antimicrobial agents in vitro, but subjective appraisal of their clinical efficacy is impossible because the agents' concentration in the vagina following dispersion is unknown (51). Both chloramine-T and phenylmercuric acetate may produce local irritation in sufficient concentration or in sensitive individuals. Because these suppositories are used for purposes similar to those for douches, the same considerations concerning benefits and risks apply.

Premoistened towelettes are used for their deodorant, cleansing, and/or cosmetic properties. Except for the propellants in sprays, ingredients of these towelettes are the same as those of spray products. Women who are sensitive to aerosol propellants might be informed of the towelette formulations. Direct irritation or sensitization from other towelette ingredients may occur.

adverse local reactions
spray application
other products

One vaginal product contains benzocaine as the local anesthetic and resorcinol for antimicrobial effects. Concentrations of benzocaine and resorcinol in this cream are not provided, so efficacy cannot be determined readily. Both ingredients may cause local irritation or sensitization (14, 29, 30). The intended purpose and use of this product present another significant hazard: the masking of vaginitis symptoms. In the presence of symptoms possibly indicating vaginitis, the pharmacist should not recommend a vaginal cream or similar local anesthetic vaginal products without concurrent recommendation by the woman's physician.

PRODUCT SELECTION GUIDELINES

The pharmacist should determine persistence, recurrence, and severity of any symptoms or ascertain signs of infection or disease before attempting to recommend a product. If infection or disease is suspected, the patient should be referred to a physician. Patient history or medication profiles may reveal predisposing factors to vaginitis such as pregnancy, diabetes, and chronic use of steroids (including oral contraceptives) or antibiotics (especially tetracyclines). If infection or other disease is suspected, a specific diagnosis and prescription products are nearly always indicated.

When satisfied that an OTC product may be used safely, the pharmacist should make the following recommendations:

- Douches used routinely in the absence of symptoms should probably be acidic or as nearly physiological as possible.
- If a douche is used to remove excessive discharge, an alkaline douche may be more effective.
- Douches and sprays should be avoided before coitus.
- Douches are not contraceptive and should be used after coitus only for cleansing. If spermicidal jelly, cream, or foam is used, douching should be delayed a minimum of 8 hours following intercourse.

- Proper application techniques should be followed.
- If irritation occurs, the product should be discontinued.
- Regardless of the reasons for seeking a vaginal product, thorough cleansing with soap and water may be equally or more effective.

SUMMARY

The benefits and hazards of vaginal cleansing and deodorant products are controversial. It is not universally accepted that these products have an advantage over cleansing with soap and water. Benefits may be largely placebo or psychological. The products may be misused in terms of frequency of use, preparation, and technique of application—perhaps the greatest problems are with the user or inadequate counseling, not the product. They also may cause direct contact irritation or allergic sensitization. The incidence of adverse effects may be small, but according to many gynecologists, potential benefits may be even smaller.

Most manufacturers state that products are evaluated extensively before marketing and that in controlled studies the products have proven safe and effective. These claims seem to be justified because the studies were controlled (especially as regards proper preparation and proper application). There is no guarantee that women in the general population prepare and apply these vaginal products properly, one important reason for the occurrence of adverse effects. With reports of questionable benefits and potential hazards, the available literature is not convincing that vaginal cleansing and deodorant products are advisable for routine use. These products should be used only on the advice of a pharmacist or physician, and their use without specific indication is unjustified. Women who prefer to use these products routinely as part of personal cleanliness habits should be fully informed of product expectations and limitations.

REFERENCES

(1) K. J. Karnaky, *Am. J. Surg.*, *101*, 456 (1961).
(2) K. J. Karnaky, *Am. J. Obstet. Gynecol.*, *115*, 283 (1973).
(3) R. Glynn, *Obstet. Gynecol.*, *20*, 369 (1962).
(4) E. A. Banner, *Med. Clin. North Am.*, *58*, 759 (1974).
(5) J. C. Hartgill, *Practitioner*, *202*, 363 (1969).
(6) G. J. Dennerstein, *Drugs*, *4*, 419 (1972).
(7) F. Sadik, *J. Am. Pharm. Assoc.*, *NS12*, 565 (1972).
(8) T. D. De and N. V. Tu, *Am. J. Obstet. Gynecol.*, *87*, 92 (1965).
(9) L. A. Gray and M. L. Barnes, *Am. J. Obstet. Gynecol.*, *92*, 125 (1963).
(10) "Summary Minutes of the FDA OTC Panel on Contraceptives and Other Vaginal Drug Products," Rockville, Md., Sept. 20–21, 1974.
(11) T. E. Swate and J. C. Weed, *Obstet. Gynecol.*, *43*, 893 (1974).
(12) J. J. Ratzan, *Calif. Med.*, *110*, 24 (1969).
(13) "Summary Minutes of the FDA OTC Panel on Contraceptives and Other Vaginal Drug Products," Rockville, Md., Feb. 7–8, 1975.
(14) "Remington's Pharmaceutical Sciences," 15th ed., A. Osol and J. E. Hoover, Eds., Mack, Easton, Pa., 1975.
(15) J. Barnes, *Practitioner*, *184*, 668 (1960).
(16) J. F. Byers, *Am. Fam. Physician*, *10*, 135 (1974).
(17) D. V. Hirst, *Am. J. Obstet. Gynecol.*, *64*, 179 (1952).
(18) J. H. Long, M. L. Carey, A. E. Hellegers, and M. P. Pentecost, *West. J. Surg. Obstet. Gynecol.*, *71*, 122 (1963).
(19) H. A. Kaminetzky, *J. Am. Med. Assoc.*, *191*, 154 (1965).
(20) L. McGowan, *Am. J. Obstet. Gynecol.*, *93*, 506 (1965).
(21) R. Glynn, *Obstet. Gynecol.*, *22*, 640 (1963).
(22) M. H. Gotlib and D. N. Adler, *Med. Times*, *96*, 902 (1968).
(23) R. S. Cohen, L. S. Polsky, C. A. Straniero, and C. Brown, *Curr. Ther. Res.*, *15*, 839 (1973).
(24) W. A. Abruzzi, *J. Am. Med. Women's Assoc.*, *21*, 406 (1966).
(25) R. J. Stock, M. E. Stock, and J. M. Hutto, *Obstet. Gynecol.*, *42*, 141 (1973).
(26) C. A. D. Ringrose, *N. Engl. J. Med.*, *295*, 1319 (1976).
(27) H. H. Neumann and A. DeCherney, *N. Engl. J. Med.*, *295*, 789 (1976).
(28) G. F. Egenolf and R. McNaughton, *Obstet. Gynecol.*, *7*, 23 (1956).
(29) F. H. Downer and C. J. Stevenson, *Adverse Drug React. Bull.*, *42*, 136 (1973).
(30) C. D. Calnan, *Proc. R. Soc. Med.*, *55*, 39 (1962).
(31) *Medical Letter on Drugs and Therapeutics*, *10*, 27 (1968).
(32) A. A. Fisher, F. Pascher, and N. B. Kanof, *Arch. Dermatol.*, *104*, 286 (1971).
(33) A. A. Fisher and M. A. Stillman, *Arch. Dermatol.*, *106*, 169 (1972).
(34) E. Schmunes and E. J. Levy, *Arch. Dermatol.*, *106*, 169 (1972).
(35) *Federal Register*, *40*, 8926 (1975).
(36) A. A. Fisher, *Arch. Dermatol.*, *108*, 801 (1973).
(37) G. Carsch, *Soap Chem. Spec.*, *47*, 38 (1971).
(38) J. Meyer-Rohn and V. Kassebart, *Kosmetologie*, *4*, 159 (1971).
(39) J. A. Cella, *Am. Cosmet. Perfum.*, *86*(10), 84 (1971).
(40) R. W. Pfirrman and P. Geistlich, U.S. Patent No. 3,574,821 (1971).
(41) G. McBride, *J. Am. Med. Assoc.*, *219*, 449 (1972).
(42) G. S. Kass, J. A. Cella, and N. H. Sloan, "Feminine Hygiene Deodorant Sprays," Paper presented at XIV International Congress of Dermatology, Venice, Italy, May 22, 1972.
(43) A. Kantner, *Am. Cosmet. Perfum.*, *87*, 31 (Feb. 1972).
(44) Y. M. Kapadia, Warner-Lambert Research Institute, personal communication, May 15, 1975.
(45) B. A. Davis, *Obstet. Gynecol.*, *36*, 812 (1970).
(46) B. M. Kaye, *J. Am. Med. Assoc.*, *212*, 2121 (1970).
(47) B. A. Davis, *Obstet. Gynecol.*, *37*, 949 (1971).
(48) J. M. Gowdy, *N. Engl. J. Med.*, *287*, 203 (1972).
(49) *Medical Letter on Drugs and Therapeutics*, *12*, 88 (1970).
(50) M. Morrison, *FDA Consum.*, *7*, 16 (1973).
(51) A. E. Elkhouly and R. T. Yousef, *J. Pharm. Sci.*, *63*, 681 (1974).

Product (Manufacturer)	Antimicrobial	Local Anesthetic/ Antipruritic/Counterirritant	Other
Betadine Douche (Purdue Frederick)	povidone-iodine	—	—
Bo-Car-Al (Calgon)	boric acid	phenol menthol methyl salicylate eucalyptol thymol	potassium aluminum sulfate
Demure (Vicks)	benzethonium chloride	—	lactic acid
Femidine Douche (A.V.P.)	povidone-iodine	—	—
Jeneen (Norwich)	—	—	lactic acid sodium lactate propylene glycol
Lysette (Lehn & Fink)	—	—	triethanolamine dodecylbenzene sulfonate alcohol, 31%
Massengill Disposable Douche (Beecham Products)	cetylpyridinium chloride	—	alcohol lactic acid octoxynol fragrance
Massengill Douche Powder (Beecham Products)	boric acid	—	ammonium aluminum sulfate berberine fragrance
Massengill Liquid (Beecham Products)	—	—	alcohol lactic acid sodium lactate octoxynol aromatics
Massengill Vinegar & Water Disposable Douche (Beecham Products)	boric acid	—	vinegar
Nylmerate II (Holland-Rantos)	boric acid	—	alcohol, 50% acetic acid polysorbate, 20% nonoxynol 9 sodium acetate
PMC Douche Powder (Thomas & Thompson)	boric acid, 82%	thymol, 0.3% phenol, 0.2% menthol	ammonium aluminum sulfate, 16% eucalyptus oil peppermint oil
Stomaseptine (Cooper)	—	menthol } 2% eucalyptol } 2% thymol } 2%	sodium perborate, 18% sodium chloride, 28% sodium borate, 25% sodium bicarbonate, 25%
Trichotine Liquid and Powder (Reed and Carnrick)	—	—	sodium perborate sodium borate aromatics sodium lauryl sulfate alcohol, 8% (liquid)
V.A. (Norcliff Thayer)	boric acid 8-hydroxyquinoline citrate	—	zinc sulfate alum
Zonite (Norcliff Thayer)	benzalkonium chloride	menthol thymol	propylene glycol buffer

Otic Products

Keith O. Miller

Chapter 18

Questions to Ask the Patient

If the patient is a child, what is the age of the patient?

How long have these symptoms been present?

Have you been swimming within the past several days?

Do you have a cold or the flu?

Have you ever had similar symptoms in the past?

Do you feel pain? Is it constant, or is it increased by chewing?

Do you have a fever?

Do you have a discharge from the ear?

Do you have loss of hearing or ringing in the ears?

Have you taken aspirin for the pain or used any fluids to rinse out the ear?

Do you have diabetes or other chronic diseases?

Ear disorders are very common and, in most cases, cause discomfort. Patients usually complain of "earache," "impacted ear," "running ear," "cold in the ear," or a combination of these symptoms. Before recommending OTC products to patients with ear disorders, the pharmacist should have a clear picture of the symptoms of ear disorders and their corresponding pathophysiology. This information will help the pharmacist understand the recommended treatment plans and permit an accurate evaluation of the patient's problem.

Ear disorders may be caused by a disease of the auricle, external auditory meatus (external ear canal), or middle ear or by a disease in another area of the head or neck. A traumatic or pathological condition of the tongue, mandibles, oropharynx, tonsils, or paranasal sinuses may cause referred pain to the ear and may appear to the patient as an "earache."

Home remedies and nonprescription drugs usually are restricted to conditions related only to the external ear. Self-medication should be reserved for minor conditions. It also may be used effectively for prophylaxis to aid the normal body defenses and to improve the integrity of the skin lining of the auricle and external auditory canal.

EAR ANATOMY AND PHYSIOLOGY

The external ear is composed of the auricle (pinna) and the external auditory meatus (Figure 1). The auricle is the external appendage consisting of cartilage (elastic type) covered by a thin layer of normal skin, except for the lobule, which is mainly fatty tissue. A thin tissue layer called the perichondrium covers both the cartilaginous auricle and the outer cartilaginous half of the external auditory canal (1). The periosteum covers the inner bony half of the external auditory canal.

The external auditory meatus is tubular and forms a channel for sound waves to pass to the tympanic membrane (drum head); it also protects the membrane from injury. In adults the external auditory canal is about 24 mm long and has a volume of about 0.85 ml (17 drops) (2). However, there are individual variations in size and shape of the auricle and external auditory canal. At about 7 mm from the tympanic membrane the channel narrows; this area is called the isthmus (3). Beyond the isthmus the canal floor dips downward to the junction of the annulus with the tympanic membrane to form a depression termed the "tympanic recess." Excess water and fluids in the tympanic recess may cause a feeling of fullness in the ear until their removal, which is accomplished easily by having the patient tilt the head on the side with the affected ear down. This position permits the excess fluid to drain out of the ear by gravity. To visualize the ear, it may be necessary to straighten the canal by applying upward traction on the auricle to permit direct visual examination of the tympanic membrane.

The auricular skin is continuous and lines the entire auditory meatus and the outer covering of the tympanic membrane (4). The skin of the cartilaginous part of the canal contains hair follicles, large sebaceous glands, which open either to the skin surface or into the hair follicle lumen, and ceruminous glands (2). There are 1000–2000 ceruminous glands in the average ear, fewer in older people (2). No hair follicles or glands (sebaceous and ceruminous) are found in the inner half of the external auditory canal.

Cerumen (earwax), the secretory product of the ceruminous glands, is derived from the watery secretions of the ceruminous glands and the oily secretions of the sebaceous glands (2). The composition of this colorless, watery fluid is a mixture of polypeptides, lipids, fatty

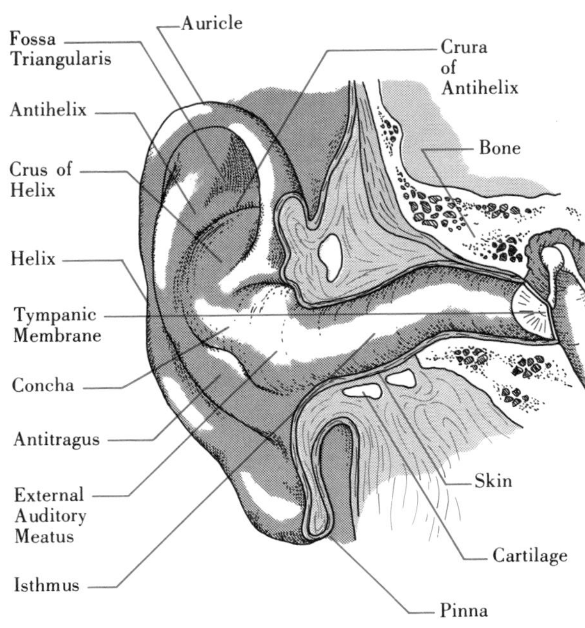

Figure 1. Anatomy of the auricle and external ear.

cerumen

tympanic membrane

disorders of the outer ear

furuncles

acids, amino acids, and electrolytes (2, 5). Cerumen is brown because it mixes with desquamated epithelial cells and dust particles. It lubricates the skin and traps foreign material entering the external auditory canal, providing a protective barrier (3, 6). Under normal conditions the cerumen forms small, round droplets and dries into a semisolid. It is then expelled unnoticed by epithelial migration, i.e., the movement of epithelial cells across the surface of the tympanic membrane and the epithelial lining of the external auditory meatus to the outside. The normal pH of the healthy external auditory meatus is between 5.0 and 7.2 (2).

The tympanic membrane is pearl-gray, egg shaped, semitransparent, and about 0.1 mm thick and 8–9 mm wide (the narrow portion is at the bottom) (2). The outer layer of its epithelium is continuous with the epidermis of the external auditory canal; the middle layer is tough, fibrous tissue; and the innermost layer is a mucous membrane continuous with the tympanic cavity lining (7). In adults the membrane forms a $\sim 45^\circ$ angle with the external meatus floor, and in infants it is almost horizontal (2). Anatomically, the tympanic membrane is considered with the external auditory canal because it is attached to the canal's medial terminal end. Functionally, it is considered with the middle ear (tympanic cavity) (3).

COMMON PROBLEMS OF THE EAR

Many disorders of the ear are minor and fairly easily resolved. However, the pharmacist should keep in mind that the pain associated with even minor disorders can be significant. Some untreated ear problems can result in hearing loss. The pharmacist can assist the patient by helping evaluate the nature of the disorder, by discussing the proper course of action, i.e., self-treatment or physician diagnosis, and by recommending an efficacious OTC product, if appropriate.

Auricle

The disorders associated with the auricle, that part of the ear not within the head, are generally minor and involve lacerations, boils, and dermatitis. These conditions are generally self-limiting.

Trauma

Lacerations, including scrapes and cuts, involving only the auricle skin usually heal spontaneously. A wound that does not heal normally should be checked by a physician. Deep wounds that may involve injury to the cartilage also require physician examination. Injury to the auricle that does not perforate the subperichondrium may cause subcutaneous bleeding and produce a hematoma. A flatulent hematoma (blood clot) requires aspiration or incision by a physician, since the red-blue swelling may obliterate normal auricular contours and frequently results in perichondritis or cauliflower ear. The swelling also can cause local pruritis and pain on touching.

Boils

Boils (furuncles) are usually localized infections of the hair follicles predisposed by irritation, pressure, friction, and scratching. Other factors suspected in recurrent lesions are diets rich in sugars and fats; states of lowered resistance such as anemia, alcoholism, diabetes mellitus, and malnutrition; poor bathing habits; and poor body hygiene.

Boils usually involve the anterior external auditory meatus. They usually begin as a red papule and may progress into a round or conical superficial pustule with a core of pus and erythema around the base. The lesion gradually enlarges, becomes firm, then softens and opens spontaneously (after a few days to as long as 2 weeks) to discharge the purulent contents. Because the skin is tightly attached, minimal swelling may cause severe pain.

Boils usually are self-limiting; however, they may be severe, autoinoculable, and multiple. Deeper lesions may lead to perichondritis. The pus-producing organism found in boils is usually *Staphylococcus.*

Usually, small boils may be treated by good hygiene combined with topical compresses and/or antibiotic ointment. Hot compresses of saline solution may be applied to the auricle and the side of the face. Antibiotic ointments do not help heal boils, but they do prevent spreading. Cases in which boils do not respond rapidly to antibiotic ointment and/or topical dressings should be referred to a physician. Recurring conditions also should be referred to rule out predisposing causes.

Perichondritis

Perichondritis is an infection involving the perichondrium, usually following a poorly treated or untreated burn, injury, hematoma, or local infection.

The onset of perichondritis is characterized by a sensation of heat and stiffness of the auricle. Pain is pronounced. As the condition progresses, an exudate forms, and the auricle becomes dark red, diffuse, and swollen. The entire auricle becomes shiny and red with uniform thickening caused by edema and inflammation (1). The lesions usually are confined to the cartilaginous tissue of the auricle and external canal. Constitutional disturbances may include generalized fever and malaise.

Perichondritis frequently results in severe auricular deformity, and atresia (a pathological closure) of the external auditory canal may occur. A patient suspected of having perichondritis symptoms should be seen by a physician.

Dermatitis of the Ear

An inflammatory condition may result from an abrasion of the auricle and, if left untreated, may develop into an infection of these skin layers. Inflammatory conditions such as seborrhea, psoriasis, and contact dermatitis (e.g., poison ivy and poison oak) also may affect the skin of the auricle and the external ear canal. Often, dermatitis of the ear is associated with seborrhea of the scalp. Contact dermatitis also may be caused by an allergic response to jewelry, cosmetics, detergents, or topical drug applications. The lesions may spread to the auditory canal, neck, and facial areas.

The symptoms of dermatitis of the ear usually include severe itching and local redness followed by vesication, weeping, and erythema. The lesions form scales and yellow crusts on the skin (7). They may spread to adjacent unaffected areas, and excessive scratching may cause them to become infected. Topical drugs should be used cautiously with dermatitis because of their potential allergenicity. Seborrheic dermatitis of the ear usually is associated with dandruff, and treatment with dandruff control shampoos is recommended. Cases that are difficult to control and generalized dermatitis around the ear should be referred to a physician.

External Auditory Canal

Boils

Boils of the external auditory canal are pathologically similar to those found on the auricle and external auditory meatus. Symptoms include pain of the infected site which usually is exacerbated by mastication. The auditory meatal opening may be partly occluded by swelling; however, hearing is impaired only if the opening is completely occluded. Edema and pain over the mastoid bone directly behind the auricle may occur. Traction on the auricle or the tragus is very painful. Patients with boils in the external auditory canal should be referred to a physician because unresolved conditions may lead to a generalized infection of the entire external auditory canal.

Otomycosis

Otomycosis, external fungal infection of the ear, is more common in warmer, tropical climates than in mild, temperate ones. *Aspergillus* sp. and *Candida* sp. are the most common causative agents (4, 8). Antibiotic treatment of a bacterial ear infection, with resultant suppression of normal bacterial flora, may predispose an individual to a mycotic external ear infection (8).

A superficial mycotic infection of the external auditory meatus is characterized by pruritus with a feeling of fullness and pressure in the ear. Pain may be present, increasing with mastication and traction on the pinna and the tragus. The fungus forms a mass of epithelial debris, exudate, and cerumen and, in the acute stage, may clog the external auditory meatus. Hearing impairment may occur. Depending on the nature of the fungus, the color of the mass may vary. *Aspergillus* sp. infections usually appear dark gray, dark brown, or black, and *Candida* sp. infections usually appear creamy-colored to gray. The skin lining the external auditory canal and the tympanic membrane becomes beefy-red and scaly and may be eroded or ulcerated (2). A scant, colorless discharge is common. Otomycosis is particularly serious in diabetic patients because of the microangiopathy and cutaneous manifestations common to diabetes mellitus (4). Mycotic ear infections must be treated by a physician.

problems associated with auditory canal

fungal infections

Keratosis Obturans

This condition is rare, and its etiology is unclear (4). Wax accumulates in the deeper parts of the external auditory canal and, with adjacent epithelial cells that contain cholesterol, forms a mass and exerts pressure on the surrounding tissue. The mass is a shiny, white, pluglike occlusion of the external auditory canal. It may cause a ring of pressure and erosion of the epithelial tissues surrounding it, forming a potential entrance for organisms to initiate a bacterial infection (1). The infection may form abscesses in the subcutaneous tissue and mastoid bone tissue.

Pain in the ear and decreased hearing are common symptoms. A discharge and tinnitus (ringing in the ear) also may occur. Mechanical removal of the obstruction is necessary and is often difficult. The removal should be reserved for a physician; patients should not attempt to remove the obstruction themselves.

Foreign Objects in the Ear

Young children often use the ear canal for inserting small items such as beans, peas, marbles, pebbles, or beads. If the objects become lodged in the ear canal, they may cause significant hearing loss. Vegetable seeds, such as dried beans or dried peas, lodged in the external auditory meatus swell when moistened during bathing or swimming and become wedged in the bony portion of the canal, causing severe pain. Furthermore, if an obstruction of the external auditory meatus is not removed promptly, it may provide a potential culture medium for organisms, resulting in acute bacterial external otitis. Insects may enter the meatus and cause distress by beating their wings and crawling.

Foreign objects lodged in the ear canal may not cause symptoms and may be found only during a routine physical examination. Usually, a hearing deficiency is observed with pressure in the ear on mastication. Pain may be present. Exudate may form because of secondary bacterial infection. Mechanical removal should be reserved for a physician because unskilled attempts at removal often result in damage to the skin surrounding the external auditory meatus.

Impacted Cerumen

The accumulation of cerumen in the external auditory meatus may be caused by any of three factors: overactive ceruminous glands, an abnormally shaped external auditory meatus, or abnormal cerumen secreted by the ceruminous glands. Overactive ceruminous glands cause cerumen to accumulate in the external auditory canal. A tortuous or small canal or abnormal narrowing of the canal may not permit normal migration of the cerumen to the outside, causing the cerumen to accumulate. Abnormal cerumen may be drier or softer than normal cerumen and may interfere with the normal epithelial migration. It is often packed deeper into the external auditory meatus by repeated attempts to remove it, which is the most common cause of impacted cerumen. In general, there usually is no cerumen in the inner half of the external auditory canal unless it has been pushed there.

wax accumulation

infections of auditory canal lining

causative organisms

swimmer's ear

In elderly persons, cerumen frequently is admixed with long hairs in the external auditory canal, thus preventing normal expulsion and forming a matted obstruction in the ear.

External Otitis

External otitis (an infection of the skin lining the external auditory canal) is one of the most common diseases of the ear. It is very painful and annoying. The external auditory canal is considered a blind canal lined with skin—a dark, warm cul-de-sac well suited to collecting moisture. Prolonged exposure to moisture tends to disrupt the continuity of the epithelial cells, causing skin maceration and fissures which provide a fertile area for bacterial growth. Additionally, this prolonged exposure to moisture tends to raise the normal skin pH, improving the growth medium for bacteria. Factors contributing to susceptibility to external otitis include race, heredity, age, sex, climate, diet, and occupational background (8). The most common causative organisms of external otitis include *Pseudomonas* sp., *Staphylococcus* sp., *Bacillus* sp., and *Proteus* sp.

There is very little subcutaneous tissue between the skin tightly bound to the perichondrium on the cartilaginous portion and the periosteum on the bony portion of the external auditory canal. Consequently, there is a disparity between the size of the visible swelling and the amount of pain associated with the condition. The lack of space available for expansion increases the tension on the skin, and inflammation causing edema provokes severe pain in the inflamed skin that is out of proportion to visible swelling. As the inflammation increases, pain may be increased significantly during mastication. Symptoms often develop following attempts to clean the ear (with cotton swabs, hairpins, matchsticks, pencils, fingers, or other objects) of foreign debris or to scratch the ear to relieve itching. The instruments may traumatize and damage the horny skin layer, forming an opening for the invasion of organisms.

A normal, healthy external auditory canal is impervious to the invasion of pathological organisms. Generally, individuals must be susceptible to bacterial infections, and the skin integrity must be interrupted before an organism can produce an infected lesion.

Another type of trauma-induced external otitis is called "swimmer's ear," or desquamative external otitis (8). Excessive moisture in the external auditory meatus may cause water to accumulate in the tympanic recess, resulting in tissue maceration and water absorption by the stratum corneum skin layer. This excessive moisture accumulation may be important in predisposing the ear canal to infection. After bathing or swimming, patients frequently attempt to clear the ear canal of water with objects that cause abrasions or lacerations of the skin lining. Also, cerumen accumulated in the external auditory meatus absorbs water, expands, and traps water, providing a basis for infection (3). Within a few hours to 1 day following exposure to excess water, symptoms of itching, pain, and possible draining from the ear with partial occlusion occur. In many cases this condition is related to climatic conditions where the relative humidity and temperature are high or where dust and sand storms occur (3).

A bacterial infection of the external auditory canal leads to inflammation and epidermal destruction of the skin lining the tympanic membrane. The infection may progress through the fibrous layer of the tympanic membrane and cause perforation and spreading of the infection into the middle ear, resulting in intense pain and discomfort. External otitis, like otomycosis, is particularly difficult to control in persons with diabetes mellitus (4, 9).

Symptoms of acute external otitis are related to the severity of the pathological conditions. There usually is mild or moderate pain that becomes pronounced by pulling upward on the auricle or by pressing on the tragus. There may be a discharge. Hearing loss may occur if the ear canal has been obstructed by swelling and edema or by debris.

Chronic external otitis usually is caused by the persistence of predisposing factors. The most common symptom is itching, which prompts patients to attempt to "scratch the ear canal" to reduce or relieve the itch. This scratching causes the skin to become obliterated or broken.

In allergic external otitis and dermatitis of the external auditory canal caused by seborrhea a common symptom is itching, burning, or stinging of the lesions. Often the complaints seem excessive compared to the visible signs.

Chronic cases and the more severe cases with symptoms of severe pain, lymphadenopathy, discharge, possible hearing loss, and fever should be referred to a physician (3). Tender nodes may be felt anterior to the tragus, behind the ear, or in the upper neck just below the pinna. Minor cases and chronic and allergic external otitis, especially "swimmer's ear" otitis, often may be treated adequately with OTC products. All progressive symptoms of disease processes pertaining to the external ear canal or auricle should be treated only under physician supervision.

Middle Ear: Otitis Media

Disorders involving the middle ear should not be treated with nonprescription otic products, but a brief overview of the common conditions involving the middle ear will aid the pharmacist in evaluating symptoms. While some symptoms of middle ear disorders are the same as those of external ear disorders, others are not. All bacterial infections of the middle ear should be evaluated and treated by a physician. The usual treatment is systemic antibiotics.

Otitis media is an inflammatory condition of the middle ear that occurs most often during childhood. Conditions that interfere with the eustachian tube function, e.g., upper respiratory tract infection, allergy, adenoid lymphadenopathy, and cleft palate, predispose individuals to otitis media. Blockage of the eustachian tube allows the oxygen in the middle ear cleft to be absorbed, leaving a relative negative pressure or vacuum which results in a transudation (movement) of fluid into the middle ear cleft. If the serous fluid in the middle ear cavity remains sterile, the condition is referred to as serous otitis media; if it becomes infected, it is called purulent otitis media.

Children often experience repeated episodes of eustachian tube obstruction caused by masses of adenoids that become edematous and block the eustachian tube openings. Adenoidectomy usually prevents future incidence. In adults, recurrent otitis media may be caused by a nasopharyngeal tumor.

The most common symptoms in the acute phase of purulent otitis media are pain, hearing loss, and constitutional disturbances such as fever—often as high as 104°F (40°C)—and malaise (10). Severity of symptoms increases as the condition worsens. Pain arises from the pressure of the fluids in the middle ear causing an outward tension on the tympanic membrane which is innervated with sensory nerves. The rapid production of fluid and tension in a short period is responsible for the acute pain, described as sharp, knifelike, and steady. It usually is not increased with mastication or when traction is applied to the auricle or tragus. Excessive nose blowing may force additional purulent mucus into the eustachian tube, perpetuating the condition. If patients are not treated promptly, the pressure may increase to the point where the tympanic membrane ruptures, resulting in a mucopurulent discharge and possibly causing secondary bacterial external otitis infection. The appearance of a discharge usually is accompanied by a lessening of pain due to the decreased tension on the tympanic membrane. The initial discharge may be bloodstained, followed by a foul-smelling, purulent, serous fluid. The tympanic membrane usually loses its pearl-gray luster and appears yellow to orange-pink, another important factor in diagnosing.

Serous otitis media symptoms include a sensation of fullness in the ear accompanied by hearing loss. The condition worsens as the fluid accumulates and fills the middle ear cleft. The feeling of fullness is associated with voice resonance, a stopped-up feeling in the ears, a hollow sound, or a popping or cracking noise in the

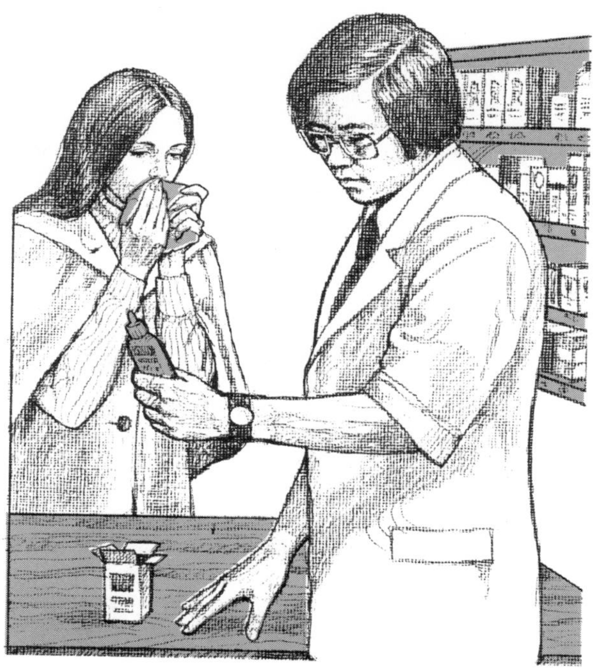

serous and purulent otitis media

mechanical deafness

hearing loss

ears, especially during swallowing or yawning. These symptoms usually are not present in external otitis.

Potential Complications

Conductive Hearing Loss

Conductive hearing loss (mechanical deafness) is a deficiency in the conduction of sound waves from the air through the tympanic membrane and ossicles to the nerve fibers in the inner ear. It may occur with external otitis, otomycosis, a foreign body in the external auditory meatus, impacted cerumen, a perforated tympanic membrane, acute serous otitis media, mastoiditis (an inflammation of the mastoid bone cleft surrounding the middle ear), and otosclerosis.

Neural Hearing Loss

Neural hearing loss usually is accompanied by tinnitus and a sensation of disequilibrium. These characteristics are very important for differential diagnosis. The condition may be caused by a viral or bacterial infection, a vascular or metabolic condition, or ototoxic drug therapy. Patients with neural hearing loss should be under a physician's care.

Chronic Otitis Media

In chronic serous otitis media the fluid in the middle ear may be thin and serous or thick and viscous ("glue ear") (4). Chronic serous otitis media occurs most often in small children. It may be caused by inadequate treatment of previous acute otitis media episodes or by recurrent upper respiratory tract bacterial or viral infections associated with eustachian tube dysfunction.

The most common symptom is impaired hearing, but the onset is often insidious, and the child may have no acute symptoms. Frequently, parents accuse the child of being inattentive and disobedient. Pain is usually absent. The tympanic membrane appears yellow or orange and lusterless, and its flexibility is lost (4). It is not perforated but often appears to be retracted.

Chronic purulent otitis media is usually secondary to a persistent tympanic membrane perforation. With exacerbation the patient may exhibit the symptoms of acute purulent otitis media as well as mucopurulent discharge.

Perforation of the Tympanic Membrane

The most common causes of traumatic perforation of the tympanic membrane are water sports, such as diving or water-skiing (7). Any corrosive agent introduced into the ear canal may produce tympanic membrane perforation. Other causes of perforation include blows to the head with a cupped hand, foreign objects entering the ear canal with excessive force, and forceful irrigation of the ear canal. At the moment of the injury, pain is severe, but it decreases rapidly. Hearing acuity will usually diminish. An untreated injury may lead to otitis media. Other complications may include tinnitus, nausea, and vertigo.

factors in diagnosis of ear disorders

symptoms of otic problems

DIFFERENTIAL DIAGNOSIS

To choose realistically between self-treatment and physician referral, the pharmacist must be able to assess the nature and severity of the patient's otic condition by evaluating the signs and symptoms (Table 1). The most common complaints may include one or more of the following symptoms: localized pain, itchiness in the ear canal, a feeling of fullness, hearing loss, lymphadenopathy, fever, and malaise.

Boils

The signs and symptoms of a boil in the ear canal include local burning pain that is increased with chewing, when traction is applied to the auricle, and when the tragus is pressed medially. A red inflamed raised lesion is observed along the ear canal. The skin around the affected area is intact and not broken providing the patient has not attempted to scratch it. The patient's subjective hearing is usually intact. If lymphadenopathy, fever, malaise, or severe pain is present, the patient should be seen by a physician.

Foreign Objects

The signs and symptoms of a foreign object in the ear usually include a feeling of fullness with hearing loss from the affected ear. Pain may be present, and increased by chewing, traction on the auricle, and pressure applied medially on the tragus. Lymphadenopathy, fever, or malaise does not occur acutely but may develop later with a foul-smelling discharge from the affected ear. Collectively, these characteristics indicate a secondary infection. All patients with foreign objects in the ear with or without secondary infection should be seen and treated by a physician.

Table 1. Symptoms of Otic Disorders

	Boil	Otomycosis	Bacterial External Otitis	Otitis Media	Impacted Cerumen
Pain[a]	often	possibly	often	rarely	rarely
Hearing deficit	rarely	possibly	possibly	possibly	often
Purulent discharge	rarely	rarely	often	rarely	rarely
Bilateral symptoms	rarely	rarely	possibly	often	rarely

[a] Pain is increased with chewing, traction on the auricle, and medial pressure on the tragus except in otitis media, where it is knifelike and steady.

External Otitis

The only conclusive means by which bacterial or fungal external otitis may be ruled out is by microbiological culture. A culture is not always practical, nor is it always needed. Pain and swelling localized in the ear canal usually are the motivating symptoms that cause the patient to seek professional help. A bacterial infection may be characterized further by increased pain with chewing, traction applied on the auricle, and pressure applied medially on the tragus. Lymphadenopathy and a feeling of fullness may be additional characteristics with possible febrile condition and associated malaise. Visualization is painful and reveals a swollen inflamed ear canal and an inflamed tympanic membrane. A purulent, foul-smelling discharge may block visual inspection of the tympanic membrane. Any foul-smelling mucopurulent discharge indicates a bacterial infection. Patients with external otitis should be referred to a physician for thorough cleaning and inspection of the ear canal.

Hearing Loss

Hearing loss is subjective unless diagnosed and evaluated by an audiologist. Acute hearing loss without pain may be due to impacted cerumen, which may be observed during direct visualization of the ear canal. Impacted cerumen in the ear canal obstructs the tympanic membrane and prevents its visualization.

Patients with impacted cerumen without secondary complications may be treated safely with OTC cerumen-softening agents. Patients with hearing loss and without pain, whose tympanic membrane is visible and not obstructed (this determination can only be inferred from answers to the pharmacist's questions), should be evaluated and treated by a physician. A perforated tympanic membrane results in decreased hearing. Usually, the patient has experienced a sharp pain of short duration at the time of the injury. Treatment for a perforated tympanic membrane includes repair and treatment to prevent infection in the middle ear.

Otomycosis

Patients with otomycosis usually complain of itching and a feeling of fullness in the affected ear. A colorless discharge may or may not be present. Pain is usually not present but may occur in severe cases. The pain is increased with chewing, traction on the auricle, and pressure applied medially on the tragus. Constitutional disturbances usually occur only in severe cases, often due to secondary bacterial infections with obstruction of the ear canal causing a hearing loss.

Otitis Media

The only conclusive means of diagnosing otitis media is a complete physical examination, using a pneumatic otoscope, and a complete patient history. Otitis media in most cases is caused by eustachian tube dysfunction. Serous otitis media refers to the accumulation of sterile nonpurulent middle ear fluid and is usually considered a noninfectious middle ear disorder. It is found most commonly in children. Patients may be asymptomatic or may complain of occasional fullness and "cracking" or a "hollow sound" in the ears. The effect is usually bilateral. Otoscopic findings are specific and may demonstrate typical changes in tympanic membrane mobility consistent with the symptoms and degree of severity of the disorder.

A complication of prolonged serous otitis media is caused by bacteria and viruses extending along the eustachian tube causing suppurative otitis media. Pneumatic otoscopic findings are specific and demonstrate a bulging, poorly resilient tympanic membrane caused by the pus and exudate that accumulate behind the tympanic membrane. The patient usually experiences discomfort with pain, dull and throbbing at first, then rapidly progressing to a sharp, knifelike, agonizing pain. These symptoms usually follow an upper respiratory infection. Constitutional symptoms include chills, fever, and malaise. A purulent discharge occurs only following tympanic membrane perforation, at which time the patient experiences sudden and welcome relief of pain. A bloody, purulent, smelly drainage flows from the ear. The fever falls rapidly to normal. Treatment is aimed at reventilating the middle ear space, reducing nasopharyngeal and eustachian tube edema, and managing the infection.

Patients with any of these symptoms should be evaluated and treated by a physician because middle ear disorders are often associated with an underlying cause and require diagnostic evaluation and treatment.

TREATMENT

Normally, the skin lining the external auditory meatus provides adequate protection against bacterial or fungal infection; cerumen provides a lubricant to the skin to maintain its integrity. The hairs help stop dust and debris from entering the meatus. Cerumen provides a continuing, self-cleaning process that removes particulate matter and debris from the external auditory meatus. An infection of the auricle or external auditory meatus is a skin infection and should be treated as such.

Progressive symptoms of otic disease processes should be evaluated and should be treated only under physician supervision. Cerumen-softening and cerumenolytic agents only soften and loosen cerumen to enable its easy removal by a physician. These agents do not remove cerumen. Effective mechanical removal by irrigation or instrumentation should be reserved for the physician. Surgical intervention may be necessary for deep cuts, bruises, or abrasions. Severe infections often require both systemic and local antibiotics. External otitis not treated properly is likely to spread to the mastoid bone or to the middle ear cavity, causing severe patient disability. Permanent hearing loss may occur.

Self-treatment of boils may be instituted by applying heat followed by an antibiotic ointment to the affected area with a soft cotton applicator over and around the boil. The antibiotic ointment may be used if the boil ruptures. The lesion is usually self-limiting and clears after several days of frequent applications. Resistant lesions require incision and drainage by a physician.

differential diagnosis and treatment

nonprescription products

Treatment of external otitis usually includes antibiotic and hydrocortisone drops applied in the ear canal. When cellulitis and lymphadenopathy are present, oral antibiotics are effective. Trauma to the ear should be avoided. The ear canals should be kept clean and dry at all times. Following swimming or bathing, the ear canals may be filled for 1–2 minutes with alcohol, glycerin, propylene glycol, or water acidified to pH of 4–5 to help restore normal acidic pH to the ear canal. An acidified aluminum acetate (Burow's) solution may be used for its astringent effect to obtain rapid resolution of edema and crusting. External otitis should be treated promptly for a satisfactory outcome.

The choice of products for prophylaxis against infection and for keeping the ear canal clean and dry at all times often depends on the availability of the ingredients. Each has been shown to be effective and safe for use in the ear canal.

Minor symptoms of otomycosis may be treated prophylactically with alcohol, propylene glycol, glycerin, or water which has been acidified. Aluminum acetate solution also may be used for its astringent effect. These ingredients have been demonstrated to be safe and effective for maintaining a clean, dry ear canal and promoting aural hygiene. The choice of the product depends on availability. Direct visualization helps the pharmacist to rule out severe infections. Patients with severe otomycosis and impacted mycotic debris should have their ear canals cleaned and treated by a physician.

Ingredients in OTC Products

Nonprescription products used for palliative treatment of auricular ear disorders should include those used to treat all topical skin disorders (see Chapter 26). Antibiotic ointments, such as neomycin and bacitracin ointments, alone or in combination with polymyxin B sulfate, are adequate for treating minor lesions of the auricle. Antibiotics cannot penetrate into abscesses because of the intrinsic tendency of abscesses to wall themselves off. Antibiotic ointments may prevent the spread of autoinoculation when they are applied to surrounding tissue. They also help keep the surrounding skin soft and moist.

ingredients in otic products

mechanisms, dosages, uses, and adverse reactions

FDA Panel recommendations

Acetic Acid Solution

Weak acetic acid solutions are used to treat mild forms of external otitis. A concentration of 2–2.5% may be made easily in the pharmacy from glacial acetic acid or from white distilled household vinegar, which is usually 5% acetic acid. A 50:50 mixture of distilled household vinegar with either water, propylene glycol, glycerin, or rubbing alcohol (70% isopropyl alcohol or 70% ethanol) may be used. (Patients should be cautioned that denaturants in 70% rubbing alcohol formulations may cause sensitization.) The mixture is conveniently made and inexpensive. Acetic acid increases the acidity of the normal skin of the external auditory canal, creating an undesirable environment for the growth of bacteria, especially *Pseudomonas* (6, 11). Alcohol is a local anti-infective and provides a local drying effect for prophylaxis against swimmer's ear (7, 12, 13).

Aluminum Acetate (Burow's) Solution

External otitis or local itching of the external ear caused by external ear dermatitis may be treated with an astringent such as 1:20 or 1:40 aluminum acetate solution (3, 11, 14, 15). One tablet or packet dissolved in 500 ml of water yields a concentration of 1:40. Aluminum acetate solution is used widely for conditions involving the external ear. Its principal value is its acidity, which restores the normal antibacterial pH of the ear canal. Applied locally as protein precipitants (15), astringents cause the affected area to become drier by reducing the secretory function of the skin glands. Contraction and wrinkling of the affected tissue may be seen; astringents also toughen the skin to prevent reinfection.

A wet compress of aluminum acetate solution may be used with a gauze dressing on the auricle (3). Drops may be instilled into the external auditory meatus. The usual dose is four to six drops every 4–6 hours until symptoms of itching or burning subside. The drops also may be used prophylactically against swimmer's ear to help clean and dry the ear canal after swimming or bathing. Aluminum acetate solution is suitable for both children and adults. Used properly, it is nonsensitizing and well tolerated. Adverse reactions are rare.

Antipyrine

The FDA OTC Panel on Topical Analgesic, Antirheumatic, Otic, Burn, and Sunburn Treatment Products concluded that antipyrine is neither safe nor effective for OTC use as a topical otic analgesic and anesthetic and should be used only under the advice and supervision of a physician. Antipyrine's clinical effectiveness and safety in treating otic disorders have not been substantiated.

Benzocaine

Benzocaine is a topical local anesthetic commonly used for pain, discomfort, or pruritis associated with skin ulcers, wounds, mucous membranes, hemorrhoids, and skin irritations, including sunburn and insect bites. Benzocaine is poorly soluble in water, very slowly absorbed through the skin, and relatively nontoxic. The localized anesthesia produced is not complete but is long acting, because of benzocaine's poor solubility and its slow absorption.

Benzocaine has been used as a local anesthetic to treat pain associated with external otitis and other disorders of the auricle and/or ear canal. Its application to weeping wounds of fulminating infections is usually not effective because adequate concentration cannot be achieved owing to drainage of body fluids away from the wound. Symptomatic pain relief in such cases may be undesirable, since it may disguise the symptoms of an exacerbating infection.

The usefulness of benzocaine or other local anesthetics for local analgesia in the ear canal is not clear. The FDA Panel concluded that benzocaine is not safe or effective for OTC use as a topical analgesic and doubts that benzocaine is effective topically as an analgesic and/or anesthetic on the tissues of the tympanic membrane and ear canal (16).

Boric Acid

Boric acid is an ingredient in several ear preparations. It is a weak local anti-infective, nonirritating to intact skin in a dilute solution of 1–5%. Supersaturated alcoholic boric acid solutions improve the antibacterial action over the alcohol itself (either 99% isopropyl or 70% ethyl alcohol). Acetic acid and boric acid increase the acidity of dosage forms, increasing the skin's normal acidity (6, 11). Because of its toxicity, boric acid should be used with caution, particularly with children and on open wounds, where the potential for systemic absorption is high.

Camphor

Camphor is used in eardrops and earwax softeners as a weak antiseptic and a mild anesthetic intended to suppress itching. However, its effectiveness in the concentrations used has not been substantiated.

Carbamide Peroxide

The antibacterial properties of carbamide peroxide (urea hydrogen peroxide) are due to its release of nascent oxygen, and its main value is to clean wounds. The effervescence caused by the oxygen release mechanically removes debris from inaccessible regions. In otic preparations the effervescence disorganizes wax accumulations. Carbamide (urea) helps debride the tissue. These actions soften the residue in the ear, and removal of the liquefied cerumen may be aided with warm water irrigation.

The FDA Panel concluded that 6.5% carbamide peroxide solution in anhydrous glycerin instilled into the affected ear is safe and effective as an earwax-softening agent for OTC use (16). The Panel recommends the solution be instilled into the affected ear and allowed to remain at least 15 minutes with the head tilted (the affected ear up) before the wax is removed by gently washing with lukewarm water and using a soft rubber syringe. The process may be repeated a second time, if necessary. It is not recommended for children under 12 years of age.

Chloroform

Chloroform is an irritant and preservative used in some eardrops. It is volatile and evaporates on exposure to the air. Its effectiveness for treating ear disorders has not been substantiated.

Glycerin

Glycerin may be used as a solvent, a vehicle, or an emollient, and also as a humectant because of its hygroscopicity. Glycerin is widely used as a solvent and a vehicle in many otic preparations (prescription-only and OTC). It is safe and nonsensitizing when applied to open wounds or abraded skin.

The FDA OTC Panel on Topical Analgesic, Antirheumatic, Otic, Burn, and Sunburn Treatment Products recommends that glycerin be used as a cerumen-softening agent in an aqueous solution containing a concentration of 95% glycerin or greater (16). Dehydrated glycerin contains no less than 99.5% glycerin. Glycerin USP contains no less than 95% glycerin; i.e., it may contain a maximum of 5% water (17).

Ichthammol

Ichthammol is a weak antiseptic and irritant with demulcent and emollient properties. Its primary contribution is as an emollient, not as an antiseptic. Ichthammol ointment (10%) is used for treating local inflammation associated with minor boils or an abscessed wound (15). Ichthammol (10%) in glycerin has been used as eardrops for treating minor inflammatory conditions of the external ear.

Menthol

Menthol, which is included in some earwax softeners, is an antipruritic and counterirritant and provides a local feeling of coolness when applied to the tissues. Menthol's clinical effectiveness in treating ear disorders has not been substantiated.

Olive Oil (Sweet Oil)

Olive oil, a fixed oil containing mixed glycerides of oleic acid (about 83%) (18), is used as an emollient and topical lubricant. Often it is instilled into the ear canal to alleviate itchiness and burning and may be used for softening earwax (11).

Phenol in Glycerin

Phenol in glycerin (5–10%) was once prescribed to treat pain caused by ear disorders (19). Presently, its use is not recommended because of its inherent dangers of necrosis and perforation of the tympanic membrane (20).

Propylene Glycol

Propylene glycol is a solvent that has preservative properties and is a useful humectant. Used in both prescription and nonprescription otic preparations, propylene glycol is a clear, colorless, nonirritating, viscous liquid. Its viscosity provides increased contact time to the tissues of the external auditory meatus. Adding acetic acid to propylene glycol increases the solution's acidity, enhancing its anti-infective properties (7, 21).

Thymol

Thymol, a phenol obtained from thyme oil, has a more agreeable odor than phenol. It has antibacterial and antifungal properties in a concentration of 1% (15). In the presence of large amounts of proteins its antibacterial activity is greatly reduced. It has been used traditionally in topical preparations partly because of its deodorant properties. Its clinical effectiveness for ear disorders has not been substantiated.

Other Cerumen-Softening Products

ingredients in otic products

uses and effectiveness

wax softening and removal

Other products used to soften earwax include light mineral oil, a mixture of warm water and 3% hydrogen peroxide (in a ratio of 1:1), and a 3% hypertonic sodium chloride solution (11). The use of undiluted 3% hydrogen peroxide and the indiscriminate use of aqueous hydrogen peroxide (1:1 ratio) instilled in the ear canal are unwise, for they may cause maceration of the skin and predispose it to infection. Cerumen-softening agents only soften the hardened, impacted cerumen. They do not and should never be expected to both soften and remove cerumen. The impacted cerumen can be removed only by irrigation or mechanical means.

Removal of the cerumen, desquamated debris, and dried secretions is often best accomplished by suction or use of a small cotton-tipped applicator. (This method should be performed only by trained personnel.) Gentle irrigation with an ear syringe or a forced water spray should be performed only if the tympanic membrane is known to be intact. Direct visualization of the ear canal is important for the patient's safety. In patients who have difficulty with hard impacted cerumen the occasional instillation of olive oil, mineral oil, glycerin, diluted hydrogen peroxide solution, or propylene glycol in the ear may soften the cerumen and promote normal removal.

The patient may irrigate the ear canal with warm water, normal saline, a mixture of 20–30% alcohol and water, or aluminum acetate solution to help prevent cerumen buildup (11). The product of choice depends on availability. Each product has been demonstrated to be effective and safe. If the tympanic membrane is perforated or if it is not known whether or not the tympanic membrane is intact, these cerumen-softening drug products should be used only under a physician's direct supervision.

More than 90% of all cases of external otitis may be treated properly with aluminum acetate solution or acetic acid (2%) in either 70% alcohol or propylene glycol, four to six drops every 4–6 hours. This treatment is preferred except in diabetic patients and in unusually severe cases of external otitis. In severe cases these solutions are often used to irrigate the debris from the ear canal to improve the effectiveness of topical antibacterial otic drops. Patients with a known tympanic membrane perforation should not use otic preparations without their physician's consent.

All nonprescription otic preparations may be contraindicated because of local irritation and hypersensitivity caused by the ingredients. Patients should be advised that if a rash, local redness, or noticeable adverse symptom occurs, the medication should be discontinued.

Other Self-Therapy Procedures

During recovery from an ear disorder, general measures are advisable to assist the natural healing process and to prevent reinfection (22).

The external auditory canal must not be exposed to water. A bathing cap should be worn while the patient is taking a shower, and swimming should be avoided during and immediately following an infection. Patients prone to recurrence should swim only after consulting a physician. If water enters the external auditory canal, the head should be tilted so that the water may drain out by gravity. If the water does not drain out, an appropriate nonprescription otic preparation may be used to help dry the external auditory canal. The auricle should be cleaned by wiping with a soft cotton cloth wrung out in soapy water, then wiped again with a damp soft cloth rinsed in clear water, and finally dried with a clean towel.

nondrug measures

assessing the disorder

consulting with the patient

PRODUCT SELECTION GUIDELINES

Patient Considerations

The pharmacist's evaluation of the patient's present health status must be based on information in the medical and drug history, including current symptoms. This information should include the presence of chronic diseases that may impair healing, e.g., diabetes mellitus (is the patient taking insulin or oral hypoglycemics?), or that may influence the patient's response to self-medication, e.g., dandruff. Other considerations include deformities or ear scars. An earache due to otitis media, secondary to an upper respiratory tract infection, should be ruled out before the pharmacist considers initiating treatment of an external ear disorder. A history of pressure in or referred pain to the ear may be caused by a tumor in the area around the ear. Recent injury or trauma in the head or neck regions also may cause referred pain to the ear. Adults with recurrent otitis media may respond very poorly to treatment.

Management of ear disorders often may be difficult because of underlying diseases or predisposing factors. The skin of patients with diabetes mellitus is more prone to infection (bacterial and fungal), especially when the diabetes is uncontrolled, and infections clear up more slowly and recur more frequently. The increased predisposition to infection is related to circulatory skin impairments, increased glucose concentrations, and abnormalities in immunological responses. Ear disorders, especially external otitis, are difficult to treat in diabetic patients. Rigid control of diabetes cannot be overemphasized for favorable outcome of treatment.

The pharmacist should ask specific questions regarding the patient's medical history, e.g., whether the patient has experienced similar symptoms previously and, if so, when and how they were treated. The pharmacist should ask the patient to describe the symptoms. The patient's history should reveal underlying disease states and predisposing factors, including allergies, which may influence the response to self-medication.

The pharmacist should first consider whether the patient can be treated appropriately with nonprescription drugs. Health professionals (pharmacists, nurses) properly trained to visualize the tympanic membrane and ear canal with a suitable otoscope and those properly instructed in aural hygiene may perform irrigation safely with an ear syringe or a forced water spray in most cases. Pharmacists may assess the severity of the otic disorder and either provide appropriate OTC medication with instructions or refer the patient to a physician. Appropriately selected nonprescription drug products often can be relied upon to provide a suitable therapeutic response. Proper selection and instruction by the pharmacist require a clear knowledge of the symptoms of the patient and the pathophysiology of the illness. Referral to medical treatment by a physician requires an ability to recognize the severity of the illness or the potential or actual complications associated with the condition.

Patient Consultation

Many physicians feel that cleansing procedures and self-medication for treating ear disorders should not be delegated to the patient or to anyone who is not properly trained. Patients must be evaluated for their ability to understand the hazards of inappropriate self-medication. The pharmacist with proper instruction in aural visualization and irrigation procedures can usually make these judgments.

The use of nonprescription drugs for the ear should be supervised like other drug products dispensed by the pharmacist. The proper use of medicine droppers for administering eardrops into the ear and ear syringes for irrigating the ear should be understood fully by the patient. Eardrops should be warmed to body temperature by holding the medication container in the palm of the hand or in a vessel of warm water for a few moments prior to administration.

A cotton plug may be inserted gently to help maintain the medication in the ear canal. Cotton wicks, however, usually require insertion with instrumentation and should be used only by trained personnel. Pulling the auricle back may allow the medication to reach a greater depth in the ear canal. Patients also must be advised that if the symptoms persist or increase in severity within a few days following the initiation of self-medication, a physician should be consulted. Symptoms usually begin to subside within 1–2 days if self-medication is useful. If symptoms persist or if an adverse reaction to the medication occurs, the patient should be referred to a physician.

SUMMARY

Otic disorders affect young and old, and their visible signs are not always proportional to the amount of pain suffered. Nonprescription products are available for treatment of disorders in both the auricle and the external auditory canal. Disorders involving the middle ear should not be treated with OTC products.

By assessing the complaint and reviewing the patient's history the pharmacist should be able to judge whether symptoms may be self-treated or referral to a physician is indicated. Pharmacists or other health professionals trained in otic procedures may examine the tympanic membrane with an otoscope and irrigate the ear canal gently with a syringe or forced water spray. This procedure should be performed only if the tympanic membrane is known to be intact and there are no underlying disorders.

advice to the patient

Objects such as hairpins, pencils, matchsticks, cotton swabs, or other sharp instruments should never touch the external auditory canal, and objects smaller than a finger draped with a clean washcloth should never enter the external auditory canal. Good personal hygiene, especially of facial and neck areas, should be maintained. Dandruff and dirty hair may be controlled with appropriate shampoos and washing. A skin infection must not be neglected, because an infection may be transferred very easily to uninfected areas.

otic products

Most OTC otic products have been shown to be safe and effective, and the choice of a specific product generally depends on availability. The pharmacist should advise the patient to consult a physician if symptoms are not ameliorated within 1–2 days after treatment is initiated or if adverse reactions occur.

REFERENCES

(1) I. Hall and B. Colman, "Diseases of the Nose, Throat and Ear," 10th ed., Williams and Wilkins, Baltimore, Md., 1973, pp. 278, 315, 324.
(2) I. Friedmann, "Pathology of the Ear," Blackwell Scientific Publications, London, England, 1974, pp. 10, 14, 15, 27.
(3) D. Deweese and W. Saunders, "Textbook of Otolaryngology," 4th ed., Mosby, St. Louis, Mo., 1973, pp. 235, 245, 272–274, 327, 328, 336, 337, 346.
(4) M. M. Paparella and D. A. Shumrick, "Otolaryngology," Vol. 2, Saunders, Philadelphia, Pa., 1973, pp. 24, 26, 29, 30, 37, 85, 103.
(5) S. Riegelman and D. L. Sorby, in "Dispensing of Medication," 7th ed., E. W. Martin, Ed., Mack, Easton, Pa., 1971, p. 908.
(6) G. L. Adams, R. L. Boies, Jr., and M. M. Paparella, "Fundamentals of Otolaryngology," 5th ed., Saunders, Philadelphia, Pa., 1978, pp. 181, 184.
(7) "Diseases of the Nose, Throat and Ear," 11th ed., J. J. Ballenger et al., Eds., Lea and Febiger, Philadelphia, Pa., 1969, pp. 505, 604, 609, 610, 612.
(8) S. R. Mawson, "Diseases of the Ear," 3rd ed., Williams and Wilkins, Baltimore, Md., 1974, pp. 218, 236, 237, 245, 251.
(9) A. Cohn, *Arch. Otolaryngol.*, *99*, 138 (1974).
(10) D. Elliott, E. Mortimer, and L. Rutledge, *Patient Care*, *5*, 20 (1971).
(11) "AMA Drug Evaluations," 3rd ed., Publishing Sciences Group, Littleton, Mass., 1977, pp. 998–999.
(12) D. Wright and F. Alexander, *Arch. Otolaryngol.*, *99*, 16, 18 (1974).
(13) D. Wright and M. Dinen, *Arch. Otolaryngol.*, *95*, 245 (1972).
(14) "Drugs of Choice 1974–1975," W. Modell, Ed., Mosby, St. Louis, Mo., 1974, p. 603.
(15) "Remington's Pharmaceutical Sciences," 14th ed., Mack, Easton, Pa., 1970, pp. 768, 775, 1191.
(16) *Federal Register*, *42*, 63556 (1977).
(17) "The United States Pharmacopeia," 19th rev., Mack, Easton, Pa., 1975, p. 223.
(18) "The United States Dispensatory," 27th ed., A. Osol and R. Pratt, Eds., Lippincott, Philadelphia, Pa., 1973, pp. 199, 804
(19) M. S. Ersner, in "Diseases of the Nose, Throat and Ear," 1st ed., C. Jackson and C. L. Jackson, Eds., Saunders, Philadelphia, Pa., 1945, p. 266.
(20) L. R. Boies, "Fundamentals of Otolaryngology," Saunders, Philadelphia, Pa., 1950, pp. 66–67.
(21) Burroughs Wellcome Co., "Medical Notes of External Otitis," 1972.
(22) R. D. Stride, *J. Laryngol. Otol.*, *73*, 48 (1959).

Otic Products

Product (Manufacturer)	Ingredients
Aquaear (Miller and Morton)	boric acid, 2.5%; isopropyl alcohol
Aqua-Otic-B (Ortega)	aluminum acetate; boric acid, 1%; acetic acid, 1%; benzocaine, 1%; propylene glycol
Aurinol (National)	acetic acid, 2%; chloroxylenol, 0.12%; benzalkonium chloride, 0.09%; propylene glycol; glycerin
Auro-Dri (Commerce)	boric acid, 2.75%; isopropyl alcohol
Auro Ear Drops (Commerce)	camphor, thymol, propylene glycol
Columbia Ear Drops (Columbia Medical)	carbamide, propylene gylcol, glycerin, chlorobutanol
Debrox Drops (International)	carbamide peroxide, 6.5%; anhydrous glycerol
Ear Drops by Murine (Abbott)	carbamide peroxide, 6.5%; anhydrous glycerin
Ear-Dry (First Texas)	boric acid, 2.75%; isopropyl alcohol
E.R.O. (First Texas)	glycerin, 95%; propylene glycol, 5%
Kerid Ear Drops (Blair)	glycerin, 30%; urea, 0.1%; propylene glycol
Oil for Ear Use (DeWitt)	cajuput oil, 1.6%; white thyme oil, 1.6%; camphor, 0.5%; menthol, 0.3%
Pfeiffer Ear Drops (Pfeiffer)	glycerin, 49.8% (v/v); propylene glycol, 49.8% (v/v); fragrances
Stall Otic Drops (Cenci)	salicylic acid, 0.5%; thymol, 0.5%; isopropyl alcohol, 70%

Ophthalmic Products

Dick R. Gourley and Michael C. Makoid

Chapter 19

Questions to Ask the Patient

Is your vision blurred? Is your eye painful as opposed to itching or stinging?

How long have these symptoms been present? What were you doing when you noticed them?

Do you have any other eye problems (e.g., double vision or twitch)?

What medications are you using? For how long?

Have you used an OTC eye product recently? Which one(s)? For what symptoms?

Are you using any other OTC products?

Do you wear contact lenses? Hard or soft lenses? What contact lens products do you use?

Do you have any allergies?

Do you have chronic diseases such as diabetes, glaucoma, or hypertension?

Have your eyes been exposed recently to irritants such as smog, chemicals, or sun glare? Have you used any pesticides or fertilizers recently?

Do you use eye cosmetics? Do you use hair spray or spray deodorants?

Have you recently had a "head cold" or "sinus" problem?

As the most available member of the health care team, the pharmacist often must deal with a patient who has ocular discomfort. In deciding between physician referral and self-medication, the pharmacist must have a thorough understanding of common eye problems. Minor symptoms may signal the beginning of a more serious problem that requires evaluation and treatment by a physician.

OTC ophthalmic products are basically safe and effective only to relieve minor symptoms such as stinging, itching, tearing, "tired eyes," or "eye strain." These problems are usually painless and self-limiting. Patients experiencing pain and/or blurred vision should be referred to a physician. They should be discouraged from self-medication when these symptoms occur or when the ocular problem has existed for 48 hours or longer.

EYE ANATOMY AND PHYSIOLOGY

The eye is divided into three general areas (1, 2): the eyelids, the external eye, and the internal eye (Figure 1).

Eyelids

The eyelids are movable folds of tissue that protect the eye and distribute tears over the surface of the globe. They are lined posteriorly with conjunctiva, a thin, transparent mucous membrane terminating at the corneal–scleral junction. Three types of glands are present in the lids, the meibomian glands and the glands of Zeis and Moll. The meibomian glands are long sebaceous glands which secrete an oily substance. This substance helps maintain the integrity of the tear film by preventing rapid evaporation. The glands of Zeis are smaller sebaceous glands associated with eyelash follicles; Moll's glands are modified apocrine sweat glands.

External Eye

The external eye, the area immediately in front of the cornea, consists of the lacrimal apparatus and the cul-de-sac which contains the lacrimal fluid. In the normal human eye, tears are constantly produced and removed, maintaining a resident volume of 7 μl (3). The lacrimal fluid keeps the cornea moist, protects the eye, and clears away foreign materials from the eye (maintains an optical surface). Once formed, tears are conveyed across the corneal surface by the movement of the eyelids, finally collecting in the lower cul-de-sac for eventual drainage into the nasolacrimal duct.

Lid movement influences the drainage rate and thus physical removal of topically instilled drugs (3). The drainage apparatus begins at the punctum and ends in the nose. The passageway is a highly vascularized mucous membrane and consequently offers an extremely facile route for systemic absorption of topically instilled drugs, giving rise to the potential for systemic side effects (4–6). Tear turnover in the precorneal area is rapid [16%/minute in humans (3)], and any additional instilled fluid also drains away rapidly, with a rate constant proportional to the volume instilled (5). This process usually accounts for the loss of more than 90% of an instilled dose (7, 8); as a result, maintaining a high drug concentration for a prolonged period in the precorneal area is difficult.

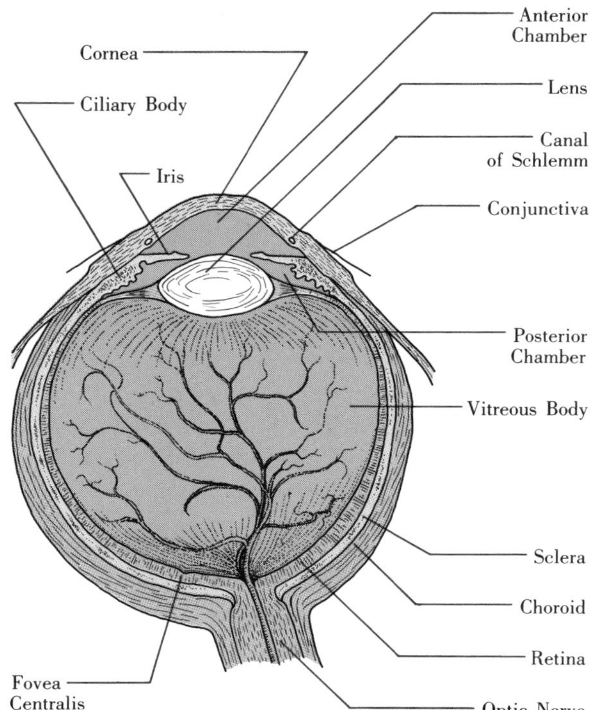

Figure 1. Horizontal cross section showing the anatomy of the eyeball.

anatomy of the eyeball

causes of eye problems

Internal Eye

The eyeball (or globe) may be considered as a three-layered sac divided into three compartments and filled with three fluids. The three coats of the eye are an outer fibrous layer, consisting of the sclera and the cornea; the middle vascular layer (uveal tract), consisting of the iris, ciliary body, and choroid; and the inner photoreceptor layer, consisting of the pigmented epithelium and retina. The three compartments are the anterior chamber, the space between the iris and the cornea; the posterior chamber, the space between the iris and the lens; and the vitreous cavity, the space dorsal to the lens. The three intraocular fluids are the aqueous humor, found in both the anterior and posterior chambers; the vitreous humor, found in the vitreous cavity; and the blood, which is in the uveal tract.

The sclera (white of the eye) makes up about 85% of the globe surface. Anteriorly, it joins with the cornea. The cornea is a smooth, nearly circular, layered membrane about 0.4 mm thick, consisting of the epithelium, Bowman's membrane, the stroma, Descemet's membrane, and the endothelium. Because the corneal epithelium forms a lipid barrier to topically applied drugs, its disruption may change drug transport. The endothelium, and to a lesser degree the epithelium, provides a barrier to excessive corneal hydration. Damage to either tissue may lead to corneal edema and impaired transparency. While all layers of the cornea are permeable to water, the epithelium and endothelium are considered lipophilic, while the stroma is hydrophilic. Unlike Descemet's membrane, Bowman's membrane does not regenerate after damage.

The iris, a thin, circular disc in front of the lens, regulates the amount of light reaching the retina, using two muscles, the sphincter pupillae and the dilater pupillae. Surrounding the globe just posterior to the limbus is the ciliary muscle. This smooth muscle influences aqueous humor dynamics and also changes the shape of the lens, enabling it to focus on nearby objects. The choroid contains the blood supply for the pigment epithelium and the visual receptors as the retinal capillary network extends to the inner nuclear layer.

The anterior chamber, the space between the iris and the cornea, is encircled by the trabecular meshwork, the outflow channel for aqueous humor via the canal of Schlemm. The meshwork consists of multiple perforated sheets (9–11). Aqueous humor is secreted from the area of the ciliary body or processes and flows from the posterior chamber through the pupillary opening into the anterior chamber.

The aqueous humor fills both the anterior and the posterior chamber. Its main functions are maintenance of the intraocular pressure and nourishment of the avascular lens and cornea. The aqueous humor turnover rate is 1–1.4%/minute, or about 2.75 μl/minute, about 80% exiting by Schlemm's canal (12–14). The bulk flow of aqueous humor is a primary means of drug removal in the internal eye (15).

Behind the lens is the vitreous cavity. Light which has passed through the cornea and lens converges in this space. The vitreous humor is a transparent jellylike substance that fills the vitreous cavity. Essentially constrained to the uveal tract, blood is primarily the nutritive source for the ocular tissues.

The retina is composed primarily of nervous tissue. It contains the retinal pigment epithelium, rods and cones, the external limiting membrane, the inner and outer nuclear layers, the inner and outer plexiform layers, the ganglion cell layer, and the nervous fiber layer.

ETIOLOGY OF OCULAR DISORDERS

Ocular inflammation and/or discomfort may be due to several conditions, including anatomical anomalies (e.g., incomplete closure of the eyelids), abnormal physiological conditions (e.g., dry eye syndrome, also referred to as keratoconjunctivitis sicca or KCS), allergic response, infection, and irritants (e.g., excessive ultraviolet radiation, drying winds, volatile chemical components of smog, and chemicals in fertilizers, pesticides, cleaning agents, and cosmetics). Table 1 provides a guide to the differential diagnosis of common causes of the inflamed eye.

Conditions due to physical causes (e.g., burns, lacerations, and concussions) or associated with specific disease states should be referred immediately to a physician.

Conditions of the Eyelids

The skin layer covering the eye is very thin and, consequently, very delicate. Patients with injured or inflamed eyelids should be referred to a physician. For

Table 1. Differential Diagnosis of Common Causes of Inflamed Eye

Parameter	Acute Conjunctivitis	Acute Iritis[a, b]	Acute Glaucoma[a, c]	Corneal Trauma or Infection[a]
Incidence	extremely common	common	uncommon	common
Discharge	moderate to copious	none	none	watery or purulent
Vision	normal	slightly blurred	markedly blurred	usually blurred
Pain	none	moderate	severe	moderate to severe
Conjunctival redness	diffuse	mainly circumcorneal	diffuse	diffuse
Cornea	clear	usually clear	steamy	may be abraded, lacerated, or ulcerated or show foreign body
Pupil size	normal	small	moderately dilated	normal
Pupillary light response	normal	poor	poor	normal
Intraocular pressure	normal	normal	elevated	normal
Conjunctival smear	causative organisms	no organisms	no organisms	organisms found only in corneal ulcer

D. Vaughan et al., *General Ophthalmology*, 4th ed., Lange Medical, Los Altos, Calif., 1965.
[a] Pharmacists should refer all patients with iritis, acute glaucoma, or corneal injury to a physician.
[b] Acute anterior uveitis.
[c] Narrow-angle glaucoma.

diagnosing an inflamed eye

inflammation and irritation

blepharitis

styes

treatment of so-called "black eye," cold compresses in the initial 24 hours after injury followed by warm applications are helpful.

Irritation

Irritation may range from slight inflammation to severe chemical burns. Chemical burns of the eyelids or external ocular tissues must be treated immediately by copious irrigation with sterile water or saline. If these are not available, tap water should be used. The important thing is to dilute and remove the offending agent quickly before extensive tissue damage occurs. Acid burns should be flushed for at least 5 minutes, and alkali burns for at least 1 hour. Under no circumstances should neutralization be attempted. Patients should be referred to an ophthalmologist as soon as possible after injury for follow-up evaluation and treatment.

Inflammation of only the lid margins (blepharitis) may result from associated seborrheic dermatitis of the scalp, contact dermatitis by chemical fumes such as smog or even the drugs used to treat inflammations, or irritation from eye strain usually caused by improper refraction. Assessment should be based on careful study of patient history. Symptoms are hyperemia of the lid margins and associated skin scaling. The main complaint is redness of the lids and burning and itching of the eyes, concomitant with conjunctivitis. Symptomatic treatment with OTC decongestants is not satisfactory, since symptoms will recur unless the cause is removed.

Infections

Hordeolum (stye) is an acute suppurative inflammation of the eyelash follicle or sebaceous or sweat gland. As with pustules anywhere in the body, the most common cause is staphylococcal. Patients should avoid spreading the infection by touching or squeezing the stye. Hordeola usually are self-limiting and respond well to hot compresses of 3% boric acid three to four times per day for 10–15 minutes (which help bring the stye to a "head," leading to drainage). Antibiotic ointment may be applied under a physician's care.

Cosmetic agents frequently become contaminated with microorganisms, and the incidence of cross-inoculation is high, particularly among adolescents (16–18). The occurrence of contamination is associated with length and frequency of use, personal habits, product formulation, and presence or absence of preservatives (16). Because cosmetics are a source of ocular infection, patients should be advised to avoid wearing eye makeup for at least 1 week prior to ocular surgery. Mascara should not be used to hide blepharitis because it may aggravate and prolong the condition. Women with signs and symptoms of blepharitis or conjunctivitis should be interviewed carefully by the pharmacist to ascertain whether eye cosmetics are used routinely.

External Ocular Disorders

Disorders affecting the external eye are chemical burn, conjunctivitis, and conditions of the lacrimal system. Since conjunctivitis may be due to causes ranging from a foreign body to an allergic reaction, careful and accurate patient assessment is essential. Many cases require physician referral. Table 2 gives a differential diagnosis of conjunctivitis.

cosmetics as factors in eye infections

types of conjunctivitis and how to differentiate them

Conjunctivitis

Conjunctivitis (inflammation of the conjunctiva) is a common external eye problem. Its symptoms are a diffusely reddened eye with a purulent or serous discharge accompanied by itching, smarting, stinging, or a scratching, "foreign body" sensation. If the patient has not experienced pain or blurred vision, conjunctivitis usually is a safe diagnosis.

Conjunctivitis may be caused by foreign bodies, contusions or lacerations, chemical irritants, allergens, bacterial or viral infections, or parasitic infestations. Most foreign bodies may be removed easily with irrigation or a cotton-tipped applicator provided no damage has occurred to deeper structures. If removal is difficult, the patient should be referred to a physician; the eye may have been irritated by rubbing, causing corneal epithelial lacerations subject to infection. Patients with contusions or lacerations of the conjunctiva should be referred to an ophthalmologist for assessment of possible trauma to the globe or conjunctiva.

Conjunctival irritation generally is treated like blepharitis caused by irritants, i.e., by removing the cause and administering OTC decongestants. A clue to chemical conjunctivitis, caused by airborne irritants such as smoke, smog, or garden sprays, is that both eyes are involved. Allergic conjunctivitis usually occurs on warm, windy days in the spring and during hay fever season. Typical symptoms—swelling, congestion, stinging, watering, and itching—also affect both eyes.

Bacterial conjunctivitis usually is self-limiting and does not impair vision. If the patient awakens with the eyelids stuck together by dried exudate or if there is discharge or signs of swelling of the preauricular lymph node, the etiology is probably bacterial. In such cases, OTC ophthalmic products have only limited efficacy (19). Referral to a physician would be in order, since recovery may be hastened with an appropriate prescription drug,

Table 2. Differential Diagnosis of Conjunctivitis

Parameter	Viral	Bacterial: Purulent	Bacterial: Nonpurulent	Fungal and Parasitic	Allergic
Discharge	minimal	copious	minimal	minimal	minimal
Tearing	copious	moderate	moderate	minimal	moderate
Itching	minimal	minimal	none	none	marked
Infection	generalized	generalized	localized	localized	generalized
Localized conjunctival lesions	none	none	frequent	frequent	none
Preauricular node	common	uncommon	common	common	none
Stained smear	monocytes	bacteria P.M.N.[a]	bacteria P.M.N.[a]	usually negative	eosinophils
Associated sore throat and fever	occasionally	seldom	none[b]	none	none

D. Vaughan et al., *General Ophthalmology*, 4th ed., Lange Medical, Los Altos, Calif., 1965.
[a] Polymorphonuclear neutrophil leukocytes.
[b] Diphtheritic conjunctivitis occurs only as a complication of diphtheria, and so the other manifestations of the disease are present also. It may be purulent.

i.e., a sulfonamide- or antibiotic-containing ophthalmic product. Without treatment, most bacterial conjunctivitis lasts 10–14 days, although *Staphylococcus* and *Moraxella* infections may become chronic. A purulent discharge characterizes the more common forms (staphylococcal or diplococcal). Corneal infections, which may exhibit symptoms similar to those of bacterial conjunctivitis, are more serious and may obliterate vision rapidly. An accurate diagnosis is important. Pinkeye, a bacterial infection caused by *Hemophilus* in warm climates and *Pneumococci* in temperate climates, is characterized by diffuse redness of the eye, photophobia, and pain and is moderately contagious.

Viral conjunctivitis may resemble chemically induced conjunctivitis; i.e., symptoms may be red, perhaps swollen, watery, itching eyes and swollen preauricular lymph nodes. Unlike chemical irritations, however, viral conjunctivitis is often accompanied by systemic symptoms. By careful patient questioning the pharmacist may discover that the patient also has influenza. The reddened eyes in such cases suggest viral conjunctivitis, which is not amenable to specific drug therapy.

Lacrimal Disorders

The therapy of dacryoadenitis (inflammation of the lacrimal gland) is determined by etiology. Assessment should be made by a physician.

Decreased tear production may be associated with aging, physical trauma, and infection (e.g., trachoma). Symptoms are burning and constant foreign body sensation and reddened and dry eyes. Treatment is tear replacement with artificial tears. There is little difference in efficacy of the different artificial tear products.

Some allergic reactions may cause excessive tearing and watery eyes. Cold water compresses and cool, clean air are beneficial for symptomatic relief, as well as OTC vasoconstrictors. If, as in hay fever, the causative agent cannot be removed, oral antihistamines may be useful.

Internal Eye Conditions

Internal eye disorders may have far graver consequences than conditions of the external eye. Early diagnosis may help prevent partial or total loss of vision. The pharmacist should emphasize the importance of physician referral.

Glaucoma

Glaucoma (19, 20) is characterized by increased intraocular pressure causing degeneration of the optic disc and defects in the visual field. It may be classified as either primary (including open-angle, narrow-angle, or hypersecretion glaucoma), congenital, or secondary. The most common form is primary open-angle glaucoma. Initial treatment of open-angle and secondary glaucoma may be medical, whereas narrow-angle and congenital glaucoma treatment is generally surgical. Most chronic open-angle glaucoma sooner or later will require surgical intervention (21).

Open-angle glaucoma is due to a decreased outflow (drainage) of aqueous humor from the anterior chamber of the eye. In patients with this disorder the chamber angles are normal, and the decreased outflow may be due to factors such as a foreign body blocking the canal of Schlemm, changes in the trabecular meshwork, ocular inflammation, ocular trauma, hemorrhage, or drug therapy.

Narrow-angle glaucoma (also called angle-closure or acute glaucoma) is characterized by a sudden onset of blurred vision followed by excruciating pain which may be accompanied by nausea and vomiting. It occurs with sudden increase in intraocular tension due to a block of the anterior chamber angle by the root of the iris, which cuts off all aqueous outflow. The chamber angle is anatomically closed. Any dilation of the pupil (e.g., from mydriatics) or swelling of the iris or lens may produce this obstruction. Pain is seen in both open-angle and narrow-angle glaucoma; however, the pain is more intense with narrow-angle glaucoma.

Uveitis

Uveitis is a general term for inflammatory disorders of the uveal tract. Causes include infection, trauma, anatomical abnormalities such as cataracts, and systemic inflammatory disease, and one or all three portions of the uveal tract may be involved simultaneously. Anterior uveitis is the term used for iritis and iridocyclitis, and posterior uveitis is the term used for choroiditis and chorioretinitis (19).

pinkeye

dacryoadenitis and other lacrimal disorders

glaucoma and uveitis

components of OTC products

TREATMENT

Most OTC ophthalmic products are promoted for relief of allergic or chemical conjunctivitis. If an irritant has not been sprayed or instilled directly into the eye and if the cornea is not abraded, OTC decongestants are useful in relieving the discomfort. It may be advisable to discontinue all topical application of medications and cosmetics.

Ophthalmologists occasionally use steroids to treat allergic conjunctivitis. Pharmacists should watch for evidence of chronic steroid use (e.g., repeated requests for prescription renewal), because long-term use may cause glaucoma and/or cataracts (2).

Patients experiencing pain or blurred vision should be referred to a physician. The pharmacist may suggest oral analgesics to relieve the pain.

Pharmaceutical Agents

In general, OTC ophthalmic products must be initially sterile and must have preservatives to maintain sterility. They should be bland, optically clear, and free from particles, filaments, and fibers. In addition, they must not contain any extraneous excipients such as agents for color or odor, and they should approximate the tonicity and pH of tears as nearly as possible.

All ophthalmic products should have an expiration date and should be used no more than 3 months from the date of opening. The hazard of introducing drug crystals into the eye is a problem associated with all ophthalmic solutions if the drug crystallizes on the lip of the bottle or the dropper tip. However, the probability of contamination is more serious. All ophthalmic solutions that are cloudy, discolored, or more than 3 months old

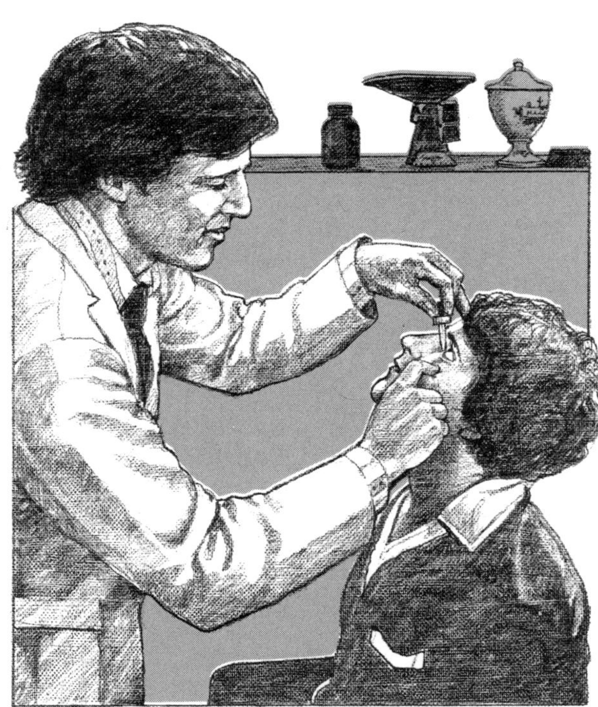

nontherapeutic ingredients of OTC ophthalmic products

from date of opening or that contain foreign particles should be discarded.

Nontherapeutic substances in OTC ophthalmic preparations include tonicity adjusters, antioxidants, stabilizers, buffers, wetting or clarifying agents, preservatives, viscosity-increasing agents, and vehicles for ointments. All were tested and reviewed by the FDA OTC Panel on Ophthalmic Drugs.

Tonicity Adjusters

Tears are isotonic, and products of 0.9 ± 0.2% sodium chloride equivalent also may be considered isotonic. The eye tolerates 0.6–1.8% sodium chloride equivalent without damage (22–26). If the instilled solution elicits excessive blinking or tearing, the product's bioavailability is severely hampered (owing to early washout by eye fluids) (15). Agents used to adjust tonicity in ophthalmic preparations are dextran 40, dextran 70, dextrose, glycerin (1%), potassium chloride, propylene glycol (1%), and sodium chloride.

Antioxidants and Stabilizers

Edetic acid (sodium salt), sodium bisulfite (0.1%), sodium metabisulfite (0.1%), sodium thiosulfate (0.2%), and thiourea (0.1%) are agents used in this category. All have been classified as acceptable by the FDA Panel. Edetic acid acts as a chelator of metal ions that catalyze redox reactions, whereas the others are oxidized preferentially instead of the active component.

Buffers

Agents used as buffers in OTC ophthalmic solutions are boric acid, potassium bicarbonate, potassium borate, potassium carbonate, sodium acetate, sodium bicarbonate, sodium biphosphate, sodium borate, and sodium carbonate. All are accepted by the FDA, although choice of a specific buffer depends on the drug being formulated.

Tears have a pH of 7.4; consequently, tear substitutes should approximate this level. The acceptable pH range for ophthalmic products is 6.0–8.0; products outside this range may be irritating. In an animal study, products outside the range of 4.0–10.0 caused corneal damage (26). Since ophthalmic products should be formulated to be approximately isotonic (0.9% sodium chloride), buffers should contribute <1% sodium chloride equivalency.

Nonionic Wetting or Clarifying Agents

Polysorbate 80 (1.0%), polysorbate 20 (1.0%), poloxamer 282 (Pluronic L-92) (0.025%), and tyloxapol (Triton WR-1339) (0.25%) are compounds used to reduce surface tension, i.e., the ability to allow water to wet the eye better. They may decrease phenylmercuric nitrate antibacterial activity. Tyloxapol is used for in situ cleaning of artificial eyes.

Preservatives

Preservatives are used to prevent growth or destroy microorganisms accidentally introduced into the container after opening. The pharmacist should discuss proper instillation technique with the patient to prevent undue inoculation.

Several preservatives have been classified by the FDA as Category I (see Table 3). Benzalkonium chloride and benzethonium chloride are accepted as preservatives, although claims such as effectiveness as cleaning agents or antibacterials are not satisfactorily proven. When concentrations of benzalkonium chloride higher than 0.013% were applied experimentally to rabbit eyes, corneal damage was reported (1).

Chlorobutanol is another commonly used preservative. This agent hydrolyzes above pH 5–6 and also permeates plastic; thus it is effectively removed from solution if stored in a plastic container.

Edetic acid is not effective alone as a preservative but enhances the action of benzalkonium chloride. It is a weak primary sensitizer, and products containing this agent have been implicated in allergic reactions.

Thimerosal should not be used with edetic acid because the chelating action of the latter can slow thimerosal's action or inactivate it altogether. The compound also may be a contact allergen due to the thio or mercuric radical. Thimerosal has antiseptic properties in ophthalmic ointments for conjunctivitis, corneal ulcer, and preventing infection following removal of foreign bodies. However, the Panel has not assessed the effectiveness of the compound for these uses in the concentrations employed.

Several other agents are being investigated by the Panel, but sufficient evidence is lacking to place them in either Category I or II. Cetylpyridinium chloride is classified in Category III because of its extensive binding capabilities.

Data are lacking on chlorhexidinium chloride be-

Table 3. Classification of Ophthalmic Product Preservatives

Compound	Concentration, %	Category
Benzalkonium chloride	0.013	I
Benzethonium chloride	0.01	I
Cetylpyridinium chloride	0.02	III
Chlorhexidinium chloride		III
Chlorobutanol	0.5	I
Edetic acid	0.1	II
Edetic acid:benzalkonium chloride	0.1:0.01	I
Parabens	0.01	II
Phenylethyl alcohol		III
Phenylmercuric acetate		III
Phenylmercuric nitrate	0.004	I
Sodium benzoate		III
Sodium propionate	0.75	III
Sorbic acid		II
Thimerosal	0.01	I

cause it is not used routinely in the United States. Parabens (methyl and propyl *p*-hydroxybenzoic acid) (aromatic preservatives) are efficient only at the limit of solubility, and at that concentration they are irritating. They are known sensitizers and a source of carbon for *Pseudomonas aeruginosa*. Phenylethyl alcohol is slow acting and potentially irritating, but it may be useful in combination with other preservatives. Sodium propionate is a fungistat and is of questionable use in ophthalmics.

Viscosity-Increasing Agents

The viscosity-increasing agents are used primarily for their physical characteristics rather than for a specific chemical action. Many of the polymers may influence interfacial tension, lowering surface tensions of saline from 72.2 dynes/cm to about 50 dynes/cm (42–66 dynes/cm) at 1% concentration. Thus they aid in wetting the eye by decreasing the contact angle of the solutions and therefore increasing the liquid's tendency to spread (27). In the concentrations used in ophthalmic products they are virtually nontoxic. Many of the polymers are film formers and may build up on contact lenses.

Agents accepted by the FDA as increasing viscosity are dextran 40, dextran 70, gelatin (1%), glycerin, hydroxyethylcellulose (HEC), hydroxymethyl propylcellulose (HMPC), lanolin, methylcellulose, petrolatum, polyethylene glycol, polyvinyl alcohol (PVA), polyvinyl pyrrolidone (PVP) (2.0%), and carboxymethylcellulose sodium. Evidence on acetylated polyvinyl alcohol is lacking, and it has been placed in Category III. Viscosity inducers may be used for their wetting, adhesive, and/or lubricating properties, specifically in dry eye treatment (artificial tears). Increased viscosity moderately increases the bioavailability of therapeutic agents by increasing retention time (8, 28).

There are no apparent differences among artificial tear products. In general, products containing viscosity agents are retained about twice as long as saline solution (several minutes). The retention time depends on the viscosity and the drainage rate, not on the concentration of the polymer (28). Methylcellulose solutions, as formulated, are more viscous than polyvinyl alcohol solutions and thus tend to form crusts on the eyelids, which may be annoying to some patients. However, the methylcellulose solutions are retained longer than the polyvinyl alcohol solutions, due to their higher viscosity for a given concentration. Products containing polyethylene glycol polymers are claimed to possess a mucomimetic property similar to gelatin and bovine mucin. In the presence of these substances the corneal surface is easier to wet.

Patients should not use alkaline borate products concomitantly with products containing polyvinyl alcohol because gel systems may form, resulting in gummy deposits.

FDA categories for preservatives

other nontherapeutic ingredients

Vehicles in Ophthalmic Ointments

ointments

Many types of vehicles (e.g., petrolatum, vegetable oils, mineral oils, lanolin, and lanolin substitutes such as polyethylene glycols) are used in ophthalmic ointments. Some of these substances are used as adjuncts to modify the product's consistency. These agents are classified in Category I for the lubrication of the eye or as drug delivery systems. Consideration must be given to the preservatives necessary to maintain sterility because the significant increase in retention time could result in corneal damage by these agents.

therapeutic ingredients in OTC ophthalmic products

Medicinal Agents

Therapeutic agents contained in OTC ophthalmic products include antipruritics, anti-infectives, astringents, and decongestants/vasoconstrictors. Few of these drugs have been proven safe and effective. Many are contraindicated in specific conditions.

Antipruritics

Antipyrine (0.1–0.4%), camphor, and menthol (peppermint oil) are present in some OTC ophthalmic medications because of their mild local analgesic and cooling effect. Such products are considered generally unsafe because foreign bodies may go unrecognized, leading to severe corneal erosions.

Anti-Infectives

There is no good OTC ophthalmic anti-infective available for treatment of minor eye infections. Boric acid is weak at best and at worst may be dangerous because of the possibility of boron toxicity, especially in small children. Silver protein products (prescription only) are effective but lack patient acceptability because of their staining properties, and the current yellow mercuric oxide products lack the active ingredient mercuric chloride due to modern manufacturing techniques. The FDA Panel is reviewing sulfacetamide (10%) (currently available only on prescription) for deregulation to OTC standing to treat surface infections of eyelids and conjunctiva. Recent indications are that sulfacetamide (10%) probably will remain a prescription product.

Astringents

Astringents are applied locally to precipitate proteins and reduce local edema and inflammation. Berberine, hydrastine, peppermint oil, and rose geranium oil are promoted as astringents in ophthalmic products, but they were judged unacceptable by the FDA Panel. Infusion of rose petals and witch hazel water (2.6%) are in Category III.

The only acceptable astringent found in eye medications is zinc sulfate (0.25%). Zinc salts have no decongestant action and are not effective as promoted. They are mild vasodilators in the concentrations used, but the only indication in ophthalmology for zinc sulfate is for a rare form of conjunctivitis caused by the gram-negative diplobacillus. This chronic conjunctivitis responds to sulfonamides.

Table 4. Classification of Ophthalmic Decongestants/Vasoconstrictors

Compound	Use[a]	Concentration, %	Category
Ephedrine hydrochloride	D	0.12%	I
Naphazoline	D	0.05%	III[b]
Naphazoline hydrochloride	D	0.03%	I
Phenylephrine	V	0.08–0.2%	I
Tetrahydrozoline	V,D	0.05–0.1%	I

[a]D, decongestant; V, vasoconstrictor.
[b]Primarily for safety considerations.

Decongestants/Vasoconstrictors

ophthalmic decongestants and vasoconstrictors and their FDA categories

factors affecting product performance

bioavailability and pharmacokinetics

Vasoconstrictors are effective in the symptomatic treatment of allergic conjunctivitis. Reddened eyes usually are rapidly whitened by vasoconstrictors, which limit the local vascular response by constricting the blood vessels. The vasoconstrictors not only affect the vascular receptors, but also stimulate other receptors such as the nerves that control pupillary size.

These agents generally are contraindicated in known narrow-angle glaucoma patients. They are designed specifically for short-term, primarily cosmetic use and should not be used on a regular basis. They are potentially hazardous in that they may mask symptoms of serious problems.

If an ophthalmic decongestant is used when there is disease of the globe interior, no relief can be expected, and complications from the lack of primary treatment may occur. Furthermore, bacterial or other infections may be masked by the use of symptomatic treatment. If an ocular condition persists, the patient should be referred to a physician.

Drugs used as decongestants/vasoconstrictors are ephedrine hydrochloride, naphazoline hydrochloride, phenylephrine, and tetrahydrozoline. Their uses, concentrations, and FDA classifications are listed in Table 4.

Ephedrine is similar to epinephrine in that it is short acting and produces rebound congestion. However, it is more stable than epinephrine.

The imidazoline derivatives, naphazoline and tetrahydrozoline, are more stable and have a longer duration of action than epinephrine. They are buffered to pH 6.2. Naphazoline is used in prescription ophthalmic solutions at 0.1%. This high concentration has been classified Category III by the FDA Panel, primarily on a safety basis. Tetrahydrozoline is used at a concentration of 0.05%.

Untoward effects occurring after imidazoline use have been reported, particularly CNS stimulation after accidental ingestion by children. Although rebound congestion was reported after intranasal use of naphazoline, it has not been reported after ophthalmic use.

Phenylephrine is the vasoconstrictor used most commonly in OTC ophthalmic products. Its relative instability accounts for its variable effectiveness. Solutions usually are effective initially, but with continued use, oxidation may reduce the product's activity significantly without discoloration. Furthermore, phenylephrine products in polyethylene containers may be less stable than those packaged in glass. The oxygen diffuses through the polyethylene and hastens oxidation of the amine unless an oxygen-resistant coating is put over the plastic bottle. Patients allergic to epinephrine may show cross-sensitivity to phenylephrine.

Rebound congestion may occur following the prolonged use of vasoconstrictors in the eye. The tissues become more congested and edematous as the vasoconstriction of the drug subsides. The phenomenon is a vicious cycle because it leads to more frequent use of the drug that causes it.

Pharmacokinetic Considerations

Properties of the drug, its formulation, and the eye itself influence the pharmacokinetics of topical ophthalmic products. Pharmacists should take these factors into consideration when recommending an OTC preparation.

The physical drug properties that probably have the most effect on transport into and through the eye are lipid solubility and water solubility (29). Protein binding of drugs in the tear fluids may further reduce the amount of free drug available for absorption and thus adversely affect its bioavailability. Metabolism in the precorneal area and sorption by tissues other than the cornea also are potential drug loss mechanisms (30–33). Because the conjunctiva and nasolacrimal duct are highly vascularized, drugs may be absorbed into the bloodstream and lost from the target site (34). Moreover, since drugs in the eye are eliminated primarily by bulk flow, elimination may be either enhanced or retarded by a drug's pharmacological effect. For example, in a glaucomatous eye the reduction of intraocular pressure brought about by increased outflow could lessen the drug's duration of action (15).

The concentration and volume instilled and the drug's contact time also are important variables which may affect a drug's ocular availability and effectiveness with some drugs. High concentrations may cause irritation, which in turn causes tearing and thus flushing of the precorneal area, removing the drug from the absorption site (15). Since the rate of nasolacrimal drainage also is a function of instilled volume, it is desirable to administer the smallest volume of product possible. In addition, patients instilling more than one medication into the eye should wait at least 3–5 minutes between drops. This is so that the first drop is not flushed away by the second drop or, conversely, the second drop is not diluted by the first. Both conditions would reduce bioavailability. (5, 35).

The eye is a unique system relative to biopharmaceutics and pharmacokinetics. Several factors not dependent on the drug molecule itself greatly influence the activity of the applied drug. The absorption and elimination rate constants used to explain the kinetics of drug transport are a compilation of the various processes going on in the whole system, dominated by an apparent parallel elimination in the precorneal area, distribution in the aqueous humor, and bulk flow from the aqueous humor (15).

PRODUCT SELECTION GUIDELINES

The following general guidelines should help the pharmacist in selecting a suitable OTC ophthalmic product:

- OTC ocular medications should not be recommended to patients who have demonstrated an allergy to any of the active ingredients, preservatives, or other agents in the product;
- Patients with narrow-angle glaucoma should not use sympathomimetics, and patients with open-angle glaucoma should use these drugs with caution;
- Patients already using a legend ophthalmic product should use OTC ophthalmic products only after consulting with a pharmacist or a physician;
- Topical anesthetics should never be instilled into the eye except by an eye care specialist;
- Pain should be treated with oral analgesics, and the patient should be referred to the patient's family physician or ophthalmologist.

The pharmacist should instruct the patient on the proper use of ophthalmic products (36). Before administration, the hands should be washed and the product inspected for expiration date, contamination, discoloration, and/or other problems.

Ophthalmic drops should be administered to the patient with the head tilted back and up. The skin below the eye just above the cheekbone should be pulled down, and the fluid dropped into the lower conjunctival sac away from the tear ducts. To avoid contamination, the dropper tip should not touch the eye or lid. Suspension fluids should be shaken well before instillation.

For ophthalmic ointments the patient should assume the same position. A thin line of ointment should be applied along the conjunctival surface of the lower lid. The patient should be instructed to close the eyes for a short period to allow the medication to be dispensed throughout the eye. Gently massaging the eye to distribute the ointment over the cornea is helpful. The tip of the ointment tube should not touch the eye, and the cap should be replaced immediately.

Eyecups should be discouraged as a method for administering ophthalmic solutions. They may harbor bacteria which can cause infections.

SUMMARY

The eye is one of the most sensitive areas of the human body and may be subject to many types of disorders. Pharmacists often are the first health care professionals to be informed of a patient's ocular condition, and the decision to recommend self-therapy with an OTC product or physician referral rests with them. Any ocular problem lasting more than 48 hours should be referred.

selecting a product

proper administration

REFERENCES

(1) F. H. Adler, "Physiology of the Eye," 4th ed., Mosby, St. Louis, Mo., 1965.
(2) D. Vaughn, R. Cook, and T. Asbury, "General Ophthalmology," Lange Medical, Los Altos, Calif., 1968.
(3) S. Mishima, A. Gasset, S. D. Klyce, and J. L. Baum, *Invest. Ophthalmol.*, *5*, 264 (1966).
(4) J. J. Greco and D. C. Kelman, *Ann. Ophthalmol.*, *5*, 57 (1973).
(5) S. S. Chrai, M. C. Makoid, S. P. Eriksen, and J. R. Robinson, *J. Pharm. Sci.*, *63*, 333 (1974).
(6) E. Epstein, *Am. J. Ophthalmol.*, *59*, 109 (1965).
(7) L. Harris and M. Galin, *Arch. Ophthalmol.*, *84*, 105 (1970).
(8) T. F. Patton, "Quantitation of Precorneal Drug Movement," Ph.D. thesis, University of Wisconsin, Madison, 1975.
(9) A. Bill and B. Svedbergh, *Acta Ophthalmol.*, *50*, 295 (1972).
(10) D. G. Cole and R. C. Tripathi, *Exp. Eye Res.*, *12*, 25 (1971).
(11) A. Bill, *Invest. Ophthalmol.*, *14*, 1 (1975).
(12) P. Ellis and D. Smith, "Handbook of Ocular Therapeutics and Pharmacology," 4th ed., Mosby, St. Louis, Mo., 1973.
(13) J. G. Daubs, *Am. J. Ophthalmol.*, *49*, 1005 (1972).
(14) E. Weigelin, F. Sayegh, W. von Klitzing, and A. Fawrmounti, *Eye Ear Nose Throat Mon.*, *54*, 13 (1975).
(15) M. C. Makoid and J. R. Robinson, *J. Pharm. Sci.*, *68*, 435 (1979).
(16) L. A. Wilson, A. J. Julian, and D. G. Ahern, *Am. J. Ophthalmol.*, *79*, 596 (1975).
(17) S. Aronson and E. Yamamoto, *Invest. Ophthalmol.*, *5*, 75 (1966).
(18) B. D. Zuckerman, *Am. J. Ophthalmol.*, *62*, 672 (1966).
(19) D. Vaughn, R. Cook, and T. Asbury, "General Ophthalmology," 7th ed., Lange Medical, Los Altos, Calif., 1974, pp. 49–53, 69–95, 192–204.
(20) F. H. Roy, "Practical Management of Eye Problems: Glaucoma, Strabismus, Visual Fields," Lea and Febiger, Philadelphia, Pa., 1975, pp. 9–17.
(21) A. M. Potts, *Am. J. Ophthalmol.*, *86*, 743 (1978).
(22) E. W. Martin, "Dispensing of Medication," 7th ed., Mack, Easton, Pa., 1971.
(23) "Biochemistry of the Eye," C. N. Graymore, Ed., Academic, New York, N.Y., 1970.
(24) J. E. Harris, in "Problems of Drug Penetration," Vol. 3, I. H. Lepold, Ed., Mosby, St. Louis, Mo., 1968.
(25) "Remington's Pharmaceutical Sciences," 13th ed., Mack, Easton, Pa., 1965.
(26) J. M. Conrad and J. R. Robinson, *J. Pharm. Sci.*, *66*, 219 (1977).
(27) M. A. Lemp and F. J. Holly, *Ann. Ophthalmol.*, *4*, 15 (1972).
(28) T. F. Patton and J. R. Robinson, *J. Pharm. Sci.*, *64*, 1312 (1975).
(29) K. D. Swan and N. G. White, *Am. J. Ophthalmol.*, *25*, 1043 (1942).
(30) S. Y. Butelho, *Sci. Am.*, *211*, 78 (1964).
(31) N. Ehlers, *Acta Ophthalmol. Suppl.*, *81* (1965).
(32) O. F. Erickson, *Am. J. Ophthalmol.*, *43*, 295 (1957).
(33) E. S. Perkins and P. Haussel, "An Atlas of Disease of the Eye," 2nd ed., Churchill Livingstone, London, England, 1971.
(34) T. F. Patton and J. R. Robinson, *J. Pharm. Sci.*, *65*, 1295 (1976).
(35) C. Asseff, R. Weisman, B. Becker, and R. Podos, *Am. J. Ophthalmol.*, *75*, 212 (1973).
(36) H. Wedemeyer and D. R. Gourley, in "Handbook for Institutional Pharmacy Practice," M. C. Smith and T. R. Brown, Eds., Williams and Wilkins, Baltimore, Md., 1978.

Product (Manufacturer)	Viscosity Agent	Vasoconstrictor	Preservative	Buffer	Other
Adsorbonac (Burton Parsons)	—	—	thimerosal, 0.004% edetate sodium, 0.1%	—	sodium chloride, 2%, 5%
Clear Eyes (Abbott)	methylcellulose	naphazoline hydrochloride, 0.012%	edetate disodium, 0.1% benzalkonium chloride, 0.01%	boric acid sodium borate	—
Collyrium Drops (Wyeth)	—	ephedrine, 0.1%	thimerosal, 0.002%	boric acid sodium borate	antipyrine, 0.4% sodium salicylate, 0.056%
Degest 2 (Barnes-Hind)	hydroxyethyl-cellulose	naphazoline hydro-chloride, 0.012%	edetate disodium, 0.02% benzalkonium chloride, 0.0067%	sodium citrate	antipyrine, 0.1%
Eye Cool (Milroy)	—	phenylephrine hydrochloride, 0.08%	edetate disodium, 0.05% thimerosal, 0.002%	sodium borate boric acid	menthol eucalyptus oil sodium chloride sodium bisulfite
20/20 Eye Drops (S.S.S.)	—	naphazoline hydrochloride, 0.012%	thimerosal, 0.005%	boric acid sodium carbonate	potassium chloride zinc sulfate
Isopto-Frin (Alcon)	hydroxypropyl methylcellulose, 0.5%	phenylephrine hydrochloride, 0.12%	benzethonium chloride	sodium citrate sodium phosphate sodium biphosphate	—
Murine (Abbott)	methylcellulose	—	benzalkonium chloride, 0.01% edetate sodium, 0.05%	mono- and dibasic sodium phosphate	glycerin
Murine Plus (Abbott)	methylcellulose	tetrahydrozoline hydrochloride, 0.05%	benzalkonium chloride, 0.01% edetate sodium, 0.1%	boric acid sodium borate	—
Naphcon (Alcon)	—	naphazoline hydrochloride, 0.012%	benzalkonium chloride, 0.01%	—	—
Ocusol Drops (Norwich)	methylcellulose	tetrahydrozoline	benzalkonium chloride	boric acid sodium borate	sodium chloride
Optigene II (Pfeiffer)	methylcellulose	phenylephrine, 0.12% (w/v)	benzalkonium chloride sodium bisulfite edetate sodium	boric acid carbonate	potassium chloride
Phenylzin (Smith, Miller & Patch)	hydroxypropyl methylcellulose, 0.1%	phenylephrine hydrochloride, 0.12%	benzalkonium chloride, 0.01% edetate disodium, 0.01%	boric acid, 1.1% sodium carbonate, 0.02%	zinc sulfate, 0.25% sodium bisulfite, 0.01% potassium chloride
Prefrin Liquifilm (Allergan)	polyvinyl alcohol, 1.4%	phenylephrine hydrochloride, 0.12%	benzalkonium chloride, 0.004%	sodium phosphate sodium biphosphate	antipyrine, 0.1%
Prefrin Z (Allergan)	polyvinyl alcohol, 1.4%	phenylephrine hydrochloride, 0.12%	thimerosal, 0.005%	sodium hydroxide sodium citrate	zinc sulfate, 0.25% sodium chloride sodium bisulfite
Soothe (Burton Parsons)	—	tetrahydrozoline hydrochloride, 0.05%	benzalkonium chloride, 0.004% edetate sodium, 0.1%	—	isotonic buffered vehicle
Tear-efrin (Smith, Miller & Patch)	hydroxypropyl methylcellulose, 0.5%	phenylephrine hydrochloride, 0.1%	benzalkonium chloride, 0.01% edetate disodium, 0.01%	—	sodium bisulfite, 0.05% sodium chloride
Vaso Clear (Smith, Miller & Patch)	—	naphazoline hydrochloride, 0.02%	benzalkonium chloride, 0.01% edetate sodium, 0.03%	—	lipiden polymeric system

Ophthalmic Decongestant Products

Product (Manufacturer)	Viscosity Agent	Vasoconstrictor	Preservative	Buffer	Other
Visine (Leeming)	—	tetrahydrozoline, 0.05%	edetate disodium, 0.1% benzalkonium chloride, 0.01%	boric acid sodium borate	sodium chloride
Zincfrin (Alcon)	—	phenylephrine hydrochloride, 0.12%	benzalkonium chloride, 0.01%	barbital barbital sodium	zinc sulfate, 0.25%

Artificial Tears Products

Product (Manufacturer)	Viscosity Agent	Preservative	Other
Adsorbotear (Burton Parsons)	hydroxyethylcellulose, 0.44%	thimerosal, 0.004% edetate disodium, 0.1%	povidone
Bro-lac (Riker)	hydroxypropyl methylcellulose	benzalkonium chloride, 0.02%	glycerin, sodium borate, boric acid
Contique Artificial Tears (Alcon)	polyvinyl alcohol, 2%	benzalkonium chloride, 0.01% edetate disodium	sodium chloride, potassium chloride, calcium chloride, magnesium chloride, sodium acetate, sodium citrate, sodium hydroxide
Goniosol Ophthalmic Solution (Smith, Miller & Patch)	hydroxypropyl methylcellulose, 2.5%	edetate disodium, 0.01% benzalkonium chloride, 0.01%	boric acid, 1.1%; sodium carbonate; potassium chloride
Hypotears (Smith, Miller & Patch)	—	benzalkonium chloride, 0.01% edetate disodium, 0.03%	lipiden polymeric vehicle
Isopto Alkaline (Alcon)	hydroxypropyl methylcellulose	benzalkonium chloride, 0.01%	—
Isopto Plain (Alcon)	hydroxypropyl methylcellulose, 0.5%	benzalkonium chloride, 0.01%	—
Lacril (Allergan)	hydroxypropyl methylcellulose gelatin	chlorobutanol, 0.5%	potassium chloride, sodium chloride, calcium chloride, magnesium chloride, sodium acetate, sodium citrate, sodium borate, acetic acid, polysorbate 80, dextrose
Liquifilm Forte (Allergan)	polyvinyl alcohol, 3.0%	chlorobutanol, 0.5%	dextrose
Liquifilm Tears (Allergan)	polyvinyl alcohol, 1.4%	chlorobutanol, 0.5%	sodium chloride
Lyteers (Barnes-Hind)	hydroxypropyl methylcellulose, 0.2%	edetic acid, 0.05% benzalkonium chloride, 0.01%	sodium chloride, potassium chloride
Tearisol (Smith, Miller & Patch)	hydroxypropyl methylcellulose, 0.50%	benzalkonium chloride, 0.01% edetate disodium, 0.01%	boric acid, sodium carbonate, potassium chloride
Tears Naturale (Alcon)	water-soluble polymeric system	benzalkonium chloride, 0.01% edetate disodium, 0.05%	—
Ultra Tears (Alcon)	hydroxypropyl methylcellulose, 1%	benzalkonium chloride, 0.01%	—

Eyewash Products

Product (Manufacturer)	Buffer	Preservative	Other
Blinx (Barnes-Hind)	boric acid sodium borate	phenylmercuric acetate, 0.004%	—
Collyrium (Wyeth)	boric acid sodium borate	thimerosal, 0.002%	antipyrine, 0.4% sodium salicylate, 0.056%

Product (Manufacturer)	Buffer	Preservative	Other
Dacriose (Smith, Miller & Patch)	boric acid sodium carbonate	benzalkonium chloride, 0.01% edetate disodium, 0.1%	potassium chloride
Enuclene (Alcon)	—	benzalkonium chloride, 0.2%	tyloxapol, 0.25%
Eye-Stream (Alcon)	sodium citrate sodium acetate	benzalkonium chloride, 0.013%	sodium chloride potassium chloride calcium chloride magnesium chloride
Lauro Eye Wash (Otis Clapp)	boric acid sodium borate	—	sodium chloride
M/Rinse (Milroy)	sodium borate boric acid	edetate disodium, 0.1% thimerosal, 0.004%	sodium chloride potassium chloride
Murine (Abbott)	boric acid potassium bicarbonate potassium carbonate	benzalkonium chloride, 0.004% thimerosal, 0.001%	hydrastine berberine glycerin
Ocusol Eye Lotion (Norwich)	boric acid sodium borate	edetate disodium, 0.05% benzalkonium chloride, 0.01%	phenylephrine hydrochloride sodium chloride
Op-thal-zin (Alcon)	—	benzalkonium chloride, 0.01%	zinc sulfate, 0.25%
Trisol Eye Wash (Buffington)	boric acid sodium borate	—	sodium chloride

Contact Lens Products

Peter P. Lamy and Ralph F. Shangraw

Chapter 20

Questions to Ask the Patient

What types of problems are you having with your lenses? Are they related to eye irritation or changes in vision?

What type of lens do you wear?

How long have you been wearing lenses?

What drugs are you currently using?

Have you become pregnant or begun using oral contraceptives since you were fitted for lenses?

How often do you clean, sterilize, or wet your lenses? Which products do you use?

How often do you renew, refresh, or clean out solutions in your lens storage containers?

How many hours per day do you wear your lenses before any problems arise?

How long ago did you see your optometrist or ophthalmologist?

Of the 90 million or so Americans who must use corrective lenses, almost 10% use contact lenses. (The term "contact lens" is somewhat of a misnomer—a properly fitted lens is never in contact with the cornea but floats freely on the precorneal fluid and mucous secretions.) Every year, approximately 1 million contact lenses are prescribed, 90% to correct vision of the healthy eye. Contact lens wearers include myopic teenagers, patients who require constant visual correction, and patients with certain ocular conditions, including aphakia (absence of the crystalline lens). Poor candidates for contact lens wear include patients lacking sufficient manual dexterity, those too young to care for the lenses properly, those with recurrent eye infections, chronic sties, chronic conjunctivitis, or insufficient tear production, patients with a high degree of astigmatism, and individuals whose work exposes them to dust, dirt, or chemical vapors (1).

Use of contact lenses and their solutions has been reviewed recently in detail (2, 3). Psychological reactions to the wearer's improved appearance are cited for the public's rapid acceptance of the lenses.

TYPES OF LENSES

In 1968 the FDA announced that all contact lenses would be classified as drugs but that hard contact lenses, owing to a history of safe use, would automatically be accepted, as would their solutions. In contrast, each soft lens system, i.e., the specific lens together with the solutions specifically designed for it, would have to be approved. Soft contact lenses (see the appendix) would have to follow the procedures set forth for new drugs.

The FDA Bureau of Devices and Diagnostics Ophthalmic Advisory Panel has requested that the FDA Commissioner consider poly(methyl methacrylate) (PMMA) lenses as "hard" lenses and all others as "soft" lenses. This classification is of considerable interest because many soft lenses in various stages of development are made of substances other than 2-hydroxymethyl methacrylate (HEMA), the material in all available soft lenses, and thus would be required to undergo scientific review.

Composition and Properties

According to the FDA OTC Panel on Ophthalmic Drugs, hard lenses are defined as being of rigid structure and usually composed of methyl methacrylate polymers having minimal or no absorptive properties. Soft lenses are flexible, have a high percentage of component substances other than methyl methacrylate polymers, and have absorptive properties capable of prolonged water, chemical, and/or drug retention.

Hard Lenses

Polymerized resins of acrylic acid and methacrylic acid esters are used in hard contact lenses (4). Poly(methyl methacrylate) (Lucite or Plexiglas), the plastic most often used, contains relatively few hydrophilic groups and many closely packed methyl groups which give the plastic its hydrophobic properties (5). Poly(methyl methacrylate) allows light transmission of 90–92%, and lenses made of this substance absorb only about 1% of water after prolonged immersion (6). The refractive index of poly(methyl methacrylate) is 1.49.

A hard lens is available (UF-9 by Vent-Air Optics) with both a quartz coating to eliminate dryness problems and an ultraviolet color to screen out sunlight. The vented design of these lenses results in a flatter edge, theoretically causing less irritation to eyelids. Hard lenses also are available as bifocal lenses and may be arranged so that the eye perceives both powers either simultaneously or alternately. In general, bifocal lenses are not very comfortable.

A "semihard" contact lens (Meso by Danker and

Wohlk) has been approved recently for use in a wide variety of visual problems such as astigmatism and hyperopia. Patients suffering decreased visual acuity from corneal edema have been helped after only a few hours of wearing the lens. The lens, previously described as "flexible but dry," is made of cellulose acetate butyrate (CAB). It is claimed to have more "wettability" than hard lenses and to exhibit improved heat transmission. The semihard lens currently is being investigated for use in extended wear, and more such lenses may be expected in the near future.

Soft Lenses

All of the common hydrophilic lenses (soft lenses) are composed of 2-hydroxymethyl methacrylate with varying degrees of cross-linking (7). Cross-linkages produce distinct chemical entities, and each lens therefore has well-defined physical and chemical properties. These differences have been described as "significant" for cosmetic use and "crucial" for therapeutic use (8).

2-hydroxymethyl methacrylate

water content

silicone lens

factors in selecting contacts or eyeglasses

Water content of soft lenses varies widely and is inversely proportional to the degree of cross-linking. The 2-hydroxymethyl methacrylate absorbs about 47% water by weight, if the water is pure, and about 30% water when immersed in normal saline solution (9). The refractive index changes from 1.53 in the dry state to 1.43 when material is fully hydrated in normal saline (10).

When it is hydrated, a 2-hydroxymethyl methacrylate lens expands about 18% in all directions (11). Oxygen exchange, although probably better than with poly(methyl methacrylate), is still insufficient to support the cornea without additional oxygen provided by tears (11). Generally, 2-hydroxymethyl methacrylate lenses are larger than the cornea and are untinted. They are comfortable only when they are at least as large as the corneal diameter, have very thin edges, and have limited movement; all of these features produce minimum contact between the lens itself and the eyelids (9). Hard contact lenses also could be manufactured to be larger in diameter than the cornea, but because they are inflexible, normal tear exchange would not occur; soft lenses flex with each blink (9).

In contrast to hard lenses, soft lenses can absorb drugs and preservatives from ophthalmic solutions (12, 13). This process may cause altered therapeutic effects and possible irritation. Some drugs may cause discoloration of soft lenses by binding to or producing oxidative breakdown of the plastic (14). All manufacturers of 2-hydroxymethyl methacrylate lenses indicate that no ophthalmic solutions or drugs, including conventional contact lens solutions, can be used by lens wearers before or while the lens is in place on the eye.

If regular soft lenses provide a poor fit, ultrathin lenses sometimes are suggested (Hydrocurve II and the Bausch & Lomb U and U3 Series). These lenses are easier to fit, are larger, flatter, and thinner (as thin as 0.07 mm) than other soft lenses, give better oxygen permeability and proper centration, do not impinge on the cornea, and cause no lid interference. Because of their extreme fragility they must be handled correctly. After being removed from the container the lens is very fragile and thus should be handled with great care. It should be air-dried for about 30 seconds before it is inserted.

A relatively new soft lens under FDA review is made of a cross-linked dimethyl polysiloxane, hydrocarbon-substituted rubber (silicone). This extremely hydrophobic lens absorbs only 0.5% water by weight—less than the conventional hard lenses—and is not permeable to most liquids. Silicone is chemically and physiologically inert, flexible, and rubbery, but it has a certain innate rigidity. It is pliable in the dry state, and fingernails can penetrate it. The lens is less flexible than the hydrogel lens, has a refractive index of 1.439, and permits light transmission of 86% in the dry state and 91% when wet (15–18). Silicone lenses currently are being investigated for their use in extended wear.

Silicone has excellent optical properties. The silicone does not conform to the cornea but maintains its shape and provides more stability than the thinner soft lenses. At least one NDA for this lens has been submitted to the FDA.

Contact Lenses or Eyeglasses

Contact lenses have gained wide patient acceptance, mainly because of their cosmetic and improved vision qualities. A few patients (high hypermetropes and high myopes) have much better vision with contact lenses than with eyeglasses, and contact lenses are essential for patients with a conical cornea or corneal scarring. The effects of corneal scars (except for loss of light transmission) often are corrected much better with contact lenses (19). Binocular vision without contact lenses cannot be achieved in cases of unilateral aphakia (cataract extraction) and anisometropia (markedly different refractive errors in each eye). Some myopic contact lens wearers perceive improved vision because the lens produces a slight magnification of the retinal image and a slight increase in light transmission. Also, contact lenses produce neither the obstruction frequently encountered by the eyeglass frame (20–22) nor the thick edges of high concave lenses.

These factors may not actually improve visual acuity, but patients have mistaken increased sensitivity to light for increased visual acuity (23). Visual acuity is, in fact, noticeably lower for many lens wearers (24). There is a considerable difference in the retinal image: the lens wearer views all objects through the optical center of the lens, whereas the eyeglass wearer observes aberrations in objects viewed through the periphery of the glasses (24).

Contact lens wearers should have an eye examination twice yearly to determine continued fit and continued corneal integrity. Myopic degeneration or detachment of the retina also should be checked at the same time. Eyeglass users need undergo eye examination far less frequently (every 2 years is an average interval). Thus the long-term overall cost of contact lenses is usually much higher than that of eyeglasses (24).

In general, there does not seem to be an appreciable difference between the effectiveness of eyeglasses and contact lenses. In a study of 3458 eyes (myopic, hyperopic, and aphakic), 3167 eyes (91.6%) achieved a visual acuity of 20/25 or better with eyeglasses, and 2881 eyes (83.3%) achieved a visual acuity of 20/25 or better with contact lenses (25).

Hard or Soft Lenses

Most patients seem to adjust well to wearing contact lenses. In a study of hard lenses in 200 patients, only 22% failed to adjust partly or completely (26). In another group fitted with soft contact lenses for errors of refraction, 57% were counted as successful (25). Published success rates vary, probably because there are no standards to which "success" can be compared. Subjective criteria such as wearing time, comfort, and vision should be considered as well as objective criteria such as ocular tissue changes and patient appearance. Using these standards, another study found 73% of 122 patients to be successful in adapting to lens wear (27).

In general, hard lenses may be worn up to 12 hours after the prescribed break-in period, although many people do not exceed an 8-hour wearing time. Soft lenses may be worn up to 18 hours. It has been suggested that a short break (at least an hour) sometime during daily wear may increase the longevity of corneal compatibility to hard lenses.

problems with hard lenses

Patients may encounter some problems initially in adapting to hard lenses:

- A slight burning sensation caused by the lack of oxygen;
- Difficulty in looking up (which disappears when eyelids learn to tolerate the "foreign body" in the eye);
- Blurred vision after lenses are removed (spectacle blur);
- Photophobia, which may be expected in the early stages of wear and may be diminished by good sunglasses;
- Flare caused by refraction from the edge of the lens (patients usually adapt to this phenomenon with time);
- Reflections (more noticeable at night);
- Redness of the eyes (caused by the eye's normal response to the "foreign body");
- Fogging of the lenses until the fluid exchange rate is adjusted;
- Excessive tearing;
- Tendency for a lens to slip off center or fall out because of excessive tearing;
- Excessive blinking (a normal reaction to the body's effort to provide a better fluid flow);
- Difficulty in focusing on nearby objects;
- Itching;
- Excessive tiredness at the end of the wearing period.

These symptoms usually disappear in time if the wearing schedule is followed conscientiously.

Another potential drawback to hard lenses is overwear. This sometimes extremely painful condition is caused by corneal irritation, which the patient usually does not notice until the lenses are removed. In most instances the corneal epithelium regenerates within 24 hours. First aid treatment might consist of eye patches (for both eyes), cold compresses, and lubricant drops. The patient should guard against infection; physicians often prescribe antibiotic drops such as those containing neomycin and polymyxin.

comparison of hard and soft lenses

Many people prefer the comfort of soft lenses to the superior vision offered by hard lenses (28). The literature indicates that soft lenses are more comfortable and more easily tolerated than hard lenses but that good visual acuity cannot be achieved by all soft lens wearers and overall visual acuity with soft lenses is not as good as that achieved with hard lenses (24). Because soft lenses conform to the cornea, they tend not to correct corneal astigmatism. Vision with soft lenses may fluctuate with lens hydration (24). When a lost or damaged soft lens is replaced by another, comfort and vision may be poorer, since reproducibility in manufacture is more difficult to achieve with soft lenses, especially those of the lathe-cut type, which are less reproducible than spin-cast lenses.

Soft lenses do present certain definite advantages. They tend to be lost less frequently than hard lenses because they are less easily dislodged (29). They are particularly good for occasional wear and sports (except swimming), do not require the disciplined daily wearing schedule of hard lenses, and do not allow dust particles to get caught easily under them.

The relative permeability of hard and soft lens material to gases has been investigated extensively because oxygen depletion may cause corneal lesions (30, 31). It appears that the soft lens causes less injury than the hard lens, but the soft lens may inhibit tear flow more (32). There may be more glucose depletion under hard contact lenses, but there is no difference in pyruvate and lactate metabolites, in the lactate/pyruvate quotient, or in concentrations of adenosine triphosphate, adenosine diphosphate, adenosine monophosphate, and glucose 6-phosphate (32, 33). An increase in corneal thickness is observed with all lens wear, but more so with hard lenses than with soft ones. The increase may be caused by an osmotic effect, a decrease in glycogen content of the cornea, or a significant decrease of transcorneal potential (34). In some cases (13 of 445 eyes), vascularization of the cornea was reported with soft lens wear (35). Increased vascularization of the cornea occurs in pathological conditions and in conditions where 24-hour lens wear is required. It is probably related to hypoxia and rarely causes significantly decreased visual acuity.

Soft lenses are apparently considerably more comfortable for the average wearer than hard lenses. They do not diminish corneal sensitivity (36). Flare, glare, and photophobia are practically nonexistent, although people with large pupils may complain of flares, particularly at dusk or at night (37). Soft lens wearers may alternate freely between lenses and eyeglasses, since they cause no "spectacle blur"; there seems to be no need for an adaptation period and no overwearing syndrome in most users. The "contact lens look" (holding the chin up, blinking frequently, restraining from quick eye movement, or avoiding looking up to the ceiling) is not seen with soft lens wearers (38). Soft lens wearers seem to complain less about atmospheric pollutants than hard lens wearers (39).

Soft lenses may be considerably more expensive than the hard ones. They may have to have a power change within 2 months of the original fitting (36). Although an average use of 2 years usually is mentioned in the literature, references to a life span of 1 year are encountered (40).

Soft lenses may be uncomfortable if debris is caught between the lens and the eye, if they are too loose, or if they are hydrated with improper solutions (38). Variable vision, caused by poor centering, and poor return of the lens after blinking may occur (36). In some cases there may be "start-up" problems; e.g., vision may be "watery." This condition usually disappears but may last as long as 2 months. Soft lenses cannot be marked "left" and "right," and a soft lens wearer who loses correct identification of the lenses may have to return to an optometrist or ophthalmologist for identification.

comparison of hard and soft lenses

Whether a hard or a soft lens is chosen, lens-induced corneal edema is one of the most serious causes of discomfort. The edema is caused by localized hypoxia, and its symptoms are photophobia, dryness, burning, and tearing (41). Patients frequently complain of seeing "halos around lights." In hot and stuffy areas, congestion and watering of the nose and reflex vasodilation in the rosacea facial areas in susceptible individuals also have been observed (42). Corneal edema increases with length of wear but disappears rapidly once the lens is removed from the eye.

In general, soft contact lenses have been proven safe and effective, although hard corneal lenses are the modality of choice for the majority of candidates for contact lens wear (43). Hard lenses continue to be recommended for the ordinary phakic wearer with no disease. Theoretically, soft lenses should be reserved for those who cannot tolerate hard lenses and for those who wish to wear lenses intermittently. However, it would appear that theory differs sharply from practice and that more and more people select soft lenses.

USE OF CONTACT LENSES

contact lens use, their indications and contraindications

Hard contact lenses are used in the therapeutic management of anisometropia (difference in refractive power of both eyes), corneal astigmatism (defective curvature), and keratoconus (conical protrusion of the cornea). There is some controversy about their use in aphakia. Scleral lenses, which cover the entire sclera of the eye, are fitted only when a patient cannot be fitted with any other type of lens. Soft lenses are used mainly for low refractive error in normal eyes, in aphakia, and as a protective membrane in many corneal disorders, e.g., recurrent keratopathy, recurrent corneal ulcers, erosion secondary to ingrown eyelashes, and epithelial defects following corneal transplantation (44, 45).

Therapeutic Indications

Contact lenses may be used in all cases of myopia and astigmatism, aphakia, anisometropia, and certain eye diseases and to control keratoconus (46). In aphakia, eyeglasses with very thick convex lenses once were the only means to correct vision, and they produced disturbing aberrations and magnification. Contact lenses minimize aberrations and reduce the size of the image to nearly that of the retinal image of the normal eye.

intraocular lenses

Efforts are being made to find new devices for the 400,000 yearly postcataract patients, but there is still no therapy safer than eyeglasses. Intraocular lenses have been used to replace the natural lens of the human eye after surgical removal, generally as a result of a cataract. These lenses came into widespread use before adequate tests were completed, and they pose questions of safety (47). Infections have been reported with intraocular lenses, particularly those sterilized with sodium hydroxide as a sterilant and sodium bicarbonate as a neutralizing solution (48). Intraocular acrylic lenses may increase the endothelial cell death rate so that the cornea may be clouded irreversibly. Medically, intraocular lenses are not yet an acceptable alternative to eyeglasses. The FDA has approved no intraocular lenses, and applications for approval will have to meet the intraocular lens investigational device regulation.

extended wear soft lenses

As an alternative to the intraocular lens implant, extended wear soft lenses have been recommended for correction of aphakia. To date, extended wear soft lenses, said to be less likely to cause complications, have been tested in 12 medical institutions. It is hoped that these lenses can be worn for periods of up to 3 months; reports from England suggest that they can be worn for as long as 2 years. The lenses present certain drawbacks: they are difficult to fit and must, initially at least, be checked several times per day; they should be suggested only when the patient has immediate access to skilled help and advice, since the patient should not handle the lenses (49, 50).

Contraindications

Corneal contact lenses are contraindicated in active intraocular or corneal pathological conditions, although they may be used in cases of open-angle glaucoma (46). They should not be used by elderly people, because of lacrimal insufficiency, or by individuals suffering from arthritis, which may restrict the movement and dexterity needed to insert the lenses. They are contraindicated in blepharitis (inflammation of the eyelid), and many people with hay fever cannot wear their lenses during certain times of the year.

Tear deficiency, excessive tear production, an obstructed nasolacrimal duct, chronic allergies, anatomical or physiological abnormalities, and various clinical conditions, such as herpes simplex, are all contraindications to contact lens use (51).

Dry spots on the cornea, often found in postmenopausal women, prevent the successful use of lenses (52). These spots, possibly caused by the absence of the precorneal film, are often identified with lacrimal insufficiency due to subclinical hypothyroidism.

The corneal topography may be altered by pregnancy or by oral contraceptives (51, 52). Microedema caused by hormonal therapy as well as premenstrual edema also are contraindications to the use of contact lenses.

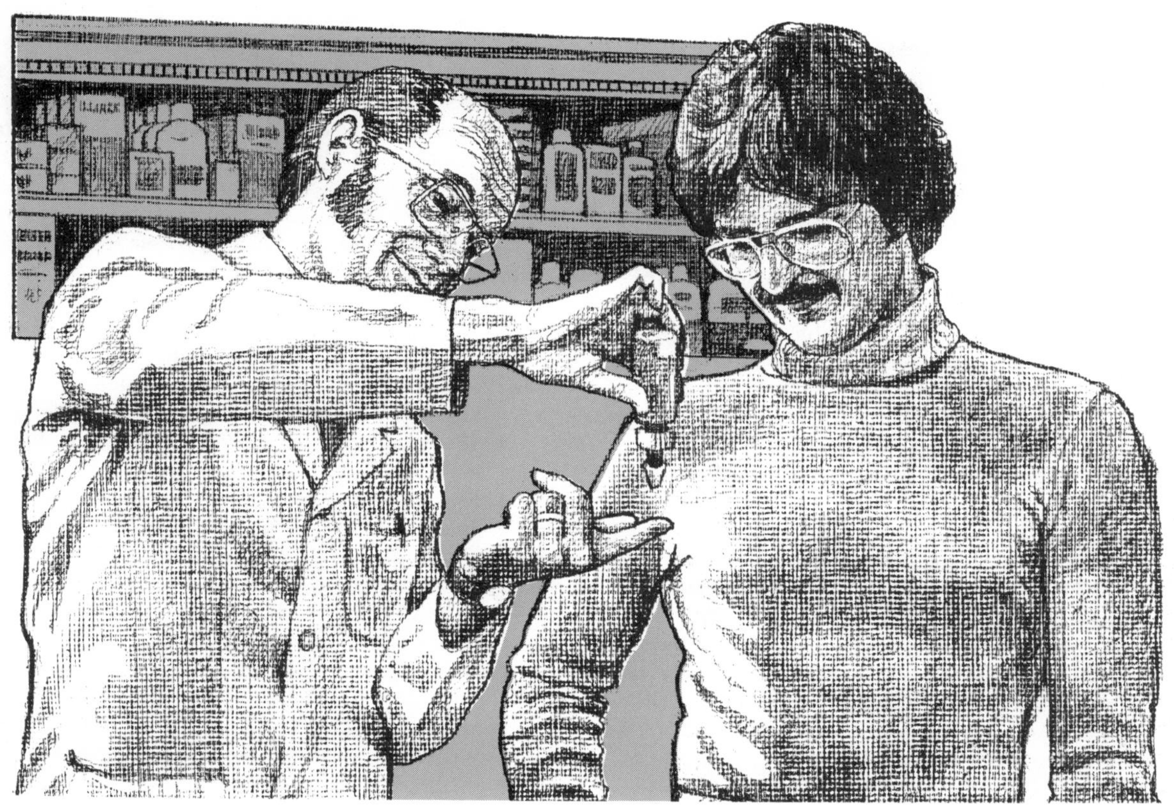

complicating factors in lens wear

lens removal procedure

Cautions

Contact lenses should be used with caution in patients with epilepsy, diabetes mellitus, high blood pressure, heart disease, or severe arthritis. Restricted use of lenses may be necessary when a person's occupation is connected with chemical vapors or dust.

Diseases secondary to contact lens wear have been described (53). Lens wearers moving from a low to a high altitude may encounter hypoxia or metabolic deficiency, resulting in irritation and corneal abrasions (54).

Many systemic medications, e.g., diuretics, affect the eyes and therefore may influence successful lens wear (55). Orally administered antihistamines and decongestants may decrease tear production and cause a mild keratitis, interfering with lens wear (56, 57).

During the adaptive period to contact lenses the eyelids may become hyperemic; this condition may lead to blepharitis, especially in the upper lid (41). Short pseudoblinks, often found with new wear of hard lenses, may cause irritation of the conjunctiva of the upper eyelid. A poor blinker or nonblinker may be helped by a fenestrated (windowed) lens (UF-9) or an otherwise adapted one (58). Chin elevation and squinting may result from irritating lenses (41).

Cosmetics must be chosen with care. Only those with an aqueous base should be used, since oil-based products may cause blurred vision and irritation if they are deposited on the lens. Powders also may be irritating if small particles become lodged under the lens. Mascara should be applied only to the very tips of the lashes. Hair sprays, in particular, must be used with caution. Irritation may occur if some of the spray particles are trapped in the tear layer beneath the lens, and some sprays may actually damage the lens. Nail polish, hand creams, and perfumes should be applied only after the lens has been inserted. Men frequently contaminate their lenses with hair preparations; special care must be taken to clean hands thoroughly before handling contact lenses.

Removal of Lenses in Comatose Patients

When blinking reflexes are absent, as in the comatose patient, a contact lens will not move enough to keep tears circulating between it and the cornea. There may be permanent corneal damage if a lens is left in place. It is probably safest to remove the lens by irrigation as described below (59):

- With the patient supine, turn the head toward the side to be irrigated and separate the lids. Irrigate gently with sterile saline solution from the nasal side, and the lens will simply float out of the eye.
- If irrigation is unsuccessful, try to remove the contact lenses by the rubber suction cup method. Wet a small contact lens suction cup with sterile saline solution and place it gently on the center of the contact lens. Pressure on the cup is then slowly released and suction will form so that the lens can be lifted from the eye. Great care must be exercised

in applying the suction cup to the contact lens; rough handling can result in permanent scarring of the cornea.

When the above methods fail or in an extreme emergency, the contact lenses can be moved temporarily onto the sclera. Gently push the lower lid against the bottom edge of the contact lens. This will slide the lens off the cornea onto the bulbar conjunctiva where it can rest safely until an ophthalmologist can remove it. Make a note on the chart that the contact lens is still in the eye, and to have it removed as soon as possible.

HARD LENS PRODUCTS

solutions and adjunctive products

ideal wetting solution

cellulose derivatives

polyvinyl alcohol

The use of hard contact lenses necessitates the concurrent use of special solutions and other adjunctive products, formulated to help the user in achieving maximum comfort and safety. In selecting or recommending a procedure for lens care, the individual's personality, temperament, physical capabilities, and characteristics should be taken into account. If a specific regimen is not suitable, it will probably be followed poorly or disregarded altogether, with possible detrimental effects (60).

Chemical composition, sterility, tonicity, pH, viscosity, stability, and, of course, effectiveness all must be considered in formulating a hard contact lens solution. The solution should have cleaning and antiseptic action and should be self-preserving. In this regard it must be actively bactericidal because viable organisms not only may cause decomposition of the solution but also may adversely affect the eye.

Standards for evaluation of preservatives in these solutions are necessary, but none have been developed that are universally acceptable. Several of 34 commercially available solutions failed to suppress microbial growth even after 24-hour contact (61).

A number of ingredients are required for buffering, adjusting tonicity, wetting, and cushioning. When the solution vehicle evaporates, a crystalline or granular residue may form, interfering with wearing comfort. An inadequately formulated solution may cause burning, stinging, excessive tearing, and possibly more serious side effects. It may exert an adverse effect on the lacrimal fluid and the eye and may cause damage to the contact lens.

Because contact lens solutions are not considered drug products, their formulations are not governed by the formulation and manufacturing restrictions placed on therapeutic ophthalmic solutions. In contrast to ophthalmic solutions, they are used over a long period, and their cumulative effect may be more severe. Contact lens solutions are used without medical supervision by inexperienced people; therefore all ingredients, including preservatives, must have a high margin of safety.

Wetting Solutions

Because hard contact lenses are hydrophobic, they resist wetting by the lacrimal fluids, producing a foreign body sensation on insertion. Tears contain protein compounds conjugated with highly hydrated polysaccharides. Although the protein components in tears give precorneal fluid a wetting effect on the lens, the wetting reaction is not immediate and may take as long as 15 minutes after insertion, resulting in severe discomfort during that time (5). For maximum wetting of hard lenses, a solution should have a surface tension of less than 39 dynes/cm^2. Normal tear fluid has a surface tension of about 46 dynes/cm^2, which accounts for the slow wetting.

A wetting solution is "an agent which coats the contact lens uniformly with a film which is intended to minimize the friction of the contact lens against the palpebral conjunctiva and cornea" (62). It should be partly retained on the lens surface after "rinsing under a stream of slowly flowing cold water for approximately five seconds" (63). The ideal wetting solution:

- Should spread over the entire surface of the lens (64);
- Should form a film that does not wash away easily;
- Should be nonirritating and nonsensitizing;
- Should not leave a residue on the lens after drying;
- Should have a cleansing and antiseptic action;
- Should be self-sterilizing;
- Should have the proper degree of viscosity for efficient lubrication (6).

Another function of a wetting solution is to provide a viscous coating that will prevent direct contact of the lens with fingers during insertion, thus avoiding transfer of oily skin deposits onto the lens. Wetting solutions are applied directly to the cornea and should act as a substitute for tears. Therefore their viscosity should approximate that of tears, so that the normal emollient action of the precorneal film is not reduced. A viscous solution also helps to stabilize the lens on the fingertip during insertion.

The wetting solution must act as a cushion between the cornea and the lens. The precorneal film has a regulated viscosity and high wetting properties which must be obtained for optical clarity. The cushion also acts as a shock absorber to prevent the lens from making sudden movements when the eyes are turned.

Because of the need for this cushioning effect, wetting solutions usually contain methylcellulose, hydroxypropyl methylcellulose, or polyvinyl alcohol (PVA) to increase the viscosity of the solution. The cellulose gums, however, do not have a wetting effect; i.e., useful concentrations of hydroxypropyl methylcellulose have a surface tension of 65 dynes/cm^2. Polyvinyl alcohol frequently is used to increase viscosity and decrease surface tension to 46–47 dynes/cm^2. Dextran 40 and dextran 70 also may be used as viscosity-inducing agents.

Excessive concentrations of viscosity-building agents may cause crusting on eyelids and storage cases and transient blurring of vision; insufficient concentrations may cause discomfort. Subjective studies have been conducted to determine the optimum level of viscosity-inducing agents (65). Solutions of varying viscosity (9–26 cP) were instilled in the subjects' eyes, and patients were evaluated subjectively. Patients complained of lack of comfort (with low-viscosity solutions) and transient blurry vision (with high-viscosity solutions). On the basis of this simple test the optimal viscosity range was found to be 15–20 cP. The viscosity of most products is not listed on the label and may vary to some extent from batch to batch because of the variability in the polymers.

The FDA OTC Panel on Ophthalmic Drugs has accepted the term "cushioning" and has defined it as providing a layer of viscid separating fluid between the contact lens and eye to lessen the sensation of placing the lens on the eye. However, the Panel continues to request data demonstrating the effectiveness of cushioning agents.

The Panel was troubled by the term "comfort" and looks for documented proof that certain agents can provide this. It has also cautioned that the term "disinfecting" should not be used simply because such an agent may have been added to a solution.

The clinical value of wetting agents has been questioned. Wetting agents, the Panel believes, are not essential to wearing contact lenses. The Panel did accept wetting agents as adjuncts for subjective improvement in wearing comfort and suggests that polyvinyl alcohol and the polysorbates are probably the only useful wetting agents. Methods have been suggested to measure wetting capability, to evaluate continued wetting action, and to evaluate a product's capability to maintain a continuous film. The Panel also suggested measurements of a product's cleaning capability, such as evaluation of cleaning with minimum friction.

Sodium chloride is used to make wetting solutions isotonic. Some solutions are made mildly hypertonic (1.1% sodium chloride) because the tonicity of tears approximates an equivalent of 1% sodium chloride. Although a mildly hypertonic solution is said to be better tolerated and to reduce superficial edema and swelling, these conclusions are questionable (66).

Wetting solutions contain a buffer system to adjust the pH and keep it at a predetermined level, optimally that of the lacrimal fluid (~7.2), since this level would cause the least discomfort. However, an investigation of 14 wetting solutions found two below pH 4.0, eight at pH 4.0–5.0, two at pH 6.0–7.0, and two above pH 7.0 (67). Solutions adjusted to a pH significantly below the physiological pH of tears should have a minimal buffer capacity so that the natural eye fluids may adjust them quickly to correct physiological pH. In adjusting pH, other factors such as the preparation's stability also must be considered. Partly acetylated polyvinyl alcohol, for example, necessitates that solutions be formulated at an acidic pH to prevent hydrolysis of the polymer.

All contact lens solutions are exposed to a high degree of contamination, and special care must be exercised in selecting a preservative. Continual application of bactericidal agents to the eye may be irritating. Wetting solutions, once they have been applied, have no germicidal activity, because the contact time is usually too short (68).

The acceptable preservatives used in contact lens solutions are limited, and they vary in their bactericidal action and sensitizing potential. Agents include a quaternary ammonium compound (benzalkonium chloride), chlorobutanol, and organic mercurials.

Benzalkonium Chloride

This compound was first proposed in 1947 as a preservative for ophthalmic solutions (69). For it to be effective, particularly against *Pseudomonas aeruginosa*, a sufficiently strong solution must be used. Too strong a solution may produce liquefaction of intercellular cement, desquamation of the epithelium, and edema. Conjunctival and corneal lesions have been found when benzalkonium chloride was used in a strength of 0.1% (70). Because the effect is cumulative, a single application may be well tolerated, but the second or third may produce irritation. Solutions of 0.02% apparently are tolerated, even when they are used three or four times per day (60). The bactericidal activity of benzalkonium chloride is reduced by compounds such as soaps, metallic ions, and rubber.

Chlorobutanol

A volatile, relatively insoluble, slow-acting bactericide, chlorobutanol seems to have no advantage over benzalkonium chloride. It usually is used at a concentration of 0.5%, although concentrations as low as 0.15% have been used. It is effective only after it permeates into the bacterial cell. Chlorobutanol is unstable in an alkaline medium and is seldom used in contact lens solutions, unless the pH is 6 or lower.

Thimerosal and Phenylmercuric Nitrate

The two most commonly used organic mercurial compounds are thimerosal and phenylmercuric nitrate. These agents have a slow rate of kill (71), and they act through the sustained release of the mercurial ion which penetrates into the bacterial cell and combines with various respiratory enzymes to inhibit metabolism. Thimerosal is a basic salt and must be used in neutral or slightly alkaline solutions. Phenylmercuric nitrate is an organic mercurial used in dilute concentrations. It differs from other organic mercurials in that it is not precipitated in an acid pH.

Other Considerations

Many wetting solutions contain a small concentration of edetate disodium which, in combination with benzalkonium chloride, chlorobutanol, or thimerosal, enhances the bactericidal properties of these agents when tested against *P. aeruginosa*. It apparently disrupts the integrity of a lipid or lipid–protein complex in the cell wall, making the cell wall's obstructing layer more permeable to the bactericidal agent (72). The FDA OTC Panel on Ophthalmic Drugs found methylparaben and/or propylparaben, used singly or in combination, ineffective if used without other preservatives present, and their effectiveness in combination with other preservative agents remains to be proven (47). This conclusion also was reached for such substances as cetylpyridinium chloride and chlorhexidine. Anionic detergents, such as sodium lauryl sulfate, are contraindicated because of their incompatibility with cationic preservatives, such as benzalkonium chloride. Organic mercurials are effective preservatives but have limited usefulness; their effect is exerted slowly, an alkaline pH is necessary for maintaining their stability

FDA Panel deliberations

cushioning

clinical value of wetting agents

sodium chloride

buffers

preservatives

other agents

in solution, and their effectiveness may be reduced by the addition of edetate disodium. Phenylmercuric nitrate activity may decrease in the presence of nonionic wetting and clarifying agents or detergents. Surfactants may inactivate preservatives by forming micelles with them.

Soaking Solutions

A soaking solution should provide hydration of the lenses to facilitate wetting and to help remove adsorbed organic substances. If these substances are allowed to remain, they inhibit antisepsis and wetting of the lens (10).

purpose of soaking solutions

Poly(methyl methacrylate) contact lenses become hydrated in contact with aqueous solutions and dehydrated on exposure to dry air (73). Hydration produces a lens of longer radius, i.e., a flatter lens. Because lenses become hydrated when they are worn, they also should be kept hydrated when not worn, so as to maintain constant dimensional stability. The average amount of precorneal fluid absorbed by dry lenses is about 30% more than that absorbed by those stored in a soaking solution (74).

Bacterial contamination and the relative effect of a wet or dry storage regimen on lens wettability have been studied extensively (67, 75, 76). Insertion of the contact lens in a dry state may cause discomfort for several minutes to an hour; wet storage may increase comfort. Soaking solutions gently soak off adsorbed material accumulated on the lens during wearing. This prevents the accumulation from drying onto the surface and into the pores of the lens, causing surface chemical change and "fogging."

The original argument against wet storage was that soaking solutions could possibly be the source of *Pseudomonas* infections (75, 77, 78). It is now known that infections may have been caused by patient failure to replace old solution with fresh soaking solution or by addition of new solution to the old one. Moreover, containers made of soft, colored plastic or those with rubber inserts may release highly irritating products which reduce the solution's bactericidal activity and alter its pH (67). To overcome this effect, it is recommended that containers not include sponge rubber pads and that they be filled daily with soaking solution for 15 minutes, after which time the solution should be discarded, new solution added to the container, and the lenses stored. Lenses stored in soaking solutions are less subject to bacterial contamination and cause less discomfort than lenses stored dry (5).

To sterilize lenses, soaking solutions usually contain benzalkonium chloride and chlorobutanol, a synergistic combination (79). Increasing the concentrations of benzalkonium chloride in soaking solutions does not seem to increase effectiveness (80, 81). Other antimicrobial agents included in soaking solutions are polymyxin B sulfate, organic mercurials, benzoic acid esters, and certain phenols and substituted alcohols (68).

Cleaning Solutions

components of cleaning solutions

Lenses must be clean for maximum hydration to occur. They absorb water from the lacrimal fluid, trapping mucus and salts on the surface which attach firmly to the lens surface, forming a thin film. An oily residue also may be left on the lens surface from the insertion procedure. These contaminants are a barrier to the wetting action of tears; they may impair vision, cause irritation, and promote infections. Cleaning solutions contain nonionic surfactants that reduce surface tension, emulsify lipids, and solubilize other debris. Lipids and proteins, often found on contact lenses, are soluble in alkaline media, but strongly alkaline solutions may decompose the plastic chemically.

All-Purpose Solutions

multipurpose solutions

These solutions, also called multipurpose or convenience solutions, are designed as a compromise between patient convenience and optimal lens care. Many formulation problems are encountered, and some of the necessary functions, e.g., wetting, may not be achieved as effectively as with an individual solution. However, it is felt that compliance often is improved with use of multipurpose solutions. Other solutions may be used on an intraocular basis (for wetting and cushioning) or on an extraocular basis (for hydration, disinfection, and cleaning) (82–84).

Artificial Tears

ingredients of artificial tears

Artificial tears are very simple solutions that provide an emollient and lubricating effect in cases of lacrimal insufficiency. They also may be used to relieve ocular irritation. These solutions are not recommended for use while the lenses are in place. They usually contain tonicity agents, such as sodium chloride; viscosity-increasing agents, such as hydroxypropyl methylcellulose or polyvinyl alcohol; and a bactericidal agent, such as benzalkonium chloride. The pH of these solutions usually is adjusted to simulate the physiological pH of tears. Calcium chloride (up to 0.05%) and magnesium chloride (up to 0.03%) may be used to modify the cation content of artificial tears.

Ocular Decongestants

conjunctivitis

Prolonged wearing of contact lenses, especially in the adaptation stage, may cause conjunctivitis. Many ocular decongestant products are available; most contain phenylephrine hydrochloride at ~0.1% concentration. There is no clinical evidence that one product is better than another. These solutions, applied after the lenses have been removed, hasten the regression of the inflammation by reducing the size of the engorged small vessels. They are not to be used with the lens in place. Decongestants affect only the symptoms (redness) and not the cause of irritation. Moreover, frequent use may lead to rebound congestion. (See Chapter 19 for a more complete discussion of these products.)

Miscellaneous Products

Many specialized solutions have been marketed for use with hard contact lenses. It is questionable whether they offer a significant advantage over the products already discussed. In many cases it seems that they are attempts at increasing product lines and sales volume.

In-the-Eye Cleaning Solutions

These solutions supposedly clean lenses while they are being worn. They contain surfactants to remove deposits (mucus and dirt) from the lens surface by surface activity and lid-wiping action.

Many agents, such as polyethylene glycol 300, propylene glycol, and polysorbate 80, have been classified as cleaning adjuncts for use outside the eye. Some were designated safe enough to be instilled directly into the eye for purposes other than cleaning, but claims for in situ cleaning cannot be made when these products are included in a formulation. Two such products are poloxamer 282 (Pluronic L-92) and poloxamer 338 (Pluronic F-108). Only one agent has been found suitable for in situ cleaning of lenses, polyoxyl 40 stearate. Benzalkonium chloride is generally used in concentrations of up to 0.013% as a preservative, and when used so, cannot be claimed to be an effective cleansing agent for contact lenses.

Preinsertion Solutions

These solutions are a variation on artificial tears. They have a high relative viscosity to enhance cushioning and reduce irritation during the "breaking-in" period. Their high viscosity may cause problems with visual acuity immediately after insertion.

Conditioners

Conditioners are recommended when tears do not supply a sufficient wetting action or cushioning effect. They also are used to clear the eye of potential debris-forming substances prior to lens insertion, and they can be applied to the eye as frequently as three to four times per day while the lens is being worn (85).

Contact Lens Remover

The DMV Contact Lens Remover is sometimes recommended to elderly patients. The pharmacist must be aware that good patient instructions are needed. The contact lens remover uses a suction cup, and if the patient places the cup on the cornea instead of the lens, corneal damage may result. Patients should be instructed to clean these removers before and after each use, since they may harbor bacteria.

Contact Lens Cases

Several devices are available for mailing, soaking, cleaning, and storing hard contact lenses. Standards for these have been recommended, and their effectiveness may be judged by the categories in Table 1 (86).

SOFT LENS SYSTEMS

Conventional contact lens solutions cannot be used with soft lenses because all chemicals, especially benzalkonium chloride, seem to bind to the soft lens material (87). Originally, the problem of lens sterility was anticipated, on the premise that bacteria and fungi would penetrate into the lens matrix. It was found, however, that the problem was not the penetration but the enzymatic degradation of the lens material by bacteria and fungi (88). Another problem, unanticipated and thus far unsolved, is that deposits of protein, particularly mucoproteins, meibomian oils, fungus remnants, and occasional calciferous deposits have been found on soft lenses. Thus separate cleaning and disinfectant cycles had to be developed for the care of soft lenses.

Cleaning Cycle

It is not yet quite clear why deposits are formed on some lenses, nor is the exact nature of these deposits known. They are probably a mixture of proteins and extraneous agents, such as cosmetics and hair sprays, introduced by the lens wearer. The rate of accumulation differs; some users may experience little difficulty with such deposits, whereas others may secrete unusually large amounts of mucus in the lacrimal fluid, causing a faster and heavier buildup of deposits. Thus dirty lenses still are the major complaint of contact lens wearers. Literature is available on cleaners and cleaning procedures of soft lenses, including concern for the basic solution used in cleaning and rinsing the lenses (89–93).

polyoxyl 40 stearate

soft lens care

Soft lenses are cleaned by placing one lens in the palm of one hand, concave side up. The lens is moistened with saline and then rubbed gently with the fingertip, using caution so as not to touch the lens with fingernails. Alternatively, the lens may be cleaned by rubbing it between thumb and index finger.

If lenses are cleaned adequately before boiling, the sterilization cycle can be fully effective, and cumulative deposits on the lens may be prevented. Rubbing followed by rinsing with normal saline solution is still the recommended procedure. If the solution is freshly prepared according to instructions, there should be no problem. A saline solution with a preservative (e.g., Lensrins) prevents microbial growth in the solution while it is not in use. The mineral and iron content of the water used to prepare the solution may cause discoloration of the lenses.

More effective cleaners, including surfactants, oxidative systems, and enzymes, have been proposed. Surfactants alone may remove deposits amenable to a reduction of interfacial tension; however, they do not remove proteins. Surfactant residue may produce a permanent coating of the lens, if the lens is subjected to repeated heat sterilization treatment.

Several prophylactic cleaners are in various stages of development and testing. A typical solution contains nonionic surfactants, edetate sodium, and, in some cases, cellulose derivatives.

The soft lens wearer must be thoroughly familiar with the type of cleaner to be used. For example, users of Soflens Tablets are cautioned to use only normal saline solutions, while other cleaners frequently contain such other ingredients as a preservative and edetate sodium or surfactant.

An enzyme cleaner is further suggested for once-weekly use with the Soflens (Bausch and Lomb). The product, containing specially purified papain and marketed in tablet form, is designed to remove protein deposits from the lens. A tablet is dissolved in a container provided for this purpose, and the lens is soaked in the

Table 1. Comparison of Some Contact Lens Cases

	Volume, ml (Two Lenses)	Cleaning Accessibility	Compartment Letter Code	Compartment Color Code	Leakproof	Patient Identification	Lens Cleaning	Lens Rinsing	Complete Lens Submersion	Lens Protection	Mirror	Absence of Metal	Lens Placement and Retrieval	Boilability	Screw, Snap, or Sliding Closure	Light Background Color	Living Hinge	Plastic Optimal Hardness
Antisept Jeweled	1.2	no	yes	no	yes	no	no	no	no	no	no	yes	no	no	yes	no	no	yes
Aquacell Mates	6.5	no	yes	yes	no	yes	no	yes	yes	no	no	yes	no	no	yes	yes	no	yes
Clean-N-Soakit	4.7	no	yes	yes	yes	no	no	yes	no	yes	no	yes	yes	yes	no	yes	no	yes
Clean-N-Stow	8.0	no	yes	yes	yes	no	no	yes	yes	yes	no	yes	yes	yes	no	yes	no	yes
Comfort Case	6.0	no	no	yes	yes	no	no	no	yes	no	no	yes	no	no	yes	yes	no	yes
Dispos-A-Kit	7.0	no	yes	no	no	no	no	no	no	no	no	yes	yes	no	yes	yes	no	yes
Guardian	6.0	yes	yes	no	yes	yes	no	no	yes	no	no	yes	no	no	yes	yes	no	yes
Hydra-Kit	5.0	no	yes	yes	no	no	no	no	yes	no	no	no	yes	no	yes	yes	no	yes
Hydra-Mat	30	no	yes	no	yes	no	yes	yes	yes	yes	no	yes	no	no	no	yes	no	yes
Ideal	5.6	no	yes	no	yes	yes	no	no	yes	no	no	yes	no	no	yes	yes	no	yes
Kelley-Hueber Mailer	1.8	yes	yes	no	no	no	no	no	no	no	no	yes	yes	no	yes	yes	no	yes
Lensine	1.8	yes	yes	no	no	no	no	no	no	no	no	yes	no	yes	yes	yes	no	yes
Multimaster	7.7	no	yes	no	yes	no	no	no	yes	no	no	yes	no	no	yes	yes	no	yes
Multi-Pack	0.8	yes	yes	yes	no	yes	no	no	no	no	yes	yes	yes	no	yes	yes	no	yes
Porta-FLOW	4.0	yes	yes	yes	yes	yes	yes	yes	yes	yes	yes	yes	yes	yes	yes	yes	yes	yes
Sentinal	7.4	yes	yes	yes	yes	yes	no	no	yes	no	yes	yes	no	no	yes	yes	no	yes
Slim Jim	0.8	yes	yes	yes	no	yes	no	no	no	no	no	yes	yes	no	yes	yes	no	yes
Tote and Soak	8.0	no	no	yes	yes	no	no	yes	no	yes	no	yes	yes	yes	yes	yes	yes	yes
Una-Pac	6.5	no	yes	yes	yes	no	no	yes	no	yes	no	no	no	yes	no	yes	no	yes
W/J B-Lens Mailer	2.8	yes	yes	no	no	no	no	no	no	no	no	yes	yes	no	yes	yes	no	yes

Adapted from J. Z. Krezanoski and J. B. Lowry, *Contact Lens Soc. Am. J.*, 7(3), 13 (1973).

cleaning soft lenses
sterilization methods

solution prepared with the tablet for no longer than 12 hours. This cleaner seems to have been formulated to satisfy those who claim that visible as well as invisible deposits may cause allergic reactions and that even apparently clean lenses may cause protein conjunctivitis, a process that may begin long before deposits are visible to the eye (94–96). However, it has been suggested that the use of enzyme cleaners may decrease the longevity of the lens.

In general, only the cleaning agents so designated should be used with a particular lens. However, there are indications that prescribers not infrequently suggest to the potential wearer solutions approved for another lens system, with apparently no ill effect to the wearer. The pharmacist at times may find difficulty in serving lens wearers appropriately, since not all pharmacies are able to stock all cleaners marketed.

Sterilization Cycle

Soft lenses are kept hydrated for patient comfort, but hydration theoretically increases the chances for microbial contamination (97). Although research shows that *Escherichia coli* and *P. aeruginosa* cannot enter the hydrogel, the FDA demands "sterilization" of the lens (39).

It has been suggested that the term "sterilization" is not really appropriate; the lens must be rendered free from (potential) pathogens, a process more accurately called "disinfecting" or, by one manufacturer of a soft lens, "asepticizing" (88).

Recent developments have given the lens wearer a choice of sterilizing methods. These methods may differ with the particular lens system chosen, and the pharmacist should stress the importance of reading the instruction booklet carefully.

Heat Sterilization

Boiling the soft lenses destroys pathogens satisfactorily but fails to kill spores. Although the effectiveness of boiling per se is not questioned, a number of factors may influence its effectiveness—the boiling cycle is tedious and inconvenient, it decreases the lens lifespan, or it may not last long enough to sterilize (98).

Another disadvantage of heat sterilization is the cumbersome containers, which may be convenient for home use but are unacceptable for travel. Distilled water may leave a residue in the container, but it can be wiped out with a paper towel (36). However, lenses that are not completely clean may be covered with proteins which could be denatured by the boiling process. This material then would have a tendency to accumulate on the lens, shortening the effective life of the lens.

Still another disadvantage to boiling is that the lens case may crack. If this happens, the case must be replaced immediately. Failure to do so may interfere with correct functioning of the boiling cycle.

An alternative to the cumbersome boiling procedure involves placing the lenses in their carrying case filled with their normal saline solution or a suitable commercially prepared solution. The carrying case is then clamped into a sterilizing unit, called an aseptor (names differ with manufacturers), provided to the patient on purchase of the lenses. The unit is filled with distilled water, which is then boiled.

A slight variation of this method involves using a much smaller heating unit. Lenses are stored in their carrying case filled with saline solution. The carrying case is then placed in the unit, which supplies dry heat; i.e., the unit itself contains no liquid. This unit is much easier to handle than the larger boiling units and may well lend itself better to travel. If the unit is not available or cannot be used for lack of electricity, lenses may be boiled in their carrying case in a pan of water for 15 minutes. Water should not be allowed to evaporate completely, as this may damage the lens.

After heat disinfection, lenses are generally ready to wear. Lens manufacturers suggest that before insertion, the lenses be rinsed with a solution such as normal saline solution. Lenses should be stored after boiling in saline solution. Hypotonic solutions or plain water makes lenses tacky and sticky and causes discomfort until tonicity is achieved by the eye. Hypertonic solutions may cause stinging, lacrimation, and hyperemia.

Cold Sterilization

Some "cold" sterilizing solutions are in various stages of development and trial. A suggested approach involves the use of an iodophore concentrate (~0.1% iodine) followed by treatment with a thiosulfate neutralizing solution. Iodine causes rapid kill and has a broad spectrum of antimicrobial activity. An advantage of this system is its color reaction. As long as a distinctive blue color persists, the disinfecting process is still going on; when solution and lenses are clear, lenses may be inserted and worn safely (98, 99). Several other solutions containing chlorhexidine gluconate, thimerosal, and edetate sodium also are being investigated (100).

Chemical disinfection of soft lenses has been approved for all approved soft lenses and bandage lenses listed in the appendix. Currently, only one manufacturer markets a series of solutions necessary for the complete cycle. These solutions provide a "cold" chemical system for cleaning and disinfecting lenses. The procedure involves cleaning with Preflex after removal of the lens from the eye, rinsing with Normol, and storing the lens for at least four hours in Flexsol. Before insertion, lenses are then wetted and lubricated with Adapettes.

methods of lens sterilization

Insertion

When soft lenses are ready for insertion, a careful process should be followed:

steps for lens insertion

- Wash the hands with noncosmetic soap, and rinse thoroughly. Dry the hands with a lint-free towel.
- Remove the right lens from its storage container.
- Squeeze the lens gently between thumb and forefinger. If the edges move toward each other, the lens is in correct position.
- Examine the lens for cleanness. If necessary, clean it again.
- Insert the lens on the right eye.
- Repeat the process for the left eye.

PRODUCT SELECTION GUIDELINES

On the basis of current information, it is difficult to recommend a particular hard contact lens solution objectively as the preferred product. A person's temperament, personality, physical characteristics, and capabilities must be taken into account. If a specific regimen is not suitable, it will probably be followed poorly or disregarded.

Ocular discomfort may be caused by lens-induced corneal edema, and removal of the lens makes the symptoms disappear. It also may be caused by a person's inability or lack of determination to follow a particular regimen. In these cases, multipurpose or all-purpose solutions may be helpful. A specific product with too high a content of total solids may cause ocular discomfort. Changing to a mildly hypertonic solution or a solution with a different viscosity-increasing agent may help. Allergic reactions to benzalkonium chloride, thimerosal, and chlorhexidine frequently have been reported by hard lens wearers.

Pharmacists should warn hard lens wearers receiving therapy involving antihistamines, oral decongestants, or diuretics that these drugs decrease lacrimal fluid production. Patients whose tears do not produce enough wetting action or who do not achieve enough cushioning with a wetting solution may be helped by a conditioner instilled while the lens is worn. Ocular irritation sometimes is relieved by use of artificial tears. If drying and irritation occur, the patient should be advised to consult an ophthalmologist.

It is not good practice to mix solutions from different manufacturers without checking contents. This procedure could lead to concurrent use of solutions with anionic and cationic agents which might inactivate one or both agents and possibly cause precipitation.

In advising patients on soft contact lens systems, the pharmacist should make sure that a solution designed for use with hard lenses is not being used on soft lenses. Moreover, the FDA-approved system for the care of particular lenses should be used; substituting one solution for another may lead to problems such as eye irritation and may damage the lens.

The pharmacist should stress that soft lens wearers should not use ophthalmic solutions or medicants, including conventional contact lens solutions, before or while the lenses are in place on the eyes. The importance of cleaning the lenses properly with the appropriate sterilization/disinfecting technique should be emphasized. Improper cleaning may lead to ocular irritation and clouded lenses.

SUMMARY

The number of contact lens wearers in the United States continues to grow. The comfort and convenience of contact lenses make them a popular choice among individuals who must wear corrective lenses to achieve visual acuity. Technological research to find the safest and most effective product continues.

Therapeutic use of contact lenses is being investigated for postcataract patients. The FDA Panel reviews all new contact lens products as drugs, and U.S. distribution depends on Panel approval. Pharmacists should attempt to keep abreast of developments in the ophthalmic field.

REFERENCES

(1) O. H. Dabezies, J. M. Dixon, and G. P. Halberg, *Patient Care, 12,* 98 (1978).
(2) R. A. Koetting, *J. Am. Pharm. Assoc., NS15,* 575 (1975).
(3) D. R. Gourley, *U.S. Pharm., 2,* 40 (1977).
(4) "Modern Plastics Encyclopedia," Vol. 1, Breskin, New York, N.Y., 1947, p. 129.
(5) O.H. Dabezies, in "Corneal and Scleral Contact Lenses," L. J. Girard, Ed., Mosby, St. Louis, Mo., 1967, pp. 347–361.
(6) H. W. Hind and I. J. Szekely, *Contacto, 3,* 66 (1959).
(7) "Soft Contact Lens," A. R. Gasset and H. E. Kaufman, Eds., Mosby, St. Louis, Mo., 1972, pp. 233–239.
(8) *Ibid.*, pp. 175–183.
(9) "Contact Lens Practice," R. B. Mandell, Ed., Charles C Thomas, Springfield, Ill., 1974, pp. 437–454.
(10) "Soft Contact Lens," A. R. Gasset and H. E. Kaufman, Eds., Mosby, St. Louis, Mo., 1972, pp. 61–71.
(11) F. B. Hoefle, *Trans. Am. Acad. Ophthalmol. Otol., 78,* OP-386 (1974).
(12) "Symposium on Contact Lenses," Mosby, St. Louis, Mo., 1973, pp. 174–180.
(13) "Soft Contact Lens," A. R. Gasset and H. E. Kaufman, Eds., Mosby, St. Louis, Mo., 1972, pp. 199–209.
(14) J. Sugar, *Arch. Ophthalmol., 91,* 11 (1974).
(15) "Symposium on the Flexible Lens," J. L. Bitonte and R. H. Keates, Eds., Mosby, St. Louis, Mo., 1972, pp. 73–79.
(16) "Contact Lens Practice," R. B. Mandell, Ed., Charles C Thomas, Springfield, Ill., 1974, pp. 519–522.
(17) A. B. Rizzuit, *Ann. Ophthalmol., 6,* 596 (1974).
(18) "Soft Contact Lens," A. R. Gasset and H. E. Kaufman, Eds., Mosby, St. Louis, Mo., 1972, pp. 126–138.
(19) C. Thranberend, *Klin. Monatsbl. Augenheilkd., 164,* 509 (1974).
(20) F. Dickenson, *Contacto, 11,* 12 (1967).
(21) C. H. May, *Contacto, 4*(2), 41 (1960).
(22) T. F. Gumpelmayer, *Am. J. Optom., 47,* 879 (1970).
(23) M. Millodot, *Arch. Ophthalmol., 82,* 461 (1969).
(24) "Contact Lens Practice," R. B. Mandell, Ed., Charles C Thomas, Springfield, Ill., 1974, pp. 83–116.
(25) J. A. Baldone, *Trans. Am. Acad. Ophthalmol. Otol., 78,* OP-406 (1974).
(26) F. B. Sannin, in "Corneal and Scleral Contact Lenses," L. J. Girard, Ed., Mosby, St. Louis, Mo., 1967, pp. 170–173.
(27) M. D. Sarver and M. G. Harris, *Am. J. Optom., 48,* 382 (1971).
(28) R. L. Sutherland and W. N. Van Leeuwen, *Can. Med. Assoc. J., 107,* 49 (1972).
(29) *Optometric Weekly, 63,* 25 (1972).
(30) I. Fatt and R. St. Helen, *Am. J. Optom., 48,* 545 (1971).
(31) D. R. Morrison and H. F. Edelhauser, *Invest. Ophthalmol., 11,* 58 (1972).
(32) L. Krejci and H. Krejcova, *Br. J. Ophthalmol., 57,* 675 (1973).
(33) R. L. Farris, Z. Kubota, and S. Mishima, *Arch. Ophthalmol., 85,* 651 (1971).
(34) S. G. El Hage, C. C. Hughes, K. R. Schauer, and R. L. Harrell, *Am. J. Optom. Physiol. Optics, 51,* 24 (1974).
(35) C. H. Dohlman, *Trans. Am. Acad. Ophthalmol. Otol., 78,* OP-399 (1974).
(36) "Symposium on the Flexible Lens," J. L. Bitonte and R. H. Keates, Eds., Mosby, St. Louis, Mo., 1972, pp. 30–32.
(37) "Soft Contact Lens," A. R. Gasset and H. E. Kaufman, Eds., Mosby, St. Louis, Mo., 1972, pp. 83–86.
(38) "Symposium on the Flexible Lens," J. L. Bitonte and R. H. Keates, Eds., Mosby, St. Louis, Mo., 1972, pp. 35–51.
(39) *Ibid.*, pp. 222–234.
(40) *British Medical Journal, 3,* 254 (1972).
(41) "Symposium on Contact Lenses," Mosby, St. Louis, Mo., 1973, pp. 1–12.
(42) *Ibid.*, pp. 65–81.
(43) W. G. Sampson, *Trans. Am. Acad. Ophthalmol. Otol., 78,* OP-423 (1974).
(44) *British Medical Journal, 2,* 655 (1977).
(45) A. R. Gasset and L. Lobo, *Ann. Ophthalmol., 8,* 843 (1977).
(46) L. J. Girard, in "Corneal Contact Lenses," L. J. Girard, Ed., Mosby, St. Louis, Mo., 1972, pp. 107–120.
(47) *Federal Register, 43,* 11759 (1978).
(48) *FDA Drug Bulletin, 7,* 7 (May–July 1977).
(49) P. S. Binder and D. M. Worthen, *Arch. Ophthalmol., 94,* 2109 (1976).
(50) H. L. Gould, *N.Y. State J. Med., 77,* 913 (1977).
(51) L. J. Girard, in "Corneal and Scleral Contact Lenses," L. J. Girard, Ed., Mosby, St. Louis, Mo., 1967, pp. 40–48.
(52) *Ibid.*, pp. 1–17.
(53) M. Ruben, *Lancet, 1,* 138 (1976).
(54) J. C. Casebeer, *Am. J. Ophthalmol., 76,* 165 (1973).
(55) H. M. Rosenwasser, *Opt. J. Rev. Optom., 100,* 41 (1963).
(56) O. W. Cole, *Contacto, 15,* 5 (1971).
(57) "Contact Lens Practice," R. B. Mandell, Ed., Charles C Thomas, Springfield, Ill., 1974, pp. 108–109.
(58) "Symposium on Contact Lenses," Mosby, St. Louis, Mo., 1973, pp. 42–52.
(59) R. F. Meyer and J. W. Henderson, *Clin. Med., 82,* 26 (Feb. 1975).
(60) *Contacto, 15,* 20 (1971).
(61) D. A. Norton, D. J. G. Davies, N. E. Richardson, B. J. Meaking, and A. Keall, *J. Pharm. Pharmacol., 26,* 841 (1974).
(62) H. L. Gould, *Eye Ear Nose Throat Mon., 41,* 359 (1962).
(63) *Contacto, 3,* 262 (1959).
(64) I. J. Szekely, *South. Pharm. J., 52,* 17 (1960).
(65) B. F. Rankin, *Optom. Weekly* (May 25, 1961).
(66) J. Z. Krezanoski, *J. Am. Pharm. Assoc., NS10,* 13 (1970).
(67) H. L. Gould and R. Inglima, *Eye Ear Nose Throat Mon., 43,* 39 (1964).
(68) "Contact Lens Practice," R. B. Mandell, Ed., Charles C Thomas, Springfield, Ill., 1974, pp. 255–284.
(69) H. W. Hind and F. M. Goyan, *J. Am. Pharm. Assoc. Sci. Ed., 36,* 33 (1947).
(70) K. C. Swan, *Am. J. Ophthalmol., 27,* 1118 (1944).
(71) S. Riegelman, D. G. Vaughan, Jr., and M. Okumoto, *J. Am. Pharm. Assoc. Sci. Ed., 45,* 93 (1956).
(72) D. R. McGregor and P. R. Elliker, *Can. J. Microbiol., 4,* 499 (1958).
(73) J. C. Neill and J. J. Hanna, *Contacto, 7,* 10 (1963).
(74) C. E. Watkins, *Optom. World* (Oct. 1964).
(75) F. M. Kapetansky, T. Suie, A. D. Gracy, and J. L. Bitonte, *Am. J. Ophthalmol., 57,* 255 (1964).
(76) H. Allen, *Arch. Ophthalmol., 67,* 119 (1962).
(77) J. M. Dixon, E. Lawaczeck, and C. H. Winkler, *Am. J. Ophthalmol., 54,* 461 (1962).
(78) M. F. Obear and F. C. Winter, *Am. J. Ophthalmol., 57,* 441 (1964).
(79) N. C. Hall and J. Z. Krezanoski, *N. Engl. J. Optom., 14,* 229 (1963).
(80) O. H. Dabezies, *Eye Ear Nose Throat Mon., 45,* 78 (Oct. 1966).
(81) O. H. Dabazies and T. Naugle, *Eye Ear Nose Throat Mon., 50,* 378 (Oct. 1971).
(82) R. E. Phares, *Contact Lens Soc. Am. J., 7,* 37 (1973).
(83) O. H. Dabezies, *Contact Lens Med. Bull., 7,* 45 (1974).
(84) G. L. Cureton, N. C. Hall, R. K. Browne, and D. E. Lauck, *J. Am. Optom. Assoc., 46,* 259 (1975).
(85) M. J. Sibley and D. E. Lauck, *Contact Lens J., 8,* 10 (1974).
(86) "Prescription Requirements for First-Quality Contact Lenses," American National Standards Institute, New York, N.Y., 1972.
(87) R. E. Phares, *J. Am. Optom. Assoc., 43,* 308 (1972).
(88) G. L. Cureton and N. C. Hall, *Am. J. Optom. Physiol. Optics, 51,* 406 (1974).
(89) J. Z. Krezanoski, *Contact Lens. Soc. Am. J., 7,* 9 (1974).
(90) J. A. Baldone, *Contact Lens Med. Bull., 4,* 9 (1971).
(91) J. Z. Krezanoski, *Ont. Optician, 5,* 9 (1974).
(92) J. Z. Krezanoski, *Int. Cont. Clin.* (in press).
(93) M. S. Favero, L. A. Carson, W. W. Bond, and N. J. Peterson, *Science, 173,* 836 (1971).
(94) M. F. Refojo and F. J. Holly, *Contact Intraocular Lens Med. J., 3,* 23 (1977).
(95) J. S. Cumming and H. Karageozian, *Contacto, 19,* 8 (July 1975).
(96) G. E. Lowther, *Am. J. Optom. Physiol. Optics, 54,* 76 (1977).
(97) "Symposium on the Flexible Lens," J. L. Bitonte and R. H. Keates, Eds., Mosby, St. Louis, Mo., 1972, pp. 205–212.
(98) W. Sagan and K. N. Schwaderer, *J. Am. Optom. Assoc., 45,* 266 (1974).
(99) H. I. Silverman, R. Pazzano, D. Korb, and R. Kluza, *J. Am. Optom. Assoc., 44,* 1040 (1973).
(100) J. Z. Krezanoski, *Ophthalmol. Opt., 12,* 1035 (1972).

APPENDIX: SOFT CONTACT LENSES

Names appearing in italics are FDA-approved systems.

- *Accusoft* (droxifilcon)
- *Ao-Soft* (tetrafilcon A; manufactured by American Optical)
- *Aquaflex* (tetrafilcon A; manufactured by UCO Optics, Inc.)
- Contaflex (manufactured by Canadian Contact Lens)
- Dominion (manufactured by Dominion Soft Lens)
- Gelflex (manufactured by Calcon)
- Hydracon (manufactured by Kontur Kontact)
- Hydralens (manufactured by Ophthalmos)
- *Hydrocurve* (hefilcon A, PHP; manufactured by Soft Lenses, Inc.)
- Hydro Marc (manufactured by Frontier)
- Jel Soft (manufactured by Invisible)
- Lacrophilic (manufactured by N & N)
- *Meso Lens* (CAB, a semihard lens; manufactured by Danker & Wohlk)
- Naturvue (hefilcon A, PHP; manufactured by Milton Roy)
- Opti Contact (manufactured by Opti-Con)
- Perma-Lens (manufactured by Cooper Laboratories, Inc.)
- *Soflens* (polymacon; manufactured by Bausch & Lomb, also U and U3 Series)
- *Softcon* (vifilcon A; manufactured by Warner-Lambert; a bandage lens)
- *Tresoft* (ocufilcon)
- Urosoft (Urocon)
- Verazel (Veracon)

Product (Manufacturer)	Suggested Use	Viscosity Agent	Preservative	Other
Adapettes (Burton Parsons)	rewetting	adsorbobase povidone	thimerosal, 0.004% edetate disodium, 0.1%	—
Adapt (Burton Parsons)	preinsertion	adsorbobase hydroxyethylcellulose	thimerosal, 0.004% edetate disodium, 0.1%	—
All-In-One (Rexall)	cleaning wetting soaking	—	edetate disodium, 0.1% thimerosal, 0.004%	—
Aqua-Flow (Smith, Miller & Patch)	rewetting	polyvinyl alcohol, 1.4% hydroxyethylcellulose	edetate sodium, 0.025% benzalkonium chloride, 0.005%	—
Blink-N-Clean (Allergan)	cleaning wetting	polyoxyl 40 stearate polyethylene glycol 300	chlorobutanol, 0.5%	—
Clean-Gel (Barnes-Hind)	cleaning	—	thimerosal, 0.004%	nonionic surfactant[a]
Cleaning and Soaking Solution (Barnes-Hind)	cleaning soaking	—	edetate disodium, 0.2% benzalkonium chloride, 0.01%	buffering and cleaning agents[a]
Clean-N-Soak (Allergan)	cleaning soaking	—	phenylmercuric nitrate, 0.004%	cleaning agent[b]
Clens (Burton Parsons)	cleaning	—	benzalkonium chloride, 0.02% edetate disodium, 0.1%	cleaning agents[a]
Clerz (Smith, Miller & Patch)	cleaning wetting	—	sorbic acid, 0.1% thimerosal, 0.001% edetate disodium, 0.1%	nonionic detergent
Contactisol (Smith, Miller & Patch)	cleaning wetting	hydroxypropyl methylcellulose	benzalkonium chloride, 0.01% edetate disodium, 0.01%	sodium carbonate boric acid potassium chloride
Contique Cleaning Solution (Alcon)	cleaning	—	benzalkonium chloride, 0.02%	—
Contique Clean-Tabs[b] (Alcon)	cleaning	—	—	cleaning agents[a]
Contique Soaking Solution (Alcon)	soaking	—	benzalkonium chloride, 0.01% edetate disodium, 0.01%	—
Contique Soak-Tabs[b] (Alcon)	soaking	—	thimerosal, 0.08% benzethonium chloride, 4%	—
Contique Wetting Solution (Alcon)	wetting	hydroxypropyl methylcellulose	benzalkonium chloride, 0.004% edetate disodium, 0.025%	—
d-Film Gel (Smith, Miller & Patch)	cleaning	—	—	nonionic detergent[a]
duo Flow (Smith, Miller & Patch)	cleaning soaking	—	edetate disodium, 0.25% benzalkonium chloride, 0.013%	—
hy-Flow (Smith, Miller & Patch)	wetting	polyvinyl alcohol	edetate disodium, 0.025% benzalkonium chloride, 0.01%	sodium chloride, 1% potassium chloride, 0.2%
Hypotears (Smith, Miller & Patch)	wetting	lipiden polymeric system	benzalkonium chloride, 0.01% edetate disodium, 0.03%	—
LC-65 (Allergan)	cleaning	—	edetate disodium thimerosal, 0.001%	cleaning agents[a]
Lensine (Smith, Miller & Patch)	cleaning	—	edetate disodium, 0.1% benzalkonium chloride, 0.01%	boric acid, 0.7% (but pH is alkaline)
Lens-Mate (Alcon)	cleaning wetting soaking	polyvinyl alcohol hydroxypropyl methylcellulose	benzalkonium chloride, 0.1% edetate disodium, 0.01%	—
Liquifilm Tears (Allergan)	wetting	polyvinyl alcohol, 1.4%	chlorobutanol, 0.5%	sodium chloride
Liquifilm Wetting Solution (Allergan)	wetting	hydroxypropyl methylcellulose polyvinyl alcohol	benzalkonium chloride, 0.004% edetate disodium	sodium chloride potassium chloride
One Solution (Barnes-Hind)	cleaning wetting soaking	NS[a]	edetate disodium, 0.1% benzalkonium chloride, 0.01%	cleaning agents[a]
Ova-Nite (Milroy)	cleaning soaking	—	benzalkonium chloride, 0.02% edetate disodium, 0.25%	nonionic surfactant[a]

Product (Manufacturer)	Suggested Use	Viscosity Agent	Preservative	Other
Pre-Sert (Allergan)	wetting	polyvinyl alcohol, 3%	benzalkonium chloride, 0.004%	—
Soaclens (Burton Parsons)	soaking wetting	—	thimerosal, <0.004% edetate disodium, 0.1%	NS[a]
Soakare (Allergan)	soaking	—	edetate disodium, 0.25% benzalkonium chloride, 0.01%	—
Soquette (Barnes-Hind)	soaking	polyvinyl alcohol	chlorobutanol, 0.4% edetate disodium, 0.2% benzalkonium chloride, 0.01%	—
Titan (Barnes-Hind)	cleaning	—	benzalkonium chloride edetate disodium	nonionic cleaner buffers[a]
Total All-in-one Contact Lens Solution (Allergan)	cleaning wetting soaking	polyvinyl alcohol hydroxypropyl methylcellulose	benzalkonium chloride edetate disodium	sodium chloride potassium chloride dextrose
Visalens Soaking/Cleaning (Leeming)	cleaning soaking	—	benzalkonium chloride, 0.02% edetate disodium, 0.10%	sodium borate/ boric acid buffer
Visalens Wetting Solution (Leeming)	wetting	polyvinyl alcohol hydroxypropyl methylcellulose	benzalkonium chloride, 0.01% edetate disodium, 0.10%	sodium chloride potassium chloride
Wet-Cote (Milroy)	wetting	polyvinyl alcohol hydroxyethylcellulose	edetate disodium, 0.25% benzalkonium chloride, 0.01%	sodium chloride potassium chloride
Wetting Solution (Barnes-Hind)	wetting	polyvinyl alcohol, 2%	edetate disodium, 0.02% benzalkonium chloride, 0.004%	sodium chloride
Wetting Solution (Rexall)	wetting	—	edetate disodium, 0.01% benzalkonium chloride, 0.004%	—

[a] Not specified.
[b] Tablet must be dissolved in water.

Product (Manufacturer)	Viscosity Agent	Preservative	Other
Adapettes (Burton Parsons)	adsorbobase povidone	thimerosal, 0.004% edetate disodium, 0.1%	—
Boil n Soak (Burton Parsons)	—	thimerosal, 0.001% edetate disodium, 0.1%	boric acid sodium borate sodium chloride, 0.7%
Flexsol (Burton Parsons)	povidone	thimerosal, 0.001% chlorhexidine, 0.005% edetate disodium, 0.1%	sodium chloride sodium borate boric acid polyoxyethylene polyoxypropylene
Lensrins (Allergan)	—	thimerosal, 0.001% edetate disodium, 0.1%	sodium chloride, 0.85%
Normol (Burton Parsons)	—	thimerosal, 0.001% edetate disodium, 0.1% chlorhexidine, 0.005%	sodium chloride sodium borate boric acid

Soft Lens Products

Product (Manufacturer)	Viscosity Agent	Preservative	Other
Pliagel (Smith, Miller & Patch)	—	antimicrobials [b]	surfactants [b]
Preflex (Burton Parsons)	hydroxyethylcellulose polyvinyl alcohol	edetate disodium, 0.02% thimerosal, 0.004%	sodium phosphate sodium chloride tyloxapol
Soflens Tablets (Allergan)	—		papain
Soft Mate (Barnes-Hind)	hydroxyethylcellulose	edetate disodium, 0.2% thimerosal, 0.004%	octoxynol sodium chloride

[a] Check label to determine type of lens to be used with.
[b] Not specified.

Sodium Chloride Solutions

Product [a] (Manufacturer)	Ingredients
Adsorbonac (Burton Parsons)	2 and 5% sodium chloride
Murocoll Methylcellulose Ophthalmic Solution (Muro)	5% sodium chloride
Muro Ointment (Muro)	5% sodium chloride

[a] These products are prescription only.

Dental Products

Richard M. Oksas

Chapter 21

Questions to Ask the Patient

How long have you been aware of the problem? Have you seen a dentist?

Is the problem painful or incapacitating? Is the pain continuous, or is it triggered by hot and cold substances?

Is the sore visible, and is there a purulent discharge? Do you have a fever?

Is the sore white in color?

Does the condition produce continuous bad breath?

Are your teeth loose? Do your gums bleed when you brush your teeth?

What are your oral hygiene habits? How do you clean your teeth (or dentures)? How often?

How often do you see your dentist? Do you use supplemental fluoride in one form or another?

Are your dentures loose? Do they cause sore spots?

Do you suffer from any chronic medical illnesses such as diabetes mellitus or rheumatic heart condition? What medication(s) are you taking?

Although there are more than 100,000 dentists in the United States, dental disease is the most common health problem of Americans. Only about 50% of children under 15 have even undergone dental examination (1), and the cavity rate of those examined is 50–70% (2), or an average of 10 cavities per child (3). Moreover, dental illness is not an age-specific phenomenon: currently, 20% of the adult population is edentulous (without natural teeth), and an additional 100 million other persons are missing at least half their teeth (4). The tragedy of these statistics is that teeth and oral tissues can remain healthy and functional for a lifetime if preventive dental techniques are followed.

The causes of this health problem are manifold. For some citizens, dental care is not considered a major health priority, and dentists are sought only in oral crisis, after the damage is done. In addition, the widespread availability and advertising claims of dental products often engender considerable confusion and make it difficult for consumers to distinguish oral health fact from fallacy.

If teeth are to be saved, patients should seek professional counsel about their mouths. Pharmacists can play a major role in promoting good oral health, since a pharmacist comes into contact with more prospective dental patients than a community dentist does during any given day (5). As a public health professional, the pharmacist should stock OTC products beneficial to oral hygiene, provide patient education on proper product usage, and make appropriate referrals to dentists. Common dental problems that the pharmacist may encounter include cavities (caries), diseased gums, halitosis, oral sores, and toothache and other oral cavity pain. The pharmacist also may be questioned about loose or broken teeth, dental work, and dentures.

ORAL ANATOMY AND PHYSIOLOGY

The oral cavity comprises both dentition (teeth) and supporting structures such as gingiva (gums) and bone. Together they perform masticatory, articulatory, and esthetic functions. Every person is supplied with two sets of teeth: 20 deciduous or primary teeth (the so-called "baby teeth," 10 in each jaw) and 32 permanent adult teeth, which begin erupting at 6 years of age.

The tooth consists of two major parts, the crown and the root. The crown (the portion visible above the gum line in a healthy mouth) appears bulbous, squat, and light-colored when properly cleaned. The root (the major portion of the tooth's body), which is not normally visible, is darker and longer and tapers to a point (apex). While the anterior or frontal teeth (incisors and cuspids) generally possess a single root, the larger posterior teeth (bicuspids and molars) are multirooted.

The crown's exposed surface is covered by a layer of enamel consisting of inorganic calcium salts (hydroxyapatite crystals), the hardest substance found in the human body. Although enamel protects the tooth from exposure to oral stress, it cannot regenerate itself when destroyed or lost. The root is covered by cementum, a softer, extremely thin (equivalent to a few cell layers in thickness) material that may wear away rapidly if the root becomes exposed. The tooth itself is composed mostly of dentin, a distinctly yellowish material consisting of solid organic substratum infiltrated with calcium salts.

Bonelike in appearance, dentin is denser than bone but softer than enamel. It surrounds the innermost tooth tissue, the dental pulp. Pulp resides within a chamber; this is the spongy "living" portion of the tooth, composed of soft vascular and neural tissues. Tooth pain occurs only when there is pulpal involvement.

The teeth cannot function properly without firm support from other oral tissue. This supportive structure, the periodontium, includes the alveolar bone, gingiva, and periodontal fibers. The tooth's root rests in a socket within the jaw bone. The alveolar (adjacent) bone and the cementum are connected by a layer of viable periodontal ligaments. Soft, pink, highly vascular gingival tissue covers the outer exposed portion of the periosteal surfaces.

ETIOLOGY OF DENTAL CONDITIONS

causes of oral problems

normal oral microbial populations

dental plaque composition

dietary factors

The etiology of oral disease is complex: enough conditions exist to warrant not only a health professional devoted solely to the oral cavity, but also specialization within that profession (e.g., periodontics, endodontics, and orthodontics). Generalized features that predispose individuals to poor oral health include endogenous (microbiological), host (habit and custom), and exogenous (diet) factors.

Endogenous Factors

In terms of microbial concentration, the mouth is perhaps the most "dirty" organ of the body; i.e., the potential for infection is greater there than elsewhere. Conditions present in the mouth, including an overabundance of nutrients, moisture, a warm ambient temperature, and oxygen, are ideal for supporting microbial growth (Table 1). Although the mouth is sterile at birth, invasion by streptococci occurs early. Microorganisms establish colonies preferentially at various anatomical sites. Anaerobes generally are late arrivals, occurring in gingival folds after tooth eruption. Because no two areas of the mouth possess an identical ratio of bacterial flora, there is relatively little value in salivary bacterial counts to determine patient propensity to caries or in vitro antiseptic effectiveness tests. Other variables significant in affecting floral patterns are oral pH, chewing and hygiene habits, time of day, and age of the patient (6).

Most kinds of oral bacteria are gram positive and facultative. Streptococci, staphylococci, and lactobacilli may be present in the lesions of oral disease. (Infections of the pulp and periodontium, however, are generally more complex and involve several types of microbes.) Under normal conditions these bacteria may be benign, but their pathological potential may be activated when stress produces an ecological microbial imbalance that causes their overgrowth and modification. Once this imbalance occurs, microbes generally become the primary agents of oral tissue destruction.

Plaque

The development of plaque is influenced by endogenous and exogenous factors. Dental plaque is a tenacious soft deposit that adheres to dental surfaces. Composed of bacteria and salivary by-products (protein, mucin, and colloidal material), plaque begins as a thin, invisible, insoluble film (pellicle), which traps more material and bacteria. Food residue after meals may be incorporated into plaque by bacterial degradation and conversion into dextran and glycoproteins. Left unchecked, the plaque thickens, and bacteria proliferate (7). Eventually, plaque around the base of the crown calcifies (calculus, or tartar) (8) via calcium salt precipitation from the saliva; calculus is removable only by professional dental cleaning. Plaque is commonly recognized as the source of microbes that cause caries and periodontitis; thus plaque buildup is related to incidence of oral disease. The best way to promote dental health is to remove plaque buildup by brushing and flossing regularly.

Exogenous Factors

Diet and other personal habits constitute other factors in maintaining oral health. Foods with a high concentration of refined sugar (sucrose) are strongly cariogenic. Sucrose is converted by bacterial plaque into volatile acids (such as lactic, pyruvic, acetic, propionic, and butyric acids) which attack, dissolve, and solubilize the calcium salts found in tooth structure (9). Unfortunately, sugar-containing foods are highly popular with the young age group in which the greatest susceptibility to caries occurs. Saccharin-containing food substitutes probably helped in this regard, but because of safety questions concerning saccharin, their future use is questionable. Other sugar substitutes may help to curb sugar-hungry appetites (10).

Excessive sugar intake is not the only source of dental caries. Other types of fermentable carbohydrates, such as fructose (found in fruit) and lactose (found in milk), also are cariogenic but to a far lesser extent than sucrose (11). Chewing gum or eating fibrous foods (e.g.,

Table 1. Bacterial Count Found in Selected Oral Locations

Area of Mouth	Total Mean Bacteria[a]	Average Aerobic Count[b]	Average Anaerobic Count[b]
Saliva, $\times 10^6$/ml	200	40	110
Gingival material (surface), $\times 10^9$/g	160	15	36
Gingival crevice (pocket), $\times 10^9$/g	130	19.7	35.2
Dental plaque, $\times 10^9$/g	250	25	46

[a] Via microscopic assay technique.
[b] Via culture media technique.

celery or carrots) does not prevent plaque accumulation or aid in its removal (12). Also, except during pregnancy and childhood, ingesting dairy products or other calcium-rich foods has little or no effect on fully developed teeth. The relationship of diet to periodontal disease is less clear because of other mechanistic factors. However, nutrition becomes more important with increasing age; geriatric patients must receive a well-balanced diet containing essential vitamins and minerals for the supportive tissue to remain viable.

Other personal habits also may influence the incidence of oral disease. Chronic exposure to irritating substances (e.g., tobacco or alcohol) may exacerbate periodontal disease (7) and eventually lead to oral cancer. The most important factors in preventing tooth and gum destruction are good personal oral hygiene habits and regular dental checkups. When missing teeth are not replaced, the resultant malocclusion (misalignment) may create a marked shift in the internal dynamics of the mouth to produce physical trauma to oral tissues which may serve as the focal point for infection.

ORAL DISEASES

The pathophysiology of oral disease is generally uniform. Tissue breakdown produced by chemical, physical, or psychological stress causes a pathogenic modification of the oral microbiology and a reduced resistance of oral tissue. Infection sets in and, because the mouth is highly vascular, produces inflammation from resultant irritation. Tissue destruction (necrosis) is facilitated by microbial by-products and inflammatory pressure; chronic halitosis (bad breath) is one of its symptoms. When the destruction becomes advanced enough, neural involvement and damage occur, creating oral pain. A possible systemic bacteremia may be dangerous to cardiac patients with rheumatic heart disease, valvular prosthesis, or congenital defects or to individuals with decreased resistance to infection from diabetes mellitus, steroid therapy, or cancer chemotherapy. The pharmacist should watch for specific signs and symptoms of common dental illness.

Caries

Dental caries afflict 95% of the public and represent the main cause of tooth loss in persons under 35. Caries generally begin on the crown's external surface or on the root if it is exposed. Tooth substance disintegrates and dissolves through action of various bacteria (*Streptococcus mutans, Actinomyces viscosus,* and *Lactobacillus*) found in dental plaque. Demineralization of the enamel progresses slowly at first, but once external dentin is reached, infection and tissue necrosis proliferate rapidly. Involvement of microtubules in the dentin leads to pulpal complications which produce the classic "toothache" (pulpitis). If endodontic (root canal) therapy is not instituted at this point in the disease, infection continues to spread from the tooth apex to the periodontal tissue, alveolar bone, and adjacent teeth.

Treatment of caries involves removing necrotic tissue, cleaning the resultant lesion, and replacing the missing substance with various restorative materials (a filling, crown, or bridge). Preventive oral hygiene aimed at avoiding plaque buildup is important in minimizing caries.

Periodontal Disease

Periodontal disease is the primary cause of tooth loss in the elderly but may affect younger persons as well if their teeth are not properly cared for. Although the tooth itself may be healthy and functional, it becomes useless when supportive tissue breaks down. Receding or swollen gums that bleed on brushing, along with tooth mobility in advanced cases, are signs of periodontal disease.

In its initial stages, periodontal disease is manifested as gingivitis, an inflammation of the gum immediately next to the neck of the dental crown. This condition frequently goes undetected because it is painless and may subside in the acute stages. Simple gingivitis is believed to be caused by irritating enzymes and toxins made by bacteria found in gingival plaque. These organisms are not related to those involved with caries, and therefore the mechanisms of the diseases differ.

common dental problems

toothache

gingivitis

trench mouth

canker and cold sores

Chronic gingivitis may result from other systemic conditions. Manifestations of gingivitis may occur in individuals with diabetes, leukemia, hypovitaminosis, or heavy metal toxicity; during pregnancy or menopause; or in association with phenytoin therapy. Any periodontal case should be referred to a dentist.

As gingivitis progresses, it produces a periodontal pocket, which continues to deepen downward along the root surface, facilitating entrapment of more debris and bacteria. As the gingival pocket increases in size, the periodontal ligament and supporting bone may become involved (periodontitis). When this happens, the root becomes visible above the gum line; periodontal debridement (surgery) is required to save the remaining supportive structure. Postsurgical patients must exercise meticulous cleaning habits to prevent disease recurrence and caries development on the susceptible exposed roots.

Other periodontal conditions include Vincent's gingivitis and periodontosis. Vincent's gingivitis (also called trench mouth and necrotizing ulcerative gingivitis) is a generalized noncontagious gingival infection caused by spirochetes and fusobacteria. It is treated by proper hygiene and diet, rest, and antibiotics. Periodontosis is extremely rare, tending to appear during adolescence, and consists of spontaneous bone loss for no known reason (possibly a genetic or autoimmune condition).

Oral Sores

Often the pharmacist is questioned about treating common canker and cold sores and other types of stomatitis of the mucosal epithelium surrounding the inner oral surface. Because sores are caused by various agents and may differ in severity and consequences, recommendations should be made only after thorough patient evaluation.

A sore may be caused by severe mechanical or chemical trauma to the exposed soft palate. When the affected area is small or the injury is minimal, the tissue usually regenerates in a few days. To prevent additional irritation to the site, an oral protectant (e.g., Orabase) may be advisable. More extensive traumatous lesions due to allergic responses or loose or malfitting dentures require a dental referral.

A sore of bacterial origin (aphthous ulcer) generally is caused by a staphylococcal infection. The sore is a raised white papule bordered by an erythematous halo. Aphthous ulcers usually occur singly inside the cheek, on the tongue, or on the soft palate (13, 14). Fever and malaise may accompany the disease in advanced stages, and antibiotic treatment may be necessary. In such instances a dental referral is recommended.

herpes virus

Herpes virus is the causative agent of true fever blisters and cold sores. This condition is often recurrent and self-limiting (lasting 14 days); by its nature, only symptomatic treatment means are available via self-medication. Herpes infections differ from aphthous ulcers in that they occur most frequently on the lips as small red papules that become vesicles (blisters), which may be painful and usually form multiple clusters. After the vesicle ruptures, the lesion becomes crusty while it heals (15, 16). Herpes is a communicable disease but seldom presents symptoms in healthy persons who come into contact with the patient. Exposure and subsequent development of infection, however, can be hazardous to very young infants and to immunosuppressed adult subjects.

fungal infections

Another potentially serious oral infection involves fungal overgrowth in the mouth (thrush or candidiasis). The fungus, of the *Candida albicans* variety, appears as a white, furry patch on the oral mucosa, tongue, and soft palate. When this white material is removed by mechanical wiping, the undersurface is inflamed and raw. Treatment requires the use of topical nystatin (17). Patients with dentures and those receiving antibiotics, steroids, or cancer chemotherapy are particularly prone to candidal (also referred to as monilial) invasion. Determining why candidiasis is present is probably as important as treating the disease itself.

Other Oral Conditions

Oral neoplasia differs from other types of sores in that it develops over a very long period and is often painless and persistent. The tumor typically appears in males over 45 years of age who have a chronic history of smoking and excessive alcohol use. It may appear anywhere in the mouth as a distinct white patch (leukoplakia) or red spot (erythroplakia). Approximately 70% occur on the tongue and floor of the mouth. As in the case of other sores that do not heal, patients should have a biopsy (18).

Oral symptoms also may arise from unrelated systemic illnesses. Infectious diseases associated with oral clinical features include anthrax, chickenpox, diphtheria, measles, mumps, several mycotic diseases, shingles, tuberculosis, and venereal disease. Malnutrition, endocrine imbalance, and hematological dyscrasia are chronic conditions that may produce gingivitis and stomatitis. Angina produces referred pain in the jaw, and neurological dysfunction may create oral paresthesia and tremor.

drug-induced oral effects

Oral drug reactions in addition to phenytoin gingival hyperplasia also may cause oral disease symptoms. Aspirin burn from using the drug as a topical anesthetic, permanent staining of dentition by tetracycline ingestion or fluoride overdosage in children, and hyposalivation (xerostomia) from anticholinergics are some drug-induced effects (19).

PATIENT ASSESSMENT

Before recommending a course of action, i.e., dental referral or self-treatment with an OTC product, the pharmacist should question the patient thoroughly as to the duration, extent, and severity of the condition. Chronic conditions generally are more serious than acute ones because the mouth has a limited capacity to repair itself and treatment often only alleviates symptoms or prevents further progression of disease or complications. The pharmacist should find out whether the area of direct damage is localized and small or generalized throughout the mouth, whether concurrent systemic symptoms such as fever are present, and whether the illness is painful or incapacitating. The answers to these questions should help the pharmacist determine the patient's immediate needs.

Pharmacists should not hesitate to refer patients to a dentist instead of recommending self-treatment. Few OTC dental products are truly therapeutic, and with the exception of herpes, most oral disease requires dental intervention. Selection of OTC products is best reserved for prevention, rather than treatment, of dental problems. Patient self-diagnosis always should be discouraged.

PREVENTIVE DENTAL CONCEPTS

brushing and flossing—the basis of prevention

Because caries and periodontal disease are caused chiefly by destruction of vulnerable tissues via microbial by-product formation, preventive dental techniques should be oriented toward ridding the mouth of plaque. The ideal method would be either to destroy disease-producing pathogens or to prevent plaque formation altogether. Research is moving in that direction through the discovery of new biochemical agents. For example, studies show that a mouthrinse containing chlorhexidine gluconate possesses both antiseptic and plaque inhibitory properties (20).

For the time being, however, a patient-motivated program of oral cleanliness and sound health habits remains the chief means of prevention. Thorough brushing and flossing on a routine basis should help prevent plaque accumulation. Caries-prone individuals should reduce sugar intake and receive supplemental fluoride to harden tooth surfaces. Periodontal irritation may be controlled by periodic professional removal of calculus and by abstinence from smoking. Problems of overhanging fillings, missing teeth, malocclusion, and improper bite should be reported immediately to a dentist for correction, because these conditions facilitate plaque accumulation that may result in periodontal disease.

Preventive techniques should start in childhood; deciduous teeth are just as important as the permanent teeth that follow. Pathologies of the so-called "baby teeth" may cause extensive damage to adult dentition as it develops below the gum line. Moreover, premature loss of primary teeth is a significant problem.

PRODUCT SELECTION GUIDELINES

Most individuals tend to purchase OTC dental products as commercial entities rather than for their therapeutic value. Because factors such as cost, palatability, and social acceptability sell products, many dental OTC preparations are formulated and promoted to fulfill cosmetic needs. As a professional health care provider, the pharmacist should know which therapeutic claims are justified and which products fall into the purely cosmetic category. The American Dental Association (ADA) Committee on Dental Therapeutics, the Consumers Union Dental Health Advisory Group, and the FDA OTC Panels on Oral Cavity Drug Products and on Dentifrices and Dental Care Agents recently issued recommendations on clinical effectiveness and safety of oral hygiene aids.

Basic Tools—Brush and Floss

There is no substitute for toothbrush and dental floss to remove plaque from teeth; some dentists believe that these two devices alone may prevent oral disease if they are used properly. Because no two mouths are alike and manipulative dexterity varies from individual to individual, no toothbrush can be considered superior to all others. The ADA makes no specific recommendations, preferring dentists to evaluate individual patient needs. However, the pharmacist should look for certain general characteristics in choosing which types to stock. According to the ADA, for general adult use the soft, polished bristle, straight-handled brush probably combines as successfully as any other the advantages of easy manipulation, efficiency, cleansibility, and structural simplicity (21). Nylon bristles are preferred over natural hog bristles because, although the latter may last longer, they are more abrasive and may damage dental surfaces and gingiva. When adults have accentuated gag reflexes, a smaller child-sized brush may be helpful.

The pharmacist may be asked what brushing technique to use and how often one should brush. Clinical studies have failed to answer these questions. Some dentists prefer a horizontal (scrub) motion, while others advocate a vertical (roll) motion. More important is the degree of thoroughness that the patient exercises while brushing. Commonly missed areas where plaque often accumulates include the gingival margin next to the base of teeth, the inner (lingual) tooth surface, interdental spaces, and posterior teeth. Proper brushing requires several minutes of effort, with equal time allotted to all portions of the mouth (including a periodic gentle cleaning of the tongue). Although a minimum of one extensive and unhurried (2–4 minutes) brushing per day may accomplish plaque removal (7), at least two brushings per day are more realistic for most people (22). Patients with particular dental problems may need to brush even more often.

Specialty toothbrushes also exist, the most prominent being the electric-powered toothbrush. Although this item cleans teeth no better than a properly used manual toothbrush, it serves more than a novelty function, because it is useful for individuals who have dexterity problems, such as the handicapped or young children (23). Electric toothbrushes accepted by the ADA include Broxident Automatic, General Electric Automatic, J. C. Penney Automatic, Sunbeam Cordless Hygienic, and Touch Tronic. Some orthodontists feel that electric brushes are contraindicated in their patients because bristles become lodged in orthodontic bands. For this reason, special orthodontic toothbrushes are available. There also are special toothbrushes for postperiodontal surgery patients (e.g., Proxabrush) and contoured brushes for denture wearers.

No toothbrush can remove calculus or clean plaque from the interproximal contact space between teeth. Dental floss or tape is used to remove plaque formation in this highly susceptible area. Floss comes in both waxed and unwaxed forms. Proper flossing technique is outlined by the American Academy of Periodontology (7):

> Cut off a long piece of floss, and lightly wrap it around your middle fingers. Insert the floss between each tooth, and holding it taut, move it gently back and forth past the point where the teeth contact each other. Move the floss with both fingers up and down five or six times on the side of each tooth, going down to the gum line but not into the gum. Repeat on the side of the adjacent tooth. When floss is frayed or soiled, one turn around the middle finger brings up a fresh section. When you have done all your teeth, rinse vigorously with water.

basic tools for plaque removal

ADA-accepted electric toothbrushes

flossing technique

toothpastes, powders, and gels

Flossing may be difficult at first, particularly if debris has not been removed previously. But with each subsequent flossing, resistance should decrease. When floss continually meets hard resistance or breaks off over a period of time, it may be a sign of calculus accumulation or an overhanging or irregular dental filling. These cases should be brought to a dentist's attention. A toothpick is not recommended as a floss substitute because it may harm gingiva, further impact food, or break off in the mouth. When brushing or flossing cannot be conducted, a thorough rinsing with water after meals is the next best thing—albeit a poor second choice.

Adjunctive Dental Aids

Additional OTC products help toothbrushes and dental floss clean the oral cavity, thereby promoting good oral hygiene and preventing dental disease. While these items are all optional from a dental point of view, their use is considered preventive and may be encouraged.

Dentifrices

Most people prefer to use a commercial dentifrice when they brush their teeth. These products come in toothpaste, toothpowder, and the newer dental gel forms. Their composition is fairly standard: a binder (to stabilize the suspension emulsion's liquid and solid phases), an abrasive (to remove debris), a sudser (to foam and froth clean), a humectant (to retain moisture), and a flavoring agent. Other active ingredients with claimed therapeutic and/or preventive properties (e.g., fluoride) also may be present. Powder dentifrices contain only abrasive and flavoring.

Because the toothbrush's mechanical action is far more important to plaque removal than the type of dentifrice selected, superior cleansing claims for the dentifrice have no scientific foundation. The properties to be considered in selecting a dentifrice are the product's abrasiveness, which, if excessive, could harm exposed dentin, and the therapeutic effectiveness of the so-called special ingredients.

In vitro studies show that dentifrices do vary greatly in abrasiveness (24). While no abrasive is harsh enough to remove enamel, some products may harm cementum and dentin; these cleansers should be avoided by individuals with periodontal disease and hypersensitive teeth. Identifying the different kinds of offending dentifrices is difficult because the interaction of inert ingredients in each formula (which changes over time) may enhance or retard the effect of abrasives in the mixture. In general, powders are more abrasive than pastes, and products that claim to be tooth whiteners often are harsher than others. Specific abrasive ingredients which may harm dentin include calcium carbonate, anhydrous dibasic calcium phosphate, and silica (25).

fluoride in caries prevention

effectiveness of various fluoride treatments

Many therapeutic claims are made about dentifrices. However, only fluoride-containing dentifrices are beneficial in preventing dental caries. Fluoride in each of its various dosage forms (Table 2) decreases the incidence of caries by converting hydroxyapatite in the enamel to a harder and less acid soluble fluoroapatite. Fluoride may be given systemically to children as sodium fluoride (during tooth development) and may be used topically in all age groups. The acidulated topical fluoride used in dental offices, the prescription and nonprescription mouthrinses, and the fluoride contained in commercial toothpaste vary in chemical form and concentration. While there has been concern regarding fluoride toxicity, it has been proven safe when used at recommended dosage levels.

The type of fluoride incorporated into the product is important to caries prevention. Dentifrices containing either stannous fluoride or monofluorophosphate are superior in that both agents are more stable in formulations. The ADA recommends that only Crest, Colgate with MFP, and Macleans Fluoride have caries-inhibiting properties (26). Consumers Union research indicates that although Gleem II contains sodium fluoride, it too produces anticaries effects (7). Nonfluoride dentifrices claiming to prevent caries by enzymatic means, acid neutralization, or incorporation of so-called antiseptic ingredients are in fact placebo.

Desensitizing toothpastes also are promoted as being therapeutically beneficial. Teeth become hypersensitive when they are exposed to variation in physical stimuli (e.g., temperature and pressure), and the condition may be due to an enamel defect or early pulpitis. Both Thermodent, which uses 1.4% formaldehyde as its active ingredient, and Sensodyne, which contains 10% strontium nitrate, are claimed to reduce the discomfort and pain of tooth hypersensitivity. Neither toothpaste has been proven clinically effective: the ADA rejects the therapeutic claims (27), and Consumers Union questions the safety of their formulation, Thermodent because of possible formaldehyde toxicity and Sensodyne because of a high degree of abrasiveness (7). In fact, any fluoride-containing dentifrice may have desensitizing effects, and some are lower in abrasion. Patients with hypersensitive teeth should be referred for dental advice.

Fluorigard (0.05% nonacidulated sodium fluoride) mouthrinse is the first nonprescription topical fluoride

Table 2. Relative Clinical Effectiveness of Various Forms of Fluoride in Caries Inhibition

Dosage Form	Type Used	Concentration per Dose	Recommended Frequency	Reported Range of Caries Inhibition, %
Systemic (in children)				
Community drinking water	sodium fluoride	1 mg	daily	60
School drinking water only	sodium fluoride	1 mg	5 days/week	35–40
Topical Application				
Fluoride treatment in dental office	acidulated sodium fluoride gel	1.23%	semi-annually	26–70
Fluoride mouthrinse	sodium fluoride	0.05%	daily	25–30
Fluoride toothpaste	stannous fluoride sodium mono-fluorophosphate	0.4% 0.76%	daily	23–34 17–38

solution on the market. Originally, it was a prescription drug product which proved beneficial in preventing caries in supervised clinical trials. Its utility in this regard as an OTC product remains unevaluated until the necessary unsupervised trials are completed. Therefore dentifrice remains as the most commonly accepted vehicle for topical fluoride.

Denture Cleansers

Like normal dentition, dentures may accumulate plaque and bacteria along their surface. Left uncleaned, these irritants may produce infections in the wearer's mouth. Dentures also may become stained and cause "denture breath."

Prosthodontists recommend that proper denture care include removing and soaking the appliance during sleep and cleaning it regularly with a denture brush. Soaking prevents dehydration of the acrylic substances in the denture itself, to avoid subsequent shrinkage and brittleness, and overnight removal allows the gums to rest.

Both chemical and mechanical cleansing aids are available. Cleansers added to overnight soak solutions include surfactants, chelating agents, and oxidizing agents such as perborates, peroxides, and hypochlorites. Because many of these products are extremely alkaline, they should be kept away from children. If swallowed, they may cause severe caustic burns of the esophagus and GI tract (28). Mechanical aids include several water soak agitation devices. After reviewing both kinds of cleansers, the ADA believes that neither type of cleanser is superior to using a denture brush for removing undesired material (29).

Denture wearers should be cautioned to avoid using undiluted washing bleach or normal formulation dentifrices to clean dentures. These substances are too harsh for such use and may damage denture material.

Disclosing Agents

Dyes are used in dentistry to reveal the location of invisible plaque and to determine the effectiveness of brushing technique in removing plaque material. Although disclosing products generally are used only on a temporary basis as oral hygiene motivators, the FDA investigated their potential carcinogenicity. Preliminary findings are that erythrosine (FD&C Red No. 3) and FD&C Green No. 3 dyes are safe when used at recommended dosage levels and expectorated (not swallowed) (30). Sodium fluorescein also is used.

Disclosing products are available in two forms: chewable tablets and dye solution. Disclosing tablets are often individually (unit dose) packaged, convenient to carry, and inexpensive. However, they may be mistaken for candy by young children. Many dentists prefer the solution type of disclosing dye for several reasons: it is quicker to apply, provides a more uniform spread of dye throughout the mouth, and may be diluted easily with water. Fluorescent dyes use sodium fluorescein as their active constituent. This substance is visible only when used with a 4800-Å (ultraviolet) light source. Because it is far more costly than other commercial disclosing products and patients may misuse ultraviolet light sources, sodium fluorescein should probably be used only in the dental office.

Oral Irrigators

Oral water irrigating devices are claimed to help remove loose debris after brushing and flossing and to provide some gingival stimulation. These products should not be mistaken for primary cleaning aids or used as substitutes for toothbrushes or floss. Their effectiveness in improving oral hygiene and preventing disease is still subject to debate (31). However, irrigators may be useful for patients who have difficulty in cleaning fixed oral appliances such as orthodontic bands or permanent bridgework.

Two types of irrigating products are available. The "pulsating" irrigators operate by an electric water pump mechanism and therefore are more costly. The main problem with this form as determined by Consumers Union is remote potential for electrocution (7). The less expensive steady stream or jet form of irrigator must be connected directly to a water faucet, sometimes requiring an adaptor or sink modification.

cleaning dentures

dyes used as plaque-locating agents

ADA-approved water sprays

hazards of denture adhesives

The list of ADA-approved irrigators includes the following brands: Dento Spray, Hydro Dent, and Pulsar (a faucet type) (29). Although Water Pik was accepted previously, the manufacturer has not provided the required data for recent re-evaluation (32).

Irrigators should never be used with high water pressures or with extremely hot or cold water. Their stream should be projected at an angle horizontal to dental surfaces because a vertical angle may further impact soft material. Finally, their use is contraindicated in certain cardiac patients (e.g., those with pathologies of rheumatic heart disease or valvular prosthesis) because bacteremias may be produced in these individuals (33, 34).

Denture Adhesives

When natural teeth are extracted, the involved area of the jaw bone decalcifies and gradually shrinks (resorption). Thus no denture, no matter how perfectly it is made, produces an ideal fit for life. The resorption rate varies from individual to individual, and denture wearers should undergo periodic dental checkups when problems are encountered.

Signs of malfitting dentures include "toast eaters syndrome" (avoidance of hard and fibrous foods in favor of soft foods such as toast and coffee) and chronic use of denture adhesives. Unfortunately, changing one's diet to prevent discomfort or nuisance and subconsciously to try to "save face" may create associated nutritional problems.

Denture adhesive products contain inert but adherent and gummy substances such as karaya, methylcellulose, ethylene oxide polymers, and petrolatum. Because many of these ingredients are water soluble, they are diluted by saliva and lose their tenacity in a few hours. The ADA Council on Dental Materials and Devices accepts certain denture adhesive products on condition that they be used either temporarily until a dentist can be consulted about denture readjustment or upon specific recommendation by a dentist. The following warning must

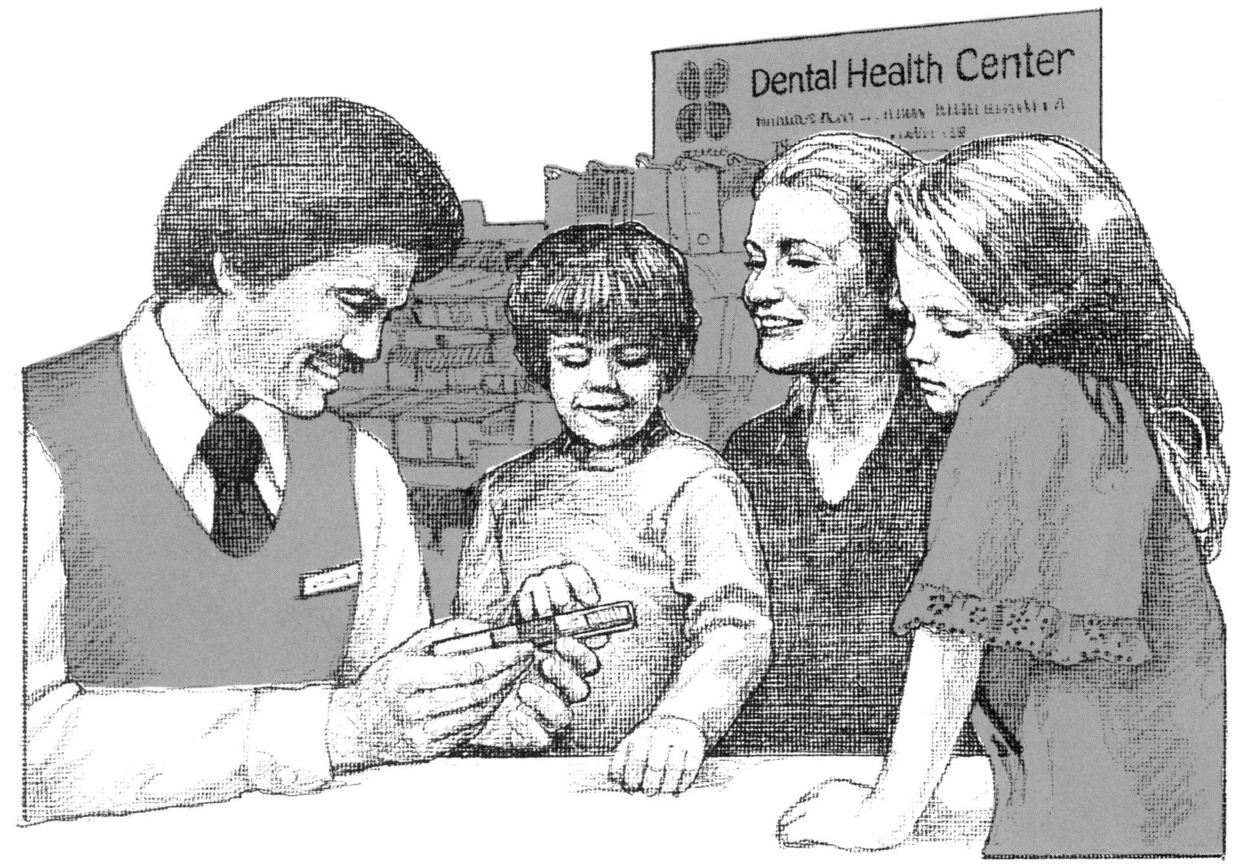

other products for temporary use

appear on the package label of ADA-accepted products (29):

> [Product name] is acceptable as a temporary measure to provide increased retention of dentures. However, an ill-fitting denture may impair your health—consult your dentist for periodic examination.

Products that currently meet ADA criteria are Benefit Denture Adhesive Powder, Corega Powder, Firmdent, Orahesive Powder, Perma-Grip Powder, Super Wernet's Denture Adhesive Powder, Wernet's Cream, and Wernet's Powder With Neoseal (26).

Unsupervised chronic denture adhesive use may cause malfitting dentures to stimulate more rapid destruction of supportive bone and produce infection or pathologies of the gingiva from irritation.

Products for Temporary Use

Denture Reliners and Cushions

A number of patients, feeling perhaps that their dentures are not fitting well or are causing irritation, resort to the use of denture reliners or cushions; they do so at great risk. A series of articles has appeared in the dental and medical literature pointing out that long-term use of such products distorts dentures, causing bite problems and jaw–joint pain (35–43). Furthermore, an unevenly fitting denture causes excessive pressure in many areas of the jaw bone, resulting in eventual bone resorption, and in some cases may actually obliterate the ridge of bone on which the denture rests. If this should happen, some drastic and expensive dental procedures will be required to remedy the situation. The following products were specifically cited in the aforementioned studies: Cushion Grip, Dentyte, Ezo Dento Cushions, and Brimms' Plasti-Liner.

One investigator has stated that anyone who finds it necessary to use an OTC denture reliner actually needs new dentures, and that these products should be totally discouraged, perhaps by making them prescription-only items (39). To discourage their home use, the ADA Bureau of Dental Health Education has published a consumer pamphlet entitled, "Don't Do It Yourself." The FDA requires that the following labeling appear on denture reliners, pads, and cushions (44):

> Warning. For temporary use only. Long-term use of this product may lead to faster bone loss, continuing irritation, sores, and tumors. For use only until a dentist can be seen.

Denture Repair Kits

A denture repair kit is another potentially dangerous OTC denture accessory. Composed of special glues and supporting materials, these items are indicated as useful in the repair of cracked or broken dentures. However, careful measurements by skilled professionals are required to align a new denture properly. Home-repaired dentures are always misaligned, a factor leading to poor fit and bone resorption (42). If items such as these are to be sold, the pharmacist should caution the patient that these products are for temporary (e.g., over the weekend) repairs only and should make certain that the patient fully understands the meaning of the following message which the FDA requires be published on the kit label (44):

> Warning. For emergency repairs only. Long-term use of home-repaired dentures may cause faster bone loss, continuing irritation, sores, and tumors. See your dentist without delay.

Products Providing Symptomatic Relief

OTC dental products in this category are of limited merit and utility, since they do not prevent or cure underlying oral pathologies. Patients should be cautioned that such preparations should be used only on a temporary basis and a dentist should be consulted if symptoms persist.

Cold Sore Products

Oral sores result from various causes, and secondary infection may occur when sores become ulcerated. Patients should be advised to seek dental treatment in cases of sores that do not heal rapidly.

Herpetic lesions (cold sores and fever blisters) take about 14 days to heal regardless of treatment, and they may recur. Herpes virus therapy should consist of making the patient as comfortable as possible and attempting to prevent further complications by cleansing with a drying agent (e.g., alcohol) and covering the area with a protective product (Orabase or a denture adhesive). Use of products such as astringents, anesthetics, antibiotics, antiseptics, and silver nitrate is irrational and may cause further irritation. The claim that *Lactobacillus*-containing preparations (e.g., Lactinex) prevent or cure herpes is unfounded (45).

Topical Anesthetics

Oral pain is a prominent sign and symptom of tissue destruction in the mouth, and it may be a powerful motivator to seeking proper dental treatment. Masking or attenuating oral pain may help make the patient feel more comfortable, but it will never stop the progression of disease that causes it.

Most commercial preparations that claim to subdue oral pain are topical anesthetics. These poultices, pastes, drops, and lotions contain ingredients such as benzyl alcohol, benzocaine, camphor, dyclonine hydrochloride, eugenol (clove oil), hexylresorcinol, menthol, and phenol. Only dyclonine and benzocaine, which are related to the local anesthetics given in dental injections, are recognized by both the ADA (46) and the FDA (47) as being safe and effective in OTC products producing local analgesia. (Some of the other ingredients may actually irritate damaged tissue.) Even these agents have limited utility in oral OTC products. Both may inhibit the gag reflex if swallowed, and poor submucosal tissue penetration does not allow them to reach the source of pain produced by teething. Benzocaine also may cause hypersensitivity (allergic) reactions (48).

In many instances, better results are achieved when oral pain is treated by short-term use of systemic antipyretic analgesics (e.g., aspirin or acetaminophen) until a dentist can be consulted. This therapy is particularly beneficial for common toothache because no topical drug can be absorbed entirely into the affected tooth pulp. Patients should not use aspirin inappropriately as a lozenge or poultice applied to the involved area. This fairly common custom not only is therapeutically irrational but may be hazardous because topical aspirin use may produce tissue traumatization via a chemical burn (49). Pharmacists should always recommend that aspirin be taken internally for dental pain.

temporary relief of oral pain

Oral Antiseptics

mouthwashes and "bad breath"

Next to toothbrushes and dentifrices, the most commonly used OTC dental products are mouthwashes. According to promotional claims, "bad breath" is a major cause of social unpopularity, and thus mouthwashes are necessary to social success. This type of cosmetic claim is harmless in itself; the danger lies in ignoring the possible cause of halitosis by masking the symptom (for example, chronic halitosis may result from oral infection or diabetes) and assuming that the "germ-killing" properties of mouthwashes will treat infections.

Most mouthwashes contain potentially antiseptic ingredients, such as alcohol, phenolic compounds, volatile oils, iodinated substances, and the newer quaternary ammonium compounds, but they are present in concentrations too small to be germicidally effective. Comparative in vitro tests with normal, nonpathogenic saliva indicate superiority of the quaternary ammonium products (50); however, in vivo studies are lacking. The ADA does not endorse any mouthwash as producing significant oral antisepsis and suggests that the use of these products to treat severe infections may be hazardous (27).

The "ideal" mouthwash should contain a high antiseptic concentration to kill the rapidly proliferating oral bacteria. Unfortunately, such a dose may be either locally irritating to tissue or systemically toxic if swallowed. In addition, nonspecificity of germicidal action may lead to microorganism overgrowth and bacterial resistance. Thus manufacturers opt for the relative safety of subtherapeutic formulations.

Occasionally, dentists recommend certain mouthwashes for specific purposes. Products containing zinc chloride are used in dental practice as astringents to decrease bleeding or irritation temporarily. Patients may gargle with saline rinses to make themselves more comfortable after dental surgery. Hydrogen peroxide (diluted with water) and similar peroxide products (e.g., Glyoxide or Proxigel) may help cleanse and debride minor wounds or sores; peroxide use, however, should be limited to 10 days because of its tissue-irritating potential.

SUMMARY

The FDA OTC Panels on Dentifrices and Dental Care Agents and on Oral Cavity Drug Products are making a concerted effort to rectify many of the problems discussed in this chapter. They have already recommended that certain toxic substances (e.g., boric acid, creosol, and mercurial compounds) be removed from oral OTC products because of high ingestion liability or topical irritation potential. They also are classifying ingredients according to effectiveness and are setting dosage and concentration ranges based on the latest clinical safety evidence. Guidelines have been suggested for the in vivo testing of controversial products such as antiseptics and anesthetics, and labeling standards are being established to ensure that product limitations are being taken into account and to avoid misleading claims.

Pharmacists may want to keep abreast of advances in the oral field, and pertinent literature is available from the American Dental Association. In particular, a pamphlet, "The Dentist and the Pharmacist," and the current edition of *Accepted Dental Therapeutics*, containing a detailed listing of ADA-approved drugs and products, may be helpful. Patient-oriented information also may be obtained for distribution.

Preventive dental care is one of the most important health issues facing Americans today, and pharmacists should be part of it. By establishing an oral hygiene center—a prominent display of oral products such as dental floss and other effective plaque-removing devices—and counseling patients on proper dental care, the pharmacist can assume the role of professional health consultant.

REFERENCES

(1) "The Health of Americans," B. Jones, Ed., Prentice Hall, Englewood Cliffs, N.J., 1970, p. 15.
(2) D. M. Wilner, R. P. Walkley, and L. S. Goerke, "Introduction to Public Health," 6th ed., Macmillan, New York, N.Y., 1973, p. 385.
(3) R. Tunley, "The American Health Scandal," Dell, New York, N.Y., 1966, p. 56.
(4) "The Health of Americans," B. Jones, Ed., Prentice Hall, Englewood Cliffs, N.J., 1970, p. 15.
(5) American Dental Association/American Pharmaceutical Association Liaison Committee, "The Dentist and the Pharmacist" (pamphlet), American Dental Association, Chicago, Ill., 1970, p. 1.
(6) "Oral Microbiology," W. Nolte, Ed., Mosby, St. Louis, Mo., 1968, pp. 9–21.
(7) Consumers Union, "The Medicine Show," Pantheon, New York, N.Y., 1974, pp. 54–75.
(8) N. Cranin, "The Modern Family Guide to Dental Health," Stein & Day, New York, N.Y., 1973, p. 72.
(9) D. A. M. Geddes, *Arch. Oral. Biol.*, *17*, 537 (1972).
(10) Council on Dental Therapeutics, "Accepted Dental Therapeutics," 37th ed., American Dental Association, Chicago, Ill., 1977, p. 242.
(11) R. G. Campbell and D. D. Zinner, *J. Nutr.*, *100*, 11 (1970).
(12) Council on Dental Therapeutics, "Accepted Dental Therapeutics," 37th ed., American Dental Association, Chicago, Ill., 1977, p. 285.
(13) D. R. Weathers and J. W. Griffin, *J. Am. Dent. Assoc.*, *81*, 81 (1970).
(14) T. C. Francis, *Oral Surg.*, *30*, 476 (1970).
(15) F. L. Horsfall and T. Tamm, "Viral and Rickettsial Infections of Man," 4th ed., Lippincott, Philadelphia, Pa., 1965, p. 892.
(16) P. N. Baer and S. B. Benjamin, "Periodontal Disease in Children and Adolescents," Lippincott, Philadelphia, Pa., 1974, p. 37.
(17) M. Krupp and M. Chatton, "Current Medical Diagnosis and Treatment," Lange Medical, Los Altos, Calif., 1976, p. 331.
(18) *Ibid.*, p. 333.
(19) K. Lewis and E. Lewis, *U.S. Pharm.*, *2*, 33 (May 1977).
(20) L. Flotra, P. Gjermo, R. Rölla, and J. Waerhaug, *Scand. J. Dent. Res.*, *7*, 180 (1972).
(21) Council on Dental Therapeutics, "Accepted Dental Therapeutics," 37th ed., American Dental Association, Chicago, Ill., 1977, p. 283.
(22) J. D. Suomi, *J. Am. Dent. Assoc.*, *83*, 1271 (1971).
(23) A. Green, S. N. Rosenstein, A. Parks, and A. H. Kutscher, *J. Dent. Child.*, *29*, 169 (1962).
(24) Council on Dental Therapeutics, *J. Am. Dent. Assoc.*, *81*, 1177 (1970).
(25) Council on Dental Therapeutics, "Accepted Dental Therapeutics," 37th ed., American Dental Association, Chicago, Ill., 1977, p. 311.
(26) *Pharmacy Times*, *43*, 74 (July 1977).
(27) Council on Dental Therapeutics, "Accepted Dental Therapeutics," 35th ed., American Dental Association, Chicago, Ill., 1973, p. 313.
(28) *Medical World News* (June 28, 1974).
(29) Council on Dental Materials and Devices, "Guide to Dental Materials and Devices," 7th ed., American Dental Association, Chicago, Ill., 1974–1975, p. 152.
(30) "Summary Minutes of the FDA OTC Panel on Dentifrices and Dental Care Agents," 8th meeting, Washington, D.C., 1974, p. 11.
(31) J. R. Elliott, *J. Periodontol.*, *43*, 217 (1972).
(32) Council on Dental Materials and Devices, *J. Am. Dent. Assoc.*, *90*, 181 (1975).
(33) A. R. Romans and G. R. App, *J. Periodontol.*, *42*, 757 (1971).
(34) M. S. Drapkin, *Ann. Intern. Med.*, *87*, 455 (1977).
(35) R. B. Lytle, *Dent. Prog.*, *1*, 221 (1961).
(36) J. B. Woelfel, J. A. Kreider, and T. Berg, Jr., *J. Am. Dent. Assoc.*, *64*, 763 (1962).
(37) J. D. Larkin, *Tex. Dent. J.*, *82*, 9 (1964).
(38) C. R. Means, *J. Prosthet. Dent.*, *14*, 623, 935, 1086 (1964).
(39) J. B. Woelfel, C. M. Winter, and R. L. Curry, *J. Am. Dent. Assoc.*, *71*, 603 (1965).
(40) J. B. Woelfel, T. Berg, Jr., A. W. Mann, and J. A. Kreider, *J. Am. Dent. Assoc.*, *71*, 23 (1965).
(41) *Journal of the American Medical Association*, *191*, 962 (1965).
(42) C. M. Winter, *Ohio Dent. J.*, *40*, 227 (1966).
(43) Council on Dental Research/Council on Dental Therapeutics, *J. Am. Dent. Assoc.*, *47*, 214 (1953).
(44) *Federal Register*, *34*, 14167 (1969).
(45) Council on Dental Therapeutics, "Accepted Dental Therapeutics," 37th ed., American Dental Association, Chicago, Ill., 1977, p. 258.
(46) *Ibid.*, pp. 106–109.
(47) "Summary Minutes of the FDA OTC Panel on Oral Cavity Drug Products," 14th meeting, Washington, D.C., 1976, pp. 3–5.
(48) Council on Dental Therapeutics, "Accepted Dental Therapeutics," 37th ed., American Dental Association, Chicago, Ill., 1977, p. 106.
(49) H. M. Clarman, *J. Am. Med. Assoc.*, *202*, 651 (1967).
(50) "Handbook of Non-Prescription Drugs," 2nd ed., APhA, Washington, D.C., 1971, p. 105.

Product (Manufacturer)	Abrasive Ingredients	Therapeutic Ingredient	Foaming Agent	Inert and Miscellaneous Ingredients
Aim (Lever Bros)	hydrated silica	stannous fluoride, 0.4%	sodium lauryl sulfate	alcohol, sorbitol, glycerin, polyethylene glycol 32, saccharin sodium, sodium benzoate, cellulose gum, flavor
Amosan (Cooper)	—	—	—	sodium peroxyborate monohydrate, sodium bitartrate
Aqua-Fresh (Beecham)	silica calcium carbonate calcium glycerophosphate	sodium monofluorophosphate	sodium lauryl sulfate	sorbitol, polyethylene glycol 8, cellulose gum
Caroid Tooth Powder (Winthrop)	not stated	—	—	papain
Chloresium (Rystan)	not stated	—	—	chlorophyll
Close-Up (Lever Bros)	hydrated silica sodium phosphate disodium phosphate	—	sodium lauryl sulfate	sorbitol, glycerin, polyethylene glycol 32, alcohol, saccharin sodium, cellulose gum, sodium benzoate, flavor
Colgate with MFP (Colgate-Palmolive)	not stated	sodium monofluorophosphate	—	not stated
Crest (Procter & Gamble)	calcium pyrophosphate stannous pyrophosphate	stannous fluoride, 0.40%	—	cellulose gum, glycerin, sorbitol, flavor
Depend (Warner-Lambert)	sodium phosphate disodium phosphate	—	—	alcohol, 23.8%; sorbitol; glycerin; polysorbate 80; saccharin sodium; caramel; flavor
Extar (Extar)	magnesium oxide calcium carbonate sodium polymetaphosphate silica gel	—	sodium lauryl sulfate	tragacanth, saccharin sodium, spralene mint, mint oil, flavor, menthol
Extar Dentifrice Powder (Extar)	sodium polymetaphosphate sodium phosphate	—	—	sequestrene, saccharin sodium
Gleem (Procter & Gamble)	calcium pyrophosphate	sodium fluoride, 0.22%	blend of anionic surfactants	glycerin, sorbitol, cellulose gum, flavor
Ipana (La Maur)	not stated	stannous fluoride	—	not stated
Listerine (Warner-Lambert)	dicalcium phosphate	—	—	not stated
Listermint (Warner-Lambert)	—	—	—	alcohol, 12.8%; glycerin; poloxamer 407; polysorbate 80; saccharin sodium; zinc chloride; saccharin; flavor
Macleans (Beecham)	dicalcium phosphate dihydrate calcium carbonate	—	—	glycerin
Macleans Fluoride Toothpaste (Beecham)	calcium carbonate, 38% magnesium aluminum silicate	sodium monofluorophosphate, 0.76%	sodium lauryl sulfate, 1.15%	glycerin, 26%
NDK Liquid (NDK Co.)	—	fluorophosphate	—	benzethonium chloride
Pearl Drops Liquid (Carter)	dicalcium phosphate aluminum hydroxide	—	—	sorbitol, carboxymethylcellulose
Pepsodent (Lever Bros)	alumina hydrated silica dicalcium phosphate	—	sodium lauryl sulfate	sorbitol, glycerin, polyethylene glycol 32, cellulose gum, titanium dioxide, saccharin sodium, sodium benzoate, flavor

Toothpaste Products

Product (Manufacturer)	Abrasive Ingredients	Therapeutic Ingredient	Foaming Agent	Inert and Miscellaneous Ingredients
Pepsodent Ammoniated Tooth Powder (Lever Bros)	sodium metaphosphate tricalcium phosphate	—	sodium lauryl sulfate	diammonium phosphate, urea, polyethylene glycol, carrageenan, saccharin, flavor
Pepsodent Tooth Powder (Lever Bros)	sodium metaphosphate dicalcium phosphate magnesium trisilicate	—	sodium lauryl sulfate	polyethylene glycol, carrageenan, saccharin, flavor
Pycopay Tooth Powder (Block)	sodium chloride sodium bicarbonate calcium carbonate magnesium carbonate tricalcium phosphate	—	—	flavor
Revelation Tooth Powder (Alvin Last)	calcium carbonate	—	soap	menthol, methyl salicylate
Sensodyne (Block)	not stated	—	—	strontium chloride
Thermodent (Leeming)	magnesium carbonate calcium carbonate sodium chloride	—	—	potassium sulfate, formaldehyde, sodium sulfate

Denture Cleanser Products

Product (Manufacturer)	Ingredients
Complete (Vicks)	calcium carbonate, glycerin, sorbitol, cellulose gum, sodium lauryl sulfate, silica, magnesium aluminum silicate, flavor
Denalan (Whitehall)	sodium peroxide, 9.5%; sodium chloride, 90%
Efferdent Tablets (Warner-Lambert)	potassium monopersulfate, 960 mg; sodium borate perhydrate, 480 mg; sodium carbonate; sodium lauryl sulfoacetate; sodium bicarbonate, 1.116 g; citric acid, 362 mg; magnesium stearate; simethicone
Effervescent Denture Tablets (Rexall)	sodium bicarbonate, citric acid, sodium perborate, sodium acid pyrophosphate, sodium benzoate, trisodium phosphate, sodium lauryl sulfate, poloxamer 188, sorbitol, silica, peppermint oil, povidone
Extar Denture Cleanser (Extar)	sodium polymetaphosphate, saccharin sodium, methylparaben, propylparaben, peppermint, sodium phosphate, sequestrene, lactose
K.I.K. (K.I.K. Co.)	sodium perborate, 25%; trisodium phosphate, 75%
Kleenite (Vicks)	sodium chloride, trisodium phosphate, sodium perborate, sodium dichloroisocyanurate dihydrate, sodium lauryl sulfate, edetate disodium, flavor
Mersene Denture Cleaner (Colgate-Palmolive)	troclosene potassium, sodium perborate, trisodium phosphate
Polident Denture Cleanser Powder (Block)	sodium perborate, potassium monopersulfate, sodium carbonate, sodium tripolyphosphate, surfactant, sodium bicarbonate, flavor
Polident Tablets (Block)	potassium monopersulfate, sodium perborate, sodium carbonate, surfactant, sodium bicarbonate, citric acid, flavor

Toothache/Cold Sore/Canker Sore Products

Product (Manufacturer)	Anesthetic	Other Ingredients
Anbesol (Whitehall)	benzocaine	iodine; glycerin; alcohol, 40%
Baby Orajel (Commerce)	benzocaine	viscous water-soluble base
Benzodent (Vicks)	benzocaine, 20% eugenol, 0.4%	hydroxyquinoline sulfate, 0.1%; denture adhesivelike base
Betadine Mouthwash/Gargle (Purdue Frederick)	—	povidone-iodine, 0.5%; alcohol, 8.8%

Product (Manufacturer)	Anesthetic	Other Ingredients
Blistex Ointment (Blistex)	—	phenol, 0.4%; camphor, 1%; ammonia; mineral oil; lanolin; petrolatum; paraffin, sodium borate; alcohol; peppermint oil; ammonium carbonate; fragrance; beeswax; polyglyceryl-3, diisostearate
Butyn Dental Ointment (Abbott)	butacaine, 4%	not stated
Cold Sore Lotion (Pfeiffer)	—	camphor, 3.6%; gum benzoin, 4.2%; phenol, 0.3%; menthol, 0.3%, alcohol, 85%; thymol; peruvian balsam
Dalidyne (Dalin)	benzocaine	methylbenzethonium chloride; tannic acid; camphor; chlorothymol; menthol; benzyl alcohol; alcohol, 61%; aromatic base
Dr. Hands Teething Gel and Lotion (Roberts)	clove oil	tincture of pellitory; menthol; hamamelis water; alcohol, 10%
Jiffy (Block)	benzocaine eugenol	alcohol, 56.5%
Kank-a (Blistex)	—	alcohol, myrrh, benzoin storax, balsa tolu, aloe
Numzident (Purepac)	benzocaine eugenol	peppermint oil, polyethylene glycollike base
Numzit (Purepac)	—	glycerin; alcohol, 10%; gel vehicle
Orabase Plain (Hoyt)	—	pectin, gelatin, carboxymethylcellulose sodium, polyethylene glycol, mineral oil
Orabase with Benzocaine (Hoyt)	benzocaine	pectin, gelatin, carboxymethylcellulose sodium, polyethylene glycol, mineral oil
Orajel (Commerce)	benzocaine	polyethylene glycollike base
Ora-Jel-D (Commerce)	benzocaine clove oil	benzyl alcohol, adhesive base
Pain-A-Lay (Roberts)	—	boric acid, cresol
Proxigel (Reed & Carnrick)	—	urea carbamide, gel vehicle
Rid-A-Pain (Pfeiffer)	benzocaine, 10%	alcohol, 7.5%
Rexall Cold Sore Lotion (Rexall)	—	phenol; benzoin; camphor; menthol; alcohol, 90%
Rexall Cold Sore Ointment (Rexall)	—	phenol; benzoin; camphor; menthol; alcohol, 30%; viscous base
Tanac (Commerce)	—	benzalkonium chloride, tannic acid
Teething Lotion (DeWitt)	benzocaine, 5.6%	propylene glycol, 44%; glycerin, 29%; benzyl alcohol, 2.5%; tincture of myrrh, 4.5%; alcohol
Toothache Drops (DeWitt)	benzocaine, 5.01% clove oil, 9.98%	beechwood creosote, 4.83%; flexible collodion (base); alcohol, 20%

Denture Adhesive Products

Product (Manufacturer)	Ingredients
Confident (Block)	carboxymethylcellulose gum, 32%; ethylene oxide polymer, 13%; petrolatum, 42%; liquid petrolatum, 12%; propylparaben, 0.05%
Corega Powder (Block)	karaya gum, 94.6%; water-soluble ethylene oxide polymer, 5%; flavor, 0.4%
Effergrip Denture Adhesive Cream (Warner-Lambert)	carboxymethylcellulose sodium, 39%; cationic polyacrylamide polymer, 10%
Effergrip Denture Adhesive Powder (Warner-Lambert)	carboxymethylcellulose sodium, 40%; cationic polyacrylamide polymer, 10%
Fasteeth (Vicks)	karaya gum, sodium borate
Firmdent (Moyco)	karaya gum, 94.6%; sodium tetraborate, 5.36%; powdered flavor essence of peppermint, 0.04%
Fixodent (Vicks)	calcium sodium poly(vinyl methyl ether maleate), petrolatum base
Orafix (Norcliff Thayer)	karaya gum, 51%; petrolatum, 30%; mineral oil, 13%; peppermint oil, 0.08%

Denture Adhesive Products

Product (Manufacturer)	Ingredients
Orafix Medicated (Norcliff Thayer)	karaya gum, 51%; benzocaine, 2%; allantoin, 0.2%; petrolatum, 28%; mineral oil, 13%; peppermint oil, 0.08%
Orafix Special (Norcliff Thayer)	cellulose gum, 25%; methyl vinyl ether–maleic anhydride and/or acid copolymer, 15%; povidone, 10%; petrolatum, 34.9%; mineral oil, 14.9%; flavor, 0.2%
Orahesive Powder (Hoyt)	gelatin, 33.3%; pectin, 33.3%; carboxymethylcellulose sodium, 33.3%
Perma-Grip Powder (Lactona)	polyethylene wax, 50.9%; carboxymethylcellulose sodium, 39.0%; cationic acrylic polymer, 10.0%; flavor
Polident Dentu-Grip (Block)	carboxymethylcellulose gum, 49%; ethylene oxide polymer, 21%; flavor, 0.4%
Poli-Grip (Block)	karaya gum, 51%; petrolatum, 36.7%; liquid petrolatum, 9.4%; magnesium oxide, 2.7%; propylparaben; flavor
Wernet's Cream (Block)	carboxymethylcellulose gum, 32%; petrolatum, 42%; liquid petrolatum, 12%; ethylene oxide polymer, 13%; propylparaben, 0.05%; flavor, 0.5%
Wernet's Powder (Block)	karaya gum, 94.6%; water-soluble ethylene oxide polymer, 5%; flavor, 0.4%

Mouthwash Products

Product (Manufacturer)	Antiseptic	Anesthetic	Astringent	Other Ingredients
Astring-O-Sol (Winthrop)	alcohol, 70%	—	zinc chloride	myrrh, methyl salicylate
Cépacol (Merrell-National)	alcohol, 14% cetylpyridinium chloride, 1:2000	—	—	phosphate buffers, aromatics
Cépastat (Merrell-National)	phenol, 1.4%	eugenol	—	menthol, glycerin
Cherry Chloraseptic Mouthwash and Gargle (Norwich-Eaton)	phenol sodium phenolate	—	—	—
Chloraseptic Mouthwash (Norwich-Eaton)	phenol sodium phenolate	—	—	—
Chlorazene Aromatic Powder (for solution) (Wisconsin Pharmacal)	chloramine-T, 5% eucalyptol	—	—	sodium chloride, 88%; sodium bicarbonate, 5%; saccharin sodium
Colgate 100 (Colgate-Palmolive)	alcohol, 15%	—	—	not stated
Fluorigard (Colgate-Palmolive)	—	—	—	sodium fluoride, 0.05%
Forma-Zincol Concentrate (Ingram)	formaldehyde	—	zinc chloride	anise oil, menthol
Gly-Oxide (International Pharmaceutical)	carbamide peroxide, 10%	—	—	anhydrous glycerin, flavor
Greenmint Mouthwash (Block)	alcohol	—	—	chlorophyll, sorbitol, surfactant, flavor
Isodine Mouthwash Gargle Concentrate (Blair)	alcohol, 35% povidone-iodine, 7.5%	—	—	—
Kasdenol Powder (Kasdenol)	available chlorine 5–6% (as oxychlorosene)	—	—	not stated
Lavoris (Vicks)	alcohol	clove oil	zinc chloride	glycerin, polysorbate 80, citric acid, flavors, poloxamer 407
Listerine (Warner-Lambert)	alcohol benzoic acid	—	—	menthol, methyl salicylate, poloxamer 407, caramel, eucalyptol, thymol
Mouthwash and Gargle (McKesson)	cetylpyridinium chloride alcohol, 14%	—	—	not stated

Product (Manufacturer)	Antiseptic	Anesthetic	Astringent	Other Ingredients
Odara (Lorvic)	phenol, 2% alcohol, 48%	—	zinc chloride	glycerin, potassium iodide, methyl salicylate, eucalyptus oil, myrrh tincture
Oral Pentacresol (Upjohn)	secondary amyltricresols, 1 mg/ml alcohol, 30%	—	—	sodium chloride, 8.61 mg/ml; calcium chloride, 0.33 mg/ml; potassium chloride, 0.299 mg/ml
Proxigel (Reed & Carnick)	carbamide peroxide, 11%	—	—	anhydrous glycerin, thickeners, flavor
Scope (Procter & Gamble)	cetylpyridinium chloride domiphen bromide, 0.005% alcohol, 18.5%	—	—	glycerin, saccharin, polysorbate 80, flavor
S.T. 37 (Calgon)	hexylresorcinol, 0.1%	—	—	glycerin
Vince Oxygenating Oral Rinse and Dentifrice (Warner-Lambert)	sodium perborate monohydrate-perborax	—	—	calcium carbonate, magnesium trisilicate, tribasic calcium phosphate

Insect Sting and Bite Products

Farid Sadik

Chapter 22

Questions to Ask the Patient

Do you have a personal or family history of allergic reactions such as hay fever?

Have you previously had severe reactions to insect stings or bites?

How extensive are the stings or bites on your body?

If the patient is not an adult, what is the age and approximate weight of the patient?

Have you developed hives, excessive swelling, dizziness, vomiting, or difficulty in breathing since being bitten or stung?

Have you ever had adverse reactions to topically applied products?

Many people die from and many more are treated for severe systemic reactions to insect stings. Accurate statistics on the number of Americans who succumb annually to insect bites and stings are lacking. However, evidence indicates that there are more yearly deaths from insect stings than from other venomous insects and animals, including snakes (1).

An insect sting or bite is an injury to the skin caused by penetration of the stinging or biting organ of an insect. The reactions that follow are produced mainly by substances contained in the venom of stinging insects or in the saliva of biting insects. Allergic reactions also may occur. Although the pain associated with skin penetration by the stinging or biting organ is brief, the aftereffects vary considerably. Reactions in nonallergic individuals usually are confined to the site of the sting or bite, whereas in allergic individuals the reaction may be local and systemic.

TYPES OF INJURIES

Stinging Insects

Stinging insects, which include bees, wasps, hornets, yellow jackets, and ants, belong to the order Hymenoptera (membranous wings). Although they are small, these insects have a venom that is, drop for drop, as potent as that of snakes and faster acting. Death caused by an insect sting results from an anaphylactic reaction and usually comes within minutes, whereas death from snake bite is usually not associated with hypersensitivity and occurs within 3 hours to several days.

The stinging insects inject the venom into their victims' bodies through a piercing organ (stinger), a specialized ovipositor delicately attached to the rear of the female's abdomen. (Males have no ovipositor and consequently are stingless.) The stinger consists of two lancets, made of highly chitinous material, separated by the poison canal. The venom flows through the canal from the venom sac attached to the stinger's dorsal section. The tip of the stinger, which is directed posteriorly, has sharp barbs, and the base enlarges into a bulblike structure. Most species of bees and wasps have two types of venom glands under the last abdominal segment. The larger gland secretes an acidic toxin directly into the venom sac; the smaller one, at the base of the sac, secretes a less potent alkaline toxin.

Honeybees

When the honeybee attacks, it attaches firmly to the skin with tiny, sharp claws at the tip of each foot, then arches its abdomen and immediately jabs the barbed stinger into the skin. Because of the barbs the stinger remains firmly embedded, and when the honeybee pulls away or is brushed off, the entire stinging apparatus (stinger, appendages, venom sac, and glands) is detached from the bee's abdomen. The disemboweled bee later dies. The abandoned stinger, driven deeper into the skin by rhythmic contractions of the venom sac's smooth muscle wall, continues to inject venom.

Other Stinging Insects

The stinging mechanism of wasps, hornets, yellow jackets, and bumblebees is basically the same as that of the honeybee. The main difference is that their stingers are not barbed. The stingers can be withdrawn easily after injecting the venom, enabling these insects to survive and sting repeatedly.

Ants

Ants use their mandibles to cling to the skin of their prey, then bend their abdomen, sting the flesh, and empty the contents of their poison vesicle into the wound (2). Because they use their mandibles, it is often believed erroneously that the bite causes the reaction.

Biting Insects

Insects such as mosquitoes, fleas, lice, bedbugs, ticks, and chiggers ("red bugs") bite (inject) their prey. They insert their biting organs into the skin to feed by sucking blood from their hosts.

Mosquitoes

Mosquitoes usually attack exposed parts of the body, face, neck, forearms, and legs, but they also may bite through thin clothing. When a mosquito alights on the skin, it starts to feed by cutting the skin with its mandibles and maxillae. A fine, hollow, needlelike, flexible structure (proboscis) is introduced into the cut and probes the tissue for a blood vessel. Blood is sucked directly from a capillary lumen or from previously lacerated capillaries with extravasated blood (3). During feeding, the mosquito injects into the wound a salivary secretion containing antigenic components, which cause the itching reaction.

various biting insects and their effects

parasites

reactions to insect attacks

Fleas

Fleas are tiny (1.5–4 mm long), bloodsucking, wingless parasites with strongly developed posterior legs used for leaping. They are found throughout the world (including Arctic regions) but breed best in warm areas with relatively high humidity. Fleas bite covered parts of the body; their bites usually are multiple and grouped and cause intense itching. Each lesion is characterized by an erythematous region around the puncture. Fleas not only are annoying, but also are responsible for transmitting diseases such as bubonic plague and endemic typhus. They may be carried into the home on pets or on clothing from flea-infested places, and they may survive and multiply without food for several weeks. In many cases, places that have been vacant for weeks are heavily infested, partly owing to the hatching of eggs.

Bedbugs

Bedbugs have a short head and a broad, flat body (4–5 mm long and 3 mm wide). Their mouth parts consist of two pairs of stylets used to pierce the skin. The outer pair has barbs that saw the skin, and the inner pair is used to suck blood and to allow salivary secretions to flow into the wound.

Ticks

Ticks are parasites that attack human and domestic animals and feed on the blood of their hosts. During feeding, the tick's mouth parts are introduced into the skin, enabling it to hold firmly. If the tick is removed, mouth parts are torn from the tick's body and remain embedded, causing intense itching and nodules. These parts should be removed by applying heat. If the tick is left attached to the skin, it becomes fully engorged with blood and remains as long as 10 days before it drops off.

Chiggers

Chiggers are prevalent in the southern part of the United States mainly during summer and fall. Only the larvae, which are nearly microscopic, attack the host by attaching to the skin and sucking blood. Once in contact with the skin, the larvae insert their mouth parts into the skin and secrete a digestive fluid which causes cellular disintegration of the affected area and intense itching.

Parasitic Infestation

Scabies

The mite causing scabies does not bite or sting. Also called "the itch," scabies is a contagious parasitic skin infestation caused by the mite *Sarcoptes scabiei,* which burrows beneath the stratum corneum. Characterized by secondary inflammation and intense itching, this infestation is associated with poor hygiene and crowded conditions. The female mite, which is responsible for causing scabies, is transmitted readily by close personal contact with an infected person. Once on the skin, the impregnated female burrows into the stratum corneum with her jaws and the first two pairs of legs, forming tunnels in which she lays eggs and excretes fecal matter. In a few days the hatched larvae form their own burrows and develop into adults. They copulate, and the impregnated females burrow into the stratum corneum to start a new life cycle. The most common infestation sites are the interdigital spaces of the fingers, the flexor surface of the wrists, the external male genitalia, the buttocks, and the anterior axillary folds. The head and neck are not affected, except in infants.

Lice

Lice are wingless parasites with well-developed legs. Each leg has a claw that helps the louse cling firmly to the skin while sucking blood. Three types of lice attack humans: head lice, body lice, and pubic lice. As their name implies, head lice usually infest the head, but they are found on other hairy parts of the body as well. The female deposits 50–150 eggs (nits), which become glued to the hair and hatch in 5–10 days. Body lice live, hide, and lay their eggs in clothing, particularly in seams and folds of underclothing, and they generally infest crowded environments. Pubic lice, commonly called crab lice because of their crablike appearance, may be encountered in patients from all social and economic strata and standards of hygiene. Crab lice infest the pubic area and armpits and occasionally eyelashes, mustaches, beards, and eyebrows.

Lice cause individuals to develop an immediate wheal around the bite. A local delayed papular reaction appears within 24 hours. Itching and subsequent scratching result in excoriation or secondary pyogenic infections.

ALLERGIC REACTIONS TO STINGS

Antigens

The immediate itching and local inflammatory reaction to an insect bite are due to vasoactive constituents in the insect venom. In susceptible individuals, subsequent allergic reactions to insect stings and bites are caused by antigenic proteins in the venom of the stinging insects and in the salivary secretions of the biting insects.

Bee venom is a combination of acidic and alkaline venom gland secretions. The secretions, which flow separately from each gland, are mixed in the stinger's venom canal before they are injected. Bee venom contains histamine and three protein fractions (4).

Wasp venom contains histamine, 5-hydroxytryptamine (serotonin), and hyaluronidase, a substance that dissolves intracellular cement to allow greater venomous penetration (5). Hornet venom contains 5-hydroxytryptamine, histamine, and acetylcholine (4). The poison of ants of the Formica family contains formic acid and 17 free amino acids.

Some species of mosquitoes have agglutinin and anticoagulant agents in their salivary secretions; others have neither (6). Many attempts have been made to identify the antigenic factors in mosquito bites by studying whole mosquito extracts. Extracts from *Aedes aegypti* were shown by paper chromatography to contain at least four fractions that can produce skin reactions (7). Chromatographic fractionation of whole extracts showed that the antigenic principle contained four constituents. Eluates of each constituent caused positive reactions in sensitized individuals (8). Eighteen amino acids have been identified in the extracts of all species of mosquitoes (9).

Sensitization

There are definite stages in acquiring sensitization to mosquito bites. An experiment with 25 volunteers who previously had not been bitten by the species *A. aegypti* divided the subjects' reactions into four stages (10).

The degree and kind of reaction depend mainly on the history of exposure to bites and on the present stage of sensitization. Stage I (incubation) begins after the first bite. The bite does not cause an immediate cutaneous reaction or itching because no previous sensitization has occurred. However, in about 24 hours a papular reaction accompanied by itching occurs at the site of the bite. As biting is repeated over time, sensitization increases. An allergic state now exists. In Stage II a reaction characterized by a wheal surrounded by erythema and accompanied by itching, heat, and pain occurs during or immediately after the mosquito has bitten. These symptoms usually subside within 2 hours. A delayed papular reaction occurs about 24 hours later. With regular exposure to bites the delayed reaction gradually starts to diminish (Stage III) and eventually disappears; however, the immediate reaction continues during or after each bite. Stage IV, which is uncommon, is marked by the absence of either immediate or delayed reaction following a bite. The stage occurs only after regular exposure to many bites over a period of years. Because desensitization is transient, Stage IV is replaced by Stage III if exposure to bites is irregular.

The reactions to other biting insects, such as fleas, bedbugs, ticks, and chiggers, resemble mosquito bite reactions.

Signs and Symptoms

The intensity of the allergic reactions to venomous insect stings varies significantly. The thrust of the stinger into the flesh causes a sharp pain. The reaction that follows may be one or more of the following: localized irritation, itching, swelling, generalized urticaria, feeling of heat and flushing of the skin, excessive perspiration, vomiting, fainting, respiratory distress, choking sensation, and loss of consciousness or death from anaphylactic shock. Temporary paralysis has occurred following tick bites (11).

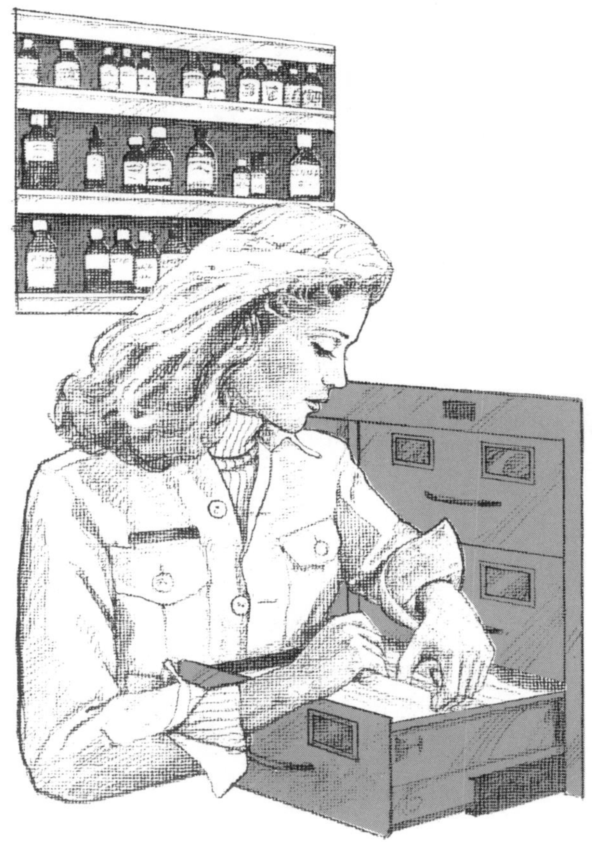

stages of sensitization

allergic reactions

The systemic reaction to injected venom begins immediately after stinging or within 20 minutes, and its intensity reaches a peak within 30 minutes. Although the pain may be acute for 1 hour or more, symptoms start to resolve and usually disappear within 3–4 hours (5).

Systemic and local allergic manifestations usually occur in individuals who have been stung or bitten previously (12). The first sting or bite is considered the sensitizing one. Each succeeding sting precipitates a reaction more severe than the preceding one. A factor that makes an insect sting potentially dangerous is that the time span between the first sting (sensitizing one) and the subsequent stings may be so long that patients forget that they are sensitive to insect venom. Another factor is that cross-sensitization may occur in individuals who have been sensitized by a member of the order Hymenoptera (12, 13). For example, a severe reaction may occur after the first ant or wasp sting in individuals sensitized to bee venom.

The reaction to ant stings generally is limited to the

area surrounding the sting bite. Immediately after a sting the skin flares and forms a wheal that lasts about 1 hour. Swelling, pruritus, papular urticaria, eczematoid dermatitis, and, in some cases, allergic systemic reactions may occur. In one report a patient experienced large white blotches surrounded by reddened areas accompanied by intense body itching, difficulty in breathing, profuse sweating, and semiconsciousness a few minutes after being stung by not more than 10 fire ants (14). In another case, following an ant sting there was an urticarial rash over the entire body, swollen eyes, labored breathing, frothy mucus expectoration from the mouth, and a near state of shock (15). In one study, biopsy specimens were obtained 6 and 30 minutes and 24 and 72 hours after volunteers were stung by ants, and the specimens were studied histopathologically (14). Epidermal intercellular edema and dermal necrosis occurred early. Pustules developed consistently at the sting site, accompanied by severe, deep necrosis. Anaphylactic reactions were reported following fire ant stings (16).

allergic reactions
anaphylactic shock
desensitization

Allergic reactions to mosquito bites vary in intensity. The formation of a wheal, erythema, papular reaction, and itching are characteristic. Scratching may cause papule and nodule formation, which may persist for a long time and lead to secondary infections such as impetigo, furunculosis, or infectious eczematoid dermatitis. The sting site may influence reaction intensity; bites are more severe on ankles and legs than on other parts of the body because of the relative circulatory stasis in the legs. Consequently, the tendency toward vesiculation, hemorrhage, eczematization, and ulceration is greater in these areas (17). Systemic reactions such as fever and malaise also are common.

Scabies symptoms usually appear after the first burrow is formed. Intense itching, especially at night, always occurs at the infestation site. The burrow (<1 cm long) is visible to the naked eye and appears as a narrow, slightly raised dark line. Unrestrained scratching may cause secondary bacterial infections (e.g., impetigo, furuncles, or cellulitis) and excoriation. Scabies diagnosis may be made by identifying the mite under a microscope and by the burrows in the skin.

When death ensues from an insect sting or bite, it is usually caused by anaphylactic shock—a result of hypersensitivity to certain proteins in the venom—rather than by the "toxicity" of the venom. A person would have to sustain approximately 500 stings simultaneously to be killed by the direct effects of venom. One researcher postulated that the severity of anaphylactic symptoms depends on the amount of the substance injected, the antigenicity of the substance, and the individual's degree of sensitivity (18). Another investigator (19) stated that "anaphylactic shock from insects is not generally known to the medical profession nor to the coroners, and cases listed as heart disease, cerebral accidents and a number of sudden deaths are sometimes due to insects."

The pathological findings in fatal cases of insect stings and bites include laryngeal obstruction and edema, pulmonary edema, dilation of the heart, epicardial hemorrhage, cerebral edema, and visceral congestion. Localized necrosis, edema, and cellular infiltration at the site of a bee sting occur in unsensitized tissue. Wasp venom also may cause necrosis of sweat glands (5).

TREATMENT

Body defenses are important in determining the intensity and kind of reaction to insect stings and bites. Some individuals acquire hypersensitivity after repeated stings or bites; others develop tolerance. Beekeepers may stop developing reactions to the stings of bees and other insects of the order Hymenoptera. Adults initially bothered by fleas may stop reacting within 1–2 years after regular exposure (17). Whether or not this result is due to a specific immunological mechanism that blocks the reaction to an injected antigen is not known.

Sensitivity to insect stings may be treated prophylactically by desensitization. Desensitization or hyposensitization is based on the concept that antibody production may be increased by subcutaneously injecting progressively increasing doses of venom or extracts of various Hymenoptera. Successful attempts have been made at desensitization by inoculations of diluted extracts from the responsible insect over a long period (20–22). Venom from the sacs of live wasps was used to diagnose and immunize against allergies to wasps (23). However, several fatalities have occurred following insect stings, despite previous desensitization therapy (24). In a recent study, insect venom immunotherapy was shown to be clinically superior to placebo or whole body extract treatment (25).

Because of the wide range of reactions to insect stings and bites, treatment usually depends on the symptoms. Nonprescription drugs are of no value in systemic reactions; such cases need the prompt attention of a physician. For local reactions an OTC product that minimizes scratching by relieving discomfort, itching, and pain may be recommended. Prophylactic products, such as insect repellents, also are available.

Physician-directed medical treatment (acute or prophylactic) is important in many cases. Because hypersensitive reactions to insect stings and bites occur rapidly and are usually severe, the sooner medical attention is given, the better the chances are for recovery. Systemic reactions caused by insect stings and bites are considered emergencies and usually are treated with one or more of the following drugs: antihistamines, corticosteroids, epinephrine hydrochloride, and isoproterenol. Respiratory support should be available, if needed; in severe cases, a tracheotomy may be necessary (26).

For hypersensitive individuals the pharmacist should advise the following procedures:

- The victim must seek medical attention immediately after an insect sting or bite.
- Basic first aid measures such as applying ice to the sting and removing the stinger are generally helpful.
- The directions and the benefits to be gained from using an insect sting emergency kit should be explained carefully. The pharmacist should emphasize that epinephrine is the drug of choice for anaphylactic reactions.

First Aid

Basic first aid measures are helpful until medical help is available. Prompt application of ice packs to the sting site helps to slow venom absorption and reduce itching, swelling, and pain (27). Removal of the honeybee's stinger and venom sac, which usually are left in the skin, is another measure that should be offered or explained, particularly to allergic individuals. The stinger should be removed before all the venom is injected; it takes about 2–3 minutes to empty all the contents from the honeybee's venom sac. The sac should not be squeezed, because rubbing, scratching, or grasping it releases more venom (26). Scraping the stinger with tweezers or a fingernail minimizes the venom flow. After the stinger is removed, an antiseptic should be applied.

Emergency Kits (Prescription Only)

emergency treatment

Insect sting emergency kits for hypersensitive individuals may be obtained by prescription. In addition to tweezers for removing the honeybee stinger, the typical kit may include the following items.

Epinephrine Hydrochloride

Because of its potent and rapid action, epinephrine hydrochloride 1:1000 injection is preferred to counteract the bronchoconstriction associated with anaphylaxis (28). It should be administered parenterally immediately after the sting. Some insect sting emergency kits have a preloaded (0.3 ml) sterile syringe. Generally, a 0.25-ml dose is injected subcutaneously, and after 15 minutes another dose may be necessary. For people who have cardiovascular disease, diabetes, hypertension, or hyperthyroidism the injection should be administered carefully.

Isoproterenol Tablets

Isoproterenol 10-mg sublingual tablets replace or complement epinephrine hydrochloride. Initially, one tablet should be dissolved under the tongue. If symptoms persist for 5–10 minutes, another tablet should be used.

Epinephrine Hydrochloride Aerosol

Inhalation of the drug relieves difficulty in breathing (28).

Antihistamines

Although they are slow in onset of action and may be ineffective in severe reactions, antihistamines often are used in conjunction with epinephrine hydrochloride. They are administered orally or parenterally.

Steroids

Steroids are slow in combating acute systemic symptoms. They usually are administered orally or parenterally with epinephrine hydrochloride.

Ingredients in OTC Products

ingredients in OTC products

Most OTC products used for symptomatic relief of insect stings and bites contain one or more of the following pharmacological agents: zinc oxide, calamine, zirconium oxide, menthol, camphor, phenol, local anesthetics, antibacterials, and antihistamines. A strong household ammonia solution or sodium bicarbonate paste applied at the site of a bee or wasp sting to relieve pain and discomfort is of little value. This treatment is based on the theory that ammonia solution and bicarbonate neutralize formic acid, mistakenly believed to be the toxic component of bee and wasp venom.

Zinc Oxide, Calamine, Zirconium Oxide

These ingredients are used in lotions, ointments, creams, and sprays for their protective and astringent properties. Zinc oxide and calamine tend to toughen the skin, reducing inflammation and oozing. Although these two compounds have been used widely, their effectiveness has not been substantiated. Zirconium oxide causes side effects when applied to the skin; deodorant antiperspirants that contain zirconium oxide have caused axillary granulomas (papular lesions). This condition may occur as a result of sensitivity to zirconium salts.

Menthol, Camphor, Phenol

These agents temporarily relieve itching. They are used empirically for their mild, local anesthetic, antipruritic, and counterirritant properties.

Benzocaine

This agent and other local anesthetics are used to relieve itching and pain. However, they are of little value in the concentrations available in most OTC products (1–2%). Some of these compounds may even be sensitizing if they are used for a long period.

Antibacterials

Benzethonium chloride and benzalkonium chloride are antibacterial agents used to prevent and treat secondary infections that may result from scratching.

Antihistamines

Topically applied antihistamines are used for their mild local anesthetic properties in relieving pruritus. The use of these compounds should be discouraged because they may cause sensitization, especially if they are applied regularly for a long period. Antihistamines are of greater value taken orally.

Scabies and Lice Treatment

Scabies and pediculosis are controlled by using gamma benzene hexachloride; benzyl benzoate is effective against scabies. Both products are available by prescription only. The patient should bathe, vigorously scrubbing the infested area. Then a 25% emulsion of benzyl benzoate or 0.5–1% cream of gamma benzene hexachloride is applied to the entire body except the face. It should remain on the skin for 24 hours, after which the patient may bathe. A second application is recommended 1 week after the first one to destroy the hatched eggs. Additional applications should be avoided because contact dermatitis may occur. If itching is not relieved immediately after treatment, a soothing lotion such as calamine lotion with menthol and camphor may be used.

Preventive Treatment: Insect Repellents

Insect repellents are chemicals that do not kill insects but keep them away from treated areas. When they are applied to the skin, repellents discourage the approach of insects and, as a result, protect the skin from insect bites. Most repellents are volatile, and when they are applied to skin or clothing, their vapor tends to discourage insects from alighting.

Oils of citronella, turpentine, pennyroyal, cedarwood, eucalyptus, and wintergreen were used for many years in insect repellent formulations. However, during and after World War II, investigations showed that these agents were relatively ineffective. Although more than 15,000 compounds have been tested as insect repellents, only a few have proven effective and safe enough to use on the skin. An insect repellent should be nontoxic, nonirritating, nonallergenic, and harmless to clothing. It should have an inoffensive odor, protect for several hours, be effective against as wide a variety of insects as possible, be able to withstand all weather conditions, and have an esthetic feel and appearance.

insect repellents
diethyltoluamide

The best all-purpose repellent is diethyltoluamide. Ethohexadiol, dimethyl phthalate, dimethyl carbamate, and butopyronoxyl are effective repellents, but they are not as effective against as many kinds of insects as diethyltoluamide. However, a mixture of two or more of these repellents is more effective against a greater variety of insects than any one repellent. Repellents may be toxic if they are taken internally. People who are sensitive to these chemicals may develop skin reactions such as itching, burning, and swelling, and repellents cause smarting when they are applied to broken skin or mucous membranes. They should be applied carefully around the eyes because they may cause a burning sensation.

PRODUCT SELECTION GUIDELINES

Medication often is requested after symptoms have appeared, and it is important to determine the nature of symptoms following the sting or bite, how soon the symptoms appeared, the severity of the symptoms, and what other drugs are being used concurrently. Personal or family history of hay fever, asthma, or contact dermatitis also is important in recommending medication for severe reactions to stings and bites. Cases of severe local reactions and systemic reactions should be referred to a physician.

OTC products are of minimal value to hypersensitive people. The pharmacist should record all information on hypersensitive individuals and should recommend that the person wear a tag or carry a card showing the nature of the allergy.

If the symptoms are minor, such as localized irritation, itching, or swelling, and there is no history of allergies, an appropriate nonprescription product may be recommended. Topical lotions, creams, ointments, and sprays are the main OTC products used for symptomatic relief of local reactions to insect stings and bites. The main considerations in product selection are reducing the possibility of additional stings or bites, providing proper protection to the affected skin, preventing secondary infection in the affected area, and relieving itching and irritation. Greasy ointments should be avoided because they may facilitate skin maceration. The best results are obtained with lotions, creams, and sprays. Local anesthetics and topical antihistamine-containing preparations should not be used excessively because they may cause sensitivity.

SUMMARY

Stings of honeybees, bumblebees, yellow jackets, hornets, wasps, and ants may cause pain, discomfort, illness, and severe local and systemic reactions. In normal individuals, stinging and biting insects cause local irritation, inflammation, swelling, and itching, which provoke rubbing and scratching. In hypersensitive individuals, anaphylactoid reactions may pose serious emergency problems. Papules or nodules from bites or stings may form and persist for months. Potential secondary infections may lead to impetigo, furunculosis, or eczematoid dermatitis. Topical OTC products may relieve or prevent these symptoms.

People sensitized to insect venom may react violently when they are stung. They need immediate, active treatment such as the administration of epinephrine hydrochloride, corticosteroids, or antihistamines. Desensitization may be accomplished by inoculating with an extract of the whole body of the responsible insect or by insect venom immunotherapy. The pharmacist can play a significant role by advising hypersensitive individuals on emergency procedures for insect stings and bites.

REFERENCES

(1) S. E. Barr, *Ann. Allergy, 29,* 49 (1971).
(2) N. A. Weber, *Am. J. Trop. Med., 17,* 765 (1937).
(3) R. M. Gordan and W. Crewe, *Ann. Trop. Med. Parasitol., 42,* 334 (1948).
(4) E. E. Buckley and N. Porges, "Venoms," Publication No. 44, American Association for the Advancement of Science, Washington, D.C., 1956, p. 171.
(5) T. K. Marshal, *Practitioner, 178,* 712 (1957).
(6) W. R. Horsfall, "Medical Entomology," Ronald Press, New York, N.Y., 1962, p. 182.
(7) J. A. McKiel and J. C. Clunie, *Can. J. Zool., 38,* 479 (1960).
(8) A. Hudson, J. A. McKiel, A. S. West, and R. K. Bourns, *Mosq. News, 18,* 249 (1958).
(9) D. W. Micks and J. P. Ellis, *Proc. Soc. Exp. Biol. Med., 78,* 69 (1951).
(10) K. Mellanby, *Nature, 158,* 554 (1946).
(11) D. S. Sax and J. Mejlszenkier, *N. Engl. J. Med., 285,* 293 (1971).
(12) J. R. Schenken, T. Tamisiea, and F. D. Winter, *Am. J. Clin. Pathol., 23,* 1216 (1953).
(13) H. L. Meuller and L. W. Hill, *N. Engl. J. Med., 249,* 726 (1953).
(14) M. R. Caro, V. J. Derbes, and R. Jung, *Arch. Dermatol., 75,* 475 (1957).
(15) C. H. Morhouse, *J. Am. Med. Assoc., 141,* 193 (1949).
(16) L. L. Brown, *South. Med. J., 65,* 273 (1972).
(17) H. V. Allington and R. R. Allington, *J. Am. Med. Assoc., 155,* 240 (1954).
(18) B. Swinny, *Tex. State J. Med., 46,* 12 (1950).
(19) J. W. Thomas, *W. Va. Med. J., 55,* 115 (1959).
(20) H. R. Prince and P. G. Secrest, *J. Allergy, 10,* 379 (1939).
(21) L. L. Henderson, *Postgrad. Med., 49,* 191 (1971).
(22) M. I. Levine, *J. Am. Med. Assoc., 217,* 964 (1971).
(23) M. J. Loveless and W. R. Fackler, *Ann. Allergy, 14,* 347 (1956).
(24) P. J. Torsney, *J. Allergy Clin. Immunol., 52,* 303 (1973).
(25) K. J. Hunt, M. D. Valentine, A. K. Soborka, A. W. Benton, F. J. Amodio, and L. M. Lichtenstein, *N. Engl. J. Med., 299,* 157 (1978).
(26) M. D. Ellis, "Dangerous Plants, Snakes, Arthropods and Marine Life of Texas," U.S. Department of Health, Education, and Welfare, 1975, p. 175.
(27) R. E. Arnold, "What to Do About Bites and Stings of Venomous Animals," Macmillan, New York, N.Y., 1973, p. 9.
(28) M. A. Passerro and S. C. Dees, *Am. Physician, 7,* 74 (1973).

Product (Manufacturer)	Application Form	Ingredients
Americaine First Aid Spray (Arnar-Stone)	spray	benzocaine, 10%; benzethonium chloride, 0.1%; alcohol, 25%
Bevill's Lotion (Bevill)	lotion	alcohol, 68%; ether, 8%; methyl salicylate, 1%; salicylic acid
Chiggerex (First Texas)	ointment	benzocaine, 2.0%; camphor, 0.008%; olive oil, 0.008%; menthol, 0.005%; peppermint oil, 0.005%; methylparaben, 0.002%; clove oil, 0.002%
Chiggertox Liquid (First Texas)	liquid	isopropyl alcohol, 53%; benzyl benzoate, 21.4%; soft soap, 21.4%; benzocaine, 2.1%
Derma Medicone (Medicone)	ointment	zinc oxide, 137.3 mg/g; benzocaine, 20.0 mg/g; 8-hydroxyquinoline sulfate, 10.5 mg/g; ichthammol, 10.0 mg/g; menthol, 4.8 mg/g; petrolatum; lanolin; perfume
Dermoplast (Ayerst)	spray	polyethylene glycol 400 monolaurate; benzocaine, 20%; methylparaben, 2%; menthol, 0.5%; polysorbate 80
Dermtex Anti-Itch Lotion (Pfeiffer)	lotion	benzocaine, 3%; benzalkonium chloride, 1:750; alcohol, 90%
Dermtex Anti-Itch Spray (Pfeiffer)	spray	benzocaine, 3%; chloroxylenol, 0.5%; alcohol, 50%
Mediconet (Medicone)	saturated medical pads	hamamelis water, 50%; glycerin, 10%; ethoxylated lanolin, 0.5%; methylparaben, 0.15%; benzalkonium chloride, 0.02%; perfume
Nupercainal Cream (Ciba)	cream	dibucaine, 0.5%; acetone sodium bisulfite, 0.37%; water-washable base
Nupercainal Ointment (Ciba)	ointment	dibucaine, 1%; acetone sodium bisulfite, 0.5%
Obtundia Surgical Dressing (Otis Clapp)	liquid	cresol–camphor complex
Pyribenzamine (Ciba)	cream ointment	tripelennamine, 2%; water-washable base (cream); petrolatum base (ointment)
Rexall First Aid Spray (Rexall)	spray	benzocaine; methylbenzethonium chloride; tyloxapol; chlorothymol; isopropyl alcohol, 4%; camphor
Surfadil (Lilly)	cream lotion	methapyrilene hydrochloride, 2%; cyclomethycaine, 0.5%; titanium dioxide, 5% (lotion)
Tucks and Tucks Take-Alongs (Parke-Davis)	saturated medical pads	hamamelis water, 50%; glycerin, 10%; methylparaben, 0.1%; benzalkonium chloride, 0.003%

Burn and Sunburn Products

James W. McFadden

Chapter 23

Questions to Ask the Patient

How old is the person who will be using the product?

What caused the burn—chemicals, sun exposure, or heat?

How severe is the burn? Is the skin broken and/or blistered?

Where is the burn? How large is the burned area?

Is the burn painful?

Which treatments have been used?

Each year in the United States, approximately 2 million burn accidents occur, causing 74,000 hospitalizations and 9000 deaths (1). Of those that die as a result of burns, about 1800 are under age 15 (2). Although these figures are high, the annual number of burn deaths has remained constant while the population has increased, and the recovery rate from serious burns is significantly higher. Care of seriously burned patients is improved, thanks to a better understanding of the pathophysiology of the burn wound, better methods of local treatment for controlling infection, and the establishment of specialized burn centers.

Confronted with a small minor burn or sunburn, the pharmacist must make the important decision whether to recommend patient self-treatment or physician referral. This chapter discusses appropriate OTC products for self-care of minor burns and sunburn, as well as medical care and complications of more severe burns.

SKIN ANATOMY AND PHYSIOLOGY

The skin is the largest organ of the human body, comprising about one-sixth of the body weight. The vascular capacity of the skin carries about one-third of the circulatory blood. There is constant fluid–electrolyte interflow between skin tissue and blood components. The skin as an organ protects underlying structures (e.g., by preventing microbial ingress), regulates temperature, serves as a reservoir of fat and vitamin D, and carries out sensory and secretory functions. Figure 1 depicts a cross-section of the skin layers in normal anatomy and in thermal damage. (See Chapter 26 for a more complete discussion of the skin.)

ETIOLOGY OF BURNS

Few bodily injuries are more traumatic than major burns. By scorching through skin and muscle, destroying nerves and blood vessels, and providing a fertile culture medium for infectious microbes, burns may cripple, disfigure, and kill.

Burns may result from several causes and, depending on their severity, may inflict minor to extensive damage to the skin or underlying tissues. Thermal trauma from flame, hot or scalding liquid, or hot objects is the most common cause. Chemicals, high-voltage electric current, and radioactive materials also cause burns.

Sunburn is common. Although sunlight includes radiation with wavelengths of 290–1850 nm, only the ultraviolet radiation of less than 300 nm produces the signs and symptoms of sunburn (3). The cause of sunburn and its attendant complaints is not fully understood; however, it is clear that preventing overexposure to the sun is more rational than treating sunburn symptoms once they occur.

PATHOPHYSIOLOGY OF BURNS

Re-epithelialization following burns depends on the depth of injury. Partial-thickness skin damage often leaves intact a viable number of appendages from which resurfacing can occur. The healing process takes 2–3 days for superficial second-degree burns and as long as 6 weeks for deep second-degree burns. Full-thickness damage causes irreversible destruction of all skin layers and appendages so that regeneration occurs only at the wound edges (see Figure 1). A uniform burn, such as that caused by scalding, may result in an injury of variable depth because of differences in skin thickness between individuals and age groups, regional differences in thickness, and the distribution and depth of skin appendages in the burned area (4). In a large deep burn (e.g., 50%, third-degree), hospitalization with massive intravenous fluid administration is necessary to correct severe shock and prevent death due secondarily to leakage of fluid and protein from the vascular compartment into the burn wound, drastically reducing blood volume (2, 5). (Death often ensues from smoke inhalation rather than the burn itself.)

Infection

Burn wound infection was at one time responsible for much late mortality in severe burns (4). Early colonization of the burn wound by gram-positive bacteria (*Staphylococci* and *Streptococci*) occurs during the first day.

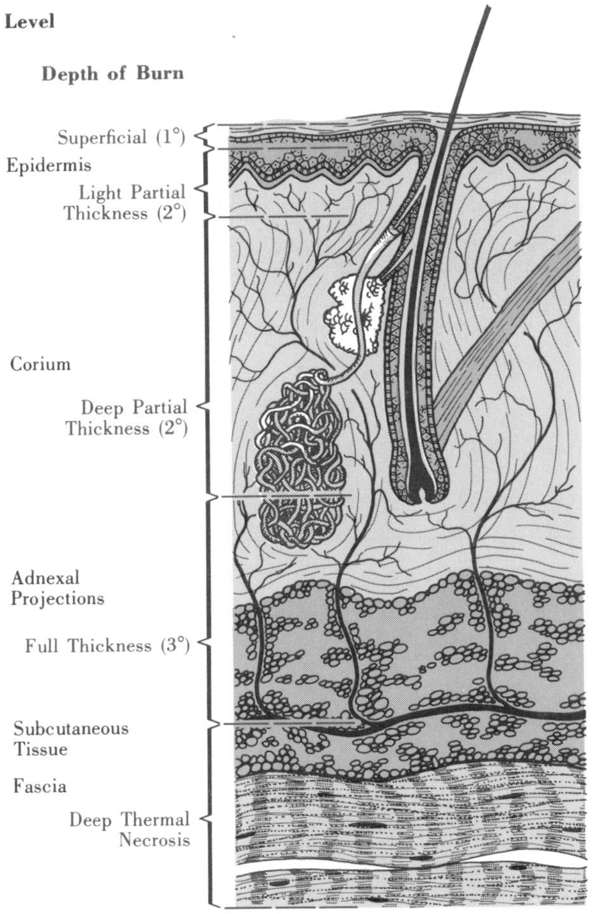

Level

Depth of Burn

Superficial (1°)
Epidermis
Light Partial Thickness (2°)
Corium
Deep Partial Thickness (2°)
Adnexal Projections
Full Thickness (3°)
Subcutaneous Tissue
Fascia
Deep Thermal Necrosis

Figure 1. Cross section of skin showing depth of burns.

role of prostaglandins in sunburn

drug photosensitivity

photoallergy

drugs with photosensitizing potential

After the third day, gram-negative bacteria (mainly *Pseudomonas aeruginosa*) predominate and may convert a second-degree burn to third-degree. The area is a luxuriant culture medium for microorganisms because there is much necrotic tissue and normal body defense mechanisms are impaired by the occluded vascular circulation. Thus topical therapy is essential and should be effective against *Pseudomonas*. Silver sulfadiazine, silver nitrate, and mafenide acetate (all prescription only) commonly are used topically for severe burns (6).

Sunburn

Dermatitis actinica is an acute inflammatory skin reaction resulting from sunburn, drug photosensitization, contact photosensitivity caused by chemicals, or unusual sensitivity to actinic rays (7). Different reactions to sunlight are caused mainly by differences in skin pigmentation. The progress of skin coloration during sun exposure seems to follow a pattern. Within the first 20 minutes, initial reddening appears, caused by oxidation of the bleached melanin; this pigmentation rapidly disappears. True sunburn erythema begins within 2–8 hours and persists for several days. Tanning usually occurs in about 2 days. Discomfort, pain, and blistering result from excessive exposure to ultraviolet radiation. If the affected area is large, malaise, nausea and vomiting, chills, and fever may occur (8).

Sunburn's delayed reaction has puzzled researchers for years. Some evidence indicates that prostaglandins are involved because prostaglandin inhibitors prevent the erythema or even blanch the reddening already present (9, 10). A 2.5% indomethacin solution (prostaglandin inhibitor) may cause blanching when applied 1.5 hours after redness is first noted. Blanched areas are cooler than the reddened areas. A fluoridated steroid preparation applied similarly has no better effect than the control vehicle. Further studies of the inflammatory consequence of sunburn may provide therapeutic prostaglandin inhibitors that can be used after excessive sun exposure and before suffering begins.

Photosensitivity

Sunburn is usually benign and self-limiting unless the burn is severe or occurs as an associated finding in a more serious disorder (e.g., porphyria, lupus, or pellagra) (7). In some patients the severity of sunburn is greater than normal for the amount of exposure. The problem may be due to drug photosensitivity. The distribution of the sunburn may be a clue; distinct boundaries of exposed areas may imply photosensitivity. Drug photosensitivity is often manifested as a phototoxic or photoallergic reaction. Phototoxic reactions may be elicited in nearly everyone if enough light energy of the appropriate wavelength is received or if appropriate concentrations of the phototoxic compound are applied topically or ingested. The reaction is characterized by an exaggerated sunburn with or without painful edema, occurring within a few hours after exposure.

Photoallergy to drugs is an acquired and altered capacity of the skin to respond to light energy in the presence of a photosensitizer. It is presumed that the reaction depends on an antigen–antibody relationship or a cell-mediated, delayed hypersensitivity response. The clinical patterns in drug-induced photoallergic reactions may range from eczematous or papular lesions, appearing 24 hours or more after sun exposure, to acute urticarial lesions, developing within a few minutes after exposure. The eruption is not localized exclusively at sun exposure sites but frequently extends beyond the areas of exposure.

Many different classes of systemic and contact chemicals and drugs may cause photosensitivity reactions (11). Causative agents include bacteriostatic components in soaps, antiseptics such as hexachlorophene and bithionol, and sunscreens such as esters of aminobenzoic acid. Reactions also may be due to substances such as brightening agents for cellulose, nylon, or wool fibers; cadmium sulfide in tattoos; essential oils in cosmetics and beauty aids; various plants used in perfumery, as flavorings, or as spices; various dyes; many drugs; and cyclamates (formerly used as artificial sweeteners). The types of drugs with photosensitizing potential are (11):

Anticonvulsants	Antineoplastics
Antihistamines	Barbiturates

Dyes
Gold and silver salts
Griseofulvin
Local anesthetics (procaine-related)
Nonsteroidal anti-inflammatories
Phenothiazine antipsychotics
Psoralen dermatologicals
Salicylates
Sex hormones
Sulfonamides
Sulfonylurea antidiabetics
Tetracycline antibiotics
Thiazide diuretics
Topical antimicrobials

ASSESSMENT

Burns are characterized and evaluated on the basis of the body area affected and the depth of penetration of the traumatized skin and underlying structures. The assessment aids in determining the treatment regimen and whether self-treatment, physician-supervised outpatient treatment, or hospitalization is required.

A convenient way to evaluate small irregular burns is to use the palm of the hand as a ruler, which can be taken to represent about 1% of body surface area (12). However, the "rule of nines" is a rapid and more sophisticated method of estimating the percentage of body surface involved in a burn wound. The body surface is divided into 11 areas, each representing about 9% of the total: the head and neck area (9%), each arm and hand (18%); the anterior trunk (18%), the posterior trunk (18%), and each leg (18%) and foot (18%). Estimates are fairly accurate for adults but less so for children and infants (Table 1). Special rapid estimating procedures have been advocated for children.

Determining burn depth is a clinical judgment. Distinctions of first, second, third, and fourth degree are clear theoretically, but the nature of the burning agent, the duration of its application, and the circumstances of the burn produce different characteristics, making experience the best guide. Depth may be estimated from certain clinical signs. A second-degree burn is red, has weeping blisters, and is painful to pinprick when evaluated within the first few hours after injury. A third-degree burn is full thickness, and the capillaries and nerve endings have been destroyed; moreover, it has the appearance of being white or charred and is insensitive to touch (12). Table 2 describes the depth classifications of burns by degree. A burn wound usually has characteristics of less severe burns on its periphery.

The American Burn Association has identified three treatment categories for burn patients (13):

- Major burn injuries: second-degree burns with a body surface area greater than 25% in adults (20% in children); all third-degree burns with a body surface of 10% or greater; all burns involving hands, face, eyes, ears, feet, and perineum; all inhalation injuries; electrical burns; complicated burn injuries involving fractures or other major trauma; and all poor-risk patients (elderly patients and those with an intercurrent disease).
- Moderate, uncomplicated burn injuries: second-degree burns with a body surface area of 15–25% in adults (10–20% in children); third-degree burns with a body surface area of less than 10%; and burns that do not involve eyes, ears, face, hands, feet, or perineum.
- Minor burn injuries: second-degree burns with a body surface area of less than 15% in adults (10% in children); third-degree burns with a body surface area of less than 2%; and burns not involving eyes, ears, face, hands, feet, or perineum; excludes electrical injuries, inhalation injuries, and all poor-risk patients.

determining size and degree of burn

"rule of nines"

percentage surface area of body parts

treatment categories for burn patients

controlling pain

TREATMENT

A major consideration in the initial treatment of all minor or moderate burns is controlling pain (12). Immediately immersing the burned area in cold water, using wet towels soaked in ice water, or submersing the burned area in cold soapy water alleviates the pain. In addition, the application of cold stops the burning insult and actually minimizes the depth of the injury (2, 12, 14). The affected part should be cooled continuously for several minutes. Local edema may be reduced even if as long as 45 minutes has elapsed before cooling is begun (15). The evidence for physiological benefit of cooling in serious burns is less than conclusive, and the lack of standardized experimental conditions makes critical clinical evaluation difficult (16). However, the subjective relief of pain by cooling is well accepted (17–19).

A minor burn usually repairs itself with or without treatment. After the initial cryotherapy (application of cold), thorough cleansing of the area is essential to promote early healing; bland soap (e.g., Ivory) and water are the best agents to use. A nonadherent and hypoallergenic burn dressing should then be applied and held in place with tape or elastic gauze; either sterile gauze, petrolatum gauze, or Adaptic serves the purpose. After 48 hours the dressing should be changed and the wound observed. If the gauze sticks to the wound surface, warm water may be used. The dressing should be soaked and removed very slowly so as not to upset any regenerating

Table 1. Surface Area (%) of Body Parts

	Years					
Surface	Birth	1	5	10	15	Adult
Head	19	17	13	11	9	7
Neck	2	2	2	2	2	2
Anterior trunk	13	13	13	13	13	13
Posterior trunk	13	13	13	13	13	13
Buttocks	5	5	5	5	5	5
Genitalia	1	1	1	1	1	1
Upper arms	8	8	8	8	8	8
Forearms	6	6	6	6	6	6
Hands	5	5	5	5	5	5
Thighs	11	13	16	17	18	19
Legs	10	10	11	12	13	14
Feet	7	7	7	7	7	7

Adapted from *Skin Xenografts*, Burn Treatment Skin Bank, Phoenix, Ariz.

Table 2. Depth Classification of Burns

Type	Tissue Affected	Characteristics
First-degree	epidermis	erythema, pain, no blistering
Second-degree	epidermis, some dermis	blisters, pain, skin regenerates
Third-degree	full skin thickness	no blisters, leathery appearance, less pain, skin grafting required
Fourth-degree and char burn	full skin thickness and underlying tissue	blackened appearance, dryness, pain, danger of deep infection

degrees of burns

ingredients in burn medications

benzocaine, lidocaine, and other local anesthetics

epithelial elements (1). After a few days, exposure is usually possible without discomfort, and barring infection, the wound heals in about 2 weeks.

A serious (i.e., moderate or major) burn needs expert medical attention to prevent complications such as shock, sepsis, scarring, and contractures. Judging whether a burn is minor or serious is not always easy. Immediately following the burn, the extent may be estimated from the nature of the injury, the painful area, and the skin's appearance. Judging burn depth is much more difficult. Even burn care specialists have problems in judging differences between second- and third-degree burns in the immediate postburn period. As the wound ages, the extent and the depth of the traumatized area become more apparent.

If there is doubt as to the burn's severity, the pharmacist should recommend physician referral after initial first aid rather than self-treatment. Patients with obviously extensive and deep burns or burns of hands, face, eyes, ears, feet, and/or perineum should be sent to a hospital burn service as soon as possible. The treatment of serious and extensive burns often requires a highly skilled team of specialists with intensive training in caring for the burned patient. The American Burn Association has formulated specific guidelines and requirements for facilities needed to handle burn victims (13).

Pharmacological Agents

As with other traumas, overtreatment of burns is a danger. Systemic antibiotics are rarely, if ever, indicated in small burns (1). A number of topical remedies may be applied; however, the routine topical use of antibacterial agents has not been found to be of value in treating minor burns (12). Surgeons often complain of difficulty in removing topical remedies applied to a patient's burn by well-meaning friends, causing added discomfort to the victim. Burn remedies containing a mixture of chemicals always involve a certain amount of risk. A burn may destroy the barrier layer of the skin and thus enhance percutaneous absorption (20). Many chemicals applied to injured skin also increase the hazard of allergic hypersensitivity reactions. If a burn is serious, the residue from the remedy may capture and protect environmental microorganisms, increasing the danger of infection. Also, the residue will have to be removed by painful procedures if a viable surface is needed for skin grafting.

Tables 3 and 4 list the various drugs commonly found in OTC burn medications, along with their FDA classifications (21).

Local Anesthetics

The advantage of the poorly soluble local anesthetic agents (e.g., benzocaine and butamben picrate) over the soluble ones (e.g., lidocaine) is the lessened danger of absorption to produce systemic toxicity. Penetration of benzocaine through the intact skin to nerve endings is slow, but concentrations as low as 5% in appropriate solution may produce local anesthesia. Commercial preparations below 20% concentration may fail to have an effect on intact or mildly sunburned skin (22). The range of benzocaine concentrations in these products is 0.5–20%. In burns that disrupt the skin barrier an effect comparable to that on mucous membranes is expected, and lower concentrations may be active.

Local anesthetics in their salt forms are water soluble; in their free base form, water solubility is low. It is the free base form that possesses local anesthetic activity. When the salt form encounters buffering body fluids, a proportion is converted to the active free base form, depending on the pKa of the base and relative buffer capacity. It was found clinically that aqueous solutions of salts are inactive on intact skin, but solutions of the free bases at similar concentrations show activity. Common water-soluble agents in burn remedies include dibucaine, lidocaine, tetracaine, and pramoxine in both salt and free base forms. A study of commercial preparations containing water-soluble agents shows no objective response on intact or sunburned skin but shows some subjective effect in sunburn (22). More effectiveness is expected on burns that destroy the barrier layer.

Acute toxicity from applied local anesthetics is rare because the short-term use in minor burns makes a systemic buildup resulting in elevated blood levels unlikely. Highly concentrated products used inappropriately on large area second- and third-degree burns may elicit toxic reactions, but these remedies generally contain low concentrations of the more toxic local anesthetics. Benzocaine has been implicated in producing methemoglobinemia in infants (23, 24) and as a skin sensitizer used topically in susceptible individuals. Of 413 patients with contact dermatitis, 6 were allergic to benzocaine as detected by patch tests (25). Because lidocaine is an amide rather than an ester type of local anesthetic, it sometimes may be substituted for other agents to which the patient is allergic; however, allergy to lidocaine is also encountered. The development of allergic reactions is less probable with short-term use of burn preparations than with preparations applied to more persistent dermatitis. Because the skin is abraded in many burns, sensitization followed by an allergic reaction to the local anesthetic is possible if the preparation is used at a later time.

Antimicrobials

Antimicrobials include quaternary ammonium compounds, iodophors, organic mercurials, phenols, and antibiotics. (See Chapter 26 for further discussion of topical anti-infectives.) Their spectra of action are variable, although most show activity against gram-positive bacteria in the laboratory. Like other skin infections, burn infections usually contain more than one kind of organism. The primary offenders in major burn sepses are *Staphylococci* (gram-positive) and *Pseudomonas* (gram-negative) bacteria.

The undesirable consequences of topical antimicrobials are that the infecting organisms may acquire a resistance to the agent or the agent may upset the ecological balance of the normal flora so that nonsensitive, resistant, and possibly more dangerous organisms predominate in the microbial population. Unless the prophylactic or therapeutic agent is specific and effective, more harm than good may result.

A group of specific topical agents essential in treating major burns is restricted to physician use. The nonprescription burn remedies generally lack the specificity and effectiveness to be recommended. Few are effective against *Pseudomonas*, and their activity against gram-positive organisms may even favor early *Pseudomonas* invasion.

The final report of the first FDA OTC Panel on Antimicrobial Products contains much useful information on antimicrobial ingredients in burn remedies (26). For many topical antimicrobials, insufficient evidence was at hand to evaluate them as Category I. To make definitive judgments, the Panel created seven new classes of antimicrobial products, three of which are potentially applicable to burn remedies:

topical antimicrobials

FDA categories for common ingredients

Table 3. FDA Category I Ingredients: Intact and Damaged Skin

Drug	Analgesic	Anesthetic	Antipruritic	Suggested Strength, %
Benzocaine	X	X	X	5–20
Butamben	X	X	X	1
Camphor	X	X	X	1–3
Dibucaine base	X	X	X	0.25–1
Diphenhydramine hydrochloride			X	1–2
Hydrocortisone			X	0.25–0.5
Juniper tar			X	1–5
Lidocaine	X	X	X	1–4
Menthol	X	X	X	0.1–3
Methyl salicylate	X			10–60
Phenol	X	X	X	0.5–2 aqueous 4 in fixed oil
Resorcinol	X	X	X	0.5–3 lotion 0.5–5 ointment
Sodium phenolate	X		X	0.5–2 aqueous
Tripelennamine hydrochloride and citrate			X	0.5–2
Tetracaine	X	X	X	0.5–1

Table 4. FDA-Classified Ingredients: Category I on Damaged Skin and Category III on Intact Skin

Drug	Analgesic	Anesthetic	Antipruritic	Suggested Strength, %
Benzyl alcohol		X		1–10
Butamben picrate	X	X		1–2
Dibucaine hydrochloride	X	X	X	0.25–1
Dimethisoquin hydrochloride	X	X	X	0.5
Diclonine hydrochloride	X	X	X	1–4
Lidocaine hydrochloride	X	X	X	1–5
Pramoxine hydrochloride	X	X	X	1
Tetracaine hydrochloride	X	X	X	1–2

- Skin antiseptic: a safe, nonirritating antimicrobial-containing preparation which prevents overt skin infection;
- Skin wound cleanser: a safe, nonirritating liquid preparation (or product to be used with water) which assists in the removal of foreign material from small superficial wounds and does not delay healing;
- Skin wound protectant: a safe, nonirritating preparation applied to small cleansed wounds which provides a protective (physical and/or chemical) barrier and neither delays healing nor favors the growth of microorganisms.

classes of antimicrobial products

status of ingredients in skin antiseptics and skin wound cleansers

skin wound protectants

Skin antiseptics are especially applicable to burn remedies. Claims must be supported by clinical studies demonstrating effectiveness. None of the examined ingredients qualified for approval. The quaternary ammonium compounds, hexylresorcinol, iodophors, phenol ($\leqq$1.5%), chloroxylenol, and triclosan were among the active ingredients for which more data were needed. Hexachlorophene, halogenated salicylanilides, phenol ($\geqq$1.5%), and tincture of iodine were judged not safe and/or effective.

Skin wound cleansers have limited use in burn wounds. They may or may not contain antimicrobials, but they must help cleanse the wound. The quaternary ammonium compounds and hexylresorcinol were judged safe and effective ingredients. Except for these agents, the ingredients requiring more data were the same as those under skin antiseptics, and active ingredients that were not safe and effective were the same.

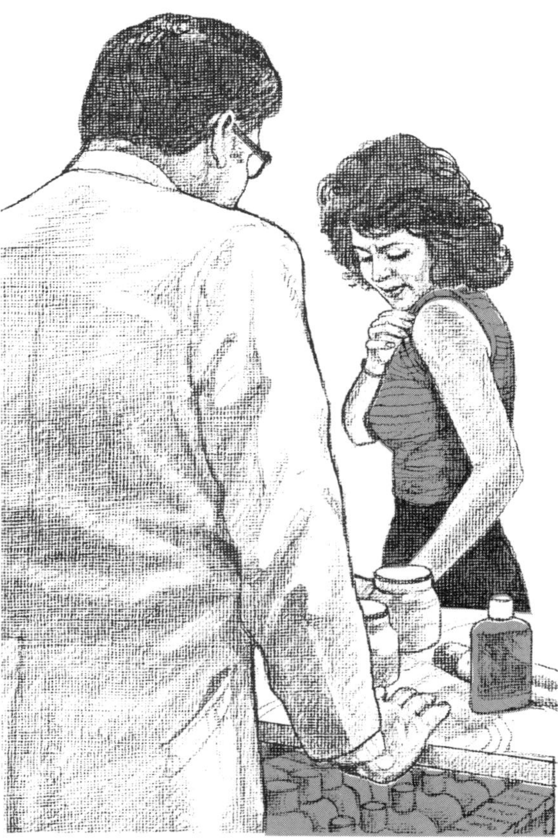

Skin wound protectants may be useful as a first aid measure in preventing wound contamination. For antimicrobials in nonprescription remedies, evaluation of suitability must be based on efficacy and possible toxicity. Specific toxicity of supposedly innocuous topical antimicrobial agents was given only minor attention prior to recent experiences with hexachlorophene. It is now recognized that absorption from topical preparations often occurs, and toxic or potentially harmful blood levels of the antimicrobial agents may be reached when the preparation is used routinely or when there is sufficient skin destruction for absorption to occur (27, 28).

Hexachlorophene has been removed from nonprescription availability largely because of its toxic effect on brain tissue when it is absorbed. Because of the production of severe, disabling photosensitivity caused by halogenated salicylanilides (e.g., tribromsalan), these ingredients have been judged unsafe for all drug and cosmetic purposes. Topical application of phenol in concentrations of 2% or more may cause CNS toxicity and gangrene (29). Accordingly, phenol concentrations of more than 1.5% (aqueous or alcoholic solution) have been judged unsafe for general use as nonprescription topical antimicrobials. Tincture of iodine is irritating to broken skin and delays wound healing. Therefore according to the Panel, it is not a safe antimicrobial for other than preparation of intact skin for surgery.

Nonprescription antibiotic preparations have not yet been evaluated by the Panel. The mixture of neomycin, polymyxin B sulfate, and bacitracin is widely used, but evaluations of the mixture have been equivocal in spite of the broad spectrum of activity and the specificity of polymyxin B sulfate against *Pseudomonas* in vitro. The absorption of toxic amounts from misuse of neomycin on large-area burns and allergic hypersensitivity reactions to neomycin have occurred (25).

Many preparations contain low antimicrobial concentrations as preservatives against spoilage. Listing an antimicrobial by name on the label may imply therapeutic or suppressant action. Unfortunately, only the names (not the amounts or concentrations) of active ingredients currently are required on OTC product labels. Preservative ingredients also are under investigation by the Panel.

Product Formulation

Few, if any, of the products claimed as being useful in minor burns or sunburn contain only one ingredient. Other components may affect the action or toxicity of the active ingredient. The FDA OTC Panel on Topical Analgesic, Antirheumatic, Otic, Burn, and Sunburn Treatment Products concluded that two or more ingredients may be combined under the following conditions (30):

- That each be present in sufficient quantity to act additively or by summation to produce the claimed therapeutic effect when the ingredients are within the effective concentration range specified for each ingredient in the monographs;

- That the ingredients do not interact with each other and one or more ingredients do not nullify the effectiveness of the other ingredients by precipitation, change in pH, or in some other manner reduce the pharmacological activity of one or more ingredients;
- That the partition of the active ingredients between the skin and the vehicle in which they are incorporated not be impeded and that the minimum effective concentration or more be delivered and the therapeutic effectiveness of each ingredient remain as claimed or not be decreased.

The Panel felt that combinations of analgesics, anesthetics, antipruritics, protectants, adsorbents, and demulcents were rational in keeping with these conditions (30). Furthermore, the Panel concluded that hydrocortisone was suitable for OTC use in the indicated concentrations, as an antipruritic for topical and otic use. According to the Panel, combinations of nonantimicrobial ingredients with antimicrobials are suitable if the antimicrobial remains safe and effective, the nonantimicrobial ingredient is safe and effective, the labeling indicates pharmacological effects of all active ingredients, the combination provides rational concurrent therapy for a significant part of the target population, and the combination meets the requirement of the definitions for the antimicrobial product category.

Burn remedies have not been subjected to this kind of examination in the past. Secondary ingredients such as volatile oils, menthol, eugenol, thymol, vitamin A, and zinc compounds will be examined to determine whether they contribute to or interfere with a claim made for a product.

In using nonprescription products for burn treatment, consideration must be given to the placebo effect of the application. Aromatic ingredients may reinforce the idea that something is being done to help this very painful condition. One surgeon reported excellent pain relief from aerosol foam shaving cream applied to the burn when the container was labeled "Special Burn Cream." If the patient saw that it was shaving cream, little relief was reported (31).

Ointments, because of their usually greasy base, are probably the least desirable form of burn treatment. Their possible misuse on serious burns may facilitate microbial contamination, and they require removal before further local treatment can be given. Creams, solutions, and aerosols are easier to remove and may, by cooling, assist other ingredients in deadening the pain. Sprays and aerosols deliver the medication in the least traumatizing manner, but there may be danger from inhalation of the suspended particles.

PRODUCT SELECTION GUIDELINES

After the burn has been assessed, the pharmacist should be able to suggest specific therapy. If the burn is minor and if the early painful phase has passed, using an unmedicated emollient preparation or simply bandaging probably is as effective as a special burn remedy. If the patient has suffered a minor but painful sunburn, preparations containing local anesthetics provide some relief. Creams or rapidly evaporating solutions or sprays may relieve pain by cooling. Wet dressings, however, may be as effective and involve little risk of further harm to the patient from irritation or allergic complications. Aspirin in therapeutic doses may be recommended if it is not contraindicated, since certain anti-inflammatory agents may modify and even prevent sunburn (9, 10) and aspirin's analgesic and antipyretic actions are beneficial.

Patient counseling should include instructions on product use. The pharmacist should explain how to apply a dressing, ointment, cream, or topical aerosol and how to use a bath (32).

Wet Dressings

FDA Panel recommendations

dosage forms

application

Any soft clean cloth, such as a cloth diaper, should be soaked in a freshly prepared solution and wrung out. The wet dressing should be applied gently to the affected area. After 3–5 minutes the cloth should be soaked in the solution again, wrung out as before, and reapplied. This process may be repeated for up to 1 hour.

If the affected skin begins to feel wrinkled or fissured (macerated), the wet dressing should be discontinued, and the patient should wait 2–3 hours before reapplying dressings soaked in a fresh solution. Depending on lesion response, this wet dressing procedure may be repeated at 2- to 6-hour intervals during waking hours.

Larger areas of the body, such as the back and abdomen, may be treated by leaving on a lightly applied larger wet dressing for about 1 hour. Care should be taken not to allow fissuring of the skin. If wrinkling or fissuring occurs, the wet dressing should be discontinued. These larger wet dressings may be applied 3–4 times a day.

Bath

The bathtub should be filled about halfway with the prescribed solution at about room temperature. If colloidal oatmeal is used, one cupful should be mixed with two cups of water before stirring into the bath water. The affected part(s) should be soaked for approximately 30 minutes, about four times per day, depending on the extent of the dermatitis and discomfort. After soaking, the inflamed area should be patted gently with a soft towel; the patient should take care not to rub or further irritate the dermatitis.

Ointment/Cream

Before any ointment or cream is applied, the affected area should be cleaned of old medication each time the dressing is changed. A thin layer of the medication always is sufficient. More ointment will not necessarily do more good—it is the medication touching the skin or wound that causes healing, not the thick layers applied. If a wound is deep or skin infection is widespread, the ointment/cream may be applied directly to the skin with a wooden tongue depressor.

After the medication is applied, it may need to be covered with a sterile gauze pad. The pad may be covered and held in place with a sterile bandage or adhesive tape. In some cases, no covering is required.

If the problem is a small one and an adhesive bandage or sterile gauze pad is used as a dressing, the ointment or cream is applied to the pad, which is then placed against the wound. A cotton-tipped applicator also may be used. To keep from contaminating the medication, the patient should avoid placing it directly on the skin from the tube.

Topical Aerosol

The container should be shaken well before using. The patient should avoid breathing the spray/mist, and in applying the product to the face should make sure not to get it into the eyes, nose, or mouth. With the container held straight up and about 6 inches (~15 cm) away from the skin, the medication should be sprayed in bursts of about 1–3 seconds, and no longer; the skin should be covered thoroughly.

SUMMARY

Pharmacists' knowledge of burn and sunburn is important. The decision whether to recommend medical care or self-therapy must be based on thorough evaluation and patient assessment. Major burns always should be examined as soon as possible by a physician. For minor burns the pharmacist should stress the usefulness of cryotherapy, decontamination, and clean dressings. Remedies containing antimicrobials also may be used on minor burns, although they are of questionable necessity. Uncomplicated cases of sunburn generally respond to the same type of therapy. First aid treatment should consist of cryotherapy or bathing the wound. A local anesthetic cream or spray may be applied if the patient insists. For both minor burns and sunburn the pharmacist may suggest therapeutic doses of salicylates, if not contraindicated, to reduce inflammation and discomfort and to promote analgesia. Whichever therapy or OTC preparation the pharmacist advises, it should do no further harm by irritation or sensitization.

REFERENCES

(1) C. P. Artz, *Med. Times, 104,* 128 (1976).
(2) C. P. Artz, *Drug Ther., 5,* 127 (1975).
(3) "The Merck Manual of Diagnosis and Therapy," 12th ed., Merck Sharp & Dohme, Rahway, N.J., 1972, p. 1492.
(4) F. D. Foley, *Surg. Clin. North Am., 50,* 1201 (1970).
(5) B. Cosman, *Hosp. Med., 7,* 55 (1971).
(6) J. A. Moncrief, *N. Engl. J. Med., 288,* 444 (1973).
(7) "Current Diagnosis and Treatment," M. A. Krupp, M. J. Chatton, and S. Margen, Eds., Lange Medical, Los Altos, Calif., 1971, p. 49.
(8) *Lancet, 2,* 30 (1973).
(9) D. S. Snyder and W. H. Eaglstein, *J. Invest. Dermatol., 60,* 110 (1973).
(10) D. S. Snyder and W. H. Eaglstein, *Br. J. Dermatol., 90,* 91 (1974).
(11) E. Stempel and R. Stempel, *J. Am. Pharm. Assoc., NS13,* 200 (1973).
(12) J. A. Moylan, *Postgrad. Med., 59,* 766 (1974).
(13) *Bulletin of the American College of Surgeons, 62,* 6 (1977).
(14) M. F. Epstein and J. D. Crawford, *Pediatrics, 52,* 430 (1973).
(15) O. J. Ofeigsson, R. Mitchell, and R. S. Patrick, *J. Pathol., 108,* 145 (1972).
(16) J. A. Moncrief, *N. Engl. J. Med., 290,* 59 (1974).
(17) H. Kravitz, *Pediatrics, 53,* 766 (1974).
(18) A. Blumefeld, *N. Engl. J. Med., 290,* 58 (1974).
(19) J. G. Appleyard, *Lancet, 2,* 1370 (1972).
(20) J. Pietsch and J. L. Meakins, *Lancet, 1,* 280 (1976).
(21) "Summary Minutes of the FDA OTC Panel on Topical Analgesic, Antirheumatic, Otic, Burn, and Sunburn Treatment and Prevention Products," June 22–23, 1976.
(22) H. Dalili and J. Adriani, *Clin. Pharmacol. Ther., 12,* 913 (1971).
(23) H. Peterson, *N. Engl. J. Med., 263,* 454 (1960).
(24) N. Goluboff and D. S. Macfayden, *J. Pediatr., 47,* 222 (1955).
(25) E. Epstein, *J. Am. Med. Assoc., 198,* 517 (1966).
(26) *Federal Register, 39,* 33103 (1974).
(27) D. L. Larson, *J. Am. Hosp. Assoc., 42,* 63 (1968).
(28) K. J. LaVelle, D. J. Doedens, S. A. Kleit, and R. B. Forney, *Clin. Pharmacol. Ther., 17,* 365 (1975).
(29) W. B. Deichman and M. L. Keplinger, in "Industrial Hygiene and Toxicology," Vol. 2, 2nd ed., Interscience, New York, N.Y., 1963.
(30) "Summary Minutes of the FDA OTC Panel on Topical Analgesic, Antirheumatic, Otic, Burn, and Sunburn Treatment and Prevention Products," Nov. 12–13, 1975.
(31) R. F. Hogarty, in "Burns: A Symposium," Charles C Thomas, Springfield, Ill., 1964, p. 74.
(32) S. Strauss, "Your Prescription and You, A Pharmacy Handbook for Consumers," Medical Business Services, Ambler, Pa., 1977.

Product (Manufacturer)	Dosage Form	Anesthetic	Antimicrobial	Other
Aerosept (Dalin)	aerosol	lidocaine	cetyltrimethylammonium bromide chloroxylenol	aromatic base
Americaine (Arnar-Stone)	aerosol ointment	benzocaine, 20%	benzethonium chloride, 0.1% (ointment)	polyethylene glycols (ointment), water-dispersible base (aerosol)
Americaine First Aid Spray (Arnar-Stone)	spray	benzocaine, 10%	benzethonium chloride, 0.1%	alcohol, 25%
Betadine (Purdue Frederick)	aerosol ointment	—	povidone-iodine, 5% (aerosol) 10% (ointment)	aqueous base (aerosol), water-miscible base (ointment)
Biotres (Central)	ointment	—	polymyxin B sulfate, 10,000 units/g bacitracin zinc, 500 units/g	—
Burn Relief Spray (Rexall)	spray	benzocaine	chlorobutanol, 0.3% benzethonium chloride	polyalkylene glycol; menthol; isopropyl alcohol, 11%
Burntame Spray (Otis Clapp)	spray	benzocaine, 20%	8-hydroxyquinoline	—
Butesin Picrate (Abbott)	ointment	butamben picrate, 1%	—	—
Dermamycin (Pfeiffer)	spray	benzocaine, 3%	chloroxylenol, 0.5%	isopropyl alcohol, 50%
Dermoplast (Ayerst)	aerosol	benzocaine, 20% menthol, 0.5%	—	methylparaben, polyethylene glycol 400 monolaurate, polysorbate 85
Foille (Carbisulphoil Blistex)	liquid ointment aerosol	benzocaine, 2%	benzyl alcohol, 4% 8-hydroxyquinoline	sulfur, bland vegetable oil
Gebauer's Tannic Spray (Gebauer)	spray	benzocaine, 0.5%	chlorobutanol, 1.2%	tannic acid, 3.9%; menthol, 0.1%
Hist-A-Balm Medicated Lotion (Columbia Medical)	lotion	diperodon hydrochloride, 0.25%	benzalkonium chloride, 0.1%	phenyltoloxamine dihydrogen citrate, 0.75%; menthol; camphor
Hyrocain (Amer. Pharm.)	cream	benzocaine dibucaine tetracaine	—	—
Kip for Burns (Young's)	ointment	—	phenol, 0.5% *o*-phenylphenol, 0.5%	spearmint oil, bay oil, methyl salicylate, salicylic acid, zinc oxide, petrolatum, paraffin, lanolin
Medicone Dressing Cream (Medicone)	cream	benzocaine, 5 mg/g	8-hydroxyquinoline sulfate, 0.5 mg/g	cod liver oil, 125 mg/g; zinc oxide, 125 mg/g; menthol, 1.8 mg/g; petrolatum; lanolin; paraffin; talc; perfume
Mediconet (Medicone)	cloth wipe	—	benzalkonium chloride, 0.02%	hamamelis water, 50%; glycerin, 10%; ethoxylated lanolin, 0.5%; methylparaben, 0.15%; perfume
Medi-Quick (Lehn & Fink)	aerosol pump spray	lidocaine	benzalkonium chloride	isopropyl alcohol, 12% (aerosol), 79% (pump)
Morusan (Beecham Labs)	ointment	benzocaine, 2%	—	cod liver oil concentrate, lanolin, petrolatum
Noxzema Medicated (Noxell)	cream lotion	—	phenol, <0.5%	menthol, camphor, clove oil, eucalyptus oil, lime water, water-dispersible base
Nupercainal Cream (Ciba)	cream	dibucaine, 0.5%	—	acetone sodium bisulfite, 0.37%; water-washable base
Nupercainal Ointment (Ciba)	ointment	dibucaine, 1%	—	acetone sodium bisulfite, 0.5%
Obtundia (Otis Clapp)	cream liquid	—	cresol–camphor complex	—

Product (Manufacturer)	Dosage Form	Anesthetic	Antimicrobial	Other
Panthoderm (USV)	cream lotion	—	—	dexpanthenol, 2%; water-miscible base
Pontocaine (Breon)	cream ointment	tetracaine hydrochloride (equivalent to 1% base) (cream) base, 0.5% (ointment)	—	methylparaben (cream); sodium bisulfite (cream); menthol, 0.5% (ointment); white petrolatum (ointment); white wax (ointment)
Pyribenzamine (Ciba)	cream ointment	tripelennamine, 2%	—	water-washable base (cream); petrolatum base (ointment)
Rexall First Aid Spray (Rexall)	spray	benzocaine	chlorothymol methylbenzethonium chloride	isopropyl alcohol, 4%; tyloxapol; camphor
Solarcaine (Plough)	cream lotion	benzocaine	triclosan	menthol, camphor
Solarcaine Spray (Plough)	aerosol spray pump spray	benzocaine	triclosan	isopropyl alcohol, 31% (pump spray)
Tanurol (O'Neal, Jones & Feldman)	ointment	benzocaine, 1%	phenol, 0.75%	tannic acid, 3%
Tega Caine (Ortega)	aerosol	benzocaine, 20%	benzyl alcohol, 2.3% chloroxylenol, 0.51%	urea, 5.38%; propylene glycol
Unguentine (Norwich)	ointment aerosol spray	benzocaine (spray)	parahydracin (ointment) benzalkonium chloride (spray) chloroxylenol (spray)	phenol, 1%; aluminum hydroxide; zinc carbonate; zinc acetate; zinc oxide; eucalyptus oil; thyme oil; menthol; eugenol (cream); alcohol, 7% (spray)
Unguentine Plus (Norwich)	cream	lidocaine hydrochloride	chloroxylenol	aluminum hydroxide, zinc carbonate, zinc acetate, zinc oxide, phenol, eucalyptus oil, thyme oil, menthol, eugenol
Vaseline First-Aid Carbolated Petroleum Jelly[a] (Chesebrough-Pond)	ointment	—	chloroxylenol, 0.5% phenol, 0.2%	petroleum jelly, lanolin
Vaseline Pure Petroleum Jelly (Chesebrough-Pond)	gel	—	—	white petrolatum, 100%
Xylocaine (Astra)	ointment	lidocaine, 2.5%	—	polyethylene glycols, propylene glycol

[a] Not meant for use over extensive body areas (e.g., sunburn).

Sunscreen and Suntan Products

George Torosian and Max A. Lemberger

Chapter 24

Questions to Ask the Patient

Is your skin extremely sensitive to the sun?

Is it difficult for you to tan?

Have you had much exposure to the sun?

Have you ever had a reaction to topical products?

Which products are you currently using? Which products have you used in the past?

Are you taking tetracycline or derivatives, a phenothiazine, diuretics, quinidine or quinine, or any sulfa drugs?

Almost everyone has experienced sunburn—the painful redness, swelling, and tenderness of the skin that are reminders of having been exposed too long to the sun's ultraviolet rays. Many people consider sunburn's effects disagreeable but relatively minor. However, the consequences of continued exposure to the sun can be significant. Long-term exposure even without severe burning causes skin to age prematurely, resulting in loss of elasticity, thinning, wrinkling, and drying. Cumulative exposure from childhood to adulthood may cause precancerous skin conditions, and skin cancer may follow.

Sunscreen and suntan products are used to prevent sunburn and/or "promote" suntan. Applied properly, they block some or all of the harmful ultraviolet rays either physically or chemically. The composition of these products varies widely; pharmacists should be aware of factors that influence effectiveness.

SUNBURN: CAUSE AND EFFECTS

A sunburn is characterized by erythema, edema, tenderness, and, in more severe cases, the formation of vesicles or bullae. The reactions, which mainly affect the epidermis (see Chapter 26 for a discussion of skin anatomy), are similar to first-degree and (when blistering occurs) second-degree burns. The burns usually are minor but may be serious if large areas blister. Sunburn is not apparent immediately. The onset of symptoms usually occurs within 1–24 hours but may be delayed for as long as 72 hours after exposure.

Ultraviolet Radiation

The ultraviolet radiation that causes sunburn and suntan is in the 290- to 320-nanometer (nm) range. Wavelengths above this range may stimulate a short-lived tan by oxidizing (darkening) melanin in the skin. Wavelengths below 290 nm are filtered out by ozone in the atmosphere (1).

The ultraviolet light alters the keratinocytes in the basal layer of the epidermis. A slight alteration results in erythema, and a severe alteration causes bullae to form from the fluid collected in the epidermis. To produce a suntan, ultraviolet light stimulates the melanocytes in the germinating layer to generate more melanin and oxidizes melanin already in the epidermis. This darkening of the skin is a normal body function that protects against further damage from sun exposure.

Skin Cancer

Basal- and squamous-cell epitheliomas are common malignancies involving alterations in keratinocyte growth. Premalignant growth of keratinocytes, called senile, or actinic, keratosis, is also common. Sunlight has been implicated as the major cause of skin cancer (2–5). The relative incidence of actinic keratosis and squamous-cell carcinomas increases with increased exposure to damaging solar rays. However, the incidence of basal-cell carcinomas seems to depend on factors other than sunlight (2).

Skin cancer is more common in fair-skinned people, less likely in dark-skinned Caucasians who are not overly exposed, and rare in the Negroid population. The frequency of skin cancer is higher in farmers, sailors, construction workers, and other individuals whose occupations require many hours of daily exposure to the sun (2–6). Skin cancer occurs more often in tropical and subtropical climates than in moderate ones because the quantity of harmful light that reaches the earth's surface is increased as the angle of the sun to a reference point on earth approaches 90° and the distance of the sun to the earth decreases (2, 5, 7–10). A constant rate of increase in the incidence of skin cancer was found in approaching the equator from north to south; the incidence approximately doubled for every 3°48′ reduction in latitude (11).

In the United States the incidence of skin cancer increases dramatically from north to south. Males are more likely to develop the disease than females, who traditionally have not experienced the occupational hazard of long exposure in the sun. The face, head, and neck areas are affected more than three times as often as sites that usually are covered. The black population shows a much lower incidence than the white population because of the natural protection afforded by darker skin (2). Skin cancer is likely to become more prevalent as the desirability of tanning continues to be popular (2); in El Paso, Texas, for example, the incidence of skin cancer per 100,000 Anglo-Americans rose from 126 in 1944 to 290 in 1960 in males and from 50 to 175 in females (12).

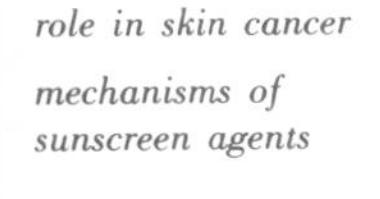

role in skin cancer

Additional studies also implicate long-term exposure to the sun as a causative factor in skin cancer. A study that found a mean annual incidence of malignant melanomas of 2.0 per 100,000 in males and 2.9 per 100,000 in females corroborated evidence for the cumulative effect of solar exposure on the development of tumors (the incidence rates appeared to increase with age), the protective properties of darkly pigmented skin, and the influence of environmental factors such as geographic location and national origin on the incidence of melanomas (13). The frequency of skin cancer in Caucasian adults in a rural Tennessee county increased with age from 0.7 per 100 (under 44 years) to 13.6 per 100 (65–74 years) for males; corresponding figures for females were 0.4 and 6.8 (6).

Thus the effects of sunlight on the skin may seem pleasant, but the end result may be extremely harmful. The problem is summarized by this statement (14): "The skin never forgets an injury. . . . The eventual condition of the skin results from a summation of all the injuries it has received."

SUNBURN PREVENTION

mechanisms of sunscreen agents

Sunscreens act either physically or chemically. Physical sunscreens provide a mechanical barrier to sunlight; for example, zinc oxide paste and titanium dioxide scatter ultraviolet light. Clothing and beach umbrellas are also effective as physical sunscreens, but ultraviolet light may be reflected from sand and water to reach under a beach umbrella and cause burning.

Chemical sunscreens absorb a specific portion of the ultraviolet light spectrum. When the light is absorbed by the sunscreen, several changes may occur in the absorbing compound (15):

- Light energy is converted to heat;
- The sunscreen molecule may dissociate into atoms or radicals;
- The molecule may be excited to higher energy levels, and its energy transferred through collision with another molecule, followed by a chemical reaction;
- The compound may become excited and lose its energy immediately by fluorescence or later by phosphorescence.

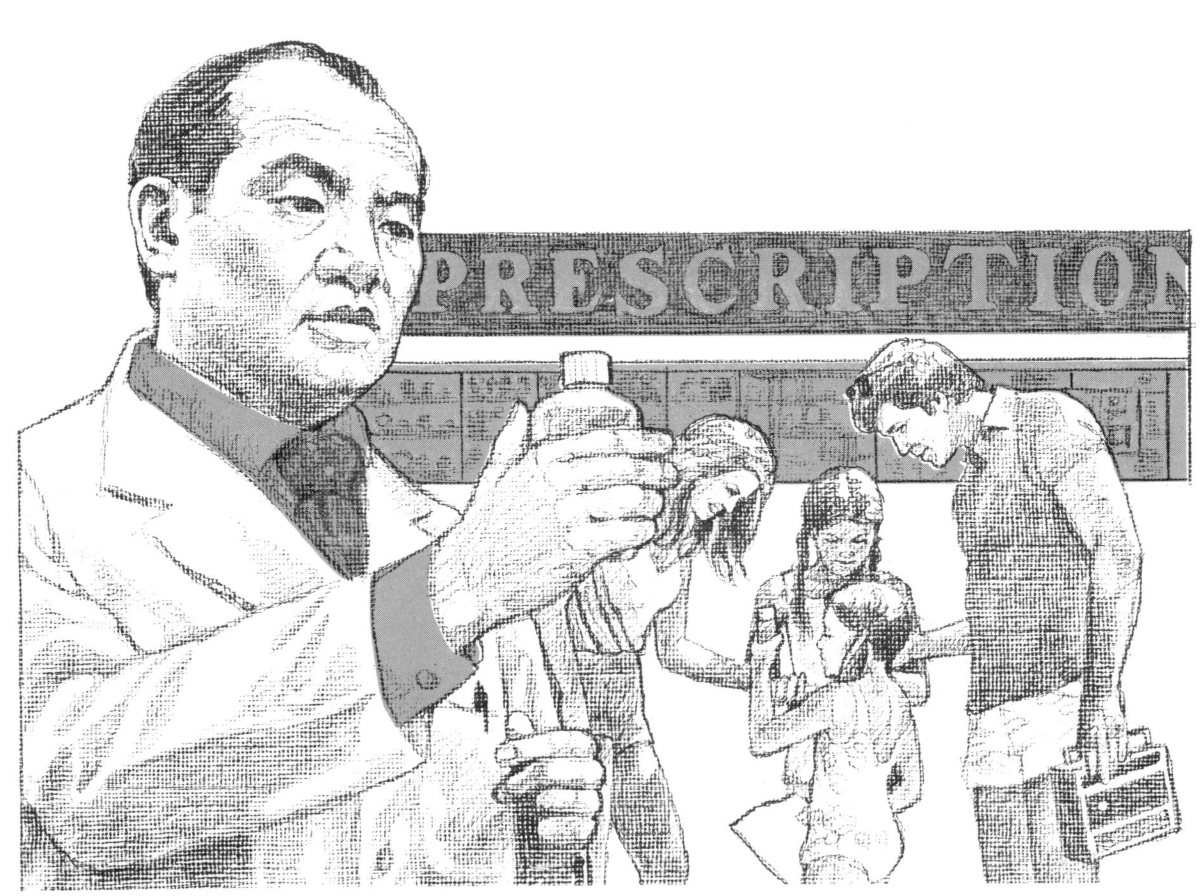

Indications for Sunscreen Use

In addition to preventing sunburn and premature aging of the skin and probably reducing actinic or solar keratosis and some types of skin cancer, sunscreen agents should be considered for protection against photosensitivity caused by certain drugs. A phototoxic reaction is one in which the chemical absorbs ultraviolet energy, the absorbed energy is transferred from the photoactivated chemical to the vulnerable cellular constituents, and cellular damage results, usually with a more or less severe sunburnlike reaction (16).

A photoallergic reaction presumably involves an immunological mechanism in which absorption of energy by the photosensitizing chemical results in the formation of a new hapten, the hapten combines with a skin protein, and this complex of the agent with the "carrier" protein initiates a hypersensitivity reaction from antigen–antibody activity in the skin. The usual clinical picture is one of an eczematous or polymorphic delayed-onset dermatitis (17).

A phototoxic reaction, or primary photosensitivity, to a given compound implies susceptibility on first exposure. A photoallergic response is characterized by a delayed onset, occurs in sensitized skin, and recurs with subsequent exposures to ultraviolet light (16, 17). Ultraviolet light above 320 nm can elicit a photoallergic response (16–18). The chemically induced sensitivity occurs with compounds such as barbiturates, chlorothiazide, chlorpromazine, demeclocycline, erythromycin, phenylsulfonylurea, promethazine, psoralens, quinidine, quinine, sulfas, and tetracycline (4, 17, 19).

The literature shows disagreement on the value of sunscreen agent protection (19). However, there is evidence that these products provide some protection, depending on the degree of photosensitization (4). A 10% sulisobenzone lotion was shown to be effective as a sunscreen agent in skin photosensitized by demeclocycline (18). Dihydroxyacetone–naphthoquinone (Duoshield) was effective in individuals photosensitized by chlorpromazine reacting to ultraviolet light between 330 and 400 nm (20). This combination also protected individuals with erythropoietic protoporphyria, when the porphyrin has an action band at 400 nm. Compounds that absorb energy throughout the ultraviolet region, such as sulisobenzone, oxybenzone, and dioxybenzone, may be the most successful for this purpose if they are used in adequate amounts.

Table 1 lists some sunscreen agents and their tentative evaluations by the FDA OTC Panel on Topical Analgesic, Antirheumatic, Otic, Burn, and Sunburn Treatment Products.

Evaluating Effectiveness of Sunscreens

Criteria are needed to judge the effectiveness of sunscreen agents. Testing the agents in humans is difficult because individuals react in varying degrees to sunlight. The minimal erythemal dose (MED), the amount of sunlight needed for a minimum perceptible erythema (redness), is used to gauge the degree of sensitivity of both protected and unprotected skin to sunlight. The protection factor (PF), the ratio of the minimal erythemal dose for protected skin to that for unprotected skin, is used to measure the relative effectiveness of sunscreens (the larger the protection factor value, the greater the protection).

Other criteria are:

- Ability to absorb in the 290- to 320-nm ultraviolet light range (320–500 nm for protection from photosensitizing drugs) (17);
- Molar absorptivity in the ultraviolet range for sunburn or photosensitization (molar absorptivity is the ability of a compound to absorb ultraviolet light—the larger the value at a specified wavelength, the better the absorption);
- Concentrations on the skin needed to absorb a desired amount of light without irritation—not all compounds that absorb in the 290- to 320-nm ultraviolet light range can be used as sunscreens; for example, salicylic acid at its effective sunscreening concentration of 5% is keratolytic and may be quite irritating.

sunscreen use as protectants in drug-induced photosensitivity

drugs eliciting photoallergic reactions

assessing effectiveness of sunscreen agents

Table 2 shows some of the more common compounds used as sunscreen agents and their molar absorptivities. The molar absorptivity values are obtained in identical solvents and conditions that allow the compounds to be compared and ranked as to their efficacy. To be most effective, the range of maximum absorption for the sunscreen agent must overlap the ultraviolet range of sunlight that produces sunburn. The larger molar absorptivity value reflects the ability of that compound to absorb ultraviolet light at the indicated wavelength.

Although the pharmacist cannot control the formulation of the various commercially available sunscreen products, a knowledge of the specific active ingredients and their concentrations helps differentiate a good product from a mediocre one. The sunscreen product that contains a sunscreen which has a larger molar absorptivity and is present at a higher concentration is the better product, provided the sunscreen agent overlays the range of ultraviolet light that produces the sunburn. In addition, sunscreen agents that have a low or intermediate molar absorptivity may be made more effective by increasing the concentration of the active ingredient. For example, if the compound isoamyl *p-N,N*-(dimethylamino)benzoate (molar absorptivity, 28,083) is used in a sunscreen product, its concentration should be at least 2.5%; if used in a suntan product, the concentration may be reduced to less than 2%, probably to 1.0–1.5%. In contrast, glyceryl *p*-aminobenzoate (molar absorptivity, 17,197) is about 59% as efficient as isoamyl *p-N,N*-(dimethylamino)benzoate and should be used at a higher concentration in sunscreen products and at a lower concentration (approximately one-half) in suntan products.

The thickness of the residual skin layer may influence the effectiveness of sunscreen products. This factor cannot be controlled pharmaceutically but can be controlled by the patient, using care to apply generous portions and to spread the product evenly over the exposed skin. Certain properties of the agent or product may contribute to its effectiveness.

FDA evaluation of effectiveness of sunscreen agents

products "promoting" suntan

Table 1. Tentative Evaluation of Sunscreen Agents

Sunscreen Agent	Dosage Range, %	FDA Category	Safety	Effectiveness
Allantoin	—	II	—	not effective
Aminobenzoic acid	5 (hydro-alcoholic), 5–15 (creams and ointments)	I	safe	effective—absorbs UV light at 290–320 nm
Cinoxate (2-ethoxyethyl *p*-methoxycinnamate)	1–3	I	safe	effective—1% solution absorbs UV light at 280–320 nm; 10% concentration absorbs UV light at 270–328 nm; maximum absorption at 310 nm
Digalloyl trioleate (mix of several derivatives of tannic acid)	2–5	I	safe	effective—absorbs UV light at 200–315 nm; maximum absorption at 297 nm
2-Ethylhexyl *p*-methoxycinnamate	2.5–5	I	no reported adverse reactions	effective—1 mg % allowed 16% transmission at 310 nm
Glyceryl *p*-aminobenzoate	2–3	I	safe—a few reported cases of contact dermatitis and photo contact dermatitis	—
Homosalate	4–15	not established	safe	prevents tanning at 15%; permits tanning at 8%
Menthyl anthranilate	—	I as sunburn protective, I as suntan preventive		absorbs UV light at 300–360 nm; maximum absorption between 332 and 345 nm

The pH

If the pH is raised or lowered, the fraction of the ionized and un-ionized sunscreen agent changes and changes the position of the peak absorbance, possibly shifting it away from the 290- to 320-nm range.

Solvent System

Various solvent systems, such as ethanol and the oil phase of an emulsion vehicle, can direct the position of the peak absorbency of the sunscreen. Shifts of the peak away from the 290- to 320-nm range may compromise the sunscreen's effectiveness.

Stability

The sunscreen must remain stable for the desired period of protection.

SUNTAN PRODUCTS

For cosmetic rather than therapeutic needs the patient may desire a suntan product. In some cases these products differ from sunscreens only by having a lower concentration of the sunscreen agent. The concentration of the active ingredient is an important factor in judging the use and effectiveness of a product. For example, SunDare Lotion, a suntan product, contains 1.75% cinoxate, but Maxafil Cream, a sunscreen product, contains 4%—about twice as much as the suntan product—and 5% methyl anthranilate, a second sunscreen. Selection of a sunscreen also may be based on the amount of ultraviolet light it absorbs. For example, some suntan products contain a sunscreen agent that blocks wavelengths of less than 320 nm but allows wavelengths of more than 320 nm to penetrate, producing a light, tran-

Table 1. Continued

Sunscreen Agent	Dosage Range, %	FDA Category	Safety	Effectiveness
p-Methoxycinnamic acid diethanolamine	8–10	III	no reported adverse reactions	effective—maximum absorption at 290 nm; 4% transmission at 25 mg %
3-(4-Methylbenzidine) camphor	1–2.5	III	safe when used as directed	effective—1% transmission at 310 nm in concentration of 13.5%; absorbs UV light at 280–310 nm
2-Mole propoxylate salt of *p*-aminoethylbenzoic acid	1–5	III	no reported adverse reactions	1, 2.5, and 5% protected at 20, 40, and 60 MED, respectively
Oxybenzone (2-hydroxy-4-methoxybenzophenone)	0.5–2	I	safe when used as directed	controls UV light at 320–400 nm; absorbs major portion of UV light at 280–320 nm
Padimate A [pentyl *p*-(dimethylamino)benzoate]	1–3.6	I	—	—
Padimate 0 [2-ethylhexyl *p*-(dimethylamino)benzoate]	1.4–4	I	does not appear to be a skin sensitizer or primary irritant	effective
2-Phenylbenzimidazole	1–4	I	safe	16% transmission at 290–310 nm
Titanium dioxide	1–15	I	safe	scatters UV light at 290–700 nm

Data from the FDA OTC Panel on Topical Analgesic, Antirheumatic, Otic, Burn, and Sunburn Treatment Products. (This table is incomplete until the panel publishes its final report.) A common method for evaluating these agents is not yet available; thus the most effective ingredient and/or product of those listed as safe and effective cannot be chosen from the information listed here. However, products containing agents listed as both safe and effective, if used in the appropriate concentrations, probably will be the more successful sunscreens. No data available for 2-ethylhexyl-4-phenylbenzophenone-2-carboxylic acid or dihydroxyacetone with lawsone.

effectiveness and FDA evaluation of sunscreen agents

sient tan. Others contain a weakly absorbent sunscreen agent, which allows a significant fraction of all the ultraviolet light to reach the skin.

Suntan products do not "promote" a tan. Some, including cocoa butter and mineral oil alone or with staining materials such as iodine or tannic acid, do not contain a sunscreen agent. None of these products provides protection from the sun. The products mainly stain and lubricate the skin and do not reverse the aging process caused by ultraviolet light. The FDA OTC Panel has stated (21) that "claims such as 'promotes tanning' for sunlight protective agents are unsubstantiated."

Some suntan products contain dihydroxyacetone and a small amount of sunscreen. Dihydroxyacetone darkens the skin by interacting with keratin in the stratum corneum. These products emphasize the cosmetic tan produced and not protection, although they may contain a small amount of a sunscreen agent and do darken the skin.

PRODUCT SELECTION GUIDELINES

Before recommending a sunscreen or suntan product, the pharmacist should know the identity of the active ingredient and its maximum absorption, molar absorptivity, and concentration (see Table 1). An in vivo evaluation also is useful in judging a product (22). The physical characteristics (molar absorptivity and maximum absorption) are available in Table 2. The identity and concentration of the active ingredients may be supplied by the manufacturer but also should appear on the label. Without this information, recommendations can be based only on intuition or personal experience. If the information is not supplied by the manufacturer, recommendations should be limited to products that indicate the identity and concentration of the active ingredients.

Studies that compare several sunscreen products in humans can serve as a basis for professional judgment. One such study evaluated 17 sunscreen products, using a mean protection factor to evaluate each product (22). Table 3 shows that products that contain 5% aminobenzoic acid are superior to those that contain aminobenzoic acid esters. However, aminobenzoic acid esters are generally used in a concentration of less than 5%. A study showed that alcoholic preparations of 5% aminobenzoic acid and preparations that contain 2.5% isoamyl *p-N,N*-(dimethylamino)benzoate were more effective than commercial products tested (23). Another product evaluation substantiates this finding in products that contain 5% aminobenzoic acid (21). Several investigators (23, 24) agree that aminobenzoic acid is more effective as a sunscreen than popular proprietary products, but they disagree that aminobenzoic acid esters are less effective than the parent compound, aminobenzoic acid. Nevertheless, 5% aminobenzoic acid seems to yield the best results as a sunscreen product. The 1978–1979 edition of *Drugs of Choice* lists products containing aminobenzoic

molar absorptivity of sunscreen agents

Table 2. Spectral Parameters for Sunscreen Agents

Compound	Molar Absorptivity	λ_{max}, nm
Aminobenzoic acid (*para*-isomer)	18,300	290
Cinoxate (2-ethoxyethyl *p*-methoxycinnamate)	19,400	306
Dioxybenzone (2,2′-dihydroxy-4-methoxybenzophenone)	11,951	282[a]
Glyceryl *p*-aminobenzoate	17,197	298
Homosalate (homomenthyl salicylate)	6,720[b]	310[b]
Isoamyl *p-N,N*-(dimethylamino)benzoate	28,083	312
Menthyl anthranilate	941[b]	315[b]
Oxybenzone (2-hydroxy-4-methoxybenzophenone)	20,381	287[a]
Sulisobenzone (2-hydroxy-4-methoxybenzophenone-5-sulfonic acid)	5,580	287[a]

All values determined in ethanol.
[a] These compounds absorb throughout the UV range.
[b] Values from A.C. Giese et al., *J. Am. Pharm. Assoc. Sci. Ed.*, *39*, 30 (1950).

Table 3. Sunscreen Protection at 305 nm

Sunscreen	Protection Factor (PF)[a] Mean MED's	SD	Range	N
Pabanol (5% aminobenzoic acid)	17.6	9.7	10–21	23
Presun (5% aminobenzoic acid)	17.6	9.7	10–21	23
Maxafil (4% cinoxate, 5% menthyl anthranilate)	9.6	5.7	6–14	23
Sea & Ski (glyceryl *p*-aminobenzoate)	8.3	4.6	5–11	13
RVPaque (red petrolatum, zinc oxide, cinoxate)	7.7	4.4	6–9	13
Solbar (3% oxybenzone, 3% dioxybenzone)	6.7	3.8	5–10	23
Sunswept (3.5% digalloyl trioleate)	6.6	3.3	5–9	23
Estee Lauder's U.V. Screening Lotion (padimate)	6.6	3.0	5–8	16
UVAL (10% sulisobenzone)	6.6	3.4	6–9	16
Afil Cream (5% titanium dioxide, 5% menthyl anthranilate)	6.3	3.5	6–8	16
Coppertone (homosalate)	6.0	2.6	4–7	17
Pan Ultra (diphenyl ketone)	6.0	2.5	4–7	17
Pabafilm (padimate)	5.9	3.4	4–9	23
Sungard (10% sulisobenzone)	5.9	3.2	3–8	17
SunDare (cinoxate)	5.9	2.4	5–7	17
Block Out (padimate)	5.5	3.1	4–7	17
RVP (red petrolatum)	3.2	2.1	2–4	18

Adapted from D.J. Cripps and S. Hegedus, *Arch. Dermatol.*, *109*, 202 (1974). SD = standard deviation, N = number of subjects.
[a] Protection factor (MED's) of 17 sunscreens applied in concentrations of 30 $\mu l/cm^2$, tested at 305-nm radiation (4-nm half-band-width.

acid, dioxybenzone, oxybenzone, and analogous products as satisfactory sunscreen products (25).

SUMMARY

Although it is possible to discourage excessive sunbathing, there is no escape from the sun. However, a preventive program using an appropriate sunscreen may prevent or minimize degenerative cutaneous changes, such as solar keratosis and skin cancer, that can result from repeated and long exposure to sunlight.

Protective habits that prevent the undesirable results of overexposure should be encouraged. These habits should be started early because the aging process caused by the sun is insidious and cumulative. If a tan is desired, short exposures to the sun, gradually extended as the sunbathing season progresses, followed by generous applications of a good sunscreen may be recommended. The sunscreen should be reapplied after bathing, excessive exercise, or sweating, at about 1- to 2-hour intervals.

Patients receiving therapy that includes photosensitizing medication should be cautioned against exposure to the sun and advised to use physical protection, such as a hat, protective clothing, and concomitant application of an effective sunscreen. Although it is an often overlooked responsibility, evaluating or selecting the proper sunscreen or suntan product is an important health service for the pharmacist to fulfill.

REFERENCES

(1) K. F. Dyer, *New Sci.*, *43*, 228 (1969).
(2) K. V. Sanderson, in "Comparative Physiology and Pathology of the Skin," A. J. Rook and G. S. Walton, Eds., Davis, Philadelphia, Pa., 1965, p. 637.
(3) D. M. Pillsbury, B. Shelley, and A. M. Kligman, "Dermatology," Saunders, Philadelphia, Pa., 1956, p. 1145.
(4) N. Tobias, "Essentials of Dermatology," 6th ed., Lippincott, Philadelphia, Pa., 1963, p. 328.
(5) M. Segi, Monograph No. 10, U.S. National Cancer Institute, Washington, D.C., 1963, p. 245.
(6) Z. W. Zagula-Mally, E. W. Rosenberg, and M. Kashgarian, *Cancer*, *34*, 345 (1974).
(7) J. Belisario, "Cancer of the Skin," Butterworth, London, England, 1959, p. 15.
(8) J. A. Elliott and D. G. Welton, *Arch. Dermatol. Syphitol.*, *53*, 307 (1946).
(9) V. A. Belinsky and L. N. Guslitzer, in "Tenth International Cancer Congress Abstracts, May 22–29," 1970, p. 109.
(10) F. Urback, S. O'Beirn, and L. Guslitzer, in "Tenth International Cancer Congress Abstracts, May 22–29," 1970, p. 109.
(11) H. Auerbach, Public Health Report, No. 76, Washington, D.C., 1961, p. 345.
(12) G. J. McDonald and E. Bubendorf, in "Tumors of the Skin," Year Book Medical, Chicago, Ill., 1964, p. 23.
(13) M. Movshovitz and B. Modan, *J. Nat. Cancer Inst.*, *51*, 77 (1973).
(14) *British Medical Journal*, *3*, 72 (1974).
(15) F. Daniels and R. A. Alberty, "Physical Chemistry," 2nd ed., Wiley, New York, N.Y., 1961, p. 654.
(16) G. Goldman and E. Epstein, Jr., *Arch. Dermatol.*, *100*, 447 (1969).
(17) D. M. Pillsbury, B. Shelley, and A. M. Kligman, "Dermatology," Saunders, Philadelphia, Pa., 1956, p. 1241.
(18) R. F. Dahlen, S. I. Shapiro, C. Z. Berry, and M. M. Schreiber, *J. Invest. Dermatol.*, *55*, 165 (1970).
(19) *British Medical Journal*, *2*, 494 (1970).
(20) J. A. Johnson, R. R. Czaplewski, and R. M. Fusaro, *Dermatologica*, *147*, 104 (1973).
(21) "Summary Minutes of the FDA OTC Panel on Topical Analgesic, Antirheumatic, Otic, Burn, and Sunburn Treatment Products," Meetings 1–6, Rockville, Md., March 1973–Jan. 1975.
(22) D. J. Cripps and S. Hegedus, *Arch. Dermatol.*, *109*, 202 (1974).
(23) M. A. Pathak, T. B. Fitzpatrick, and E. Frenk, *N. Engl. J. Med.*, *280*, 1461 (1969).
(24) I. Willis and A. M. Kligman, *Arch. Dermatol.*, *102*, 405 (1970).
(25) "Drugs of Choice, 1978–1979," W. Modell, Ed., Mosby, St. Louis, Mo., 1978.

Product (Manufacturer)	Sunscreen Agent	Other
A-Fil Cream (Texas Pharmacal)	menthyl anthranilate, 5%	titanium dioxide, 5%
Block Out (Sea & Ski)	octyldimethyl-aminobenzoic acid, 8%	alcohol, 70%; moisturizers; fragrance
Coppertone Lipkote (Plough)	homosalate	—
Coppertone Nosekote (Plough)	homosalate, 7% oxybenzone	—
Coppertone Shade Lotion (Plough)	homosalate, 8% oxybenzone, 3%	—
Coppertone Suntan Foam, Lotion, Oil, and Spray (Plough)	homosalate, 8% (foam, lotion) 9% (oil, spray)	—
Coppertone Super Shade Lotion (Plough)	oxybenzone padimate	—
Coppertone Tanning Butter and Butter Spray (Plough)	homosalate, 6% (butter) 8% (spray)	cocoa butter, coconut oil
Dark Tanning Butter (Sea & Ski)	—	acetylated lanolin, cocoa butter, mineral oil, moisturizers, emollients
Dark Tanning Oil (Sea & Ski)	padimate, 1.1%	mineral oil, emollients, moisturizers
Eclipse (Herbert)	glyceryl *p*-aminobenzoate, 3% padimate O, 3%	alcohol, 5%; oleth-3 phosphate; petrolatum; synthetic spermaceti; glycerin; mineral oil; lanolin alcohol; cetyl stearyl glycol; lanolin oil; triethanolamine; carbomer 934P; benzyl alcohol, 0.5%; perfume
Florida Tan Tanning Oil and Dark Tanning Oil (Florida Tan)	aminobenzoic acid	cocoa butter, coconut oil, aloe, almond, lanolin, banana, fragrance
Golden Tan Lotion (Sea & Ski)	octyldimethyl-aminobenzoic acid, 1.7%	cocoa butter, mineral oil, lanolin, alcohol
Indoor/Outdoor Foam and Lotion (Sea & Ski)	padimate, 1.05%	dihydroxyacetone, 4%; lanolin; glycerin (foam); mineral oil
Maxafil Cream (Texas Pharmacal)	menthyl anthranilate, 5% cinoxate, 4%	—
Mentholatum Stick (Mentholatum)	padimate A	petrolatum, menthol, camphor, essential oils
Natural Woman Suntan Lotion (LaMaur)	oxybenzone dioxybenzone	—
Pabafilm (Owen)	isoamyl *N,N*-dimethylaminobenzoate, 2.5%	alcohol, 70%
Pabagel (Owen)	aminobenzoic acid, 5%	alcohol, 57%
Pabanol (Elder)	aminobenzoic acid, 5%	alcohol, 70%
Paba Sun Lotion (Amer. Pharm.)	aminobenzoic acid	allantoin, cocoa butter, vitamins A, D, and E, sesame oil, avocado oil
Palmer's Cocoa Butter Formula (Browne)	benzophenone 3, 0.5%	cocoa butter; vitamin E, 0.1%; allantoin, 0.1%; mineral oil; microwax
Post Sun (Westwood)	—	mineral oil, propylene glycol, glyceryl stearate, polyethylene glycol 40 stearate, lanolin, methylparaben, propylparaben, fragrance, triethanolamine
Pre Sun (Westwood)	aminobenzoic acid, 5%	alcohol, glycerin, choleth-24, hydroxyethylcellulose
Q. T. Quick Tanning Foam and Lotion (Plough)	homosalate, 8%	dihydroxyacetone
RVPaba Stick (Elder)	aminobenzoic acid red petrolatum	—
RVPaque (Elder)	cinoxate red petrolatum	zinc oxide
RVP Cream (Elder)	red petrolatum	hydrocarbon oil, ointment base
RVPlus (Elder)	red petrolatum titanium-coated mica platelets	—

Product (Manufacturer)	Sunscreen Agent	Other
Sea & Ski Lotion (Sea & Ski)	octyldimethylaminobenzoic acid, 2.5%	glycerin, mineral oil, lanolin, sesame oil
Snootie (Sea & Ski)	padimate, 2.5%	glycerin, stearic acid, dimethicone
Solar Cream (Doak)	aminobenzoic acid, 4%	titanium dioxide, 12%; water-repellent cream base, 84%
Solbar (Person & Covey)	dioxybenzone, 3% oxybenzone, 3%	—
Sudden Tan Foam and Lotion by Coppertone (Plough)	homosalate, 6.25%	dihydroxyacetone, caramel
Sunbrella (Dorsey)	aminobenzoic acid, 5%	alcohol, 50%
SunDare Clear (Texas Pharmacal)	cinoxate, 1.75%	alcohol, 51.8%
SunDare Creamy (Texas Pharmacal)	cinoxate, 2%	lanolin derivative
SunGer Extra Protection (Plough)	homosalate oxybenzone	—
SunGer Sun Block (Plough)	padimate oxybenzone	—
SunGer Weather and Tanning Stick (Plough)	homosalate	—
Sunswept (Texas Pharmacal)	digalloyl trioleate, 3.5%	—
Super Shade Lotion by Coppertone (Plough)	aminobenzoic acid, 5%	—
Tan Care by Coppertone (Plough)	—	glycerin, stearic acid, glyceryl monostearate, isopropyl myristate, polyethylene glycol 75, lanolin
Tega-Tan Foam (Ortega)	glyceryl *p*-aminobenzoate	emulsifier, alcohol, aromatics
Tropic Sun Oil and Butter (Sea & Ski)	padimate, 1.1% (oil)	cocoa butter, coconut oil, almond oil, mineral oil, lanolin
Uval Sun'n Wind Stick (Dorsey)	padimate A, 3%	—
Uval Sunscreen Lotion (Dorsey)	sulisobenzone, 10%	—

External Analgesic Products

Paul Skierkowski and Nancy Burdock

Chapter 25

Questions to Ask the Patient

Is the pain in a joint or in the muscle?

How long have you had the pain?

Is the pain a result of an accident or overwork?

(If the pain is in a joint) Is the joint red, swollen, or warm to the touch? Is the pain worse when you get up in the morning, and does it tend to subside as the day goes on?

Have you experienced abdominal pain, nausea, or pain when urinating?

Does the pain radiate to other areas?

Do you have a fever or other "flu" symptoms?

What treatments have you tried? How well did they work?

Analgesics are used externally to treat conditions such as burn, sunburn, dental pain, hemorrhoids, and muscular pain. This chapter deals with the use of external analgesics for skeletal muscle pain. (For additional information, see Chapter 9 on internal analgesics.)

ETIOLOGY OF MUSCULAR PAIN

Pain receptors are present in most areas of the body, including skeletal muscles. Stimuli activating these receptors cause sensory impulses which are translated into a pain perception. The threshold of response varies greatly among individuals (1).

Skeletal muscle pain is quite common, especially in an urban society where people are not accustomed to strenuous exertion. When people do strain themselves, their muscles become sore and painful to move. Muscle pain also may occur as a result of prolonged, fixed, and stressful positions such as bending over for long periods. Tension and anxiety also may induce prolonged tonic contraction of muscle, causing pain (2).

Because of its location and structure, the shoulder area is subject to more stress and strain than any other articulation of the body. In addition to all its other activities, its pendulum structure makes it continuously subjected to gravitational pull. A painful shoulder is more prevalent among elderly persons but frequently occurs in athletes and with certain occupations, such as house painting, where the arms are used vigorously and repetitively (3).

Acute, temporary stiffness and muscle pain also may result from cold, dampness, rapid temperature changes, and air currents. In some cases, internal stimuli such as tension, constipation, GI distention, and other minor disorders are reflected as shoulder pain. These episodes are likely to be acute and self-limiting, and elimination of the cause and symptomatic treatment generally provide relief. Poor posture is also a frequent cause of skeletal muscle pain.

Bursitis, an inflammation of the bursae of the body, is a common cause of shoulder pain. It may be acute, due to trauma, or chronic, in which case other causes such as infection should be suspect. Bursitis is characterized by localized pain, tenderness, and swelling. Limited motion of adjacent joints is common (4).

Arthritic pain is caused by swelling of joints. When the joint is at rest, the pain usually is relieved; when the joint is in use, especially in a twisting motion, the pain is more persistent. Stiffness is also a constant symptom, most prominent on first arising. Although arthritis is a chronic systemic disease, local treatment of painful joints may give temporary symptomatic relief.

In counseling patients about pains thought to be associated with skeletal muscles, the pharmacist should inquire into activities that may have brought on the condition. This information may eliminate other organic problems possibly misinterpreted as skeletal muscle pain. For example, a posteriorly perforating duodenal ulcer or gas accumulation in the colon may cause pain radiating into the back, and spinal disease may cause radial pain in the thigh muscle. However, if the pain developed after the patient spent the day weeding a garden or painting a ceiling, it generally can be relieved with external and/or internal analgesics.

The pharmacist should be particularly cautious in assessing patient complaints of arthritic-type pain. Although external analgesics are useful adjuncts in treating such disorders, they are not indicated as the sole treatment. Only after a definitive diagnosis has been made and proper drug therapy has been instituted should external analgesics be used. Failure to follow this procedure may lead to progressive joint destruction.

TREATMENT OF MUSCULAR PAIN

The topical OTC products for the symptomatic relief of pain due to sprains, strains, sore muscles and joints, neuralgia, rheumatism, arthritis, and similar disorders contain counterirritant agents. Counterirritants are applied locally to produce a mild, local, inflammatory reaction with the object of affecting another site, usually adjacent to or underlying the irritated surface. The skin's intensity of response depends not only on the nature of the irritant employed, but also on its concentration, the solvent in which it is dissolved, and the period of contact with the skin (5).

The counterirritant drug is applied to the skin where pain is experienced. Pain is only as intense as it is perceived to be, and the perception of other sensations from application of the counterirritant, such as massage and warmth, crowds out perception of the pain. Several theories have been proposed to explain the mechanism of action of the irritant drugs (6):

counterirritants

mechanism of action theories

nerve fibers

- Stimulation of sensory nerve endings, producing vasodilation in a remote area because of reflexes acting through the cerebrospinal axis;
- Stimulation of sensory nerve endings, producing localized vasodilation of the skin due to axon reflexes;
- A summation of painful stimuli due to the local inflammatory insult produced by counterirritants.

There is no unanimity of opinion concerning these theories.

Reflexes mediated through the cerebrospinal axis, originating from sensory nerve fiber stimulation, produce efferent stimuli that elicit a vascular dilator response in the viscera. The afferent sensory nerve fibers from the skin synapse in the spinal cord with efferent vasomotor fibers to the viscera (Figure 1). Stimulation of the skin by a counterirritant increases the number of afferent stimuli passing to a segment of the spinal cord from which arise many visceral efferent fibers.

The axon reflex hypothesis suggests that sensory nerves are connected directly with the arteriolar nerve network. For example, stimulation of the skin's sensory nerves by a counterirritant causes a stimulus to pass along the nerves and then to the branches of the arterioles. This action produces an increase in the blood flow to the muscles which, with concomitant waste disposal and other chemical changes, leads to recovery (7).

Counterirritants also may produce a summation of pain stimuli. The classical signs of cutaneous and subdermal inflammation are heat sensations, redness, pain, and swelling. In producing these effects the counterirritants also may relieve visceral pain by causing intense stimulation of the areas of pain interpretation of the brain, partly abating visceral pain stimuli. According to this theory of their action, stimuli originating in the viscera or muscles are transmitted over fibers in a common pathway along with sensations from the skin. Stimuli from the viscera or muscles are referred to the same area of the spinal cord as the stimuli from the skin. If the intensity of the stimulation from the skin is increased by a drug's irritant action, the character of the visceral or muscle pain becomes modified. With intense skin stimulation, the visceral pain stimuli may be partly or completely obliterated insofar as the sensorium is concerned. The patient's attention is diverted from the diseased visceral structure by the application of the counterirritant drug (5).

An additional effect of some products is to produce an irritant response. These drugs, known as rubefacients, produce active or passive hyperemia, and it is hypothesized that this increase in blood pooling and/or flow is accompanied by an increase in localized skin temperature. The degree of irritation must be controlled, however, as stronger irritation may cause blistering. The increase in localized skin temperature then may act by the counterirritant effect. This positive thermal response for some agents has been documented by thermography (8).

Undoubtedly, the action of counterirritants in relieving pain has a strong psychological component. However, the therapeutic merits, based on established empirical observation, are well recognized. Whatever their mechanism of action, the judicious use of the counterirritant drugs has a place in medical practice.

Ingredients in OTC Products

Many ingredients in external analgesic products were reviewed extensively by the FDA OTC Panel on Topical Analgesic, Antirheumatic, Otic, Burn, and Sunburn Treatment Products. Most of the products used as counterirritants are volatile substances. These agents include allyl isothiocyanate, camphor, menthol, methyl salicylate,

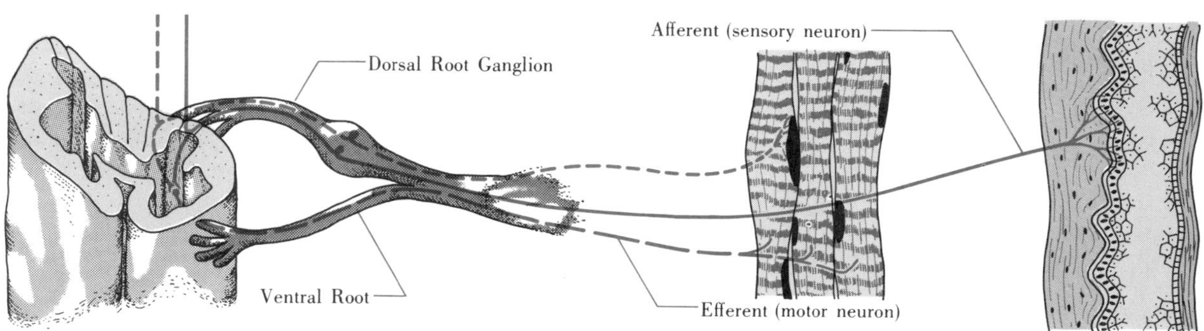

Figure 1. Reflex pathways showing the afferent (sensory) fibers, efferent (vasomotor) fibers, and their synapse in the spinal cord. Adapted from F.H. Netter, *The Ciba Collection of Medical Illustrations,* Ciba Pharmaceutical Company, New York, N.Y., 1962, p. 65.

oils of clove, cinnamon, wormwood, myristica (nutmeg), chenopodium, eucalyptus, turpentine, and thymol. Some formulations may include aspirin, histamine dihydrochloride, methacholine chloride, or triethanolamine salicylate as additional active ingredients.

Methyl Salicylate

Methyl salicylate, occurring naturally as wintergreen or sweet birch oil, is the most widely used counterirritant. When it is rubbed on the skin, it produces mild irritation and is absorbed to an appreciable extent (5). Systemic analgesic effects due to the absorption of the salicylate component are possible; however, there is no clinical evidence to support this hypothesis.

The effective range of concentrations for methyl salicylate is 10–60%, and this product has been placed in Category I as a counterirritant–rubefacient. Unfortunately, methyl salicylate's pleasant odor and taste may induce ingestion of the substance, especially by children—as little as one teaspoonful may be fatal (9). Federal law requires that liquid preparations containing more than 5% of methyl salicylate be dispensed only in child-resistant containers with warnings to use only as directed for external use and to keep out of children's reach.

Camphor

Camphor is used for its local action as a rubefacient when rubbed on the skin. When it is not applied vigorously, however, it may produce only a feeling of coolness. Camphor also has a mild local anesthetic action, and its application to the skin may be followed by numbness. The recommended concentration for external use is 1–3%, but it is used in various preparations in concentrations as high as 9%. Camphor and camphorated oil have been placed in Category I with a limitation on size for camphorated oil. Because of CNS stimulant effects, camphor and camphorated oil are highly toxic if ingested.

Menthol

Menthol is a natural product from Japanese mint oil or is prepared synthetically. It is applied topically, in concentrations as high as 16%, for its mild anesthetic and counterirritant properties.

Menthol has the particularly outstanding property of producing a feeling of coolness, quite noticeable in the respiratory tract when low concentrations of menthol are inhaled, as in many medicinal inhalant preparations and even in topical application. This sensation is caused by the selective stimulation of nerve endings sensitive to cold (6). Menthol has been classified in Category I.

Thymol

Thymol is a natural phenol which may be produced by synthesis. It is used in various liquid and ointment preparations as an analgesic and also for its antifungal and antibacterial properties. Effective in concentrations between 1 and 2%, thymol has been placed in Category I.

Turpentine Oil

Turpentine oil is used for its counterirritant properties either full strength or as a component of various liniments. It is effective in a concentration range of 10–50% and is in Category I. Many accidental poisonings occur by ingestion of an excessive amount of this substance (10).

Allyl Isothiocyanate

Allyl isothiocyanate, volatile oil of mustard, is a powerful local irritant. Applied in excessive concentrations for extended periods, it may produce severe vesication and even perforation of the skin with danger of subsequent infection. It is found most often as a minor component of ointment preparations but is also available in a plaster. The effective concentration range is 0.5–5%, and it has been placed in Category I.

Clove Oil

Clove oil, which contains eugenol as its main constituent, is also an ingredient in various ointment preparations and is widely used as a component of toothache preparations. It has strong counterirritant action.

components of external analgesic products

actions, concentrations, and toxicity

FDA classifications

Capsicum Oleoresin

Capsicum oleoresin, an irritant product of cayenne pepper, produces a feeling of warmth without vesicant action when it is applied to intact skin. It is generally used in concentrations of less than 1%, and it is classified as a Category I item.

Other Ingredients

Methacholine chloride in a concentration of 0.025% and histamine dihydrochloride and methyl nicotinate in concentrations of 0.1–1% are used for their local vasodilator properties. These agents produce sensitivity reactions in some individuals.

Some of the other volatile oils commonly found in OTC preparations are wormwood and eucalyptus oils. Eucalyptus oil is effective in concentrations of 0.5–15% and is classified in Category I. Wormwood oil is in Category III.

Triethanolamine salicylate in a concentration of 10% acts as an analgesic without counterirritant properties. It also is absorbed readily (11). The salicylates have been placed in Category III as topical analgesics because of insufficient data concerning their effectiveness following absorption after topical application. The Panel recognized that salicylates are present in the body tissues after topical application but found no conclusive correlation between blood and urine salicylate levels and analgesia (12).

Dosage Forms

The OTC external analgesics usually are available as liniments, gels, lotions, and ointments.

Liniments

Solutions or mixtures of various substances in oil, alcoholic solutions of soap, or emulsions are called lini-

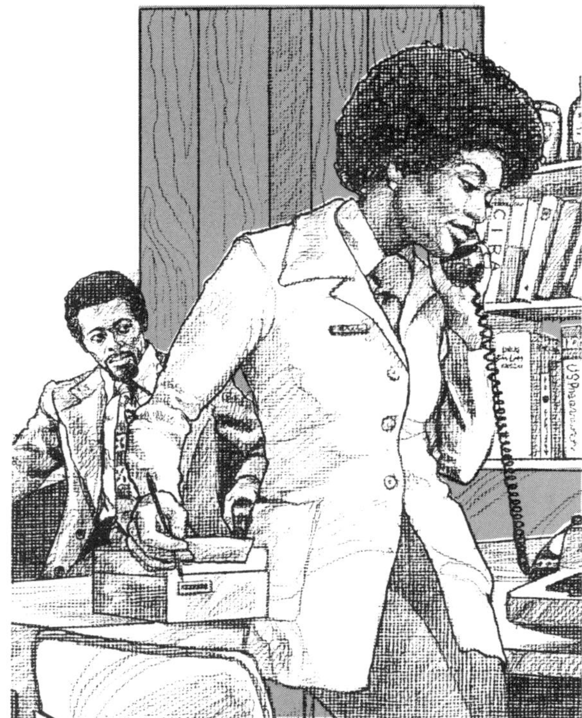

dosage forms

mechanism of absorption through the skin

role of the vehicle and humidity

ments. These products are intended for external application and should be so labeled. They are applied to the affected area with friction and rubbing of the skin, the oil or soap base providing ease of application and massage. Liniments with an alcoholic or hydroalcoholic vehicle are useful in instances in which rubefacient, counterirritant, or penetrating action is desired; oleaginous liniments are used primarily when massage is desired. By their nature, oleaginous liniments are less irritating to the skin than alcoholic liniments.

Liniments generally are not applied to broken or bruised skin areas because excessive irritation or infection may result. The vehicle for a liniment should be selected on the basis of the kind of action desired (rubefacient, counterirritant, or massage) and on the solubility of the desired components in the various vehicles (13).

Gels

Gels used for the delivery of topical analgesics are more appropriately called jellies because they are generally clear and of a more uniform, semisolid consistency. A greater sensation of warmth may be experienced with the gel than with equal quantities of the same product in a different dosage form such as a lotion. Therefore patients should be advised against using excessive amounts of the gel formulation, since an unpleasant burning sensation may be experienced.

Lotions

These liquid preparations are used for the protective or therapeutic value of their constituents. Depending on the ingredients, they may be alcoholic or aqueous and are often emulsions. Their fluidity allows rapid and uniform application over a wide surface area. Lotions are intended to dry on the skin soon after application, leaving a thin coat of their active ingredients on the skin surface.

Ointments

These dosage forms are particularly desirable for external analgesics because percutaneous absorption may occur more readily than from other bases. Balms are aromatic ointments often containing balsam.

Percutaneous Absorption

Active ingredients are included in locally applied products for one of the following reasons:

- To be effective in the product itself as it is applied to the skin (e.g., sunscreen);
- To be released for action at or on the skin surface (e.g., anti-infective);
- To be absorbed into the skin (e.g., local analgesic or local anesthetic).

Except under the first condition, active ingredients must leave the base (release) to exert their effect or to be absorbed.

The active ingredient's tendency to leave the base and enter the skin depends partly on the partition coefficient between the base and the skin (the relative lipophilic attraction of base and skin to the active ingredient). An oleaginous base tends to retain and thus slow release of active ingredient to the skin. However, the drug release rate increases as its concentration in the base increases. Furthermore, the rate of absorption into skin is enhanced by skin hydration.

Percutaneous absorption is the absorption of substances from the skin surface to areas beneath the skin (nerve endings), including entrance into the bloodstream. The medication is not usually intended to enter the general circulation. However, once the drug substance has penetrated the skin, it is close to blood capillaries that feed subcutaneous tissue, and absorption into the general circulation is possible. Fortunately, most of the substances for topical use as counterirritants are nontoxic in the amounts generally absorbed.

Selecting the vehicle is as important as selecting the drug. The choice depends on the solubility, stability, and ionization of the active ingredient (14). Staining properties, tackiness, or consistency may influence the patient's choice of a product. The lipophilic nature of the base, the active ingredient, and the concentration of active ingredient determine the rate and degree of penetration. These factors vary with different drugs and vehicles.

Humidity has a definite influence on the absorption of substances through the skin. Skin hydration may be achieved by covering or occluding the skin with plastic sheeting to prevent loss of moisture from the skin or by using oleaginous vehicles such as petrolatum (15). Thus practically speaking, ingredient absorption into skin is enhanced when the product is applied in an oleaginous base, owing to its hydrating effect.

Among the most widely used vehicles are petrolatum, mineral oil, lanolin, and anhydrous lanolin. Preparations with these vehicles are greasier than creams and contain little or no water. "Greaseless" vehicles are oil-in-water formulations, usually preferred for daytime use (14).

Petrolatum, a purified mixture of semisolid hydrocarbons obtained from petroleum, has protective and emollient properties when applied to the skin. Anhydrous lanolin differs from lanolin in that it contains practically no water. Because both are obtained from the fatlike substance in sheep's wool, many individuals are allergic to them (16).

The site of application, the amount of rubbing, and the length of time for which the medication is permitted to remain in contact with the skin also influence percutaneous absorption. Percutaneous absorption seems more effective when the drug is applied to skin with a thin epidermis. Absorption from sites such as the palms of the hands and soles of the feet, which have thick layers of epidermis, is comparatively slow.

The longer the period of rubbing, the greater the absorption. The massaging action produced by rubbing also may produce some increased circulation at the application site. Most preparations instruct the patient to "gently massage" the preparation into the skin. When products containing counterirritants and local anesthetics are applied with massage, they enhance relief of skeletal muscle pain (17). The anesthetic agent is absorbed and acts on nerve endings, potentiating analgesia (18).

The longer the medication remains in contact with the skin, the greater the amount of drug absorbed. The preparations may be applied as often as needed. There seems to be little agreement on how often the preparations should be applied for optimal results.

Untoward Effects

Hypersensitivity

Hypersensitive reactions either to active volatile oil components or to the vehicle are not uncommon. Reactions may be manifested as a generalized eruption at the application site. Some patients manifest idiosyncrasy to salicylates (19).

Toxicity

Ingestion of substances such as camphor, methyl salicylate, and turpentine oil has resulted in death. The mean lethal dose of turpentine in adults is probably 120–180 ml; ingestion of 2 g of camphor generally produces dangerous effects in adults. The amount of these substances that may be absorbed percutaneously is assumed to be small enough that there is little danger of toxicity (10).

Camphorated oil is toxic when ingested. There are numerous reports of systemic toxicity where camphorated oil was mistaken for castor oil and ingested. As little as one teaspoonful (750 mg to 1 g of camphor) caused the death of a child (20, 21); camphor poisoning has resulted from the application of camphorated oil to the chest of a 2.5-year-old child (22).

Cautions

External analgesics are intended for use on intact skin and should not be applied to broken skin or raw surfaces. Their application to skin areas devoid of the normal barrier may lead to rapid absorption into the bloodstream with consequent toxicity. These preparations should not be applied to sensitive mucous membranes, such as those inside the nose or mouth. They should not be used on children (unless the label on the preparation specifically states that the product is intended for this use) because percutaneous absorption is greater in children than in adults. Most package inserts available to the patient warn that for conditions affecting young children, a physician should be consulted.

The following precautions and warnings apply to topical analgesic products (23):

- Keep out of eyes and mucous membranes;
- Do not apply to wounds or abraded skin;
- Do not use on infants or small children;
- For local application only: do not apply to large areas of the body;
- Discontinue use if untoward reactions occur;
- Frequency of application should be mediated by concentration, other ingredients, the vehicle, and directions for administration;
- Contraindicated in individuals displaying an idiosyncrasy to salicylates.

vehicles used for external analgesics

side effects and precautions for use

nondrug approaches

Adjunctive Measures

Although OTC preparations have merit of their own as therapeutic agents, they may be inferior to simple physical measures. Applying either moist or dry heat is an effective method of easing muscular pain and promoting circulation and muscle relaxation.

Moist heat not only promotes circulation but also supplies moisture to the area of application, thereby offering a more penetrating sensation. There are several methods of applying moist heat. The most simple method is the use of towels soaked in hot water. Hot water bottles, moist electric heating pads, and steam packs are available in pharmacies as alternative methods that may be suggested. Patients should be advised to use steam packs carefully until they become familiar with the heat characteristics. Towels should be layered carefully between the skin and the steam packs to prevent skin burn.

Heating pads, hot water bottles, and heat (infrared) lamps are all safe means of applying dry heat if they are used judiciously. The degree of heat should be such as to produce a comfortable and soothing sensation of warmth. Towels may be placed next to the skin to absorb perspiration and also to prevent overheating, especially of the bony prominences. Hot objects should never be applied to patients who are asleep or unconscious. A patient receiving heat from an infrared lamp should never be left alone without easy access to the switch in case of overheating. Automatic timers are helpful in keeping treatment within safe limits.

Severe burning or blistering of skin areas may occur from using a counterirritant and a heat source simultaneously. An advantage of external analgesic preparations over heat treatments is that they are less trouble to use and allow the patient freedom of movement while giving symptomatic relief.

SUMMARY

If the use of an OTC external analgesic is indicated, the pharmacist should advise the patient about its proper use, with appropriate advice concerning safety. The patient also should be advised that the preparation is intended only for temporary and symptomatic relief. A minor muscular pain may be caused by a more serious problem that cannot be ameliorated by an OTC preparation. If the condition persists, a physician should be consulted.

REFERENCES

(1) T. S. Szasz, *Arch. Neurol. Psychiatry, 74,* 174 (1955).

(2) "Cecil-Loeb Textbook of Medicine," 13th ed., P. B. Beeson and W. McDermott, Eds., Saunders, Philadelphia, Pa., 1971, p. 153.

(3) J. L. Hollander, "Arthritis and Allied Conditions," Lea and Febiger, Philadelphia, Pa., 1966, p. 1233.

(4) "Handbook of Medical Treatment," M. J. Chatton et al., Eds., Lange Medical, Los Altos, Calif., 1970, p. 361.

(5) "Krantz and Carr's Pharmacologic Principles of Medical Practice," 8th ed., D. M. Aviado, Ed., Williams and Wilkins, Baltimore, Md., 1972, pp. 891–893.

(6) "The Pharmacological Basis of Therapeutics," 5th ed., L. S. Goodman and A. Gilman, Eds., Macmillan, New York, N.Y., 1975, p. 951.

(7) B. S. Post, *Arch. Phys. Med. Rehabil., 42,* 791 (1961).

(8) D. W. Lewis and P. J. Verhonick, *Appl. Radiol., 6,* 114 (1977).

(9) R. H. Dreisbach, "Handbook of Poisoning," Lange Medical, Los Altos, Calif., 1971, p. 252.

(10) R. E. Gosselin, H. C. Hodge, R. P. Smith, and M. N. Gleason, "Clinical Toxicology of Commercial Products," 4th ed., Williams and Wilkins, Baltimore, Md., 1976, p. 157.

(11) "Facts and Comparisons," Facts and Comparisons, Inc., St. Louis, Mo., 1975, p. 503.

(12) "Summary Minutes of the FDA OTC Panel on Topical Analgesic, Antirheumatic, Otic, Burn, and Sunburn Treatment Products," 19th Meeting, Rockville, Md., May 21–22, 1975.

(13) J. B. Sprowls and H. M. Beal, "American Pharmacy," Lippincott, Philadelphia, Pa., 1966, p. 268.

(14) "Drugs of Choice, 1978–1979," W. Modell, Ed., Mosby, St. Louis, Mo., 1978. pp. 700–701.

(15) R. B. Stoughton, *Arch. Environ. Health, 11,* 551 (1965).

(16) "Remington's Pharmaceutical Sciences," 15th ed., Mack Publishing, Easton, Pa., 1975, p. 1532.

(17) E. E. Gordon and A. Haas, *Ind. Med. Surg., 28,* 217 (1959).

(18) "Report From Biological Sciences Laboratories," Foster D. Snell, Inc., Elizabeth, N.J., Aug. 8, 1972.

(19) K. L. Melmon and H. F. Morrelli, "Clinical Pharmacology: Basic Principles in Therapeutics," Macmillan, New York, N.Y., 1972, p. 576.

(20) J. M. Arena, "Poisoning," 3rd ed., Charles C Thomas, Springfield, Ill., 1974, p. 368.

(21) A. G. Smith and G. Margolis, *Am. J. Pathol., 30,* 857 (1954).

(22) G. D. Summers, *Br. Med. J., 4,* 1009 (1947).

(23) "Summary Minutes of the FDA OTC Panel on Topical Analgesic, Antirheumatic, Otic, Burn, and Sunburn Treatment Products," 4th Meeting, Rockville, Md., Sept. 27–28, 1973.

Product (Manufacturer)	Application Form	Counterirritant	Other
Absorbent Rub (DeWitt)	lotion	camphor, 1.6%; menthol, 1.6%; methyl salicylate, 0.7%; wormwood oil, 0.6%; sassafras oil, 0.5%; capsicum, 0.03%	isopropyl alcohol, 69%; green soap, 11.6%; pine tar soap, 0.9%; *o*-phenylphenol, 0.5%; benzocaine, 0.5%
Absorbine Arthritic (W. F. Young)	lotion	methyl salicylate, menthol, methyl nicotinate	greaseless, stainless emulsion base
Absorbine Jr. (W. F. Young)	lotion	wormwood oil, thymol, menthol, chloroxylenol	acetone
Act-On Rub (Keystone)	lotion	methyl salicylate, menthol, camphor, eucalyptus oil, mustard oil	isopropyl myristate, balm base, lanolin
Analbalm (Central)	lotion	methyl salicylate, 5%; camphor, 2.5%; menthol, 0.5%	greaseless nonstaining emulsion base
Analgesic Balm (Lilly)	ointment	methyl salicylate, 15%; menthol, 15%	hydrocarbon waxes, lanolin, petrolatum, sorbitan sesquioleate, water-soluble base
Antiphlogistine (Roberts)	poultice	methyl salicylate, eucalyptus oil, salicylic acid	glycerin, kaolin, boric acid, peppermint oil
Arthralgen (Robins)	ointment	methyl salicylate, 15%; thymol, 1%; menthol, 10%; methacholine chloride, 0.25%	polyethylene glycol base
Aspercreme (Thompson)	lotion cream	triethanolamine salicylate	greaseless base
Banalg (Cole)	lotion	menthol, methyl salicylate, camphor, eucalyptus oil	greaseless base
Baumodyne (North American)	gel	menthol	—
Ben-Gay (Leeming)	lotion	methyl salicylate, 15%; menthol, 7%	greaseless base
Ben-Gay Extra Strength Balm (Leeming)	ointment	methyl salicylate, 30%; menthol, 8%	greaseless base
Ben-Gay Gel (Leeming)	gel	methyl salicylate, 15%; menthol, 7%	hydroalcoholic gel base
Ben-Gay Greaseless/ Stainless Ointment (Leeming)	ointment	methyl salicylate, 15%; menthol, 10%	greaseless base
Ben-Gay Original (Leeming)	ointment	methyl salicylate, 18.3%; menthol, 16%	oleaginous base
Braska (Keystone)	lotion	methyl salicylate, menthol, camphor, monoglycol salicylate, methyl nicotinate, salicylamide	isopropyl alcohol
Counterpain Rub (Squibb)	ointment	methyl salicylate, 10.2%; menthol, 5.4%; eugenol, 1.4%	—
Dencorub (Roberts)	lotion	methyl salicylate, menthol, camphor, eucalyptus oil	—
Doan's Rub (Purex)	cream	methyl salicylate, 25%; menthol, 10%	—
Emul-O-Balm (Pennwalt)	lotion	menthol, 22.45 mg/ml; methyl salicylate, 22.45 mg/ml; camphor, 11.22 mg/ml	ribbon gum tragacanth, 8.37 mg/ml; methylparaben, 1.50 mg/ml; propylparaben, 0.30 mg/ml
End-Ake (Columbia Medical)	liniment	methyl salicylate, eucalyptus oil, menthol, camphor	—
End-Ake Cream (Columbia Medical)	cream	methyl nicotinate, dipropylene glycol salicylate, capsicum oleoresin	salicylamide, histamine dihydrochloride
Exocaine Plus (Kirk)	ointment	methyl salicylate, 30%; menthol crystals, 2%; clove oil, 1%	benzocaine, 5%
Exocaine Tube (Kirk)	ointment	methyl salicylate, 30%; clove oil, 1%	benzocaine, 5%
Heet (Whitehall)	lotion spray	methyl salicylate, capsicum, camphor, menthol (spray), methyl nicotinate (spray)	alcohol, 53%
Icy Hot (Searle)	ointment	methyl salicylate, 29%; menthol, 8%	—
Infra-Rub (Whitehall)	cream	methyl nicotinate, histamine dihydrochloride, capsicum oleoresin	glycol monosalicylate, lanolin

Product (Manufacturer)	Application Form	Counterirritant	Other
Lini Balm (Arnar-Stone)	aerosol foam	methyl salicylate, 15%; camphor, 2%; eucalyptus oil, 2%; menthol, 1%	polyoxyalkalene lanolin
Mentholatum (Mentholatum)	ointment	camphor, 9%; menthol, 1.35%	aromatic oils, petrolatum base
Mentholatum Deep Heating (Mentholatum)	ointment lotion	methyl salicylate, 12.7% (ointment), 20% (lotion); menthol, 6%; eucalyptus oil (ointment); turpentine oil (ointment)	lanolin, greaseless base
Minit-Rub (Bristol-Myers)	ointment	methyl salicylate, 10%; menthol, 3.54%; camphor, 4.44%; eucalyptus oil, 1.77%	anhydrous lanolin, 4.44%
Musterole Deep Strength (Plough)	ointment	methyl salicylate, menthol, methyl nicotinate	—
Musterole Regular, Extra, and Children's Strength (Plough)	ointment	camphor, menthol, methyl salicylate, mustard oil, glycol monosalicylate	—
Neurabalm (S.S.S.)	lotion	methyl salicylate, menthol, eucalyptus oil, cajuput oil, camphor, chlorothymol	alcohol, 54%; acetone; benzocaine
Oil-O-Sol (Mosso)	lotion	castor oil, 40.8%; camphor oil, 6.8%; hexylresorcinol, 0.1%	corn oil
Omega Oil (Block)	lotion	methyl salicylate, methyl nicotinate, capsicum oleoresin, histamine dihydrochloride	isopropyl alcohol, 50%
Panalgesic (Poythress)	lotion spray	methyl salicylate, 55%; camphor, 4%; menthol, 0.25%	emollient oils, 19%; alcohol, 17%; aspirin, 5%
Rid-A-Pain (Pfeiffer)	ointment	methyl nicotinate, glycol monosalicylate, methyl salicylate, capsicum oleoresin, menthol, camphor	washable base
Rumarub (Pfeiffer)	lotion	methyl salicylate; camphor; oils of sassafras, origanum, cassia, cajuput, clove; oleoresins of capsicum; ginger; menthol	propylene glycol, alcohol
Sloan's (Warner-Lambert)	liniment	turpentine oil, 46.76%; pine oil, 6.74%; camphor, 3.35%; methyl salicylate, 2.66%; capsicum oleoresin, 0.62%	kerosene, 39.88%
Soltice Hi-Therm (Chattem)	cream	eucalyptus oil, 10 mg/g; methyl salicylate, 50 mg/g; menthol, 70 mg/g; camphor, 70 mg/g	greaseless base
Soltice Quick Rub (Chattem)	cream	eucalyptus oil, 10 mg/g; methyl salicylate, 50 mg/g; menthol, 50 mg/g; camphor, 50 mg/g	greaseless base
SPD (Amer. Pharm.)	cream lotion	methyl salicylate, 10%; menthol; camphor; methyl nicotinate, 1%; capsicum oleoresin, 0.5% (cream)	washable greaseless base
Stimurub (Otis Clapp)	ointment	menthol, methyl salicylate, capsicum oleoresin	—
Surin (McKesson)	ointment	methyl salicylate; menthol; camphor; methacholine chloride, 0.25%	greaseless base
Yager's Liniment (Yager)	liniment	turpentine oil, 8%; camphor, 3.1%	aqua ammonia, 1.4%; ammonium oleate
Zemo Liquid (Plough)	lotion	methyl salicylate, thymol, eucalyptol, menthol, phenol	sodium salicylate; sodium borate; benzoic acid; boric acid; alcohol, 35%
Zemo Liquid Extra Strength (Plough)	lotion	methyl salicylate, menthol, thymol, eucalyptol, phenol	sodium salicylate; sodium borate; benzoic acid; boric acid; alcohol, 40%
Zemo Ointment (Plough)	ointment	methyl salicylate, menthol	triclosan, zinc oxide, boric acid, benzoic acid

Topical Anti-Infective Products

Paul Zanowiak

Chapter 26

Questions to Ask the Patient

What area of the skin is affected? How extensive is the area involved?

Is the skin broken?

How long have you had this condition? Have you had it before? Are other members of your family also affected?

Has the condition developed as the result of a previous rash or skin disorder?

Do you have a fever or other flulike symptoms?

Do you have diabetes? Have you been checked for it?

What treatments have you tried for this condition? Were they effective?

Are you presently using any medications?

Topical anti-infectives are products used to counteract infection on local tissue. The active ingredients of these products are antimicrobials; most are antibacterial or antifungal. Because this product classification is so broad, discussion is limited to antimicrobial products for use in prevention and self-treatment of skin infections. (See Chapters 27–31, which deal with specific and localized skin conditions.)

SKIN ANATOMY AND PHYSIOLOGY

Normal skin thickness is 3–5 mm, the thickest skin being on the palms and soles and the thinnest on the eyelids and parts of the genitals. The skin is divided into three main layers (Figure 1). The outermost layer (epidermis), which is quite compact and nonvascular, consists of stratified squamous epithelial cells. The next layer (dermis or corium) is formed of vascular connective tissue. These two layers are not similar in composition but adhere firmly to each other. The hypodermis is the innermost layer.

The epidermis is composed of several distinct layers. The innermost, in close association with the dermis, is the stratum germinativum, which consists of columnar/cuboidal epithelial cells. Above this is the prickle cell layer (stratum spinosum), composed of layers of polygonal epithelial cells. This layer is thicker in the palms than in hairy skin.

These two epidermal layers are involved in mitotic processes toward epidermal regeneration and repair. The prickle cells contain keratinocytes, the pigment-forming melanocytes that contain melanin precursors and melanin granules, which are produced by cellular division. As the keratinocytes migrate to the skin surface, they change from living cells to dead, thick-walled, flat, nonnucleated cells that contain keratin, a fibrous protein.

Above the prickle cell layer is the granular layer (stratum granulosum), which is actually several layers of flattened, polygonal cells. These cells contain granules of keratohyaline, which are changed to keratin in the outermost skin layer (stratum corneum, or horny outer layer). The stratum lucidum, present only in areas of thick skin, is between the granular layer and the stratum corneum. It is a narrow band of flattened, closely packed cells believed to contain eleidin, a possible derivative of keratohyaline. The stratum corneum is composed of flat, scaly dead (keratinized) tissue. Its outermost cells are flat (squamous) plates that are constantly shed (desquamated).

The dead cells lost from the outer surface of the epidermis are replaced by new cells generated by the mitotic processes of the stratum spinosum and stratum germinativum. The newer cells push older ones closer to the surface. In the process they become flattened, lose their water content, fill with keratin, and gradually die, taking their place on the skin surface.

The dermis, which supports the epidermis and separates it from the lower fatty layer, consists mainly of collagen and elastin embedded in a mucopolysaccharide substance. Fibroblasts and mast cells are found throughout. The dermis also contains a network of nerves and capillaries that are the neurovascular supply to the dermal appendages, i.e., hair follicles, sebaceous glands, and sweat glands. The main sublayers of the dermis are the papillary and reticular layers. The papillary layer, adjacent to the epidermis, is very rich in blood vessels, and the papillae probably act as conduits to bring blood nutrients near the avascular epidermis. The reticular layer, below the papillary layer, contains coarser tissue which connects the dermis with the hypodermis.

The hypodermis, composed of relatively loose connective tissue of varying thicknesses, provides necessary pliability for the skin. In most areas this layer also

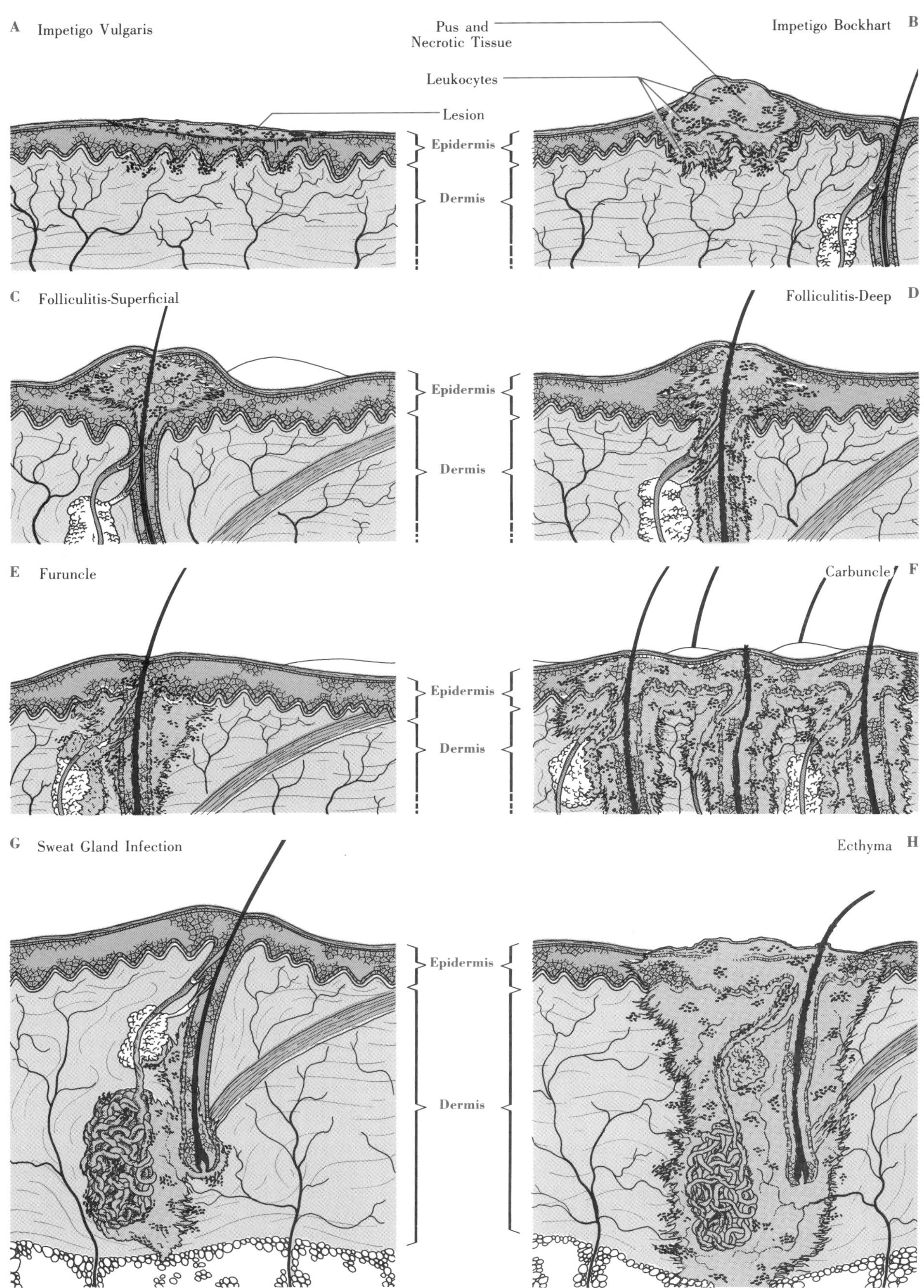

Figure 1. Cross section of common pyodermas.

includes a layer of fat (panniculus adiposus) which is involved in thermal control, food reserve, and cushioning or padding.

Skin Appendages

Hair Follicle

A hair shaft is generated by a hair germ at the base of a hair follicle. The follicle basically is an inward tubular folding of the epidermis into the dermis. The hair within the follicle is a fiber of keratinized epithelial cells that grow as a result of multiplication of cells in the hair germ.

Sebaceous Glands

Most sebaceous, or sebum-producing, glands are located in the same areas as hair, since they are usually appendages of the hair follicles. The ducts of these glands are lined with epithelial cells that are continuous with those of the basal layers of the epidermis. The sebaceous glands are holocrine, because the gland cells from which sebum is derived are destroyed in its production. Not all sebaceous glands are associated with hair follicles. They also are found in genital areas, around the nipples of the breast, and on the edges of the lips.

Sweat Glands

Sweat glands develop from epithelial cells that proceed downward from the epidermis. Independent of hair follicles, they are long, hollow tubes that reach into dermal and hypodermal areas in most of the body. Their secretory parts are in the hypodermis. The excretory ducts ascend through the epidermis as wavy or curved channels. Sweat is an eccrine secretion: no part of the gland cell is destroyed.

Eccrine Sweat Glands

These glands are cholinergically innervated, although the nerve fibers are sympathetic. The heat regulation centers of the hypothalamus control overall secretion of the sweat glands. Emotional stress as well as heat can produce sweating. Sweat is basically a saline solution with some electrolytes, but it is devoid of carbohydrates, fats, or proteins. Much more sweat is produced by the true sweat glands (several liters per day) than by the apocrine glands.

Apocrine Glands

These glands, erroneously called "sweat" glands, are located in the axillae, areolae of the nipples, and perianal and genital areas. Larger and deeper in the skin than true sweat glands, they produce a milky secretion that appears in very small amounts on the skin and has a characteristic odor.

The apocrines generally are attached to a hair follicle by a duct leading down into the coiled, secretory glandular tubules, which are covered by myoepithelium. This covering allows contraction to adrenergic stimulation. Thus stimulation, as in stress, releases the secretion, which is odorless until the skin bacteria utilize the fats present. This process results in the characteristic pungent odor of apocrine "sweat." In the absence of apocrine secretions, such as in prepuberty, sweat is odorless.

Nails

The nails are modifications of the keratinized layer of the epidermis. The nail bed on which the nail plate lies derives from the basal epidermal layers. The body of the plate, at its periphery, is surrounded by the nail root. The root is derived from the nail groove, which is a process of the basal epidermal unit. The white area at the base is called the lunula, and the part of the nail groove that enfolds the plate at its margin is the eponychium. The hyponychium is a thick layer of stratum corneum immediately beneath the plate of the nail's distal tip.

Normal Skin Function

glands associated with skin layers

skin as a barrier

water content of skin

The skin acts as a barrier between the environment and the body, protecting the body from harmful external agents, e.g., pathogenic organisms and chemicals (1, 2). The skin also contributes to sensory experiences. It is involved in temperature control, development of pigment, and synthesis of some vitamins. It is important in hydroregulation because it controls moisture loss from the body and moisture penetration into the body.

Except for the stratum corneum, the skin is living tissue and requires nutrition, including oxygen. The cells of all the layers use nutrients and excrete water and carbon dioxide. Most oxygen is supplied from the blood; a small amount is supplied from the air. Similarly, carbon dioxide is taken away from the tissues mainly by the blood, but some is "exhaled" directly to the atmosphere.

Dermal Hydration

The skin's water content is important to its normal health. If the corneous layer becomes significantly dehydrated, its elasticity is affected negatively. Returning water to the skin is the only means by which induced brittleness can be reversed. The stratum corneum may be hydrated by water transfer from lower layers or by the water accumulation (perspiration) caused by occlusive coverings, e.g., bandages and oleaginous pharmaceutical vehicles, at the surface. The accumulation of moisture by occlusive coverings seems to "open" the compactness of the stratum corneum, facilitating penetration of this area by drug molecules (3).

Sebum

The skin surface is covered with sebum, a mixture of fatty substances whose constituents include free fatty acids (mainly palmitic and oleic), triglycerides, waxes, cholesterol, squalene, and other hydrocarbons and traces of fat-soluble vitamins (4). Sebum is a product of the sebaceous glands. It lubricates the skin surface to ensure suppleness and acts as a surface barrier to moisture loss from the deeper skin layers because of its fatty nature. Chemically, it prevents skin penetration by other substances, and it has some antiseptic and antifungal properties. Sebum also is an emulsion of sweat and surface waste products of cutaneous cells (5).

Skin Surface pH

The secretions that accumulate at the skin surface are weakly acidic (pH of 4.5–5.5) (the acid mantle) (6). The pH varies slightly from individual to individual and among different areas of the body; it is somewhat higher in areas where perspiration evaporates slowly (1).

The acid mantle has been postulated to be a protective mechanism because microbes tend to grow better at pH of 6–7.5 and infected areas have comparably higher pH values than normal skin (1). Several fatty acids (propionic, caproic, and caprylic) found in sweat specifically inhibit microbial and fungal growth (7). Thus the importance of the "acid mantle" concept is not solely in the inherent pH, but more likely in the specific compounds responsible for the acidity. The ingredients of sebum also have fungicidal and bactericidal properties (8, 9).

the acid mantle

normal skin microorganisms

skin infections

pyodermas

The buffer capacity of skin surface secretions is another protective mechanism—when the pH is raised or lowered, the skin can readjust effectively to its normal pH (1). People whose skin takes longer to revert to a normal value may be prone to skin diseases (10).

Skin Flora

Various microorganisms live on the surface of healthy, intact skin (11). The individual species that make up the flora exist in a normal ecological balance. The flora act as a defense mechanism to control the growth of potential pathogenic organisms and their possible invasion of the skin and body.

Infection by pathogenic organisms is related to the breakdown of the skin's "disinfecting," protective mechanism or to the development of an abundance of colonies of pathogenic organisms (6). A breakdown in the normal ecological balance may be potentiated by alterations in the skin's other defense mechanisms.

Normally, the stratum corneum has only about 10% water content, which ensures elasticity but is generally below that needed to support luxuriant microbial growth (6). An increase in moisture content may allow microbial growth, leading to infection. A break in the intact surface has a deleterious effect on the skin's defensive properties, allowing large numbers of pathogenic organisms to be introduced into the inner layers.

Infection may be caused by excessive scrubbing of the skin (especially with strong detergents), excessive exposure to water, occlusion, increasing the skin temperature, excessive sweating, excessive bathing, and injury (6, 12–14). Thus the presence and extent of a microbial skin infection generally depend on the extent of breakdown of the skin and its defense mechanisms, the number of pathogenic organisms present, and the supportive nutrient environment for such organisms (6).

The flora of various skin areas are diverse, including aerobic and anaerobic microbial organisms, staphylococci and corynebacteria, sarcinae, and occasional gram-negative rods (15). The number of organisms on the various areas of the skin differs. Changes in kind and number of organisms occur in these constituent populations during different periods of life and during different seasons of the year (6). Flora population varies; some persons have a constantly high microbial population (15).

CUTANEOUS INFECTIONS

Cutaneous infections may be caused by bacteria, fungi, viruses, or parasites. Fungal and viral infections are covered in detail in Chapter 28. Many, but not all, bacterial infections are amenable to topical therapy. Careful assessment of the condition must be made before appropriate treatment can be recommended.

Bacterial Infections

Bacterial skin infections are classified as pyodermas (Figure 2) because pus usually is present. They are caused principally by β-hemolytic streptococci and hemolytic staphylococci (16). The lesions result from external infection or reinfection, and they may be superficial or involve deeper dermal tissue. These pyodermic infections are primary (where no previous dermatoses exist) or secondary (where a predisposing dermal problem already exists). Other organisms also may be present in secondary pyodermas, including gram-negative bacteria (e.g., *Pseudomonas aeruginosa*), which are especially prevalent on warm, moist skin, such as the axillae, ear canals, and interdigital spaces.

The main pyodermic infections are impetigo, folliculitis, furuncles (boils), carbuncles, erysipelas, sweat gland infections, ecthyma, and pyonychia (16–18).

Impetigo

Impetigo vulgaris (caused by streptococci, staphylococci, or both) probably is the most superficial of the pyodermas, mainly involving surface areas. Direct contact with lesions or infected exudate generally is required for its transmission. Scrupulous hygiene is necessary to avoid reinoculation by spreading the exudate. Thus soiled dressings should not touch unaffected areas, and transport of exudate by clothing should be prevented. The patient's hands and nails should be kept clean, and scratching the lesions should be avoided.

Lesions initially are small red spots (19), which evolve rapidly into characteristic vesicles (tiny sacs or blisters) filled with amber fluid. Exudate collects and forms yellow or brown crusts on the surface. Direct spreading occurs rapidly when the exudate is not carefully removed. The eruptions may be circular with clear central areas and may occur in groups. The exposed parts of the body are most easily affected, but no area of the skin is immune if autogenous reinfection is not controlled. Impetigo is most common in children, where it is highly contagious.

Furfuraceous impetigo (pityriasis simplex faciei) is a superficial streptococcal infection found almost exclusively in children. The lesions, scaly, red, round patches of varying sizes, occur most often on the face. This impetigo seems to occur more often in cold weather, and depigmentation of the patchy areas may occur in previously affected areas.

In primary impetigo the responsible bacteria cause the infection directly (e.g., impetigo vulgaris). Some forms, however, occur secondarily to the presence of

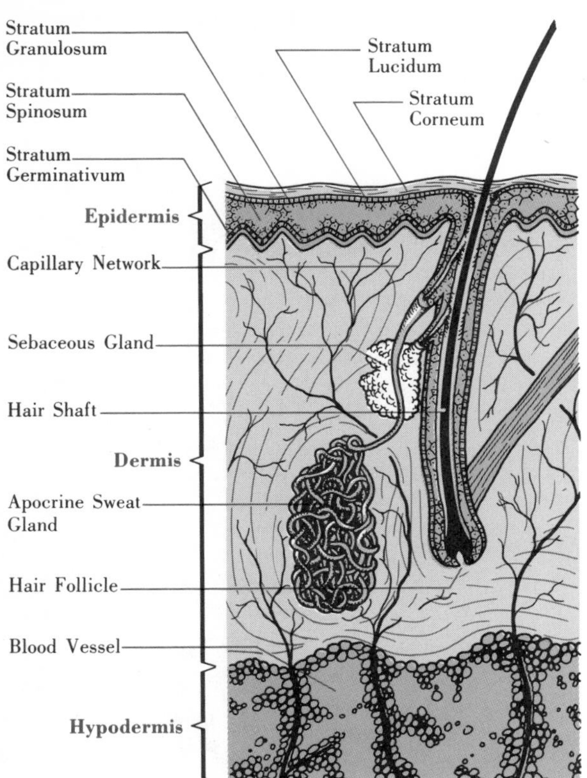

Figure 2. Cross section of human skin.

other infections, injury, or general breakdown in skin defenses. Thus impetigo Bockhart usually occurs as a secondary infection to another condition (furuncles, discharging ears, or wounds). Lesions characteristically are tiny follicular pustules around hair shafts and may be encircled by narrow, red rings (areolae).

Folliculitis

Follicular pustules are superficial or deep, depending on the pathogen and on the site involved. They involve only the hair shafts; surrounding tissue is not affected. Usually, the superficial forms are very similar to impetigo Bockhart, and they may be secondary infections. Skin areas regularly exposed to water, grease, oils, tars, and other contaminants seem most easily affected.

Furuncles and Carbuncles

These pyodermas are generally staphylococcal infections located in or around hair follicles. The lesion may start as a superficial folliculitis but develops into a deep nodule. The fully established furuncle has elevated swelling, is erythematous, and is very painful. Furuncles are most common in males. Hairy areas and areas subject to maceration and friction (e.g., collar, waist, buttocks, and thighs) seem most vulnerable. The initial erythema and swelling stage is followed by thinning of the skin around the primary follicle, centralized pustulation, destruction of the pilosebaceous structure, discharging of the core (plug), and central ulceration. Scarring often occurs. Chronic furunculosis is common, with new lesions appearing intermittently for months or years.

Furuncles may be secondary infections to other dermatoses or diseases. Diabetes mellitus and agammaglobulinemia may predispose a person to furuncles or carbuncles. Chronic cases of these pyodermas should be referred for urinalysis and blood glucose and glucose tolerance tests.

Carbuncles involve clusters of follicles with deeper and broader penetration over a larger area than furuncles. Furuncles may develop into carbuncles by infiltration or infection of adjacent follicles.

Sweat Gland Infections

These staphylococcal infections originate in sweat and related apocrine glands; they may look like furuncles. Axillary apocrine sweat glands are the most common site, but other apocrine glands (e.g., perianal, perimammillary, and genital) also are vulnerable. Sweat gland infections may result as a secondary infection to an irritant; deodorant/antiperspirant products may produce an initial dermatitis. People with chronic skin conditions (e.g., acne or folliculitis) may be predisposed to sweat gland infections (16).

staphylococcal infections in hair follicles and sweat glands

pyogenic infection of the nails

Infants are subject to superficial infections (periporitis) and deeper and multiple abscesses of these glands. Generally, infants in poor health are more prone to such infections, which occur mainly as secondary infections to other skin disorders. Sweat gland abscesses in the axillae (hidradenitis axillaris) occur in adolescents and adults with an endocrine disorder.

Sweat gland infections begin as small, superficial, very tender pustules. They rapidly develop into hard, tender, bluish-red elevated swellings. There can be many such abscesses. Within several days, softening usually occurs, and the abscess ruptures, exuding pus, blood, and serous fluid.

Ecthyma

Ecthyma is similar to impetigo but deeper. Lesions begin as pustules and form deep crusts with red margins. Removal of the crusts results in purulent, ulcerous wounds. This condition often occurs as a secondary infection to minor traumas (scratches). People with poor circulation seem predisposed to ecthyma, because the lower part of the legs is a common site.

Erysipelas

This infection, caused by a β-hemolytic streptococcus, is a cellulitis characterized by a rapidly spreading, red, and edematous plaque. Erysipelas is superficial and has sharply established borders and a glistening surface (19). It occurs most often on the scalp and face and is usually accompanied by elevated temperature, chills, and malaise.

Pyonychia

Pyonychia is a pyogenic infection of the nails with swelling and tenderness of surrounding tissue. Moderate pressure may force a pus exudate, and the nail may develop with irregularities. It is important that this condition be recognized accurately to avoid confusion with candidal or other fungal infections which can also affect nails.

Infectious Eczematoid Dermatitis

This name refers to any chronic eczematous skin condition with an infectious component. Originally, it was used to describe any secondary infection arising on the skin adjacent to an area of primary infection, and it is also applied in some cases of contact dermatitis caused by topical agents. Thus this term is too general and confusing and probably should be avoided (see Chapter 28).

Otitis Externa

external ear infections

This inflammation of the external ear may be a secondary infection (e.g., to seborrheic scaling of the scalp) involving bacteria and fungi. Although it is essentially an inflammation, microbial pathogens may be found in its exudate. Lesions are characterized by redness, edema, crusts, and oozing. Real pus is rare, unless a true infection also is present in the ear canal. Because of the ear's warmth, darkness, and moisture, microorganisms flourish as secondary contributors to the original dermatitis. (See Chapter 18 for a complete discussion of otitis externa.)

Fungal Infections

dermatomycoses

Fungal infections, often called dermatomycoses, are among the most common cutaneous disorders (16, 17). Characteristically, they exhibit single or multiple lesions that may have mild scaling or deep granulomas (inflamed nodules). Superficial infections (tinea, ringworm, and dermatophytosis) affect hair, nails, and skin, and are caused mainly by three genera of fungi: *Trichophyton, Microsporum*, and *Epidermophyton. Candida* also may be involved (16). Fungal infections of hairless skin generally are superficial, and the organisms are found in or on the uppermost skin layers. In fungal infections of areas covered with heavy hair the organisms are much deeper because of hair follicle penetration.

Tinea Pedis

athlete's foot

This infection, known popularly as athlete's foot or ringworm of the feet, is caused by several species of fungi. Its severity depends on the degree of host resis-

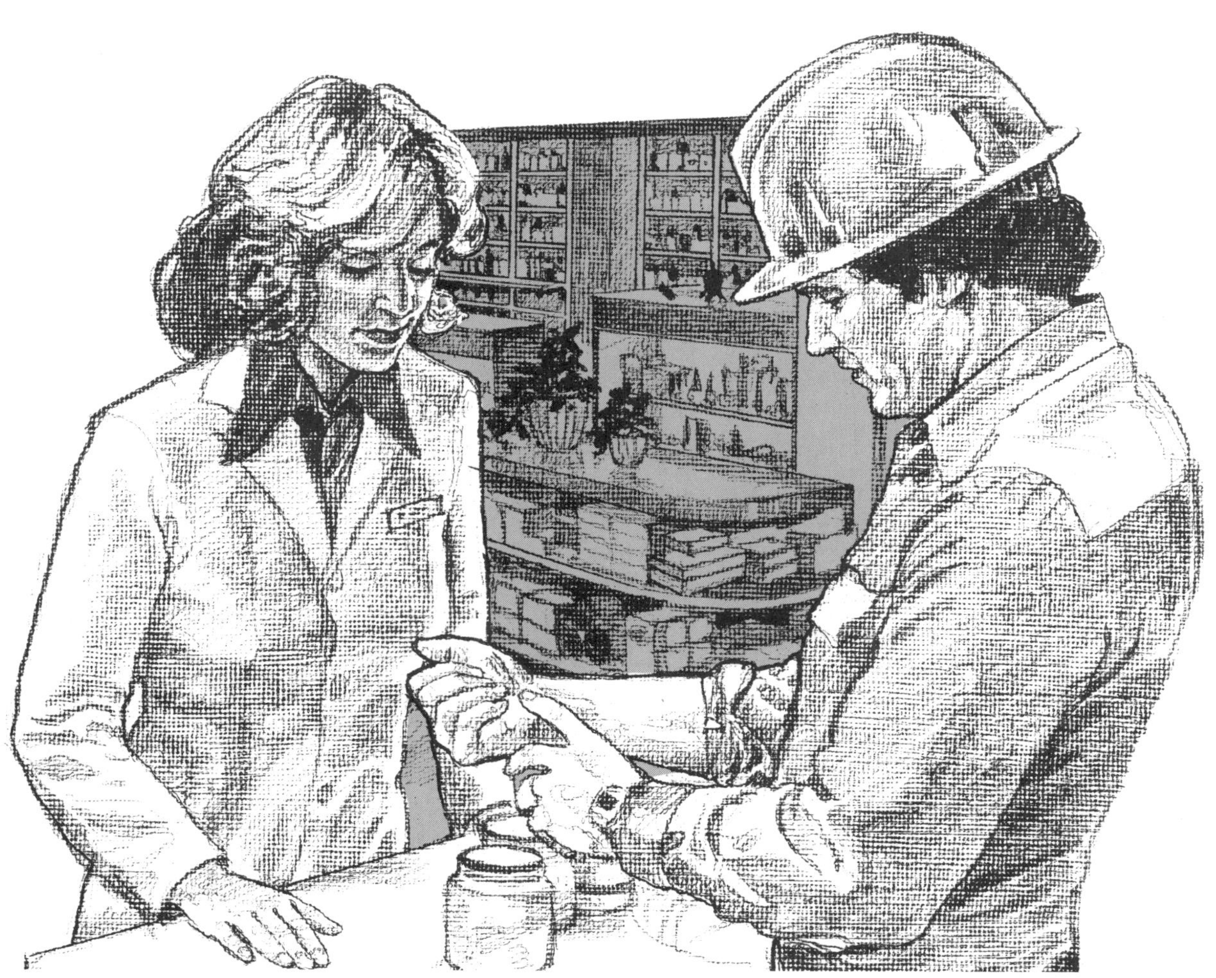

tance and the specific causative organism. The lesions may be characterized by an erythematous and scaly dermatitis (*E. floccosum*), exudation and maceration with defined borders ringed with tiny vesicles (*C. albicans*), acute vesicular formation between toes and on the soles of the feet with maceration and fissures (*T. mentagrophytes*), and hyperkeratolytic thickening of the skin with few or no vesicles and inflammation (*T. rubrum*). (See Chapter 31 for a complete discussion of athlete's foot.)

Tinea Capitis

Transmitted by direct contact with infected people or animals, this infection is caused by *Microsporum* and *Trichophyton*. The lesions are small papules infiltrated by broken hairs. The papules enlarge and form scaly, red patches. Inflammation, varying degrees of alopecia, and soft and wet deeper lesions may occur.

Tinea Cruris

This infection, caused by *E. floccosum*, *C. albicans*, and species of *Trichophyton*, occurs on the medial and upper parts of the thighs and the pubic area (jock itch). The lesions have specific margins that are slightly elevated and more inflamed than the central parts; small vesicles are found at the margins. Acute lesions are bright red and turn brownish in chronic cases, and they may scale. This condition is generally bilateral with severe pruritus.

Tinea Corporis

Species of *Trichophyton* and *Microsporum* are the causative organisms of this condition. The lesions involve glabrous skin and begin as small, circular, erythematous, scaly areas. They spread peripherally, and the borders may contain vesicles or pustules. Tinea corporis easily may be mistaken for an "eczema," because lesions may resemble eczematoid conditions.

Other Fungal Infections

Moniliasis, caused mainly by *C. albicans*, usually occurs in intertriginous areas, such as the groin, axillae, interdigital spaces, under breasts, and the corners of the mouth; moisture and friction accelerate the condition (20). Involvement of the mucous membrane appears as "thrush," vaginal candidiasis, and pruritus ani. Candidal paronychia is most common in people whose activities involve routine immersion of the hands in water. Systemic diseases such as diabetes, infection, or malignancy may lower general resistance and allow *C. albicans* infections to flourish. Certain drugs, e.g., antibiotics used locally in the GI tract, also may contribute to infection. Pregnancy is often a predisposing cause of vaginal candidiasis.

Other fungal skin infections include tinea barbae (barber's itch or ringworm of the beard); tinea manum (hands); tinea versicolor, where the lesions are brown in color; tinea circinata, generally ringed, red lesions that can agglomerate into polycyclic configurations; tinea unguium (onychomycosis), where the nail may become hypertrophic, discolor, and scale; and erythrasma (in axillary or pubic areas) (16, 18).

Viral Infections

Viruses are responsible for dermal diseases such as herpes simplex, herpes zoster, and verrucae (warts) (19). A complete discussion of warts is given in Chapter 31.

Herpes Simplex

Herpes simplex is a viral infection of the skin and mucous membrane. The causative agent is a fairly large virus, herpesvirus hominis (HVH) (20). It has two strains—Type 1, common to herpes labialis, and Type 2, generally involved in genital herpes lesions and transmitted by sexual contact (21).

Herpes simplex (Type I) is manifested as groups of tiny vesicles filled with straw-colored fluid after an incubation period of 5 days (19). The vesicles develop into blisters and plaques. The area may be reddened, slightly edematous, and uncomfortable—malaise, headache, and initial itching, stinging, and burning may accompany the lesions. Most occurrences heal spontaneously in about 10 days; however, there is a marked tendency for lesions to recur (19). Lymph nodes of the area may be tender. The lesions usually appear on the lips and nose (as fever blisters or cold sores), fingers, and genital areas (18).

jock itch

moniliasis

herpes viral infections

shingles

Herpes Zoster (Shingles)

This viral infection, neurotropic in humans, is caused by a virus similar to that which causes chickenpox (18, 22). Lesions appear suddenly and acutely along the course of a nerve or group of nerves on one side of the body as reddened, swollen, round plaques, ranging in size from about 0.5 cm to areas larger than a hand; the spinal ganglia seem to be the primary site. The plaques may be painful after lesions form, and it is possible for them to appear as successive "showers" or crops over several days (18). The lesions develop into fairly large blisters, which become crusty in 2–14 days as they dry. The regional lymph nodes generally are tender. An episode is followed by a lasting immunity; recurrent cases are extremely uncommon.

EVALUATION

Before recommending a topical product for self-medication of adverse cutaneous conditions, the pharmacist should ascertain what type of condition exists. The pharmacist also should be aware of the clinical manifestations and therapy of skin disorders other than infection (e.g., contact dermatitis or psoriasis) as well as drug-induced eruptions (23). Antimicrobial products should be considered only in cases of true infection.

The pharmacist can prevent erroneous self-medication by advising medical attention if the condition calls for it or by suggesting a more appropriate OTC product. Incorrect self-medication may cause a delay in healing, possible deleterious progression of the disease, toxicity, obvious discomfort, and unnecessary cost. The following circumstances warrant medical attention:

- The condition has lasted for more than a few days;
- Appropriate treatments have not been successful, and the condition is getting worse;

- Applications of drug products have been used for several days over large areas, especially on denuded skin (checking for systemic toxicities), drainage is excessive and has occurred for several days, and improper cleaning of infectious exudate has led to widespread infection;
- There is predisposing illness, such as diabetes or systemic infection, or symptoms of such illness;
- Fever or malaise occurs;
- An unrecognized primary dermatitis (e.g., allergic dermatitis or primary irritation due to agents such as soap or chemicals) exists and has caused a secondary infection (such infections are generally difficult to treat with nonprescription drugs);
- Lesions are deep and extensive;
- Lancing to aid drainage is necessary (because this process requires good technique and timing, it must not be done by the patient);
- There is doubt as to the causative organisms (bacteria versus fungi, for example).

circumstances requiring medical attention

indications for topical antibiotic preparations

Probably the best approach to follow is to limit the use of OTC topical antimicrobial products to superficial conditions that involve minimal areas, when no predisposing or actual illness exists. Thus self-administered topical products should be viewed as extensions of supportive treatment (e.g., proper cleaning, proper hygiene, and clean bandaging), not as "miracle" treatments. An anti-infective drug in an appropriately designed vehicle or base (i.e., with a proper rate of drug release) should be used to ensure bioavailability and appropriate skin penetration. Proper drug use with a regimen of cleanliness should then achieve therapeutic success and keep the infection from spreading while normal anti-infective defenses combat the infecting organisms so that tissue can regenerate normally.

Medical attention should be sought in all but the most superficial, uncomplicated skin infections, especially if it appears that systemic medication is needed. Deep-seated and complicated secondary infections must have medical attention. Improper lancing as self-treatment may cause scarring and spreading of the condition by infected exudate; secondary infections may complicate the situation further. Scars subsequent to chronic carbuncles in children are a result of improper self-treatment.

TREATMENT

In general, most uncomplicated surface infections may be treated with topical anti-infectives once the acute stage has subsided. Many deep-seated lesions cannot be reached by topically applied products; in such cases, systemic treatment is required. The pharmacist should recommend physician referral if the condition is widespread or recurrent.

In secondary infections, effective treatment must include attention to the primary disease. Development of a predisposing illness, e.g., diabetes mellitus in patients with recurring carbuncles, must be watched for, diagnosed medically, and treated appropriately.

Adjunctive therapy including proper hygiene is important in preventing infection from spreading. Many drugs used topically for cutaneous infections are available by prescription only, and there are strong indications for their exclusive use in such conditions. The therapeutic efficacy of nonprescription products for other than the most superficial cutaneous infections is at best questionable.

Indications for OTC Product Use

Certain conditions are more amenable than others to treatment with OTC topical anti-infective agents. In evaluating patient symptoms the pharmacist should narrow down as closely as possible the specific pathogen, fungus, or virus involved.

Bacterial Infections

The effectiveness of topical agents in treating impetigo and other bacterial skin infections depends on the drug's specific antimicrobial spectrum, supportive hygienic measures, the extent of lesions, and the manner in which the drug is used. Since the pharmacist cannot know the exact pathogen involved in a particular infection, it is helpful to know which general antibiotics are useful.

Following the acute stage, bacitracin and neomycin ointments, which are available as OTC products, are usually effective in treating impetigo vulgaris, impetigo Bockhart, folliculitis, sweat gland infections, and ecthyma. Bacitracin is less sensitizing than neomycin. Polymyxin B sulfate in combination with other agents also has been used. To promote better penetration of the drug, the lesion's crust should be removed carefully following thorough softening with moist cream compresses before the ointment is applied at the base of the lesion.

Ammoniated mercury ointment (5–10%) has some effectiveness in treating impetigo vulgaris (17) but is not recommended. Other agents, including gentamicin, iodochlorhydroxyquin ointment and cream, precipitated sulfur, salicylic acid, and ichthammol in petroleum as compounded prescriptions, have been used with varying degrees of success but are not recommended.

In conditions requiring systemic treatment to destroy deep-seated pathogens, e.g., carbuncles and furuncles, topical antibiotics may be applied to prevent the lesions from spreading across the skin surface. Patients with erysipelas and pyonychia should be referred to a physician for treatment with systemic antibiotics.

Proper use of topical antibiotics should cure the infection in 14–21 days (24). Ointments should be applied at least three times per day to ensure continuous medication; intermittent applications can prolong the infection. Infected areas should be cleaned and patted dry after unaffected areas are cleaned (17). If lesions recur after topical management is stopped, a physician should be consulted for systemic antibiotic therapy.

Some physicians claim that systemic antibiotics are the only therapy for impetigo and feel that their topical use should be discouraged (25). One investigator recommends that topical antibiotics be discouraged in treatment of impetigo because these products are ineffective, they trigger dermatoses, and they render systemic drugs ineffective (25). The last criticism seems unduly restrictive. The pharmacist may recommend topical antibiotic preparations for localized, uncomplicated impetigo.

Fungal Infections

Treatment for these conditions varies according to the degree of inflammation, the organism involved, and the site of infection. For example, superficial tineas due to *Trichophyton*, *Microsporum*, or *Epidermophyton* are treatable with topical OTC preparations; *Candida* infections are not. However, tinea infections involving the scalp or bearded areas may penetrate the hair shaft and be difficult to reach with topical antifungal agents. Similarly, fungal infections involving the nail areas of the hands or feet cannot be treated effectively with topical agents. Another problem is differential self-diagnosis between tinea infections and *Candida* and nonfungal dermatoses (e.g., psoriasis, contact dermatitis, and seborrhea) in their acute or chronic states.

The pharmacist must exercise care in recommending OTC medication. In general, if the problem is a mild flare-up of a suspected tinea infection of the foot or groin, conservative self-medication should provide relief of symptoms in a few days. Suspected tinea infection of other body areas should be diagnosed by a physician.

indications for use of topical antifungal preparations

Desiccation and exposure to light and cooler temperatures are supportive procedures for cutaneous fungal infections. Griseofulvin, orally administered, probably is the most effective antifungal medication. However, this is not an OTC drug. In various superficial tinea infections (cruris, pedis, and capitis), griseofulvin elicits rapid results but is not effective against infections caused by *C. albicans* or against tinea versicolor (26). Tinea cruris responds to iodochlorhydroxyquin (3% cream or suspension) (20). Preparations containing undecylenates have some use in superficial dermatomycoses (e.g., athlete's foot) but are weakly effective for more extensive use (27). Tolnaftate is effective topically against the organisms that cause tinea and ringworm but ineffective against candidal organisms (27). It is used topically in conjunction with oral griseofulvin to provide effective therapy for chronic lesions.

exfoliation

Peeling the stratum corneum (exfoliation) helps ameliorate some fungal infections. Sulfur and salicylic acid ointments, dilute iodine solutions, carbol–fuchsin solution (Castellani's paint), and benzoic acid and salicylic acid ointment help soften the skin for peeling (19, 20). Triacetin (spray, powder, or cream) has been used to treat superficial fungal infections. Sodium propionate and undecylenic acid in combination with zinc salts of triacetin have achieved some popularity as fungistatic agents (24).

Cutaneous candidiasis is usually found in areas of chafing. Greasy products should be avoided; creams, powders, and lotions are preferred. Iodochlorhydroxyquin (3% cream or lotion) and nystatin are suggested for these infections (20).

In treating onychomycoses, oral griseofulvin is suggested for *Trichophyton* or *Epidermophyton* infections, and nystatin cream is effective for monilial infections (28). If the invading organism is *C. albicans*, exposure to water must be avoided; 2–4% thymol in chloroform (nail paint) has been reported to be beneficial (29).

Viral Infections

treating viral infections

Because herpes simplex is self-limiting, generally clearing up in about 10 days, a "therapeutic nihilism" approach to medication, i.e., palliative treatment only to counter discomfort, has been suggested (see Chapter 28) (18). Topical use of lidocaine (2.5% ointment, an OTC drug) is sufficient to ameliorate the discomfort of herpes simplex; emollients (petrolatum) may be used for the cracking and crusting (26). Thymol iodide powder, a 2–5% tannic acid solution, or zinc oxide paste also may be used to ease discomfort. For itching, mentholated petrolatum or camphor spirit has been used with varying degrees of success. Secondary bacterial infections should be treated with systemic antibiotics. Products that contain sunscreens could be useful for cases triggered by sunlight. Such infections, if close to the eyes, need ophthalmological consideration (31).

For herpes zoster, only symptomatic treatment is possible with OTC medication (e.g., simple dusting powders, drying and cooling lotions, cool oatmeal baths, and anesthetic ointments) (18, 31). Medical attention is always required for herpes zoster, or the patient may be permanently scarred.

Percutaneous Absorption Factors

physical–chemical factors in absorption

A drug must be released from its vehicle if it is to exert an effect at the desired site of activity (either the skin surface, the epidermis, or the dermis). The release of a topical drug from its base occurs at the interface between the skin surface and the applied layer of product. The physical–chemical relationship between the drug and the base determines the rate and the amount of drug released. Considerations such as the solubility of the drug in the base, its diffusion coefficient in the base, and its partition coefficient into sebum and the stratum corneum therefore are important. A drug with a strong affinity for the base will be released less readily than one whose solubility in the base is lower. Likewise, a drug with a proper balance of polar and hydrocarbon moieties, i.e., a partition coefficient approaching 1, will penetrate the stratum corneum more readily than drugs that are either highly polar or highly lipoidal, since that portion of the skin possesses both hydrated proteins and lipids. Other factors influencing drug release include the degree of hydration of the stratum corneum, the pKa of the drug, the pH of the base and of the skin surface, the drug concentration, the thickness of the applied layer, and the temperature. These factors are applicable to drug release from all topical dosage forms: medicated powders, ointments, pastes, emulsified cream or lotion bases, gels, suspensions, and solutions.

transport considerations

Percutaneous absorption is the transport of substances from the skin surface to the general circulation. Minor routes of such transport involve passage between the keratinized units of the stratum corneum and through the skin's appendages, i.e., hair follicles and sweat and sebaceous glands. The major route is by direct penetration through the stratum corneum, followed successively by transfer though the deeper epidermal layers and the papillary dermis (3). Since the epidermis is not vascularized, the drug will not enter the blood or lymphatic system until it reaches the capillary network of the dermis.

After application of a topical drug product, the transport of its drug(s) cannot begin until the surface of the stratum corneum is "charged" with the drug(s) (3). A delay period occurs while a drug is transferring from its vehicle or base into and through the sebum (where present), and then to the stratum corneum.

Depending on the physical–chemical properties of a drug vis-à-vis those of sebum and the various skin layers, the drug movement into and through the skin meets with varying degrees of resistance. The sebum, when present, is a minor barrier to drug transfer. The stratum corneum is the rate-limiting barrier to percutaneous absorption, i.e., provides the greatest resistance. Since it is nonliving tissue, the stratum corneum may be viewed as having the general characteristics of an artificial, semipermeable membrane, molecular passage through which is completely passive (bulk diffusion) (32). Once a molecule has crossed the stratum corneum, there is much less resistance to its transfer across the rest of the epidermis into the dermis (32). When the corneum is hydrated extensively, drug diffusion in general is accelerated (32). Occlusion increases the hydration of the stratum corneum from within the skin, fostering the transfer of all drugs. This action occurs because the hydration swells the stratum corneum, loosening its normally tight, dense packing arrangement and thereby making diffusion easier for all molecules. The increased amount of water present under such conditions probably further enhances the transfer of polar molecules.

absorption and transport of active ingredients from vehicle

drug transfer

components of topical anti-infective products

OTC antibiotics—their spectrum of activity and side effects

Greasy, hydrocarbon bases, e.g., petrolatum, are occlusive, promote stratum corneum hydration, and generally increase molecular transport. Hydrous emulsion bases are less occlusive; water-soluble bases, e.g., polyethylene glycols, are nonocclusive. The latter, in fact, may attract water from the stratum corneum to minimize such transport. Powders with hydrophilic ingredients also decrease hydration, since they promote evaporation from the skin by sorbing available water and increasing its surface area.

Drug absorption through wounds, burns, chafed areas, and the lesions of various dermatoses, i.e., where the integrity of the stratum corneum has been altered, is essentially uncontrolled (33). Such conditions result in artificial shunts of the percutaneous absorption process, leading to potentially dangerous levels of absorption. Absorption increases as the area of medicated application increases. Extreme care must be used in applying topical medications to areas of damaged skin (3).

Ingredients in OTC Products

Various drugs are used for topical application to prevent or treat infection (15, 16, 19, 26, 34–38). The major classes of drugs used are antibiotics, antifungal agents, and antiseptics.

Antibiotics

The major topical OTC antibiotics are bacitracin, gramicidin, neomycin, and polymyxin B sulfate, alone or in combination. The rationale for their use in combination is to ensure a broad spectrum of antibacterial activity through additive spectra of the individual component antibiotics.

Bacitracin

Bacitracin is a polypeptide antibiotic that prevents the completion of synthesis of bacterial cell membranes. Its main action is against gram-positive and gram-negative pathogens. It can be used topically (for bacterial infections) and parenterally because it is not absorbed through GI mucosa. Because it is nephrotoxic, excessive topical use, especially in vehicle bases that promote percutaneous absorption, should be avoided. Resistance to it is rather uncommon, and hypersensitivity is rare. It is unstable in aqueous solution and when it is exposed to light.

Gramicidin

Gramicidin is a polypeptide antibiotic effective against gram-positive bacteria. It cannot be absorbed after oral administration and has significant systemic toxicity (hemolysis and kidney and liver damage) that precludes parenteral use.

Neomycin

This aminoglycoside antibiotic is effective against gram-positive bacteria by its intervention in protein synthesis. Of the topical antibiotics, it is the one most likely to sensitize. Neomycin is used orally for GI tract infections and to "sanitize" the bowel before intestinal surgery. As such, it is minimally absorbed. However, if sufficient levels are reached in the blood, kidney damage and ototoxicity may result. Therefore its major use is in topical treatment of cutaneous infections, where the chance for such toxicity is rare.

For topical use, neomycin is available in cream and ointment forms. Staphylococci and coliform bacilli may develop resistance to neomycin. To prevent this occurrence, neomycin generally is used in combination with polymyxin or bacitracin.

Polymyxin B Sulfate

Polymyxin B sulfate is effective against gram-negative bacteria but not against gram-positive bacteria or fungi. It alters membrane permeability of bacteria and is not absorbed from the GI tract. Polymyxins do not readily develop resistant strains of bacteria but may cause renal damage and paresthesia if sufficient concentrations reach the blood. In topical use such toxicity is rare.

Antifungal Agents

Many topical antifungal products (31, 36) are covered in detail in Chapter 28. Agents used for cutaneous skin infections are found in ointments, creams, powders, and aerosols.

Benzoic Acid and Salicylic Acid Ointment

This ointment (Whitfield's ointment) is used in treating cutaneous fungal infections because of its keratolytic effect. It peels the skin and removes the debris on which organisms can grow, making deeper infections accessible to specific topical antifungal compounds.

Dyes

Gentian violet and carbol–fuchsin solutions have been used for superficial fungal skin infections. However, they are not significant antifungal agents and have the distinct disadvantage of staining. More effective antifungal agents, e.g., tolnaftate, have replaced these dyes in treatment of topical fungal infections.

Fatty Acids

Sweat has antifungal properties probably caused by its fatty acid content. Sodium propionate, a fatty acid derivative used as a topical antiseptic, has mild fungistatic activity. It has been used in topical products in concentrations of as much as 10% and with undecylenic acid. Undecylenic acid has the greatest antifungal activity of the fatty acids. It may cause irritation and sensitization and should be discontinued if these effects occur. It is basically fungistatic, needing long exposure at high concentrations to achieve a fungicidal effect. It is used in combination with its zinc salt in ointment, cream, powder, and aerosol forms (5% acid, 20% salt) for an additive antifungal effect.

Salicylanilide

Salicylanilide is a fungistatic agent used mainly for tinea capitis (5%, ointment). Its derivatives are used in antiseptic soaps.

Selenium Sulfide

Selenium sulfide is effective in the treatment of tinea versicolor and seborrheic dermatitis of the scalp. It is also used in OTC topical products to control dandruff, usually as a detergent–suspension. Contact with the eyes and sensitive skin areas should be avoided because of its potential as an irritant. Although not absorbed to a significant degree through the skin, it is hazardous if swallowed, producing CNS effects and respiratory and vasomotor depression.

Tolnaftate

Tolnaftate is a topical OTC antifungal agent effective against all species of fungi (except *C. albicans*) that cause cutaneous infections, including tinea. Complete clearing of cutaneous lesions may take several months. Nevertheless, tolnaftate is probably the most effective OTC topical antifungal available. Fungal infections of the nails, palms of the hands, and soles of the feet are not very responsive to tolnaftate or any topical treatment. Combination therapy in such cases is appropriate, i.e., oral therapy (griseofulvin) with tolnaftate (27).

Triacetin

Triacetin in aerosol (15%), cream (25%), or powder form (33%) is used in treating superficial fungal infections. Because its activity depends on the slow release of acetic acid, triacetin probably is best viewed as effective only in the most superficial of cutaneous fungal skin infections.

Antiseptics

A number of substances are used as antiseptics in OTC anti-infective products (34, 36). Not all are recommended as safe and effective.

Acids

Acids are used in topical preparations because they kill or inhibit bacterial growth.

Acetic acid. This acid has been used as a bactericide. *Pseudomonas* appears particularly vulnerable to it, and it has been used for surgical dressings. Dilute solutions (e.g., 5%) also are used for otitis externa and otitis media ("swimmer's ear").

Boric acid. This weak acid has been used as a topical antiseptic and eyewash. The aqueous solution (2.5%) inhibits bacterial growth, but it does not kill many forms of bacteria. Boric acid is an extremely dangerous systemic poison. Boric acid powder or solutions used on abraded skin may be absorbed readily to cause severe systemic poisoning: nausea, vomiting, diarrhea, exfoliative dermatitis, kidney damage, and acute circulatory failure may result. The minor therapeutic value of this compound, in comparison with its potential as a poison, has led to the general recommendation that it no longer be used as a therapeutic agent.

agents for treating cutaneous fungal infections

agents used as antiseptics in topical products

possible mechanisms and indications

Alcohols

Ethanol (70%) and isopropyl alcohol are included in topical anti-infective products for their bactericidal effect.

Ethanol. Ethanol (70%) has good bactericidal activity and acts relatively quickly but has little residual effect. It rapidly denatures cellular protein of microorganisms, lowers the surface tension of bacteria to help in their removal, and has a solvent effect on sebum. However, it is not an effective antiviral agent, nor does it kill spores. It is not a desirable wound antiseptic because it irritates already damaged tissue. The coagulum formed may, in fact, protect the bacteria.

Ethanol may contain denaturants. It is not a recognized skin sensitizer. However, excessive exposure in high concentrations can dehydrate the corneum. Systemic ingestion produces usual alcoholic intoxication and severe GI distress. Denaturants cause the GI symptoms to become exacerbated.

Isopropyl. Isopropyl alcohol ("rubbing alcohol") has somewhat stronger bactericidal activity and lower surface tension than ethanol. In general, it is used like ethanol solutions for cleaning and for its antiseptic effect on the skin. It can be used undiluted or as 70% aqueous solutions. Denaturants are not added because isopropyl alcohol itself is not potable. Isopropyl alcohol has a greater potential for "drying" the skin because its lipid solvent effects are stronger than those of ethanol. It may be gently swabbed over the ear to prevent otitis externa, when conditions may precipitate it, e.g., after swimming.

agents used as antiseptics in topical products

coal tar dyes

possible mechanisms and indications for topical antiseptics

Dyes

The coal tar dyes are synthetic organic compounds, some of which have antiseptic properties (36). Several have wound-healing properties, and others are used in various diagnostic procedures.

Acridine dyes. The acridine dyes are yellow flavines. Proflavine and acriflavine are used therapeutically as topical antimicrobial agents. Their strongest antibacterial action occurs in alkaline media on gram-positive organisms at dilutions of 1:1000 to 1:10,000. These agents have not become popular for topical use.

Gentian violet. This methylrosaniline dye kills gram-positive organisms and many fungi. It is used in concentrations of 1:1000 to 1:5000.

Methylene blue. This dye is a bacteriostatic agent. It is used as a urinary antiseptic, but rarely, if ever, as a topical agent.

Scarlet red. This azo dye is used more for its positive healing effect on wounds than as an antiseptic. It stimulates cellular proliferation and is used to treat burns and other dermal lesions. The azo dyes (5%, ointment) are not recommended as topical antimicrobials.

Halogenated Salicylanilides/Related Compounds

Tribromsalan (TBS), dibromsalan (DBS), fluorosalan, triclocarban (TCC), and cloflucarban are antimicrobial agents used in soaps. The FDA has curtailed the use of several halogenated salicylanilides, including tribromsalan and dibromsalan, because of their potential as photosensitizers (39). Safer alternative agents exist, and the FDA feels that the risk-to-benefit ratio is improper for continued use of these chemicals in soaps. People sensitized to antimicrobial soaps should be cautious about using soaps not labeled explicitly (40).

There is concern that the widespread use of antimicrobial soaps may lead to disruption of the skin's normal flora. In general, the agents in the soap kill gram-positive flora, and effective and long-term reduction of the microbes may cause the pathogenic gram-negative species to proliferate (41–43). Extensive use of anti-gram-positive agents in hospitals and nursing homes may produce a large increase in gram-negative infections (44). However, absolute proof of antimicrobial agents in soaps as the causative agents for gram-negative cutaneous infections has not been shown.

Halogen Compounds

These antiseptics include sodium hypochlorite and iodine-containing compounds.

Iodine. Solutions of elemental iodine or those that release iodine from chemical complexes are used as presurgical skin antiseptics and as wound antiseptics. Their antimicrobial effect is attributed to their ability to oxidize microbial protoplasm. Caution must be taken that strong iodine solution USP (Lugol's) not be used as an antiseptic. Iodine solution USP (2% iodine, 2.5% sodium iodide) is used as an antiseptic for superficial wounds. Iodine tincture USP (2% iodine, 2.5% sodium iodide, about 50% ethanol) is less preferable than the aqueous solution (2%) because it is irritating to tissue.

In general, bandaging should be discouraged after iodine applications to avoid tissue irritation. Iodine solutions stain skin, are irritating to tissue, and may cause sensitization in some people.

Iodoform. Iodoform has minimal antibacterial activity in itself. However, the slow liberation of free iodine, when it is exposed to body secretions, exerts an antiseptic effect. Although it has been used on gauze for topical treatment of abscessed cavities, this application has questionable therapeutic efficacy and should be discouraged.

Povidone-iodine. Povidone-iodine is an organic complex used in topical nonprescription antiseptics to treat minor infections of mucous membranes and cutaneous tissue and as a preoperative antiseptic. Percentage of the active ingredient varies according to product type from 1% in ointments to 0.75% in shampoos and skin antiseptics. As an antiseptic it is less effective than iodine solutions but effectively controls minor infections. Organic iodine compounds usually are less irritating, less toxic, and less sensitizing than inorganic sources, but they are somewhat less effective as antiseptics. However, the organic iodine complexes generally have better patient acceptance than solutions of elemental iodine, since they are nonstinging and nonstaining. Their efficacy in combating cutaneous infection, although less than that of elemental iodine solutions, is recognized.

Sodium hypochlorite. The antimicrobial effect of sodium hypochlorite results from liberation of elemental chlorine. Concentrated solutions (5%) are very irritating to tissue and are used as disinfectants (e.g., for utensils and swimming pools). Dilute solutions (0.5% or less) (Modified Dakin's) have been used as topical antiseptics with varying degrees of success.

Hexachlorophene

Hexachlorophene previously had wide success as a topical antiseptic. It was restricted to prescription use when it was shown that the agent was absorbed through the skin of infants, causing nerve damage. Emulsions that contain 3% hexachlorophene are effective antiseptic/cleansing products used for hand washing of hospital personnel, surgical hand scrubs, and preoperative skin preparations (38). Because hexachlorophene has a substantive (binding) property, repeated use leaves an antimicrobial residual film on the skin.

Ichthammol

Ichthammol (ammonium ichthosulfonate) is a sulfonated and neutralized (ammonia) derivative of the distillate of bituminous rock or schists (36). It has little value as a topical antiseptic or as a "drawing salve" for boils. A viscous, brownish-black semiliquid with a characteristic bituminous odor and an emollient effect, this agent is used less commonly now than it was in the past.

Iodochlorhydroxyquin

This antibacterial and antifungal agent is available in nonprescription products as a cream or ointment (3%) and as vaginal inserts and powders (36). It is considered an effective compound.

Mercurial Compounds

Several mercurial compounds have antiseptic/disinfectant properties. In general, however, they are considered poor antiseptics for wounded skin because serum and tissue proteins reduce their antimicrobial potency. If these compounds are used extensively or on large areas of abraded skin, mercury may be absorbed and may become a systemic poison; therefore their use should be discouraged.

Inorganic salts of mercury are tissue irritants. Such toxic properties are reduced when the mercury is incorporated into an organic compound. Some investigators believe that the alcoholic component of mercurial tinctures has greater antimicrobial effect than the mercurial component (31).

Several organic mercurials are incorporated into OTC topical antimicrobial products. These compounds may cause rashes because they are contact sensitizers.

Merbromin. Merbromin is less effective as a skin antiseptic than the other organic mercurials. However, it is used as a preoperative germicide (2%, aqueous). Serous fluids reduce its antimicrobial potency.

Nitromersol. Nitromersol is more effective as an antiseptic than soluble inorganic compounds of mercury but less effective than alcohol. It is not a serious tissue irritant, and it is available as a tincture in a dilution of 1:200.

Phenylmercuric salts. These salts inhibit growth of gram-positive and gram-negative bacteria and topical fungi. As skin antiseptics, however, they are not as effective as ethanol. Their activity is not reduced, as is that of ethanol, in the presence of serum proteins or soaps, which may cause deactivation of some antiseptics by coagulation or precipitation.

Thimerosal. Thimerosal has antibacterial and antifungal properties, but it is also less effective than ethanol. It is found in several types of topical products, including aqueous solutions, tinctures, ointments, creams, and aerosols. Systemic toxicity occurs less frequently with thimerosal than with other mercurials because the mercury in thimerosal is tightly bound to the organic configuration. The usual concentration is 0.1%.

Oxidizing Agents

The oxidizing agents used as antiseptics in topical preparations include hydrogen peroxide, potassium permanganate, and potassium chlorate.

Hydrogen peroxide. Hydrogen peroxide (3% solution) is the most widely used of these compounds; sodium and zinc peroxides also are used. Enzymatic release of oxygen from hydrogen peroxide occurs when it comes into contact with blood and tissue fluids. The mechanical (fizzing) release of the oxygen has a cleansing effect on a wound, but organic matter reduces its effectiveness. The duration of action is only as long as the period of active oxygen release. Using peroxide on the intact skin is of doubtful value, because release of the nascent oxygen is too slow. This compound must be used only where the released gas can escape; therefore it should never be used in abscesses, nor should bandages be applied too soon after its use.

Potassium chlorate. Potassium chlorate solutions have been used for treatment of mucous membranes of the mouth. However, this agent's potential toxicity overshadows its usefulness.

Potassium permanganate. Potassium permanganate is a strong oxidizing agent, but it rapidly decomposes in the presence of organic material. Its use as an antiseptic is questionable.

Phenolic Compounds

In very dilute solutions, phenol is an antiseptic and disinfectant. It is bacteriostatic at a 1:500 concentration and both bactericidal and fungicidal at a 1:50 concentration, but it is ineffective against spores. Phenols and substituted phenols precipitate and denature cellular proteins. Their antimicrobial activity continues in the presence of organic matter.

Liquefied phenol. A solution of phenol crystals dissolved in 10% water is used locally like trichloroacetic acid to "peel down" lesions. It should be used with a coating of petrolatum around the lesion to protect healthy, intact skin from its caustic effect.

mercurial, oxidizing, and phenolic compounds as topical antiseptics

concentration ranges and side effects

Phenol. Phenol has local anesthetic activity and is claimed to be an antipruritic in concentrations of 1:100 to 1:200, as in phenolated calamine lotion. In aqueous solution of more than 1%, it is a tissue irritant and should not be used on skin.

Mixtures of phenol and camphor in oily solutions are "old favorites" as nonprescription antiseptics for use on minor cuts and burns, insect bites, athlete's foot, fever blisters, and cold sores. However, if they are applied to moist areas, lesions may occur because these products contain relatively high amounts of phenol, e.g., 4%. These products should be used with caution.

Substituted phenols. Substituted phenols, including the halogenated phenols (e.g., hexachlorophene) and the alkyl substituted phenols, have more bactericidal effects than phenol. Halogenation of a phenolic compound increases the antiseptic properties. Dihalogenated and trihalogenated forms have greater potency but are less water soluble than monohalogenated phenols.

Cresols are alkyl derivatives of phenol. Three isomers, the *ortho, meta,* and *para* forms, all have similar disinfectant properties. They are used mainly as disinfectants of inanimate surfaces and objects. Cresol is more potent than phenol but has a greater potential for toxicity.

Resorcinol is somewhat antibacterial and antifungal but is much less potent than phenol; its systemic effects are the same as those of phenol. As an ointment (2% or more) it has been used in treating ringworm and several dermatoses. However, other topical agents (e.g., tolnaftate) are more effective in treating ringworm. Resorcinol monoacetate exerts even milder but longer action because it releases resorcinol slowly. Both resorcinol and the monoacetate are used in acne preparations, mainly for their keratolytic effect; their antiseptic effects are best described as mild or minor.

Hexylresorcinol (0.1% dilution) is a general antiseptic, but it is irritating and may produce sensitivity. Thymol and chlorothymol are also alkyl derivatives of phenol with minor antibacterial and antifungal properties.

Silver Compounds

The silver ion has an antiseptic effect because of its ability to precipitate the protein of cellular components of microorganisms. Soluble inorganic silver salts and organic silver compounds have been used as topical antiseptics. However, except for silver nitrate, most silver compounds are used less and less with the advent of more effective antiseptic agents. In general, silver salts are precipitated relatively quickly by chloride in cell components. The organic silver compounds are less irritating to tissue than the inorganic salts but are less effective as antimicrobial agents.

Silver nitrate. Silver nitrate is a fairly potent bactericide at a concentration of 1:1000; at 1:10,000 it is bacteriostatic. Aqueous solutions (0.5%) are used on dressings for second- and third-degree burns to prevent infection. Extensive use, however, may deplete chloride ions and cause electrolyte imbalance.

other topical antiseptics

benzethonium and benzalkonium chlorides and other surfactants

nondrug measures

Toughened silver nitrate. Toughened silver nitrate pencils may be used to cauterize minor wounds (shaving) and to treat warts. Mild silver protein and colloidal silver iodide are other nonprescription forms of silver. However, they have minimal antiseptic efficacy.

Surfactants

Soaps and quaternary ammonium compounds are sometimes included in topical anti-infective products. In addition to their antiseptic properties, these agents are used for their cleansing properties.

Quaternary ammonium compounds. These compounds are cationic surfactants that have antimicrobial activity on gram-positive and gram-negative bacteria but not on spores. Gram-negative bacteria are more resistant than gram-positive ones; thus they need a longer period of exposure. Quaternary ammonium compounds emulsify sebum and have a detergent effect to remove dirt, bacteria, and desquamated epithelial cells. Their antimicrobial activity is caused by disrupting membranes and denaturing lipoproteins. These compounds are inactivated by anionic ones (e.g., soaps and base/vehicle ingredients such as viscosity builders).

Nonprescription quaternary ammonium compound products include benzalkonium chloride, benzethonium chloride, and methylbenzethonium chloride. These compounds are formulated as creams, dusting powders, and aqueous or alcoholic solutions. Concentrates are available for dilution to proper concentration for topical use. If mistakenly used undiluted, these concentrates may cause serious irritation. Quaternary compounds are irritating to the eyes, and caution must be used in this regard. For use on broken or diseased skin, concentrations of 1:5000 to 1:20,000 should be used; on intact skin and minor abrasions a concentration of 1:750 is useful.

Methylbenzethonium chloride is effective against microorganisms that split urea to form ammonia. Thus it is used as a diaper rinse and for application to areas subject to irritation from ammonia formation, e.g., groin, thighs, and buttocks.

Soaps. Soaps are anionic surfactants. They are used as supportive treatment (cleansing) in preventing skin infections. Their actual antiseptic properties are minimal.

Sulfur

Sulfur alone is not antiseptic. It has been speculated that its mild germicidal effect is caused by the formation (by microorganisms or cutaneous tissue) of hydrogen sulfide and pentathionic acid. It is used in topical medications more for its keratolytic properties, which are useful for treatment of various dermatoses (36). However, used topically, sulfur may promote comedo formation.

Supportive Procedures

Supportive procedures common to the treatment of all skin infections also have been documented (17). Because skin infections are triggered by external infection and reinfection, precautions should be taken to prevent their continuation or extension through self-reinoculation. Soiled bandages or clothing should not touch unaffected areas (infected clothes should be washed separately); such areas should be cleaned regularly or protected by suitable antiseptic products. The hands should be kept very clean. Direct contact with others should be avoided. In children, a special effort must be made to prevent manipulation of the lesions. Irritants such as drug products, tight clothing, or bandaging make the skin vulnerable to further spread of the infection; drying or lubricating powders may be used in these areas to minimize chafing.

Scrubbing or prolonged soaking of the lesions should be avoided to prevent extension of the pathogens by maceration of the area. General cleaning with water and nonirritating soap usually is adequate. Mild antiseptic soaps may be helpful in preventing pyodermas but are not very effective in treating them (45). These soaps may be used prophylactically to control skin bacteria, but they are not effective against bacteria deep in the epidermis. Certain halogenated salicylanilides incorporated into these soaps have been shown to cause contact dermatitis or photodermatitis (6).

The pharmacist should advise on the proper use of bandaging. Bandages are occlusive; they foster hydration of the epidermis and therefore increase drug penetration. Different types of bandages produce different degrees of occlusiveness; plastic wrappings are the most effective. Processes that can cause maceration (e.g., occlusive wet dressings and adhesive bandages) must be avoided except to promote "pointing" or "coming to a head" for drainage of pus, as with carbuncles (17), or to soften the crusty scab in impetigo to facilitate its removal before applying antibiotic ointment. Hot compresses, applied without injury, promote "pointing."

In addition to treating dermal infections, certain topical antimicrobial agents are used to prevent skin infection. Deodorant soaps that include these agents are popular, although their efficacy has not been proven. Skin antiseptic products also are available for general prophylactic use.

PRODUCT SELECTION GUIDELINES

Once the pharmacist has evaluated the patient's condition, an appropriate treatment must be selected.

Self-medication with topical anti-infectives and supportive procedures should be reserved for superficial, uncomplicated skin infections. More serious cutaneous infections should be referred to a physician for systemic therapy. Proper use of the patient medication profile may help the pharmacist by signaling known allergens, possible cross-sensitization and general skin sensitivity, potential drug interactions, and possible predisposing illnesses. The profile along with the patient interview also is useful in narrowing down reasons for long-lasting or recurring infections (e.g., poor bandaging practices).

FDA Recommendations

Another guideline the pharmacist may consider is the recommendations of the two FDA OTC Panels on Topical Antimicrobials. The initial recommendations of the Antimicrobial I Panel were published in September 1974 as a proposal to establish a monograph for the safety and efficacy of topical drugs used in seven types of OTC products: antimicrobial soaps, health care personnel handwashes, patient preoperative skin preparations, skin antiseptics, skin wound cleansers, skin wound protectants, and surgical hand scrubs (38).

The proposal generated significant comment and additional data, necessitating further FDA deliberation and resulting in the publication of a "tentative final" order (January 1978) for these compounds (46) (Table 1). In response to comments and requests concerning that document, the FDA Commissioner has decided to reopen the administrative record for the drugs reviewed in it (47). Further comments will be solicited, followed by publication of yet another "tentative final" monograph. Eventually, a final, regulatory monograph for these compounds will be completed.

Initial recommendations of the Antimicrobial II Panel were published in April 1977 as a proposal to establish a safety and efficacy monograph for topical OTC antibiotic drugs (48). Table 2 summarizes these recommendations for products used as skin wound antibiotics and skin wound protectants. Examples of the latter product type include antibiotics added to increase the product's effectiveness by "preventing the continuation of a wound with organisms introduced from the environment or by preventing the growth of organisms in the formulation"; whereas the former includes those used to "prevent or treat overt skin infections" (48). The Panel also will review topical OTC antifungal drugs and acne medications. Certain miscellaneous topical antimicrobial products, e.g., mercurials, alcohols, and medicated bandages, have been assigned to the OTC Miscellaneous External Panel (47).

An early concern of the OTC Antimicrobial I Panel centered around the use of certain halogenated salicylanilides as ingredients in topical drug and cosmetic products (39). Such compounds, e.g., tribromsalan, dibromsalan, and tetrachlorosalicylanilide (TCSA), had been used as active or inactive ingredients in various OTC drug products and cosmetics, mainly antibacterial soaps. They were assessed by the Panel to be potent photosensitizers and cross-sensitizers. Since safer, alternative antimicrobial agents are available, the FDA (September 1975) (49) ruled that these compounds are not generally recognized as being safe and effective (39). Any drug product containing them would be considered a new drug entity, requiring a new drug application (NDA). Also, any cosmetic product including these as ingredients would be deemed adulterated.

The OTC Antimicrobial I Panel was concerned also that antimicrobial soaps could upset the normal flora on the skin surface, leading to infection by surviving pathogenic "residents" (39). However, the Panel did acknowledge that more data on the relationships of concentration, contact time of antimicrobial agents with the skin, number of exposures, and the total microbial population of the flora were needed.

Under these circumstances the Panel recommended caution in the use of these compounds/products and advised that the concentration of such ingredients in soaps be adjusted to levels that reduce the flora only enough to produce a deodorant effect. The Panel's report noted that experts have estimated that a 70% "kill" of normal flora yields a deodorant effect (39). Some antimicrobial soap bars, however, were found to reduce 90% or more of gram-positive organisms; so powerful an activity was deemed potentially harmful.

FDA Panel recommendations

factors in selecting an effective product

importance of proper use

Pharmacist Considerations

Having selected a therapeutic agent, the pharmacist must choose the proper drug product type—powder, solution/tincture, ointment, cream, lotion, or aerosol. The advantages and disadvantages of creams and ointments must be weighed for each case. Similarly, the use of lotions or suspensions rather than semisolid dosage forms must be determined. Powders, for example, may be used for chafed, moist areas of superficial infections but not on open lesions; occlusive ointments for hydration of the skin; and water-washable creams or lotions for hairy areas or when occlusion is not appropriate. The pharmacist also must select the most appropriate base for the degree of skin penetration desired.

The pharmacist should be aware of possible allergens in the product's base formula. Hypoallergenic cosmetics may provide a useful parameter in this regard; perfumed products and those that contain ingredients recognized as sensitizers (lanolin derivatives and some preservatives, e.g., parabens and emulsifying agents) should be avoided. If a quaternary ammonium antiseptic is used, the pharmacist should caution against concomitant use of products that could render the compound ineffective, such as an anionic agent.

The pharmacist also should advise on the proper use of the suggested product. For infections, intermittent applications are considered poor therapy; regular applications are preferable. However, overmedication may lead to irritation and possible systemic absorption and toxicity. An appropriate "thickness" of application should be suggested to avoid overmedication and to ensure therapeutic concentrations at the lesions. The need for cleanliness and avoidance of all situations that could cause reinfection must be stressed to the patient. Also, bandaging and its effects on the infection should be explained.

FDA categories for components of topical anti-infective products

Table 1. FDA-Classified Compounds

Use	Compound	Category
Antimicrobial soap	benzalkonium chloride[a]	II
	benzethonium chloride[a]	II
	chloroxylenol	III
	cloflucarban	III
	hexylresorcinol[a]	II
	iodine complexed with phosphate ester of alkylaryloxypolyethylene glycol[a]	II
	iodine tincture[a]	II
	methylbenzethonium chloride[a]	II
	nonylphenoxypoly(ethyleneoxy)ethanol-iodine[a]	II
	phenol > 1.5% aqueous/alcoholic	II
	phenol ≦ 1.5% aqueous/alcoholic	III
	poloxamer-iodine	II
	povidone-iodine	III
	triclocarban[b]	III
	triclosan[b]	III
	triple dye[a]	II
	undecoylium chloride-iodine	II
Health care personnel handwash	benzalkonium chloride	III
	benzethonium chloride	III
	chloroxylenol	III
	cloflucarban[b]	II, III
	hexylresorcinol	III
	iodine complexed with phosphate ester of alkylaryloxypolyethylene glycol	II, III
	iodine tincture	II
	methylbenzethonium chloride	III
	nonylphenoxypoly(ethyleneoxy)ethanol-iodine	II, III
	phenol > 1.5% aqueous/alcoholic	II
	phenol ≦ 1.5% aqueous/alcoholic	III
	poloxamer-iodine	II, III
	povidone-iodine	III
	triclocarban[b]	III
	triclosan	II
	triple dye[a]	II
	undecoylium chloride-iodine	III
Patient preoperative skin preparation	benzalkonium chloride	III
	benzethonium chloride	III
	chloroxylenol	III
	cloflucarban	II
	hexylresorcinol	III
	iodine complexed with phosphate ester of alkylaryloxypolyethylene glycol	III
	iodine tincture[c]	I
	methylbenzethonium chloride	III
	nonylphenoxypoly(ethyleneoxy)ethanol-iodine	III
	phenol > 1.5% aqueous/alcoholic	II
	phenol ≦ 1.5% aqueous/alcoholic	III
	poloxamer-iodine	III
	povidone-iodine	III
	triclocarban	II
	triclosan	II
	triple dye[a]	II
	undecoylium chloride-iodine	III
Skin antiseptic	benzalkonium chloride	III
	benzethonium chloride	III
	chloroxylenol	III
	cloflucarban	II
	hexylresorcinol	III

Table 1. Continued

Use	Compound	Category
Skin antiseptic (cont.)	iodine complexed with phosphate ester of alkylaryloxypolyethylene glycol	III
	iodine tincture	III
	methylbenzethonium chloride	III
	nonylphenoxypoly(ethyleneoxy)ethanol-iodine	III
	phenol > 1.5% aqueous/alcoholic	II
	phenol ≦ 1.5% aqueous/alcoholic	III
	poloxamer-iodine	III
	povidone-iodine	III
	triclocarban	II
	triclosan	III
	triple dye[d]	II, III
	undecoylium chloride-iodine	III
Skin wound cleanser	cloflucarban[b]	II, III
	chloroxylenol	III
	hexylresorcinol[e]	I
	iodine complexed with phosphate ester of alkylaryloxypolyethylene glycol	III
	iodine tincture	III
	nonylphenoxypoly(ethyleneoxy)ethanol-iodine	III
	phenol > 1.5% aqueous/alcoholic	II
	phenol ≦ 1.5% aqueous/alcoholic	III
	poloxamer-iodine	III
	poloxamer 188[f]	I
	povidone-iodine	III
	quaternary ammonium compounds[g]	I
	triclocarban[b]	II, III
	triclosan	III
	triple dye[a]	II
	undecoylium chloride-iodine	III
Skin wound protectant	benzalkonium chloride	III
	benzethonium chloride	III
	chloroxylenol	III
	cloflucarban	II
	hexylresorcinol	III
	iodine complexed with phosphate ester of alkylaryloxypolyethylene glycol	III
	iodine tincture	III
	methylbenzethonium chloride	III
	nonylphenoxypoly(ethyleneoxy)ethanol-iodine	III
	phenol > 1.5% aqueous/alcoholic	II
	phenol ≦ 1.5% aqueous/alcoholic	III
	poloxamer-iodine	III
	povidone-iodine	III
	triclocarban	II
	triclosan	III
	triple dye[a]	II
	undecoylium chloride-iodine	III
Surgical hand scrub	benzalkonium chloride	III
	benzethonium chloride	III
	chloroxylenol	III
	cloflucarban	II
	hexylresorcinol	III
	iodine complexed with phosphate ester of alkylaryloxypolyethylene glycol	III
	iodine tincture	II
	methylbenzethonium chloride	III
	nonylphenoxypoly(ethyleneoxy)ethanol-iodine	III
	phenol > 1.5% aqueous/alcoholic	II
	phenol ≦ 1.5% aqueous/alcoholic	III
	poloxamer-iodine	III

FDA categories for components of topical anti-infective products

Table 1. Continued

Use	Compound	Category
Surgical hand scrub (cont.)	povidone-iodine	III
	triclocarban	III
	triclosan	II
	triple dye[c]	II
	undecoylium chloride-iodine	III

[a]Placed in Category II due to a physical and/or chemical incompatibility in formulation.
[b]Category III only when formulated in a bar soap to be used with water.
[c]2% iodine, 2.5% sodium iodide, 50% ethanol.
[d]Category II for use outside the neonatal nursery.
[e]≦ 1/1000.
[f]In aqueous 20–40% solution.
[g]E.g., methylbenzethonium chloride, benzethonium chloride, and benzalkonium chloride, ≦ 1/750 in water.

FDA categories for topical antibiotics

Table 2. FDA-Classified Antibiotic Compounds

Use	Compound	Category
Skin wound antibiotic	bacitracin	III
	chlortetracycline hydrochloride	III
	gramicidin D	III
	neomycin sulfate	III
	oxytetracycline hydrochloride	III
	polymyxin B sulfate	III
	tetracycline hydrochloride	III
Skin wound protectant	bacitracin	I
	chlortetracycline hydrochloride	I
	gramicidin D	III
	neomycin sulfate	III
	oxytetracycline hydrochloride	I
	polymyxin B sulfate[a]	I
	tetracycline hydrochloride	I

From *Federal Register*, *42*, 17642 (1977).
[a]Only when used in combination with bacitracin, tetracycline hydrochloride, chlortetracycline hydrochloride, or oxytetracycline hydrochloride.

The condition's progress should be monitored. If other eruptions or dermatitis, indications of irritation or maceration, spreading or "deepening" of the lesions, or denuding of the skin by the product occurs, self-medication should be stopped and medical attention sought. Likewise, if the condition does not respond positively in a reasonable period, a physician should be consulted.

SUMMARY

Topical antimicrobials are used to treat and prevent cutaneous infections caused by bacteria, fungi, and viruses. Knowledge of design and formulation aspects of topical antimicrobial products is important in selecting appropriate therapeutic agents and products. The patient interview is essential in ascertaining whether self-medication or professional medical attention is indicated. If OTC products are appropriate, the pharmacist should instruct the patient on their use and on supportive procedures.

A review of the FDA OTC Antimicrobial I and II Panel viewpoints on topical antimicrobial and antibiotic products (39, 46) emphasizes the need for constant evaluation of therapeutic efficacy and safety of nonprescription drug products. The pharmacist should keep current with the regulations resulting from the recommendations of these OTC Panels.

REFERENCES

(1) J. S. Jellinek, "Formulation and Function of Cosmetics," 2nd ed., Wiley, New York, N.Y., 1970, pp. 4–14.
(2) J. A. A. Hunter, *Br. Med. J.*, *4*, 340, 411 (1973).
(3) B. Idson, *J. Pharm. Sci.*, *64*, 901 (1975).
(4) A. M. Kligman, "The Epidermis," Academic, New York, N.Y., 1964, p. 387.
(5) S. M. Blaug, in "Prescription Pharmacy," 2nd ed., J. B. Sprowls, Jr., Ed., Lippincott, Philadelphia, Pa., 1970, pp. 230–239.
(6) F. G. Weissmann, *Drug Intell. Clin. Pharm.*, *8*, 535 (1974).
(7) S. M. Peck and W. R. Russ, *Arch. Dermatol. Syphilol.*, *56*, 601 (1947).
(8) S. Rothman, A. Smiljaric, A. L. Shapiro, and A. W. Weitkamp, *J. Invest. Dermatol.*, *8*, 81 (1947).
(9) J. M. L. Burtenshaw, *J. Hyg.*, *42*, 184 (1942).

(10) V. W. Burckhardt and W. Baumle, *Dermatologica*, *102*, 294 (1951).
(11) A. M. Kligman, in "Skin Bacteria and Their Role in Infection," H. I. Maibach and G. Hildrick-Smith, Eds., McGraw-Hill, New York, N.Y., 1965, pp. 13–31.
(12) M. T. Hojyo-Tomoka, R. R. Marples, and A. M. Kligman, *Arch. Dermatol.*, *107*, 723 (1973).
(13) L. F. Montes and W. H. Wilborn, *Br. J. Dermatol.*, *81*, 23 (1969).
(14) R. R. Marples, in "Skin Bacteria and Their Role in Infection," H. I. Maibach and G. Hildrick-Smith, Eds., McGraw-Hill, New York, N.Y., 1965, pp. 33–42.
(15) "Drugs of Choice, 1978–1979," W. Modell, Ed., Mosby, St. Louis, Mo., 1978, pp. 144–148.
(16) E. L. Laden, in "Modern Dermatologic Therapy," T. H. Sternberg and V. D. Newcomer, Eds., McGraw-Hill, New York, N.Y., 1959, pp. 374–377, 386–403.
(17) M. B. Sulzberger and J. Wolf, "Dermatology: Diagnosis and Treatment," 2nd ed., Year Book Medical, Chicago, Ill., 1961, pp. 277–356.
(18) *Ibid.*, pp. 417–453.
(19) B. M. Barker and F. Prescott, "Antimicrobial Agents in Medicine," Blackwell Scientific Publications, London, England, 1973, pp. 18–149.
(20) E. T. Wright, in "Modern Dermatologic Therapy," T. H. Sternberg and V. D. Newcomer, Eds., McGraw-Hill, New York, N.Y., 1959, pp. 404–420.
(21) "The Merck Manual," 12th ed., D. N. Holvey, Ed., Merck, Rahway, N.J., 1972, pp. 33–37.
(22) H. Blank and G. Rake, "Viral and Rickettsial Diseases," Little, Brown, Boston, Mass., 1955, pp. 71–96.
(23) W. Bruinsma, "A Guide to Drug Eruptions," Excerpta Medica, Amsterdam, Netherlands, 1973, pp. 45–48, 87–103.
(24) H. C. W. Stringer, *Drugs*, *6*, 413 (1973).
(25) W. C. Duncan, *Postgrad. Med.*, *52*, 96 (1972).
(26) R. C. V. Robinson, in "Pharmaceutical Therapeutics in Dermatology," M. Waisman, Ed., Charles C Thomas, Springfield, Ill., 1968, pp. 49–64.
(27) "AMA Drug Evaluations," 3rd ed., Publishing Sciences Group, Littleton, Mass., 1977, pp. 821–839.
(28) J. M. Hasegawa, *Postgrad. Med.*, *47*, 239 (1970).
(29) J. W. Wilson, *Arch. Dermatol.*, *92*, 726 (1965).
(30) C. M. Davis, *Postgrad. Med.*, *52*, 109 (1972).
(31) "Drugs of Choice, 1978–1979," W. Modell, Ed., Mosby, St. Louis, Mo., 1978, pp. 698–744.
(32) P. Brisson, *Can. Med. Assoc. J.*, *110*, 1182 (1974).
(33) I. H. Blank, R. D. Griesemer, and E. Gould, *J. Invest. Dermatol.*, *30*, 187 (1958).
(34) F. H. Meyers, E. Jawetz, and A. Goldfien, "Review of Medical Pharmacology," Lange Medical, Los Altos, Calif., 1970, pp. 512–515.
(35) "AMA Drug Evaluations," 3rd ed., Publishing Sciences Group, Littleton, Mass., 1977, pp. 790–797.
(36) "The Pharmacological Basis of Therapeutics," 4th ed., L. S. Goodman and A. Gilman, Eds., Macmillan, New York, N.Y., 1970, pp. 1032–1066.
(37) P. S. Herman and W. M. Sams, Jr., "Soap Photodermatitis," Charles C Thomas, Springfield, Ill., 1972, pp. 17–61.
(38) "AMA Drug Evaluations," 3rd ed., Publishing Sciences Group, Littleton, Mass., 1977, pp. 883–894.
(39) *Federal Register*, *39*, 33102 (1974).
(40) A. A. Fisher, "Contact Dermatitis," 2nd ed., Lea and Febiger, Philadelphia, Pa., 1973, pp. 197–216.
(41) W. R. Markland, *Nord. Briefs*, *465*, 3 (1975).
(42) N. J. Ehrenkranz, D. Taplan, and P. Butt, in "Antimicrobial Agents and Chemotherapy—1966," G. L. Hobby, Ed., American Society for Microbiology, Ann Arbor, Mich., 1966, pp. 255–264.
(43) R. A. Amonette and E. W. Rosenberg, *Arch. Dermatol.*, *107*, 71 (1973).
(44) J. N. Braun and C. O. Solberg, *Br. Med. J.*, *2*, 580 (1973).
(45) R. R. Leonard, *Arch. Dermatol.*, *95*, 520 (1967).
(46) *Federal Register*, *40*, 50527 (1975).
(47) *Federal Register*, *43*, 1210 (1978).
(48) Personal communications, Jan. 1979: W. L. Guess, Chairman, FDA OTC Panel on Topical Antimicrobials II; A. M. Welch, Special Assistant to the Director, Division of OTC Drug Evaluation, FDA; L. Geismar, Chief, Analgesic, Antiperspirant, and Antimicrobial Branch, Division of OTC Drug Evaluations, FDA.
(49) *Federal Register*, *42*, 17642 (1977).

Product (Manufacturer)	Antiseptic	Antifungal Agent	Antibiotic	Other
Achromycin Ointment (Lederle)	—	—	tetracycline hydrochloride, 3%	—
Aftate Antifungal Spray Liquid, Spray Powder, Powder, and Gel (Plough)	—	tolnaftate, 17%	—	—
Alu Wets (Stiefel)	aluminum chloride hexahydrate	—	—	—
Argyrol Stabilized Solution (Smith, Miller & Patch)	silver protein, 10 and 20%	—	—	edetate calcium disodium, 1.1%
Aureomycin Ointment (Lederle)	—	chlortetracycline, 3%	—	—
Baciguent Ointment (Upjohn)	—	—	bacitracin, 500 units/g	—
Bacimycin (Merrell-National)	—	—	bacitracin, 500 units/g neomycin, 3.5 mg/g	petrolatum base
Bactine (Miles)	benzalkonium chloride	—	—	alcohol, 3.17%
Baximin Ointment (Columbia Medical)	—	—	polymyxin B sulfate, 5000 units/g bacitracin, 400 units/g neomycin sulfate, 5 mg/g	—
Betadine Solution, Microbicidal Applicator, Swab Aid, Swab Sticks, Gauze Pads, and Whirlpool Concentrate (Purdue Frederick)	povidone-iodine, 10%	—	—	—
Betadine Surgical Scrub, Surgi-Prep Sponge Brush, and Shampoo (Purdue Frederick)	povidone-iodine, 7.5%	—	—	detergents
B.F.I. Powder (Calgon)	4-pentyloxyphenol	—	—	bismuth formic iodide zinc phenolsulfonate bismuth subgallate aluminum potassium sulfate boric acid eucalyptol menthol thymol
Clorpactin WCS 90 Powder (Guardian)	available chlorine, 3–4%	—	—	—
Clorpactin XCB (Guardian)	available chlorine, 4–4.9%	—	—	—
Cruex Medicated Cream (Pennwalt)	chloroxylenol, 3%	zinc undecylenate, 20%	—	—
Cruex Powder (Pennwalt)	—	calcium undecylenate, 10%	—	—
Cuprex (Beecham)	—	—	—	copper oleate tetrahydronaphthalene
Desenex Liquid (Pennwalt)	—	undecylenic acid, 16%	—	alcohol, 40%
Desenex Powder and Ointment (Pennwalt)	—	zinc undecylenate, 20% undecylenic acid, 5% (ointment) 2% (powder)	—	—
Drest (Dermik)	alkylisoquinolinium bromide, 0.15% benzalkonium chloride, 0.125%	—	—	alcohol, 14.1% protein greaseless gel povidone
Epi-Clear Antiseptic Lotion (Squibb)	benzoyl peroxide, 5 and 10%	—	—	—

Product (Manufacturer)	Antiseptic	Antifungal Agent	Antibiotic	Other
Ergophene (Upjohn)	phenol, 7.5 gr	—	—	sodium borate, 1.66 gr fluidextract ergot, 45 minims zinc oxide, 22.5 gr
Isodine Antiseptic Skin Cleanser (Blair)	povidone-iodine, 7.5%	—	—	—
Isodine Antiseptic Solution and Ointment (Blair)	povidone-iodine, 10%	—	—	—
Lubraseptic Jelly (Guardian)	*o*-phenylphenol, 0.1% *p-tert*-pentylphenol, 0.02% phenylmercuric nitrate, 0.007%	—	—	—
Mercresin (Upjohn)	secondary amytricresols	—	—	*o*-hydroxyphenyl-mercuric chloride acetone alcohol
Merlenate Ointment (North American)	phenylmercuric nitrate, 1.15%	undecylenic acid, 5%	—	—
Myciguent Cream and Ointment (Upjohn)	—	—	neomycin sulfate, 5 mg/g	—
Mycitracin (Upjohn)	—	—	polymyxin B sulfate, 5000 units/g bacitracin, 500 units/g neomycin sulfate, 5 mg/g	—
Neo-Polycin Ointment (Dow)	—	—	polymyxin B sulfate, 5000 units/g bacitracin zinc, 400 units/g neomycin (as sulfate), 3.5 mg/g	fuzene base polyethylene glycol dilaurate polyethylene glycol distearate light liquid petrolatum synthetic glyceride wax white petrolatum
Neosporin Ointment (Burroughs Wellcome)	—	—	polymyxin B sulfate, 5000 units/g bacitracin zinc, 400 units/g neomycin sulfate, 5 mg/g	white petrolatum
Obtundia (Otis Clapp)	cresol–camphor complex	—	—	—
Ova Nite (Milroy)	benzalkonium chloride, 0.02%	—	—	nonionic surfactant edetate disodium, 0.25%
Polysporin Ointment (Burroughs Wellcome)	—	—	polymyxin B sulfate, 10,000 units/g bacitracin zinc, 500 units/g	white petrolatum
Prophyllin (Rystan)	—	sodium propionate, 1% (solution) 5% (ointment)	—	chlorophyll, 0.0025% (solution) 0.0125% (ointment)
Quin III (Pfeiffer)	iodochlorhydroxyquin, 3%	—	—	—
Quinalor Compound Ointment (Squibb)	halquinols, 0.5% benzoyl peroxide, 10%	—	—	methyl salicylate polyethylene glycol mineral oil eugenol menthol
Rid-A-Pain (Pfeiffer)	chloroxylenol	—	—	alcohol, 50% benzocaine, 3%

Product (Manufacturer)	Antiseptic	Antifungal Agent	Antibiotic	Other
Sea Breeze (Sea Breeze)	—	benzoic acid	—	alcohol, 43% peppermint oil clove oil eucalyptus oil eugenol boric acid camphor
SeptoDyne Solution (Winthrop)	poloxamer-iodine	—	—	—
SeptoDyne Surgical Scrub (Winthrop)	poloxamer-iodine	—	—	detergents
Spectrocin Ointment (Squibb)	—	—	neomycin, 2.5 mg/g gramicidin, 0.25 mg/g	polyethylene glycol mineral oil
Sperti Ointment (Whitehall)	phenylmercuric nitrate, 1:10,000	—	—	shark liver oil, 3% yeast cell derivative, 67 units skin respiratory factor/g
S.T. 37 (Beecham)	hexylresorcinol	—	—	glycerin
Terramycin Ointment with Polymyxin B Sulfate (Pfipharmecs)	—	—	oxytetracycline hydrochloride, 30 mg/g polymyxin B sulfate, 10,000 units/g	—
Triple Antibiotic Ointment (North American)	—	—	polymyxin B sulfate, 5000 units/g bacitracin, 400 units/g neomycin sulfate, 5 mg/g	—
Vaseline First Aid Carbolated Petroleum Jelly (Chesebrough-Pond)	chloroxylenol, 0.5%	—	—	petroleum jelly lanolin phenol, 0.2%
Vioform Ointment and Cream (Ciba)	iodochlorhydroxyquin, 3%	—	—	petrolatum base (ointment) water-washable base (cream)
Zea Sorb Powder (Stiefel)	chloroxylenol, 0.5%	—	—	microporous cellulose, 45% aluminum dihydroxyallantoinate, 0.2%
Zemo Soap (Plough)	triclocarban	—	—	—
Zephiran Chloride Solution and Spray (Winthrop)	benzalkonium chloride, 0.13%	—	—	—
Zephiran Towelettes (Winthrop)	benzalkonium chloride chlorothymol	—	—	alcohol, 20% perfume

Acne Products

Raymond E. Hopponen

Chapter 27

Questions to Ask the Patient

How old are you?

How long have you had acne?

Are the blemishes hot, red, swollen, or painful?

Are the blemishes only whiteheads and blackheads or are there also closed cysts under the skin?

Does the problem seem to be localized to areas of external irritation, e.g., where clothes rub?

What types of cosmetics and/or hair preparations do you use?

What types of medications are you currently using?

What treatments have you used? How effective were they?

Are you now or have you been under a physician's care for this condition?

Acne vulgaris is a chronic skin condition characterized mainly by comedones (whiteheads and blackheads). In severe cases, inflammation, pustules, cysts, and scarring may occur. Acne occurs most commonly on the face, back, and chest. Although it does not pose a severe physical threat, it should not be ignored, since it may cause a great deal of emotional stress and anguish. Acne occurs most often in adolescence, a period in which many physiological, social, and psychological adjustments are made and when personal appearance and peer acceptance are important. Acne may occur in older persons as well.

Studies of the incidence of acne in adolescents indicate that it is nearly universal in this group. A study of 1555 young people 8–18 years of age found 100% recognizable acne at the ages of maximum incidence—14 years for girls and 16 years for boys (1). Moreover, 50% of the girls and 78% of the boys had acne severe enough to be termed clinical. Subclinical lesions were noted in about one-third of the 8- to 9-year-old group. Another study found that only 10–11% of a studied group of high school students had sought medical help for acne, but about 60% were self-medicating (2).

The widespread incidence of acne in adolescence, its remissions and recurrences, and its variability in response to treatment have prompted many theories implicating personal habits, diet, personality, and physiology as contributing factors. The role of diet, however, remains controversial (3). For example, although several studies demonstrated that chocolate does not affect acne (4), some clinicians remain unconvinced and suggest that it be removed from the diet. No convincing evidence has been presented to implicate nuts, fats, colas, or carbohydrates, and many clinicians feel that dietary restrictions for individuals with acne are unwarranted. Iodides and bromides are secreted in the sweat and may cause acne-like eruptions when they are ingested in substantial amounts as in therapeutic agents containing these ions. The amount of iodine in seafoods or iodized salt is not significant.

ETIOLOGY

Acne vulgaris commences in the pilosebaceous units in the dermis (Figure 1). These units, consisting of a hair follicle and the associated sebaceous glands, are connected to the skin surface by a duct (the infundibulum) through which the hair shaft passes. On the smooth skin of the body the hair may be very fine or entirely absent. Because the sebaceous glands are most common on the face, back, and chest, acne tends to occur most often in these areas. The sebaceous glands produce sebum, a mixture of fats and waxes, which serves to maintain proper hydration of skin and hair. The sebum passes to the skin surface via the infundibulum and then spreads over the surface to retard water loss.

Noninflammatory Acne

The cause of acne is increased activity of the sebaceous glands and of the epithelial tissue lining the infundibulum. This increase is induced by the greater production of hormones, especially androgenic hormones, as puberty approaches. The glands produce more sebum, causing increased skin oiliness. The epithelial tissue, an extension of the surface epidermis, forms the lining of the infundibulum and becomes thinner as it extends into the deeper portions of the duct. Normally, it continually sheds cells which are carried to the skin surface by the flow of sebum. In acne, however, the shed epithelial cells are more distinct and durable, sticking together to form a coherent horny layer that blocks the follicular channel (5). This impaction plugs and distends the follicle to form a microcomedo.

As more cells and sebum are added, the comedo becomes visible (whitehead) and is called a "closed"

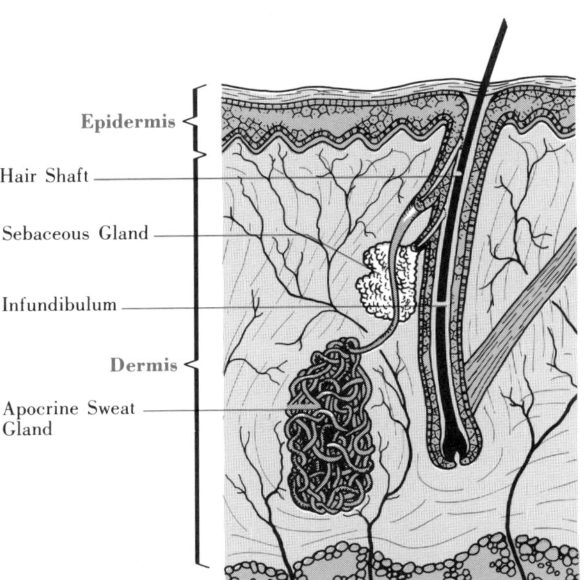

Figure 1. Normal pilosebaceous unit.

characteristics of inflammatory and noninflammatory acne development

relationship between acne and menstrual cycle

comedo; i.e., its contents do not reach the surface of the skin (Figure 2). It is not expressed easily with a comedo extractor and may need to be lanced with a surgical blade before the plug can be extruded. If the plug enlarges and protrudes from the orifice of the follicular canal, it is called an "open" comedo; i.e., its contents are open to the surface. The tip of the plug may darken (blackhead) because of the accumulation of melanin produced by the epithelial cells lining the infundibulum (6). Open comedones may be expressed easily with a comedo extractor. Although sebum still is produced, the sebaceous glands tend to shrink during comedo formation. Acne characterized by the presence of closed and open comedones is called "noninflammatory" acne.

The hair in the follicles may play an important role in the development of comedones. If it is thin and small, it may not be able to maintain an open channel, and it then becomes entrapped in the plug. The heavier hair of the scalp and beard may push the developing plug to the surface, thus preventing comedo formation.

Inflammatory Acne

"Inflammatory" acne is characterized by inflammation (surrounding the comedones), papules, pustules, and nodulocystic lesions. It is more likely to cause permanent scarring than noninflammatory acne. Inflammatory acne typically begins in closed comedones, rarely in open comedones. As the microcomedo develops, it distends the follicle, so that the walls become thin. At this stage a primary inflammation of the follicle wall may develop with disruption of the epithelial lining and lymphocyte infiltration into and around the follicular wall (7). The process may stop with healing of the lesion in 7–10 days.

However, if the follicle wall ruptures and the contents are discharged into the surrounding tissue, a more severe inflammatory reaction results. The epithelial cells, the sebum, and any microorganisms present all represent foreign substances capable of eliciting an inflammatory reaction. The result is an abscess, which in the process of healing may cause scars or pits to form. Fingering or picking at inflamed follicles or attempting to express closed comedones may produce inflammatory lesions by rupturing the follicle wall.

Current theories explaining the development of inflammatory acne suggest that the initial inflammation of the follicle wall results from the presence of free fatty acids derived from the sebum (7). Normal sebum does not contain free fatty acids and is nonirritating. However, in the presence of lipolytic enzymes, triglycerides of the sebum are split, releasing the fatty acids. The normal bacterial flora of the sebaceous duct are the source of the enzymes responsible for splitting the triglycerides.

The main microorganisms found in the sebaceous duct are an anaerobic rod, *Corynebacterium acnes*, and one or two species of cocci. These organisms are the predominant flora that normally inhabit the skin. They are not considered pathogens and rapidly die off if the follicle wall is ruptured and they are released into the surrounding tissues. *C. acnes* generally is regarded to be the source of the lipolytic enzymes responsible for free fatty acid formation in the sebum. The effectiveness of oral tetracycline in treating inflammatory acne is due to its ability to suppress the normal bacterial population of the sebaceous duct and so reduce the concentration of free fatty acids (8).

The presence of pustules or cysts indicates inflammatory acne, a type that should be treated by a physician. Treatment requires prescribed medication and possibly excision and drainage of lesions. Because of the danger of permanent scarring in this type of acne, medical help should be sought.

Aggravating Factors

Many women with acne experience a flare-up of symptoms during the premenstrual part of their cycle. The flareup cannot be explained on the basis of hormone levels alone, although the change in the progesterone level has been implicated. Changes in sebaceous activity also have been claimed to be responsible. It was suggested that the premenstrual flareup, which occurred in 60–70% of women with acne, is caused by a reduction in the size of the orifice of the pilosebaceous duct (9). Measurements of orifice diameters during the complete cycle showed that the size was markedly reduced during the premenstrual phase.

Hydration also decreases the size of the pilosebaceous duct orifice, a change that is reversible (10). This reduction explains the exacerbation of acne in high humidity or in conditions where frequent and prolonged sweating occurs.

Local irritation or friction may increase the incidence of acne symptoms. Rough or occlusive clothing, headgear straps, and pieces of equipment used in athletics often aggravate acne. Resting the chin or cheek on

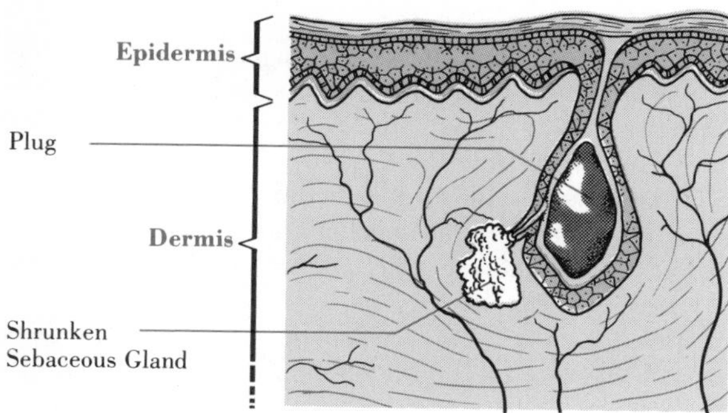

Figure 2. Closed comedo.

the hand frequently for long periods creates localized conditions conducive to pustule formation in acne-prone individuals.

"Acne cosmetica," a condition resembling noninflammatory acne vulgaris, was found in about one-third of adult women who were examined, but not in adult men (11). The lesions of acne cosmetica are typically closed, noninflammatory comedones and cannot be distinguished from similar lesions of acne vulgaris. The condition was attributed to cosmetics because a comparable condition was not noted in men. Furthermore, half the cosmetic cream bases used by these women were comedogenic in rabbit ear tests and on the skin of human volunteers. The condition responded readily to treatment with tretinoin.

TREATMENT

Acne cannot be cured. In most cases, however, with currently available therapeutic regimens, symptoms may be reduced, and permanent scarring minimized. Because acne persists for long periods, frequently from adolescence to the early twenties, treatment must be long-term. Periods of remission or reduction in severity of lesions may occur, especially in summer, but treatment should be resumed when necessary.

Treatment of acne with OTC products involves removing excess sebum from the skin, preventing closure of the pilosebaceous orifice, minimizing conditions conducive to acne, and avoiding covering lesions with cosmetics. Controlling inflammation and infection, suppressing or altering hormonal activity, and correcting destructive effects should be left to a physician (12).

Removal of Excess Sebum

The preferred method for removing excess sebum from the skin is a conscientious program of daily washing. The affected areas should be washed thoroughly three times per day with warm water, soap, and a soft washcloth. Scrubbing should be gentle to avoid damage and should be done for several minutes to work the lather thoroughly into the skin. The purpose of the washing is to produce a mild drying of the skin and, perhaps, mild erythema (3). Washing causes barely visible peeling which can loosen comedones. If washing produces a feeling of tautness in the skin, the intensity and frequency of washings should be reduced.

Ordinary facial soaps usually produce satisfactory results. Soaps containing antibacterial agents have been suggested for use in controlling acne, but no conclusive evidence has been presented to indicate their value over nonmedicated soap. There is little rationale for using soaps that contain sulfur, salicylic acid, or resorcinol. If the affected area is rinsed properly, these added medications are washed away. Soap substitutes that contain surfactants (ionic or nonionic) have been suggested for use in acne because they are less drying to the skin. However, because a mild degree of drying is desirable, an ordinary facial soap should be tried first. Some cleansing preparations contain pumice, polyethylene, or aluminum oxide particles to add abrasive action to the cleansing effect. However, these products are more expensive than soap, and it is doubtful whether they are more advantageous than soap and a soft washcloth. If it is inconvenient to wash during the day, a cleansing pad that contains alcohol, acetone, and a surfactant may be used.

role of cosmetics in acne

treatment objectives—reducing symptoms and minimizing scarring

Because acne treatment is aimed at removing excess sebum from the skin, other topically applied fats and oils should be eliminated, e.g., cosmetics that contain fats. Hair dressings in excessive amounts should be avoided; those used should contain a minimum of oil. "Pomade acne," manifested by comedones on the forehead and temples, was reported to be caused directly by the long-term use of hair dressings that contain petrolatum or liquid petrolatum (13). Frequent hair shampooing should be encouraged because acne is usually accompanied by an oily scalp.

Preventing Pilosebaceous Closure

Topical agents that cause irritation and desquamation are used to prevent closure of the pilosebaceous orifice. The irritant effect of these peeling agents causes an increased turnover rate of the epithelial cells lining the follicular duct (3). Peeling agents also cause keratolysis, which reduces the cohesiveness of the follicular lining. The net effect is to reduce the tendency to form new comedones and to loosen the structure of formed comedones and aid in their extrusion.

Ingredients in OTC Products

The mildest agents—the ones usually tried first—are sulfur, resorcinol, and salicylic acid.

Sulfur

Sulfur generally is used in the precipitated or colloidal form at 2–10% concentrations. The higher concentrations produce a more intense effect. Other forms of sulfur such as zinc sulfide and sodium thiosulfate are milder in action. Some evidence suggests that although sulfur does help to resolve comedones, it also may promote the development of new ones (14). Sulfur (but not thiosulfate or sulfide) was comedogenic in rabbit ear tests and, on long exposure, on the backs of human subjects (14), although recent evidence refutes this observation (15). Sulfur generally is accepted as being an effective agent for promoting the resolution of acne lesions, and its overall effect is one of improving the condition.

Resorcinol and Salicylic Acid

Resorcinol usually is used in concentrations of 1–4%. Resorcinol monoacetate is milder in action and may be used at higher concentrations. Resorcinol may produce a dark brown scale on some darker-skinned individuals, and they should be forewarned (15). The reaction is reversible when the medication is discontinued.

Salicylic acid is used in 0.5–2% concentrations. A combination of resorcinol and salicylic acid in an alcoholic solution is advantageous because it dries quickly and does not leave a visible film. Resorcinol and salicylic acid often are added to sulfur-containing preparations to increase activity.

components of acne products

mechanisms and effectiveness

antibiotics in acne treatment

tretinoin and zinc

Benzoyl Peroxide

Benzoyl peroxide is a primary irritant that increases epithelial cell growth rate, leading to an increased sloughing rate. This increase results in a looser structure of the follicular plug and promotes resolution of comedones (17). Benzoyl peroxide is used in concentrations of 5–10% (the lower concentration is suggested at the beginning of treatment). It is applied at night after the affected area is washed with soap and water. Fair-skinned individuals may find it advantageous to leave it on for only 2 hours at a time until the skin becomes conditioned to the treatment.

Benzoyl peroxide produces a feeling of warmth, slight stinging, and reddening of the skin. If the stinging or burning is excessive after an application, the preparation should be removed with soap and water and not reapplied until the next day. Because benzoyl peroxide is highly irritating, it should be kept away from the eyelids, lips, and neck. Other sources of irritation, such as sun lamps, should be discontinued, and it may be necessary to reduce the vigor and frequency of washing. Benzoyl peroxide is an oxidizing agent and may bleach colored fabrics, so care should be used to avoid spillage onto clothing. Its potential explosiveness has been eliminated in commercial preparations by combining it in a 35:65 ratio with dicalcium phosphate.

Antibacterials

It should be remembered that acne is not an infection. The inflammation found in some cases is the result of a foreign body reaction to follicular contents. The only microorganisms involved are the nonpathogenic normal flora found deep within the follicles out of the reach of the usual antibacterial agents applied to the skin surface. Therefore it is not surprising that topically applied antibacterial agents generally have not been found valuable in treating acne. Exceptions to this statement, however, have been noted in the case of fat-soluble derivatives of erythromycin, tetracycline, and clindamycin (18, 19). These derivatives, applied as dilute solutions in organic solvents, presumably are effective because of their ability to diffuse through the fatty contents of the sebaceous follicle to reach the *C. acnes* located in the lower segments of the follicle. There they suppress the activity of these organisms and so reduce the production of comedogenic free fatty acids from the sebum.

Oral tetracycline, which requires a prescription, is effective in treating inflammatory acne. It has been recognized by an ad hoc study committee of the American Academy of Dermatology as a rational, effective, and relatively safe drug for use in this condition (20). It is not effective for the resolution of noninflammatory comedones.

Other Treatments

Tretinoin (vitamin A acid), a prescription drug, is a topical medication proven effective in treating acne characterized primarily by the presence of comedones. Like benzoyl peroxide, tretinoin acts by its irritant effect to increase epithelial cell proliferation.

Exposure to sunlight often is beneficial in acne, and consequently, improvement often is noted during the summer. The improvement is believed to result from the irritant properties of the ultraviolet wavelengths of sunlight, which stimulate increased proliferation of the epithelium. Ultraviolet lamps produce the same effect, but they generally are not recommended because of the difficulty in determining and regulating the amount of limited exposure necessary to produce the required mild erythema. If a sunlamp is used, care must be taken to protect the eyes adequately from the light's damaging effect. It also may be wise to have a second person time the exposure to avoid the danger of falling asleep under the lamp.

An interesting development in acne treatment has been the observation that the oral administration of zinc sulfate may result in significant improvement (21). The postulation is that zinc is necessary for maintaining proper levels in the body of retinol-binding protein, a vitamin A transport protein, which carries vitamin A from the liver to target tissues. Acne victims showed lowered serum levels of the protein and zinc (22). However, in a double-blind controlled clinical trial, no statistically significant differences were noted between a zinc-treated (411 mg/day) and placebo group of patients (23).

Treatments that have been abandoned as not being effective include oral vitamin A, laxatives, bacterial vaccines, and digestive aids such as pancreatin, pepsin, bile salts, and acidophilus bacterial cultures.

Secondary Formulation Factors

Suspensions, lotions, creams, and gels are the vehicles generally used to carry antiacne medications to the skin. Lotions and creams should have a low fat content so that they do not counteract drying and peeling. Ethyl or isopropyl alcohol added to liquid preparations and gels hastens their drying to a film. On the other hand, nonfatty gels, in particular, are slow drying if formulated in a completely aqueous base.

Thickening agents in preparations should not dry to a sticky film. The solids of most preparations leave a film that is not noticeably visible and does not need coloring to blend with the skin. Some products, however, are intended to hide blemishes by depositing an opaque film of insoluble masking agents such as zinc oxide on the skin. These products need tinting to improve their cosmetic effect.

PRODUCT SELECTION GUIDELINES

Only noninflammatory acne should be self-medicated. Individuals exhibiting characteristics of inflammatory acne should be referred to a physician. The pharmacist should examine the patient's medication history, including previous measures taken to control the acne, which medications were used, when, and for how long, and the degree of success and personal acceptance of the preparation tried. Subjective data on a person's attitude toward treatment and willingness to participate actively in a skin care program should be determined to assist the pharmacist in deciding what treatment course to recommend.

The success of a program to control acne depends on patient willingness to devote the time and effort required to carry out a continued daily regimen of washing the affected areas and applying medication. A clear explanation of the acne process should be given, and misconceptions should be corrected. The pharmacist should advise on scalp and hair care, the use of cosmetics, and, above all, the need for long-term, conscientious care. Positive moral support is sometimes necessary to reduce patient concern.

Claims made for OTC products for acne relief must be studied carefully for their accuracy. Various creams, lotions, antiseptics, and skin peels are available, and formulas should be examined carefully before a value judgment is made.

If a medication previously has not been used consistently, one of the milder peeling agents should be recommended. Resorcinol, salicylic acid, or sulfur preparations should be suggested first. These preparations along with conscientious washing with soap, water, and a washcloth may control the acne in many cases. If a milder agent was tried conscientiously without success, benzoyl peroxide should be tried. However, the cautions on its very irritating properties should be observed. Cases of acne that continue to be resistant to control should be referred to a physician.

SUMMARY

Acne vulgaris occurs almost universally in young adults from early teens to middle twenties and occasionally appears in older people. Acne generally is not amenable to a cure, but it may be controlled to improve appearance and to prevent the development of severe acne and its resultant scarring. With sympathy, understanding, and reassurance, acne sufferers may be made to understand that the condition is not irreparable and that care must be given to the affected areas for a long time for improvement to occur.

REFERENCES

(1) J. L. Burton, W. J. Cunliffe, I. Stafford, and S. Shuster, *Br. J. Dermatol.*, *85*, 119 (1971).
(2) R. J. Schachter, E. S. Pantel, G. M. Glassman, and I. Zweibelson, *N. Y. State J. Med.*, *71*, 2886 (1971).
(3) R. M. Reisner, *Pediatr. Clin. North Am.*, *20*, 851 (1973).
(4) J. E. Fulton, G. Plewig, and A. M. Kligman, *J. Am. Med. Assoc.*, *210*, 2071 (1969).
(5) A. M. Kligman, *J. Invest. Dermatol.*, *62*, 268 (1974).
(6) D. Blair and C. A. Lewis, *Br. J. Dermatol.*, *82*, 572 (1970).
(7) R. K. Freinkel, *N. Engl. J. Med.*, *280*, 1161 (1969).
(8) R. K. Freinkel, J. S. Strauss, S. Y. Yip, and P. E. Pochi, *N. Engl. J. Med.*, *273*, 8350 (1965).
(9) W. J. Cunliffe and M. Williams, *Lancet*, *2*, 1055 (1973).
(10) M. Williams, W. J. Cunliffe, and D. Gould, *Br. J. Dermatol.*, *90*, 631 (1974).
(11) A. M. Kligman and O. H. Mills, *Arch. Dermatol.*, *106*, 843 (1972).
(12) S. B. Frank, "Acne Vulgaris," Charles C Thomas, Springfield, Ill., 1971, p. 175.
(13) G. Plewig, J. E. Fulton, and A. M. Kligman, *Arch. Dermatol.*, *101*, 580 (1970).
(14) O. H. Mills and A. M. Kligman, *Br. J. Dermatol.*, *86*, 620 (1972).
(15) J. S. Strauss, P. H. Goldman, S. Nacht, and E. H. Gans, *Arch. Dermatol.*, *114*, 1340 (1978).
(16) S. B. Frank, "Acne Vulgaris," Charles C Thomas, Springfield, Ill., 1971, p. 184.
(17) P. Vasarenish, *Arch. Dermatol.*, *98*, 183 (1968).
(18) J. E. Fulton, *Arch. Dermatol.*, *110*, 83 (1974).
(19) S. B. Frank, *Postgrad. Med.*, *61*, 92 (1977).
(20) Ad Hoc Committee on the Use of Antibiotics in Dermatology, *Arch. Dermatol.*, *111*, 1630 (1975).
(21) G. Michaelsson, L. Juklin, and A. Vahlquist, *Arch. Dermatol.*, *113*, 31 (1977).
(22) G. Michaelsson, A. Vahlquist, and L. Juklin, *Br. J. Dermatol.*, *96*, 283 (1977).
(23) L. Orris, A. R. Shalita, D. Sibulkin, S. J. London, and E. H. Gans, *Arch. Dermatol.*, *114*, 1018 (1978).

Product (Manufacturer)	Application Form	Sulfur	Resorcinol/ Salicylic Acid	Other
Acnaveen (Cooper)	bar	2%	salicylic acid, 2%	colloidal oatmeal, 50%
Acne-Aid (Stiefel)	cream lotion	2.5% (cream) 10% (lotion)	resorcinol, 1.25% (cream)	alcohol, 10% (lotion) chloroxylenol, 0.375% (cream)
Acne-Aid Detergent Soap (Stiefel)	cleanser	—	—	sulfated surfactants hydrocarbon hydrotropes, 6.3%
Acnesarb (C&M)	solution	—	salicylic acid, 3%	isopropyl alcohol, 63% boric acid, 2% methylbenzethonium chloride, 0.08%
Acnomel (Smith Kline & French)	cream cleanser	8% (cream) 4% (cleanser)	resorcinol, 2% (cream) 1% (cleanser)	—
Acnotex (C&M)	lotion	8%	salicylic acid, 2.25%	methylbenzethonium chloride, 0.08% propylene glycol powder base acetone isopropyl alcohol, 22% perfume
Acnycin (Columbia Medical)	cream	5%	resorcinol, 2%	zinc oxide
Benoxyl (Stiefel)	lotion	—	—	benzoyl peroxide, 5 and 10%
Bensulfoid (Poythress)	lotion	colloidal, 2%	resorcinol, 2%	alcohol, 12% zinc oxide, 6% thymol, 0.5% hexachlorophene, 0.1% perfume
Betadine Skin Cleanser (Purdue Frederick)	cleanser	—	—	povidone-iodine, 7.5% detergents
Brasivol (Stiefel)	cleanser	—	—	aluminum oxide neutral soap detergents (fine, medium, rough)
Cenac (Central)	lotion	colloidal, 8%	resorcinol, 2%	isopropyl alcohol, 30%
Clear and Easy (Thompson)	sponge	—	—	triclocarban, 1% soapless detergent
Clearasil Antibacterial Acne Lotion (Vicks)	lotion	—	—	benzoyl peroxide, 5%
Clearasil Medicated Cleanser (Vicks)	cleanser	—	salicylic acid, 0.25%	alcohol, 43% allantoin, 0.1%
Clearasil Regular, Tinted, and Stick (Vicks)	cream stick	8%	resorcinol, 2% (cream) 1% (stick)	bentonite, 11.5% (cream) 4% (stick) alcohol, 10% (cream)
Clearasil Vanishing Formula (Vicks)	cream	3%	resorcinol, 2%	bentonite, 10% alcohol, 10%
Contrablem (Texas Pharmacal)	gel	5%	resorcinol, 2%	alcohol, 9.5%
Cuticura (Purex)	ointment	precipitated	—	8-hydroxyquinoline petrolatum mineral oil mineral wax isopropyl palmitate synthetic beeswax phenol pine oil rose geranium oil
Cuticura Acne Cream (Purex)	cream	—	—	benzoyl peroxide, 5% alcohol, 1%

Product (Manufacturer)	Application Form	Sulfur	Resorcinol/ Salicylic Acid	Other
Cuticura Medicated Soap (Purex)	soap	not stated	—	triclocarban, 1% oxyquinoline soap base
Dry and Clear Acne Cream (Whitehall)	cream	2%	salicylic acid	benzoyl peroxide, 10% benzethonium chloride
Dry and Clear Acne Medication (Whitehall)	lotion	—	salicylic acid	benzoyl peroxide, 5% benzethonium chloride
Dry and Clear Cleanser (Whitehall)	liquid	—	salicylic acid	benzethonium chloride benzoic acid alcohol, 50%
Drytergent (C&M)	cleanser	—	—	lecinol alkyl-aryl surfactant
Drytex (C&M)	lotion	—	salicylic acid	alcohol, 40% methylbenzethonium chloride acetone polysorbate 20 fragrance
Epi-Clear (Squibb)	lotion	10%	—	alcohol, 10% benzoyl peroxide, 10%
Epi-Clear Scrub Cleanser (Squibb)	cleanser	—	—	aluminum oxide, 38% (fine) 52% (medium) 65% (coarse)
Epi-Clear Soap for Oily Skin (Squibb)	cleanser	—	—	sulfated surfactants, 6.3% hydrocarbon hydrotropes
Finac (C&M)	lotion	2%	—	methylbenzethonium chloride, 0.08% powder base isopropyl alcohol, 8% perfume
Fostex (Westwood)	cream cleanser soap	2%	salicylic acid, 2%	—
Fostril (Westwood)	lotion	2%	—	laureth-4 zinc oxide talc
Ionax Foam (Owen)	aerosol foam	—	—	benzalkonium chloride, 0.2% polyoxyethylene ethers soapless surfactant
Ionax Scrub (Owen)	paste	—	—	benzalkonium chloride, 0.2% granular polyethylene polyoxyethylene ethers alcohol, 10%
Klaron (Dermik)	lotion	colloidal, 5%	salicylic acid, 2%	alcohol, 13.1%
Komed (Barnes-Hind)	lotion	—	resorcinol, 2% salicylic acid, 2%	isopropyl alcohol, 22% sodium thiosulfate, 8% menthol camphor colloidal alumina
Komex (Barnes-Hind)	cleanser	—	—	sodium tetrahydrate decahydrate granules
Liquimat (Texas Pharmacal)	lotion	5%	—	alcohol, 22% tinted bases

Product (Manufacturer)	Application Form	Sulfur	Resorcinol/ Salicylic Acid	Other
Listerex Golden Lotion (Warner-Lambert)	cleanser	—	salicylic acid, 2%	thymol, 0.16% polyethylene granules surface-active cleansers menthol eucalyptol
Listerex Herbal Lotion (Warner-Lambert)	cleanser	—	salicylic acid, 2%	polyethylene granules surface-active cleansers
Loroxide (Dermik)	lotion	—	—	chlorhydroxyquinoline, 0.25% benzoyl peroxide, 5.5%
Lotio Alsulfa (Doak)	lotion	colloidal, 5%	—	colloidal clays, 95%
Lotioblanc (Arnar-Stone)	lotion	—	—	zinc sulfate sulfurated potash
Lowila (Westwood)	soap	—	—	nonmedicated
Medicated Face Conditioner (MFC) (Mennen)	liquid	—	salicylic acid, 1%	alcohol, 55%
Microsyn (Syntex)	lotion	—	resorcinol, 2% salicylic acid, 2%	sodium thiosulfate, 8% colloidal alumina menthol camphor
Multiscrub (Bristol-Myers)	cream	2%	salicylic acid, 1.5%	soapless detergents polyethylene resin granules, 26%
Noxzema Antiseptic Skin Cleanser (Noxell)	cleanser	—	—	alcohol, 65% aluminum chlorhydroxy allantoinate
Oxy-5 (Norcliff Thayer)	lotion	—	—	benzoyl peroxide, 5%
Oxy-10 (Norcliff Thayer)	lotion	—	—	benzoyl peroxide, 10%
Pernox Lotion (Westwood)	lotion	2%	salicylic acid, 1.5%	surfactants polyethylene granules
Pernox Regular and Lemon (Westwood)	cleanser	2%	salicylic acid, 1.5%	surfactants polyethylene granules
Persadox (Texas Pharmacal)	lotion cream	—	—	benzoyl peroxide, 5%
Persadox HP (Texas Pharmacal)	cream lotion	—	—	benzoyl peroxide, 10%
pHisoAc (Winthrop)	cream	colloidal, 6%	resorcinol, 1.5%	alcohol, 10%
pHisoDerm (Winthrop)	cleanser	—	—	entsufon sodium petrolatum lanolin
piSec (Owen)	cream	3.14%	—	benzalkonium chloride, 0.2% polyoxyethylene ether
Postacne (Dermik)	lotion	microsize, 2%	—	alcohol, 29%
Quinalor Compound (Squibb)	ointment	—	—	benzoyl peroxide, 10% halquinols, 0.5% menthol methyl salicylate polyethylene glycol mineral oil eugenol
Resulin (Schieffelin)	lotion half-strength lotion	8%	resorcinol, 4%	alcohol, 32%
Rezamid (Dermik)	lotion	microsize, 5%	resorcinol, 2%	alcohol, 28.5% chloroxylenol, 0.5%
Saligel (Stiefel)	gel	—	salicylic acid, 5%	hydroalcoholic gel
Sastid Al (Stiefel)	cleanser	1.6%	salicylic acid, 1.6%	aluminum oxide surfactants

Product (Manufacturer)	Application Form	Sulfur	Resorcinol/ Salicylic Acid	Other
Sastid Plain (Stiefel)	cleanser	1.6%	salicylic acid, 1.6%	soapless surfactants
Sastid Soap (Stiefel)	cleanser	10%	salicylic acid, 3%	—
Seale's Lotion (C&M)	lotion	6.4%	—	sodium borate zinc oxide acetone bentonite
Seba-Nil (Texas Pharmacal)	solution	—	—	alcohol, 49.7% polysorbate 80
Seba-Nil Cleansing Mask (Texas Pharmacal)	cleanser	—	—	polyethylene granules
Spectro-Jel (Recsei)	gel	—	—	isopropyl alcohol, 15% methylcellulose, 1.5% glycol–polysiloxane, 1% cetylpyridinium chloride, 0.1%
Stri-Dex Medicated Pads (Lehn & Fink)	medicated pads	—	salicylic acid, 0.5%	sulfonated alkylbenzenes citric acid alcohol
Sulfoil (C&M)	cleanser	not stated	—	sulfonated castor oil propylene glycol
Sulforcin (Texas Pharmacal)	lotion	5%	resorcinol, 2%	alcohol, 11.65%
Sulfur Soap (Stiefel)	cleanser	precipitated, 10%	—	—
Teenac (Elder)	gel	1.5%	—	mercuric sulfide, 0.5% urea
Therac (C&M)	lotion	colloidal, 4%	salicylic acid, 2.35%	bentonite perfume
Therapads (Parke-Davis)	pads	—	salicylic acid, 1.5%	alcohol, 50%
Therapads Plus (Parke-Davis)	individual wipes	—	salicylic acid, 1.5%	alcohol, 70% sodium alkyl aryl polyether sulfonate, 0.1%
Thylox Medicated Soap (Dent)	cleanser	magnetic, 8.8%	—	—
Topex (Vicks)	lotion	—	—	benzoyl peroxide, 10%
Transact (Westwood)	gel	2%	—	laureth 4, 6% alcohol, 40%
Tyrosum Packets (Summers)	cleanser	—	—	alcohol acetone polysorbate
Vanoxide (Dermik)	lotion	—	—	benzoyl peroxide, 5% chlorhydroxyquinoline, 0.25%
Xerac (Person & Covey)	gel	4%	—	isopropyl alcohol, 44%
Zinc Sulfide Compound Lotion (Upjohn)	lotion	22 gr	—	zinc, 12.3 gr boric acid sodium borate aluminum hydroxide

Dry Skin, Dandruff, Seborrhea, Psoriasis, and Eczema Products

Joseph R. Robinson

Chapter 28

Questions to Ask the Patient

How long have you had this condition?

Which area of the skin is affected? Is the condition patchy or uniformly distributed?

Is the condition stable or does it fluctuate greatly? Can you relate the fluctuation to a cause?

Is your skin exposed to detergents or chemicals? At home, at work? What types of cosmetics do you use?

Is there a family history of skin disease, asthma, or hay fever?

Have you consulted a dermatologist? What was recommended?

What treatments have you used? How effective were they?

Considering the extent of exposure of the skin to a wide variety of chemicals and environmental insults, it demonstrates remarkable resiliency and recuperative ability. (See Chapter 26 for a complete discussion of the anatomy and physiology of the skin.) Cosmetic and OTC drug advertisements have been able to create the impression that many normal physiological processes are in fact abnormal or at least undesirable. There are, of course, metabolic, bacterial, fungal, viral, and other skin abnormalities that should be treated with drugs. Conditions such as dry skin, dandruff, seborrhea, psoriasis, and eczema must be considered from both the cosmetic and the pathological points of view so that the pharmacist can advise patients on the use of OTC products.

DRY SKIN

Almost everyone has had dry or chapped skin. In some people it is a seasonal or acute occurrence; in others the condition is chronic. Although dry skin is not life threatening, it is annoying and uncomfortable because of the attendant pruritis and, in some cases, pain and inflammation. In addition, dry skin is more prone to bacterial invasion than normal skin.

Dry skin is characterized by one or more of the following signs and symptoms: roughness and flaking, loss of flexibility and elasticity, fissures, hyperkeratosis, and inflammation.

Factors in Skin Hydration

The cardinal characteristic of a dry skin condition is inadequate moisture content in the stratum corneum. This water content may be influenced by several factors.

Dry skin occurs commonly in elderly individuals. As skin ages, the entire epidermal layer thins and the hygroscopic substances decrease, so that ability to retain moisture decreases. The reduced hormonal level lowers sebum output and with it skin lubrication (1). In addition, keratin cross-linking induced by long-term exposure to ultraviolet radiation causes skin to harden. This cross-linking also is associated with increased surface dryness and general pruritis.

A number of skin conditions may lead to extensive water loss. In psoriasis a significant increase in transepidermal water loss occurs from the affected skin but not from neighboring skin (2).

Relative humidity is important in maintaining normal hydration. Keratin (the horny skin layer) softens when moisture content is about 10% (60% relative humidity). In a normal indoor climate, moisture content is 10–15%; at 95% relative humidity it increases to 65%. With low temperature and relative humidity, however, the outer skin layer dries out (3, 4), becomes less flexible, and may crack when flexed, increasing the rate of moisture loss. High wind velocity also causes this condition.

One theory states that water retention depends on the presence of hygroscopic substances within the corneum cells (5). These substances are contained by cell membranes permeable to water but not to electrolytes. Physical disruption, extraction of lipids with solvents, or prolonged detergent use may damage the cell membranes, allowing the hygroscopic substances to be lost and reducing the corneum's ability to retain water (6–9).

Moisture is diffused rapidly to the keratin from lower layers, about 50–100 times faster than it is lost from the epidermal surface to the environment. However, water movement through the keratin is relatively slow. A hydrophilic substance called natural moisturing factor (NMF) may influence keratin moisture retention (10). Several components of this substance, e.g., lactate, polypeptides, hexosamines, pentoses, urea, pyrrolidine, carboxylic acid, and inorganic ions, have been isolated and identified, but their mechanism of action is unknown (11–13). However, when they are applied to the skin surface, only temporary hydration results.

water content of skin

To maintain normal skin hydration, the water content of the stratum corneum must remain at about 10%. Water is lost from the skin through perspiration (as much as 2 liters/hour under extreme thermal stress) and transepidermal diffusion, a relatively constant process. Because human skin is such an effective barrier, only about 120 ml of water/day is lost from the average adult skin surface (20,000 cm^2) (14). Removal of the stratum corneum barrier increases the water loss rate about 50 times (15, 16).

Physical damage to the stratum corneum itself increases the transepidermal water loss rate dramatically, but within 1–2 days a temporary parakeratotic barrier provides 50% of the normal function, and total function is restored in 2–3 weeks.

Treatment

raising moisture level

The main objectives in treating dry skin are to raise the stratum corneum moisture level and to re-establish its integrity. Water is the only true plasticizer for human corneum (10), but simply adding water to the skin is not a useful approach, unless the corneum can retain it. If hydrated skin is not covered immediately with an occlusive substance, such as petrolatum or plastic, it will become dehydrated quickly.

Several approaches in treating a dry skin condition are available (17):

- Lubricating the skin;
- Moisturizing, i.e., hydrating and thus thickening the skin;
- Chemically softening the keratinous epidermal layer.

Lubricating the Skin

This is more of a psychological approach—the skin feels smooth but is not necessarily hydrated or back to normal. Various OTC cosmetic products in an assortment of vehicles are available to correct a dry skin condition, or at least help temporarily to alleviate some discomforting aspects.

Moisturizing Agents

An ideal moisturizer should fulfill certain conditions (13). It should regulate and maintain the stratum corneum water level above the critical level (10%) but not to such a degree as to induce superhydration or maceration. Superhydration of the stratum corneum reduces its barrier efficiency, making it more susceptible to invasion by microorganisms, irritants, and allergens. In addition to this most important characteristic, the effectiveness of a moisturizing agent should be independent of environmental changes, and continued application should not cause damage to the stratum corneum by the removal of or interference with its natural moisturizers. The product should be nonirritating and nonsensitizing, and stable in cosmetic formulations. The agents used most commonly as nonprescription moisturizers are glycerin and fatty acid esters.

Glycerin

humectants

Humectants such as glycerin are used in dry skin products for their moisturizing properties. The humectant is absorbed into the skin to help replace the missing hygroscopic substances, or, if absorption does not occur, the humectant on the skin surface attracts water from the atmosphere and serves as a reservoir for the stratum corneum.

Although products containing 50% glycerin (e.g., glycerin and rose water) often are used to treat a dry skin condition, glycerin does not penetrate into the skin, and high humidity is needed for it to attract water from the environment. (The incidence of dry skin is lowest when relative humidity is high.) Glycerin also increases the transepidermal moisture loss rate, an effect opposite to what is desired. Despite these drawbacks, glycerin is effective in treating dry skin.

A partial explanation for the drug's mechanism of action is that it accelerates moisture diffusion from the dermal tissue to the surface and holds water in intimate contact with the skin. In this manner, it brings moisture to the parched stratum corneum from the dermal region into and through the horny layer. In addition, glycerin provides lubrication to the skin surface.

Hormones

estrogenic creams

Topical application of estrogenic creams improves the water retention capacity, proliferation of cells, plumpness, and overall appearance of the skin. However, the FDA limits the amount of hormone that can be contained in a cosmetic hormone product, and hormone products have no reported beneficial effect on the course of a dry skin condition over and above that of the vehicle containing the hormone. Although most hormone-containing products are in oleaginous or semi-oleaginous vehicles, it is difficult to separate the contribution of the base from that of the hormone. Most, if not all, cosmetic hormone cream effects, i.e., plumping of the skin, disappearance of the tiny crow's feet lines, and alleviation of the dry skin condition, are due to the vehicle rather than the hormone.

Occlusive Agents

emollients

These agents, called emollients, are used in combination with a hygroscopic moisturizer in dry skin formulations. Although an occlusive barrier alone does prevent water evaporation from the skin, some researchers believe that the moisture thus retained is not sufficient to maintain normal hydration (13). Others feel that prolonged occlusive action (e.g., a plastic film used 6–14 nights) enhances the metabolic rate in the epidermis, thereby increasing production of protein and low molecular weight, water-soluble materials that become part of the stratum corneum (18). Substances that restore damaged keratin quickly are preferable to occlusives with long-term action.

Frequency of application of these products depends on severity of the dry skin condition as well as the hydration efficiency of the occlusive agent. Care must be exercised to avoid excessive hydration or maceration. In addition, although most commercial formulations generally are bland, contact with the eye or with broken or abraded skin should be avoided because irritation from formulation ingredients is possible in these cases. This is especially true with emulsion systems because the surfactants in these systems can cause proteins to be denatured.

Because sebum and skin surface lipids contain a relatively high concentration of fatty acid glycerides, vegetable and animal oils (e.g., avocado, cucumber, mink, peanut, safflower, sesame, and turtle) have been used to treat dry skin. Their inclusion in dry skin products is presumably due to their unsaturated fatty acid content. These oils contribute to skin flexibility, but their occludent effect is less than that of petrolatum. Although there is a great psychological appeal to products containing these oils, their actual value in treating a dry skin condition is not documented.

mineral oil and other oil products

Mineral oil products are adsorbed better than vegetable oil products (19). Adsorption onto and absorption into the skin increase with increases in temperature and concentration of the oil. Bath oils, which are applied at a high temperature but unfortunately at a low oil concentration, are moderately effective in improving a dry skin condition. Part of their effect is due to the slip or lubricity they impart to the skin, which may be more important to the patient than the occlusive properties. Bath oils applied as wet compresses are effective in treating dry skin (20). However, except for bath oils there is a general lack of consumer appeal for applied oil products. In most cases, the emulsion system products are the ones that are preferred.

Oil-in-water emulsions are preferred over water-in-oil emulsions or pure oil products because they feel less greasy. Oil-in-water emulsions help alleviate the pruritis associated with dry skin by virtue of their cooling effect as the water evaporates from the skin surface. There is sufficient oil in most oil-in-water emulsions to form a continuous film on the skin surface so long as waxes, gums, and other formulating agents provide an occlusive film after the water evaporates (21). The thickness of the oil film on the skin from an oil-in-water emulsion is less than that from a water-in-oil emulsion because there is less oil. However, other ingredients in the product may contribute to correcting the dry skin condition. It is not agreed whether one emulsion form is safer and more effective than the other (6, 22).

Petrolatum seems to be the most effective occlusive agent. Unfortunately, it is not well accepted by the consumer because of its greasiness and staining properties. Mineral oil is not as efficient a barrier as petrolatum, and silicones are even less efficient than mineral oil (23, 24).

other components of dry skin products

Squalene

Attempts have been made to formulate products that duplicate the normal oil mantle of the skin as a means of treating dry skin. However, sebum is not an effective barrier against moisture loss from the skin. It helps protect the horny layer from drying and helps reduce friction so that the skin remains flexible and smooth, aiding in the prevention of chapping. Squalene is a normal component of skin lipids and is a reasonably effective barrier.

Vitamin A

Topical application of vitamin A has little beneficial effect on a dry skin condition other than its occlusive properties. Vitamin A is extremely oil soluble and penetrates the skin only at high concentrations. Vitamin A acid, or retinoic acid, is more water soluble than vitamin A and has been used topically to treat acne, psoriasis, and other conditions involving accelerated mitosis. Other oil-soluble vitamins such as E and D also have occlusive properties but no specific indication for the dry skin condition.

Keratin-Softening Agents

Chemically altering the keratin layer softens the skin and cosmetically improves its appearance. This approach does not need substantial addition of water, but all of the attendant dry skin symptoms may not be alleviated unless water is added to the keratin layer. Agents used as softeners in OTC dry skin products are urea and allantoin (17).

Urea

Urea (10–30%) is mildly keratolytic and increases water uptake in the corneum, giving it a high water-binding capacity (25, 26). Urea accelerates fibrin digestion at about 15% concentration and is proteolytic at 40%. It is considered harmless and has been recommended for crusted necrotic tissue. Concentrations of 10% have been used on simple dry skin, and 20–30% systems have been used for difficult dry skin conditions, such as in podiatry. Animal or human urine has been used for centuries in treating dry skin, presumably because of the urea content.

Allantoin

Allantoin (0.3%) and allantoin complexes also are claimed to soften keratin by disrupting its structure. Allantoin is considered a relatively safe compound but is apparently less effective than urea.

DANDRUFF

incidence of dandruff

Dandruff is a chronic, noninflammatory scalp condition characterized by excessive scaling of scalp tissue (27). Subjective estimates of its incidence range widely (2.5–70% of the population) (28, 29). However, on the basis of visual observation and objective corneocyte count, about 18% of the population has moderately severe dandruff or worse, and 18% has mild dandruff (30, 31).

Dandruff is not a disease but rather a normal physiological event much like growth of hair and nails, except that the end product is visible on the scalp and thus has substantial cosmetic and social impact. It appears at puberty, when many skin activities are altered, reaches a peak in early adulthood, levels off in middle age, and declines in advancing years. The process correlates very well with the proliferative activity of the epidermis.

Signs and Symptoms

Dandruff is characterized by accelerated epidermal cell turnover (epidermopoiesis), an irregular keratin breakup pattern, and the shedding of cells in large flakes. There seems to be only one visible manifestation of dandruff—scaling. It is normal for epidermal cells on the scalp to slough off continually just as on other parts of the body. However, the epidermal cell turnover rate in normal individuals is greater on the scalp than on other parts of the body (32) and involves the infundibulum of the hair follicle (33). Dandruff flakes often appear around a hair shaft due to the epithelial growth at the base of the hair, which restricts the elimination of sloughed keratin.

dandruff characteristics

epidermal turnover rate

distinguishing dandruff from other skin conditions

selenium sulfide

zinc pyrithione

In dandruff patients the epidermal cell turnover rate is about twice that in normal individuals. The visible scaling is a result of an increased rate of horny substance production on the scalp and the sloughing of large scales (squamae). Dandruff flakes appear white because of air in the clefts between the cellular fragments. This phenomenon does not occur in the normal condition, because the horny substance breaks up in a much more uniform fashion (27). Scalp horny layer in normal individuals consists of 25–35 fully keratinized, closely coherent cells arranged in an orderly fashion. However, in dandruff, the intact horny layer usually has fewer than 10 cells, and nonkeratinized cells are common. With dandruff, crevices occur deep in the stratum corneum, resulting in cracking, which generates large flakes. If the large clumps or flakes can be broken down to smaller units, the visibility of dandruff decreases.

As the rate of keratin cell turnover increases, the number of incompletely keratinized cells (parakeratotic cells) increases. Parakeratosis is characterized by retention of nuclei in keratin layer cells. The number of these cells helps distinguish dandruff from psoriasis or seborrhea; there are more cells in seborrhea and psoriasis than in the dandruff condition. Parakeratotic cells in dandruff appear in clusters, possibly as a result of tiny inflammation foci which are incited when capillaries squirt a load of inflammatory cells into the epidermis, causing accelerated epidermal growth in a small area (34). These microfoci are found in all scalps but are increased proportionately in dandruff.

The specific cause of this accelerated cell growth is unknown. It is not due, as had been theorized, to microorganisms. For many years it was assumed that dandruff was a result of elevated microorganism levels, particularly of the yeast *Pityrosporon ovale*, on the scalp (29, 35). However, the presence of these organisms does not lead to dandruff, nor does their elimination influence the condition. Their accelerated growth does occur as a result of the dandruff condition, which provides a favorable growth medium.

Dandruff is a trivial medical problem, and treatment is fairly straightforward. Some characteristic features may help the pharmacist in distinguishing dandruff from other, more serious, skin conditions (30):

- Dandruff is seasonal; it is mild in the summer months and most severe from October through December.
- Unlike seborrhea and psoriasis, dandruff is uniform and diffuse. Patchiness probably results from brushing the hair, which dislodges adherent flakes.
- Poor hygiene does not cause dandruff in a nondandruff patient, but it exacerbates existing symptoms.
- Dandruff is a very stable process and is not subject to sudden shifts in severity from week to week. It is less subject to outside stress than psoriasis and seborrhea.

Treatment

There is no cure for dandruff, only control of the condition. Total removal of hair eliminates the dandruff condition, but this approach is obviously rather drastic and generally unacceptable. Cleaning the hair and scalp frequently, perhaps daily, often is sufficient to control dandruff. OTC dandruff products contain specific ingredients to reduce epidermal turnover rate, dissolve keratin flakes, and disperse the scales into smaller subunits.

Cytostatic Agents

Using cytostatic agents is the most direct approach to controlling dandruff. By increasing the time necessary for epidermal turnover, it is possible to bring about a dramatic decline in visible scurf. Selenium sulfide and zinc pyrithione at concentrations of 1–2% reduce cell turnover rate significantly. This cytostatic activity is not restricted to conditions where the rate of epidermal turnover is great but also is observed in normal skin, where application of these compounds proportionately lengthens turnover time. Zinc pyrithione is considered by some to be slower acting than selenium sulfide, but this theory has not been proven (30, 33). Both products at OTC concentrations are effective in controlling dandruff.

Their effectiveness is influenced by a number of factors. Zinc pyrithione is strongly bound to both hair and skin, and the extent of binding correlates with clinical performance (36). The drug's adsorption increases with contact time, temperature, concentration, and frequency of application. Zinc pyrithione is bound to the external skin layers and does not penetrate into the dermal region.

In general, cytostatic toxicity is minimal. However, skin burns, particularly under the fingernails, and some cases of conjunctivitis have been noted with selenium sulfide. Pharmacists should caution against using these agents on broken or abraded skin. Selenium sulfide is highly toxic if ingested orally.

Keratolytic Agents

Keratolytic agents are used in dandruff products to dissolve or lyse keratin and facilitate its removal from the scalp in smaller particles. There are many types of keratolytics, with distinctly different modes of action. Resorcinol is presumed to act as a keratolytic by its irritant effect, which causes vesicle formation in the stratum corneum. Sulfur is believed to function by an inflammatory process, causing increased sloughing of cells. Salicylic acid lowers skin pH, causing increased hydration of keratin and thus facilitating its loosening and removal.

Vehicle composition, contact time, and concentration are important considerations to the success of a keratolytic. Salicylic acid functions best as a keratolytic when used in an oil-in-water emulsion base (37–40), whereas sulfur shows its best activity in a nonemulsion base. Contact time is minimal in a shampoo, since significant absorption/adsorption of the agent by the skin cannot occur during the brief period of contact while shampooing. Ointments applied a few times per day and left on are naturally much more effective. However, ointments and pastes are difficult to use on the hairy scalp, and thus aqueous and alcoholic preparations are preferable.

The concentration of keratolytics in OTC scalp products is not sufficient to impair the normal skin barrier but does affect the abnormal parakeratotic stratum corneum (41). Salicylic acid at a concentration of 10–15% showed a keratolytic effect in 2–3 days; 3–5% concentrations took 3 days; and 1% concentrations (the usual concentration in OTC pastes and ointments is 1–2%) took several days. Sulfur behaved similarly. A 10–20% concentration is keratolytic after 1–2 days, 5% in 3 days, 3% in 7 days, and 1% in 10 days.

Keratolytic agents have a primary irritant effect, particularly on mucous membranes and the conjunctiva of the eye. They have the potential of acting on hair keratin as well as skin keratin, and hair appearance may suffer as a result. Toxic manifestations after application of resorcinol to abraded skin have been reported (42, 43).

Scale-Dispersing Agents

Dispersing the scales into smaller subunits decreases their visibility (30). For mild forms of dandruff, vigorous washing with a bland shampoo at frequent intervals may control excess scaling. Many bland shampoos leave a detergent residue on the scalp which perhaps interrupts the lipid–horny cell layer structure at the keratin layer surface, causing subsequent sloughing of keratin in smaller, less visible subunits.

Medicated shampoos also are available. Because their activity increases with longer contact time, these shampoos should be left on the scalp for 5–10 minutes before rinsing. It is important to rinse the hair thoroughly after shampooing: soaps and other components of medicated products sometimes act as a "glue," joining together small flakes to make larger, more visible ones. The agents used most commonly in OTC dandruff shampoos are detergents, chelating agents, and coal tars.

Detergents such as sodium lauryl sulfate often are found in dandruff shampoos. Tars may have been ancient dandruff medications that depended on dispersion for their activity (30). Coal tars are traditional dermatological agents, but they have undesirable side effects such as photosensitivity and retardation of wound healing. Coal tar products probably should not be recommended for dandruff unless the condition is refractory. The value of antiseptics such as quaternary ammonium compounds in dandruff may be due more to dispersion of the flakes than to other activity. Quaternary ammonium compounds are known surfactants and can function in this capacity to reduce the size of the horny scale.

SEBORRHEA

Seborrheic dermatitis is a general term for a group of eruptions that occur predominantly in the area of greatest sebaceous gland activity. The most common form is seborrhea capitis, which is characterized by greasy scales on the scalp, frequently extending to the middle one-third of the face with subsequent eye involvement. The distinctive characteristics of seborrhea are its common occurrence in the hairy skin (specifically the scalp), the appearance of well-demarcated, dull yellowish red lesions, and the associated presence of greasy scales (44).

Etiology

The cause of seborrhea is unknown; many factors, e.g., allergies, stress, and diet, cause or aggravate the condition. The characteristic accelerated cell turnover and enhanced sebaceous gland activity give rise to the prominent scale displayed in the condition, although there is no quantitative relationship between the degree of sebaceous gland activity and susceptibility to seborrhea. Hence predisposing factors are complex.

It is almost universally accepted that seborrhea capitis is merely an extension of dandruff. Some researchers, however, dissent from this view, offering evidence that seborrhea is a separate condition from simple dandruff (30). For example, they point out that the nucleocytes (parakeratotic cells) commonly make up 15–25% of the corneocyte count in seborrhea dermatitis but rarely exceed 5% in dandruff. This evidence and other distinguishing features of the two conditions are shown in Table 1.

Diagnosis and Treatment

Fortunately, misdiagnosis of the seborrhea condition as dandruff is not of great consequence because both involve accelerated epidermal turnover with scaling as the principal manifestation. Hence treatment is generally the same in both cases. However, some aspects of seborrhea capitis are worth noting. Dandruff is considered a relatively stable condition, whereas seborrhea fluctuates in severity, often as a result of stress. Involvement of eyebrows and eyelashes with associated eyelid problems such as blepharitis is common in seborrhea but not in dandruff. Special precautions for eyelid involvement require control of the scalp condition as well as specific ophthalmic agents (see Chapter 19).

PSORIASIS

Psoriasis, which accounts for approximately 5% of all visits to dermatologists in the United States (44), is a papulosquamous skin disease, characterized by well-defined pink or dull red lesions covered with silvery scales (44, 45). The edge of the lesion is sharply delineated, and gentle scraping of the lesion produces micalike scales. Psoriatic lesions have a marked predilection for

resorcinol, sulfur, and salicylic acid

detergents, chelating agents, and coal tars

differentiating dandruff and seborrhea

characteristics of psoriasis

distinguishing features of dandruff, seborrhea, and psoriasis

characteristics of psoriasis

guttate psoriasis in children

Table 1. Distinguishing Features of Dandruff, Seborrhea, and Psoriasis

Characteristic	Dandruff	Seborrhea	Psoriasis
Location	scalp	scalp and other areas of the body, e.g., axilla	scalp and other areas of the body, particularly those prone to stress (the folds of the elbows and knees, scalp, and face)
Influence of external factors	generally a stable condition, does not fluctuate from week to week	influenced by many external factors, notably stress	influenced by irritation and other external stress
Inflammation	absent	present	present
Epidermal hyperplasia	absent	present	present
Epidermal kinetics	turnover rate is two times faster than normal [a]	turnover rate is about five to six times faster than normal [a]	turnover rate is about five to six times faster than normal [a]
Percentage of parakeratotic cells	rarely exceeds 5% of total corneocyte count [b]	commonly makes up 15–25% of corneocyte count [b]	commonly makes up 40–60% of corneocyte count [a]

[a] Adapted from K. J. McGinley et al., *J. Invest. Dermatol.*, *53*, 107 (1969).
[b] Adapted from A. M. Kligman et al., *J. Soc. Cosmet. Chem.*, *25*, 73 (1974).

certain areas of the body such as the scalp, the folds of the elbows and knees, and the genitoanal region. The condition is unpredictable in its course but has a tendency to be chronic and relapsing.

Signs and Symptoms

There seems to be an inherited predisposition to psoriasis because in more than one-fourth of psoriatic patients there is an associated family history. No age is exempt from the condition; most cases develop in individuals 10–50 years old. Psoriasis is rarely found in Afro-Americans, Japanese, and American Indians. It is distributed almost equally between men and women (46).

Skin in the psoriatic plaque is characterized by accelerated epidermopoiesis, proliferation of capillaries in the dermal region, extensive infolding of the epidermal–dermal junction, and invasion of the epidermis by polymorphonuclear leukocytes (44). The greatly expanded surface area of the epidermal–dermal junction by infolding and the presence of two or three basal cell layers lead to a greatly exaggerated mitotic growth and epidermal thickness. Normal epidermal turnover is 25–30 days; in psoriatic plaque skin, it is ≦3–4 days (46). At this rapid rate, the keratin produced has many parakeratotic cells, and the granular layer is absent in severe cases.

Although much research has been done recently on the cause(s) of psoriasis (47–52), the specific biochemical event triggering psoriatic skin formation remains unknown. It is possible that cyclic adenosine 3′,5′-monophosphate (cAMP) mediates the regulation of epidermal proliferation and that there is a defect in the adenylcyclase–cAMP system in psoriatic skin (53–55).

Psoriatic lesions frequently develop in sites of vaccination, scratch marks, surgical incisions, or skin tests and have been reported to be produced by shock and noise. In fact, the response to skin trauma is so predictable (Koebner's phenomenon) that it can be used in diagnosis. For example, when scaling is not evident, making diagnosis difficult, scales may be induced by light scratching. It has been shown that both epidermis and dermis must be damaged before the reaction occurs, and the response generally occurs in 6–18 days following injury (56, 57). Endocrine factors also have been implicated frequently in psoriasis. The condition often improves or clears during pregnancy but may reappear after parturition.

Psoriasis in children is usually of the guttate variety. When these small lesions coalesce, they form large characteristic plaques. "Pustular psoriasis," which may or may not be a form of psoriasis, is localized on the palms and soles. Pitting of the nails is common and frequently can be used as a diagnostic aid.

Acute guttate psoriasis attacks often occur at puberty, following childbirth, or after respiratory infections. This condition, which is characterized by many small lesions distributed more or less evenly over the body, accounts for about 17% of psoriatic patients. Various systemic illnesses may precipitate psoriatic attacks. For example, psoriasis onset in children commonly follows streptococcal tonsillitis. Hot weather and sunlight improve the condition, and cold weather worsens it.

A relationship exists between psoriasis and inflammatory polyarthritis (distinguished from rheumatoid arthritis by its onset, which is usually subacute and occurs in only one joint). Approximately 4% of all patients with polyarthritis also have psoriasis, the skin manifestation of psoriasis preceding the arthritis by many years. A more telling statistic is that psoriasis is found in the families of 40% of polyarthritic patients. The cause of this relationship is unknown, but there is a difference in the time course of psoriasis between patients with and without polyarthritis. For example, psoriasis of the nails occurs in 80–90% of patients with arthritis as compared to 30–40% of patients without arthritis (38).

The duration of psoriasis is variable. A lesion may last a lifetime, or it may disappear quickly. The course of the disease is marked by spontaneous exacerbations and remissions. When the psoriatic condition is initiated by a guttate attack, the disease carries a better prognosis than that of a slower and more diffuse onset. When lesions disappear, they may leave the skin either hypopigmented or hyperpigmented.

Diagnosis

Diagnosis usually is straightforward for simple psoriasis. Sites of involvement, the dry silvery appearance of the scale, and a small area of bleeding (Auspitz sign) after scale removal are characteristic. The bleeding puncta is the top of the capillary loop in the skin. Precipitating factors such as a recent vaccination, disease, pregnancy, or trauma are useful evidence in a preliminary diagnosis.

It is important not to confuse psoriasis with other diseases that may have similar symptoms but call for different treatment methods. When the scalp or the flexural and intertriginous areas are involved, psoriasis must not be mistaken for seborrhea or moniliasis. Psoriasis of the scalp generally produces dry, patchy, adherent scales; seborrhea is usually manifested as a yellowish, oily scale (seborrhea oleosa) and tends to be more diffuse. If lesions are present in the groin, axilla, and inframammary region, diagnosis based on visual inspection may be difficult. Identifying the fungal organism from lesion scrapings proves the presence or absence of moniliasis. Seborrhea and psoriasis sometimes are distinguishable by their scale color and appearance. In psoriasis the plaque has a full, rich, red color with a particular depth of hue and opacity not normally seen in eczema and seborrhea. In dark-skinned races this color quality is lost. More elaborate histological and pathological diagnosis may be done by a physician (58–60).

Other skin diseases whose symptoms resemble those of psoriasis are localized neurodermatitis, particularly in the genitoanal regions, and fungus conditions with circular or annular lesions. When psoriasis alternates with or is complicated by other diseases, such as seborrhea, diagnosis is much more difficult.

Treatment

There is no cure for psoriasis, only a reduction in severity. Different stages of the disease are treated by different methods. Acute psoriatic onset characterized by severely erythematous lesions calls for soothing local therapy such as a bland, nonmedicated cream. As the acute process subsides and the usual thick-scaled plaques appear, more potent therapy, e.g., keratolytics, may be used. Many patients respond well to simple measures, whereas others are refractory to the most formidable treatment.

There is consensus that "guerrilla tactics are better than a frontal assault," with the more powerful agents held in reserve (43). In eruptive or unstable forms of the disease, even mild sunlight may provoke a Koebner-type exacerbation. In general, therapy should take the following approach:

- Discussion with the patient as to the nature of the condition (acceptance of the disease may reduce stress or emotional instability);
- Rest, mild sedation, and simple local measures such as sunlight (ultraviolet light in suberythemal doses) and mild keratolytic products;
- Tar products and weak topical corticosteroids in combination with ultraviolet light.

Topical Agents

Drug penetration of diseased skin is facilitated if the psoriatic plaque is removed before therapy or if an occlusive bandage is used after the drug is applied. Psoriatic skin loses water 8–10 times faster than normal skin. In fact, when large areas of the body surface are involved, whole body skin water loss may be as much as 2–3 liters/day, in addition to normal perspiration loss. Evaporation of this volume of water requires over 1000 cal. For this reason, psoriatic patients may show increased metabolic rates and are prone to peptic ulcer formation.

Because psoriatic skin is more permeable to many substances than normal skin, the barrier that normally prevents drug penetration through skin is disrupted in psoriasis, causing rapid drug entrance. Thus in the early stage the disorder responds rapidly to local treatment, and then the improvement rate slows as the skin barrier approaches normalcy.

The agents used most commonly in topical psoriasis treatment preparations are keratolytics and tar products, either individually or in combination. In general, the combination therapy consists of using a keratolytic during the day and applying coal tar at night.

Keratolytics

Salicylic acid (2–10%) is commonly used for psoriasis. Because it is an irritant, there is concern about worsening of the psoriatic condition. Salicylic acid in concentrations of 0.5–10% in a petroleum jelly base does not affect the proliferation rate of psoriatic epidermal cells (61). Many patients respond to salicylic acid (2%) in cream or ointment form, applied several times per day. Keratolytics should be applied at a low concentration initially, and the dose should be increased as patient tolerance develops.

Tar Products

Like many dermatological diseases, psoriasis improves significantly during the summer, especially during periods without stress. Tar and ultraviolet light therapy has been used since 1925 (62). For many years the therapeutic response with this form of therapy was be-

relationship of psoriasis and arthritis

psoriasis diagnosis

precipitating factors

reducing severity of psoriasis

therapeutic strategy

commonly used keratolytics

lieved to be caused by phototoxicity, but this theory has been challenged (63, 64). Ultraviolet light alone may be helpful for the condition, but the activity is enhanced significantly with coal tar. The combination is better than either agent alone.

Recent work has shown the combinations of 1% crude coal tar and long-wavelength ultraviolet light and of 6% crude coal tar with ultraviolet light to be equally effective (65). Hence only modest levels of coal tar are needed. Moreover, crude coal tar from high- and low-temperature sources seems equally effective (66).

Combinations of coal tar and keratolytics are useful. Bathing in coal tar or using a tar soap also may be effective. However, some patients show a worsening of the condition when exposed to coal tar products.

Others

ammoniated mercury, anthralin, colchicine, and psoralens in psoriasis treatment

Ammoniated mercury with or without a keratolytic has been used. Its beneficial effect is doubtful, and its propensity toward causing sensitivity and potential systemic toxicity should restrict its use seriously.

Occlusion with a plastic film reduces the skin cell metabolic rate and allows reformation of the granular layer in the psoriatic plaque.

Anthralin (dithranol) is an effective topical agent but has considerable burning and staining properties. A derivative of anthralin, triacetoxyanthracene, lacks the burning and staining effects of anthralin but is less effective.

Application of colchicine (1%) in hydrophilic ointment for several weeks has been tried. This approach is still experimental, but the preliminary results are encouraging (67).

An increasingly important mode of therapy is the use of systemic or topical psoralens in combination with ultraviolet light (68–73). Side effects from systemic use of the psoralens appear modest and can be reduced further by topical application. Moreover, by using an oleaginous vehicle to minimize reflection of the ultraviolet light, debridement of the lesion is unnecessary (68).

Internal Agents

orally administered agents

Antihistamines

The attendant pruritis of psoriasis may be alleviated with systemically administered antihistamines. The sedation properties of antihistamines also are useful where an associated emotional factor is involved. Some patients respond to minor tranquilizers in small doses or to sedatives such as phenobarbital. Topical application of antihistamines is of questionable value.

Vitamin A

Vitamin A is believed to be involved in epidermal activity, but the consensus is that it is ineffective in treating psoriasis. Preliminary results on topically applied tretinoin (vitamin A acid) are encouraging, but additional work is needed.

Others

Cyanocobalamin has been found to be generally ineffective. Vitamin D helps in cases complicated by hypocalcemia.

Alternate Therapy

The most direct approach to treating psoriasis is to reduce epidermal activity by means of prescription-only cytostatic agents such as corticosteroids and systemically administered methotrexate. Corticosteroids, such as hydrocortisone, have a significant suppressive effect on psoriasis, but the danger of rebound limits their use. Other concerns with this form of therapy, in addition to systemic absorption of these potent steroids, are local atrophy, which may result from prolonged use of these agents, and reduced tolerance to other agents. Relapse occurs more quickly after topical corticosteroids than after tar or anthralin therapy. In addition to the normal side effects of systemically administered corticosteroids, high doses cause involution of the condition, but after therapy is stopped, the disease is almost certain to be worse than it was initially (45). Thus the systemic use of these agents usually is contraindicated in all but the most severe forms of psoriasis.

The serious potential side effects and toxicity of methotrexate therapy are well known. Strict supervision of patients receiving methotrexate, including frequent blood analysis and regular liver biopsy, is essential (74). Results of a recent survey of dermatologists showed that methotrexate, hydroxyurea, and azarabine were used as chemotherapy for psoriasis by 50%, 10%, and 2% of the dermatologists polled (75). Despite this relatively high usage of methotrexate, only a small percentage of the patients were given liver biopsy and creatinine clearance tests.

Some physicians used to recommend special diets for psoriatic patients, but this approach proved to be of no benefit. The major point in diet control was to lower the cholesterol level, which is altered in many psoriatic patients. Other diet modifications included low protein and low tryptophan.

ECZEMA

symptoms of eczema

Eczema is a noninfectious, inflammatory dermatosis in which the affected skin is erythematous. It is a pattern of skin manifestations rather than a specific disease and can be either acute or chronic.

The term "eczema" was used formerly for a large group of skin disorders of unknown etiology, many of which are now called by more specific names. When the cause of a particular skin condition was elucidated, the disease was given a different name, and the eczema nomenclature was dropped or modified. Today, most dermatologists define eczema as "skin inflammation from whatever cause," and the term is synonymous with dermatitis.

Signs and Symptoms

The main symptoms of eczema are pruritis and weeping of the skin. The itching may convert to pain over time, and the weeping may diminish, giving way to a scaly condition; at no time does the epidermal tissue appear normal. Symptoms may include papules, vesicles, edema, and patches. In the acute stages there is a uniform pattern of papular vesicles on an erythematous base. In the chronic form the weeping may be absent, but epidermal thickening and scaling are present. Excoriations, crusting, and secondary infections may occur as sequelae to the pruritis (76).

Eczema may be precipitated by external (exogenous) or internal (endogenous) sources.

Exogenously Induced Eczema

The conditions of exogenously induced eczema are grouped under the general heading of contact dermatitis (Table 2). The offending substance irritates the skin on first or multiple exposure or may generate an allergic response. In either case the result is skin inflammation.

Irritant Dermatitis

Many agents have a propensity to irritate. A primary irritant generally elicits a response on first exposure; secondary irritants cause an inflammatory response only if certain ancillary circumstances are met or if the agent is applied again.

The symptoms of irritant dermatitis range from mild erythema accompanied by pruritis to actual necrosis and skin ulceration. Primary irritants cause pruritic erythema or perhaps ulceration; secondary irritants, which frequently generate a low-grade inflammation for a long period, tend to produce symptoms more closely related to chronic eczema (Table 2).

In general, the factors influencing skin irritation are the substance itself, the climate, and biological variation in the host. The degree of skin irritation from an applied substance is a function of the intrinsic irritation potential of the test material, its concentration, and its ability to remain bound to the skin.

Applying a strong acid or base to the cutaneous skin surface causes irritation and a subsequent inflammatory reaction. Likewise, the irritant properties of topical drugs such as camphor, menthol, coal tar, and resorcinol are well known, but classification of these agents as primary or secondary irritants is a function of their concentration. Very high camphor concentrations are needed to produce the same degree of irritation as that achieved with relatively low coal tar levels. Agents such as bithionol and hexachlorophene, which are bound to the epidermal layer, cause irritation with repeated application. Some substances used to treat other skin conditions, e.g., psoriasis, may be irritating to eczematous skin.

Environmental conditions play a role in skin texture and its resistance to irritant substances. High humidity allows greater skin hydration and thus faster penetration. Occlusion also keeps the skin hydrated.

Factors such as age and skin color also are influential in irritant dermatitis. Aged skin is less prone to irritation than youthful skin, presumably because drug penetration is more difficult. Darker skinned races seem to be less susceptible than lighter skinned individuals, although the evidence to prove this observation is scant.

precipitating factors in eczema

characteristics of exogenously induced eczema

types of dermatitis

Concomitant administration of more than one substance may induce skin irritation. A secondary irritant that is not irritating to the skin when applied alone may cause irritation in combination with an agent that promotes absorption, such as a surfactant. Damaged skin also encourages skin irritation.

Allergic Dermatitis

Allergic reactions are classified as immediate (anaphylactic), intermediate (Arthus), cytotoxic, and delayed (tuberculin) (Table 3). Some individuals react abnormally, with appropriate skin manifestations, to common substances such as mushrooms, strawberries, or shellfish, but the changes do not appear to be mediated by antibodies or delayed sensitivity, and they usually occur on first exposure to the substance. Thus they are not allergies

Table 2. Exogenously Induced Eczema

Characteristic	Weak or Secondary Irritant Dermatitis [a]	Irritant Dermatitis [b]	Allergic Dermatitis [c]
Mechanism	abrasion, desiccation, trauma, dryness, soreness, and fissuring precede eruption	direct insult to tissue, no preceding dryness or fissuring	immunological, initial contact sensitizes, subsequent contact elicits a response, no preceding eruption
Onset	slow, over days, months, or years	sudden, response in 30 min to several days after exposure	sudden, response in 24–48 hours after exposure
Symptoms	hyperkeratosis, erythema, vesicles, and fissuring	erythema, vesicles, exudation, and sometimes necrosis	erythema, vesicles, edema, and necrosis
Usual location	hands	hands	hands and face
Patch test	negative	positive	positive

[a] Cumulative insults are required. [b] Single exposure to an offending agent. [c] Multiple exposures are usually required.

Table 3. Types of Allergic Reactions in the Skin

	Anaphylaxis	Arthus Reaction	Cytotoxic Reaction	Delayed Reaction
Response mediator	sensitizing antibody	precipitating antibody	antibody or cell	cell
Skin test	immediate wheal or flare	Arthus reaction with polymorph infiltration, appearing in 2–4 hours but may progress to necrosis for hours or days	immediate wheal and flare, granulomatous lesions with or without polymorphs, first appearing in 2–6 hours	delayed, tuberculin response
Clinical manifestation	erythema	serum sickness	eczema	eczema
Skin or vascular changes	urticaria; angioneurotic edema	allergic vasculitis; nodular vasculitis	purpura; homograft rejection	contact dermatitis; homograft rejection

[a] Adapted from W. E. Parrish, *An Introduction to the Biology of the Skin*, Blackwell Scientific Publications, Oxford, England, 1970.

allergic reactions in the skin

possible mechanisms and characteristics

therapeutic approach

but rather idiosyncrasies caused by an intrinsic factor or defect in the tissues. Not all symptoms of allergic dermatitis respond equally to drug therapy.

Immediate (anaphylactic) reaction. In this case the antibody sensitizes the tissue cells passively. Administration of exogenous antigen reaches the sensitized cells, causing cell injury and release of pharmacological agents. These agents cause further local changes, which usually include contraction of smooth muscle, increased vascular permeability, and edema. The cell injury from this type of reaction is transient, and most of the cells recover. Antihistamines suppress or modify the tissue changes in species of animals in which histamine is the most active pharmacological agent. They do not prevent the antigen–antibody reaction but do prevent histamine release if given prophylactically.

Atopic dermatitis or eczema is sometimes associated incorrectly with anaphylactic allergy. Affected individuals show positive skin tests and develop allergic signs after exposure. However, normal treatment for allergy such as avoiding contact with allergens and administration of antihistaminic drugs seldom brings relief.

Intermediate (Arthus) reaction. In this reaction the antigen combines with the antibody in tissue spaces or in the circulation to produce a type of complex, which causes secondary changes to the tissue, depending on concentration and composition. The main change is massive infiltration of the extravascular tissues, which usually occurs 2–4 hours after the antigen is administered. Administration of corticosteroids suppresses full development of the Arthus reaction.

Cytotoxic reaction. A cytotoxic reaction is one in which cells are damaged. In the allergic classification it is restricted to cell damage caused by delayed sensitivity specific for the antigen in the susceptible target cell. The lysis of red cells by antibodies specified for the red cells is an example of reaction of an antibody to an antigen acquired by the cell. The cell that has adsorbed the antigen is usually damaged.

Delayed (tuberculin) reaction. This type of reaction takes a number of hours to reach a maximum response and occurs in the absence of demonstrable globulin antibody. The lesion produced is a diffuse reaction characterized by accumulation of fluid (edema). The allergic response may be inhibited by corticosteroids but is not altered by antihistamines.

The essential features of the delayed sensitivity reaction are its mediation by cells only and its passive transfer to normal subjects by cells only. No circulating antibodies can be detected.

Infective Dermatitis

Infective dermatitis is a skin condition caused by the presence of microorganism toxins, not by the organism's specific pathogenic activity. The mechanism of action for this type of eczema has not been established, but it is known that inoculating the skin of susceptible individuals with a bacterial culture or filtrate produces an eczematous condition. It is presumed that bacterial toxins or antigens elicit the unfavorable response. The condition responds favorably to systemic antibiotics.

Endogenously Induced Eczema

Atopic and asteatotic eczema and neurodermatitis are conditions due to internal sources. Symptoms generally last longer (years) than those of exogenously induced eczema.

Atopic Eczema

This skin disease occurs primarily during childhood and early adulthood, usually in folds of arms or knees. It may begin shortly after birth and last many years, or it may last only 1–2 years and disappear. The symptoms are erythema, scaling, and weeping, accompanied by severe pruritis. Unfortunately, secondary or associated infections are common, making diagnosis and treatment difficult. The etiology of the condition is unknown, but patients often have associated asthma or hay fever. Because skin sensitivity to a wide range of agents is common, skin tests are not very beneficial as diagnostic aids.

Asteatotic Eczema

This eczema is characterized by dry and fissured skin and by scantiness or absence of the sebaceous secretions. It occurs mainly during the dry winter weather and in elderly individuals.

Neurodermatitis

This chronic form of eczema is found more often in women, generally localized in the nape of the neck, legs, genitoanal region, and forearms. The areas of involvement are highly lichenified and become worse when continually rubbed or scratched. Emotional stress plays a role in this condition (77).

Diagnosis

Because some forms of eczema respond differently to different drugs, the distinction between endogenous and exogenous patterns is important in initiating proper therapy. In most cases of contact dermatitis, an accurate diagnosis is made readily on the basis of the eczematous character, configuration, and location of the rash and itching. Eczema of the backs and sides of the fingers and hands, eyelids, genitoanal region, wrists, forearms, and feet suggests contact eczema. Occupational and leisure activities, family history, and recently used topical medicaments and cosmetics also are useful diagnostic aids (78–80).

In some cases of eczema (especially eruptions of the hands) there is a mixture of infectious eczematoid, atopic, and contact dermatitis. With contact dermatitis, once the skin reacts to one substance, it may be more vulnerable to other substances, making diagnosis and treatment more complicated. Allergic or primary irritant dermatitis may be a secondary eruption caused by an agent used in therapy, complicating one of the other forms of eczema.

The duration of the eruption can also be helpful. For example, atopic dermatitis lasts for months or years; contact dermatitis does not.

Treatment

Eczema therapy must be approached cautiously to prevent deterioration of the condition. In some forms of eczema the patient is sensitive to a wide variety of agents, and therapeutic entities may aggravate already inflamed skin. In contact eczema, drug therapy is needed for only a short time because withdrawal of the allergen or irritant ameliorates the condition. However, in atopic dermatitis, therapy is needed for long periods. Minor tranquilizers, sedatives, and especially counseling are useful in treating neurodermatitis.

For most forms of eczema it is worthwhile to protect the lesions from clothing and fingernails, especially in small children. A bland dressing often helps without resorting to additional drugs.

Particularly in acute eczema, the patient should be instructed to avoid soap and water (or use sparingly), friction from wool and rough clothing, heavy exercise, known irritants and allergens, and self-testing to identify a suspected allergen (81, 82).

Ingredients in OTC products for eczema are antiseptics, astringents, cooling agents, keratolytics, and protectants.

Antiseptics

Antiseptics are necessary in infective dermatitis but should be used cautiously in the more general forms of eczema. Many of these agents have considerable sensitizing and irritating potential, particularly when they are used chronically. For example, neomycin should not be used for maintenance treatment of hypostatic or genitoanal eczema (80).

Astringents

Astringency is sometimes needed to reduce the extent of weeping. Baths or local compresses (15–30 minutes each) a few times per day help dry the weeping areas. So as not to aggravate the eczema, more potent astringents should be reserved until the erythemal inflammation of the acute phase subsides. Calamine lotion and other powder-based substances that dry weeping through water adsorption or astringency should be avoided. These agents have a tendency to crust, and removing the crusts causes bleeding and potential infections.

eczema therapy

components of OTC products

indications for use

Cooling Agents

Cooling the skin surface reduces the extent of pruritis. In the acute phase of eczema, soothing lotions applied as wet compresses are helpful, but aromatic substances such as menthol and camphor should be used cautiously so as not to exacerbate the condition. The cooling effect of an infrequently applied lotion or emulsion is only transitory. Orally administered antihistamines may be used for their sedative and antipruritic effects. Topically administered antihistamines should not be recommended or used because of their questionable efficacy and their significant tendency to become sensitizers. Antihistamines and corticosteroids act prophylactically to prevent further inflammation. They have no effect on existing inflammation, and hence improvement in the condition should be evaluated accordingly.

Keratolytics

Keratolytics usually are avoided in eczema unless extensive lichenification has occurred. These agents and those that reduce the mitotic activity of the epidermis, such as tars and anthralin, should be used cautiously.

Protectants

To protect small areas of eczematous skin, zinc oxide (Lassar's) paste, zinc oxide ointment, or paste-impregnated bandages may be used. Some of these topical products are astringents as well as protectants. For larger areas, soaking in aluminum acetate solution or water reduces the weeping. Covering the lesions or applying a drug with an occlusive barrier increases the degree of tissue maceration and also may prevent heat loss. This effect may contribute to discomfort of the affected area.

PRODUCT SELECTION GUIDELINES

During 1977, sales for medicated shampoos were more than $142 million (83). Advertisements not only have created persona non grata status for the dandruff sufferer, but also have attempted to obliterate the difference between dandruff, a nonpathological condition, and psoriasis and seborrhea, which are pathological conditions. Thus the pharmacist's most important consideration in recommending a product for treating a skin condition is proper identification of the disorder.

The principal skin conditions that exhibit symptoms similar to dandruff—psoriasis and seborrhea capitis—also involve an accelerated keratin production rate, but psoriasis and seborrhea are distinct from dandruff. Many people consider dandruff an extension or mild form of seborrhea, but evidence shows this theory to be questionable (30). Fortunately, an incorrect diagnosis is not serious because the agents used to treat all of these conditions are similar, except in severe cases.

Table 1 lists distinguishing features of dandruff, seborrhea, and psoriasis. In addition to these rather general differences, there are more elaborate cytological differences (84). For the pharmacist without access to extensive laboratory diagnostic aids, the site of the condition, the influence of external factors, and the overall severity of the condition are often useful in distinguishing the conditions.

Some agents in OTC dandruff products possess antibacterial and antifungal activity. This approach to dandruff control is used because of the abnormally elevated flora in the dandruff patient. However, reducing the microbial count does not reduce dandruff unless these agents have a surfactant effect to disperse scales or reduce dandruff in another manner (85). The questionable statement "to prevent secondary infections" is not altogether acceptable as a rationale for inclusion of these agents.

In other skin disorders, overtreatment or improper treatment often exacerbates the condition. For example, pruritis is a constant feature of eczema, and thus a counterirritant may be indicated; however, application of a counterirritant for psoriasis may aggravate the condition, particularly in its early stages.

SUMMARY

The causative mechanisms of skin diseases such as psoriasis and most types of eczema are unknown, or at best speculative. Even without a precise mechanistic understanding, sophisticated analytical techniques are available so that pathological changes in the skin can be described in great detail. This advance permits a more rational approach to therapy, even though it is, in many respects, empirical. It is important that patients suffering from these dermatological problems have proper diagnosis before attempting treatment with home remedies or OTC preparations. The pharmacist can perform a valuable service by helping patients determine the nature of their problem and the best course to follow to alleviate it.

REFERENCES

(1) R. M. Handjani-Vila, B. Rondot, and F. Lachampt, *Cosmet. Perfum.*, *90*, 39 (1975).
(2) G. Rajka and P. Thune, *Br. J. Dermatol.*, *94*, 253 (1976).
(3) R. H. Wildnaur, J. W. Bothwell, and A. B. Douglass, *J. Invest. Dermatol.*, *56*, 72 (1971).
(4) J. D. Middleton and B. M. Allen, *J. Soc. Cosmet. Chem.*, *24*, 239 (1973).
(5) J. D. Middleton, *Br. J. Dermatol.*, *80*, 437 (1968).
(6) M. Mezei, W. Sager, W. D. Stewart, and A. L. DeRuyters, *J. Pharm. Sci.*, *55*, 584 (1966).
(7) H. Baker, *J. Invest. Dermatol.*, *50*, 283 (1968).
(8) J. D. Middleton, *J. Soc. Cosmet. Chem.*, *20*, 399 (1969).
(9) I. H. Blank and E. B. Shapiro, *J. Invest. Dermatol.*, *25*, 391 (1975).
(10) I. H. Blank, *J. Invest. Dermatol.*, *18*, 433 (1952).
(11) O. K. Jacobi, *Proc. Sci. Sect. Toilet Goods Assoc.*, *31*, 22 (1959).
(12) K. Laden, *Am. Perfum. Cosmet.*, *82*, 77 (1967).
(13) S. J. Strianse, *Cosmet. Perfum.*, *89*, 57 (1974).
(14) A. M. Kligman, in "The Epidermis," W. Montagna and W. C. Lobitz, Jr., Eds., Academic, New York, N.Y., 1964.
(15) D. Spruit and K. W. Malton, *J. Invest. Dermatol.*, *45*, 6 (1952).
(16) D. Monash and I. H. Blank, *Arch. Dermatol.*, *78*, 710 (1958).
(17) R. L. Goldenberg, *Skin Allerg. News*, *5*, 20 (1974).
(18) R. L. Anderson, J. M. Cassidy, J. R. Hansen, and W. Yellin, *J. Invest. Dermatol.*, *61*, 375 (1974).
(19) E. A. Taylor, *J. Invest. Dermatol.*, *37*, 69 (1961).
(20) I. I. Lubowe, *West J. Med.*, *1*, 45 (1960).
(21) E. M. Seiner, S. Bieser, R. Guidice, I. O. Kawat, E. Kaplan, B. Kauth, and D. Stone, *J. Am. Podiatr. Assoc.*, *63*, 571 (1973).
(22) S. Rothman, "Physiology and Biochemistry of the Skin," University of Chicago Press, Chicago, Ill., 1954, p. 26.
(23) G. Barnett, in "Cosmetics: Science and Technology," 2nd ed., M. S. Balsam and E. Sagarin, Eds., Wiley, New York, N.Y., 1972.
(24) G. K. Steigleder and W. P. Raab, *J. Invest. Dermatol.*, *38*, 129 (1962).
(25) H. Ashton, E. Frank, and C. J. Stevenson, *Br. J. Dermatol.*, *84*, 194 (1971).
(26) D. P. Nash, *J. Am. Podiatr. Assoc.*, *61*, 382 (1971).
(27) A. B. Ackerman and A. M. Kligman, *J. Soc. Cosmet. Chem.*, *20*, 81 (1969).
(28) S. Bourne and A. Jacobs, *Br. Med. J.*, *1*, 1268 (1956).
(29) F. C. Roia and R. W. Vanderwyk, *J. Soc. Cosmet. Chem.*, *20*, 113 (1969).
(30) A. M. Kligman, R. R. Marples, L. R. Lantis, and K. J. McGinley, *J. Soc. Cosmet. Chem.*, *25*, 73 (1974).
(31) K. J. McGinley, R. R. Marples, and G. Plewig, *J. Invest. Dermatol.*, *53*, 107 (1969).
(32) H. Goldschmidt and A. M. Kligman, *Arch. Dermatol.*, *88*, 709 (1963).
(33) G. Plewig and A. M. Kligman, *J. Soc. Cosmet. Chem.*, *20*, 767 (1969).
(34) A. M. Kligman, *Cosmet. Perfum.*, *90*, 16 (1975).
(35) F. C. Roia and R. W. Vanderwyk, *J. Soc. Cosmet. Chem.*, *15*, 761 (1964).
(36) T. Okumura, S. Hayashi, F. Tokiwa, and S. Horin, *Cosmet. Perfum.*, *90*, 101 (1975).
(37) E. Strokosch, *Arch. Dermatol. Syphilol.*, *47*, 16 (1943).
(38) *Ibid.*, 216.
(39) E. Strokosch, *Arch. Dermatol. Syphilol.*, *48*, 384 (1943).
(40) *Ibid.*, 393.
(41) "Textbook of Dermatology," Vol. 1, 2nd ed., A. Rook, D. S. Wilkinson, and F. J. G. Ebling, Eds., Blackwell Scientific Publications, London, England, 1972, p. 253.
(42) "United States Dispensatory and Physicians' Pharmacology," 26th ed., Lippincott, New York, N.Y., 1967.
(43) K. W. Chesterman, *J. Am. Pharm. Assoc.*, *NS12*, 576 (1972).
(44) "Textbook of Dermatology," Vol. 2, 2nd ed., A. Rook, D. S. Wilkinson, and F. J. G. Ebling, Eds., Blackwell Scientific Publications, London, England, 1972, pp. 1192–1234.
(45) G. M. Lewis and C. E. Wheeler, "Practical Dermatology," 3rd ed., Saunders, Philadelphia, Pa., 1967, pp. 207–218.
(46) G. Weinstein, *Br. J. Dermatol.*, *92*, 229 (1975).
(47) K. Aso, E. K. Orenberg, and E. M. Farber, *J. Invest. Dermatol.*, *63*, 375 (1975).
(48) G. Mahrle and C. E. Orfanos, *Br. J. Dermatol.*, *93*, 495 (1975).
(49) P. D. Mier and J. van Den Hurk, *Br. J. Dermatol.*, *94*, 219 (1976).
(50) J-J. Guilhou, J. Clot, J. Meynadier, and H. Lapinski, *Br. J. Dermatol.*, *94*, 501 (1976).
(51) J-J. Guilhou, J. Meynadier, J. Clot, E. Charmasson, M. Dardenne, and J. Brochier, *Br. J. Dermatol.*, *95*, 295 (1976).
(52) G. Mahrle and C. E. Orfanos, *Br. J. Dermatol.*, *95*, 591 (1976).
(53) J. J. Voorhees and E. A. Duell, *Arch. Dermatol.*, *104*, 352 (1971).
(54) R. K. Wright, S. H. Mandy, K. M. Halprin, and S. L. Hsia, *Arch. Dermatol.*, *107*, 47 (1973).
(55) M. M. Mui, S. L. Hsia, and K. M. Halprin, *Br. J. Dermatol.*, *92*, 255 (1975).
(56) L. Stankler, *Br. J. Dermatol.*, *81*, 534 (1969).
(57) J. S. Comaish and J. S. Greener, *Br. J. Dermatol.*, *94*, 195 (1976).
(58) "Dermal Pathology," J. H. Graham, W. C. Johnson, and E. B. Helwig, Eds., Harper and Row, New York, N.Y., 1972, pp. 325–332.

(59) M. Gordon, W. C. Johnson, and C. F. Brugoon, Jr., *Arch. Dermatol.*, *95*, 402 (1967).
(60) E. J. Van Scott and T. M. Ekel, *Arch. Dermatol.*, *88*, 373 (1963).
(61) H. Pullman, K. J. Lennartz, and G. K. Steigleder, *Arch. Dermatol. Forsch.*, *251*, 271 (1975).
(62) W. H. Goeckerman, *Northwest Med.*, *24*, 299 (1925).
(63) L. Tanenbaum, J. A. Parrish, M. A. Pathak, R. R. Anderson, and T. B. Fitzpatrick, *Arch. Dermatol.*, *111*, 467 (1975).
(64) L. Tanenbaum, M. A. Pathak, and J. A. Parrish, *Arch. Dermatol.*, *111*, 395 (1975).
(65) A. R. Marisco, W. H. Eaglstein, and G. D. Weinstein, *Arch. Dermatol.*, *112*, 1249 (1976).
(66) R. S. Chapman and O. A. Finn, *Br. J. Dermatol.*, *94*, 71 (1976).
(67) K. H. Kaidbey, J. W. Petrozzi, and A. M. Kligman, *Arch. Dermatol.*, *111*, 33 (1975).
(68) H. Schaefer, K. Vivell, V. Kentsch, W. Schella, and S. Jenny, *Br. J. Dermatol.*, *94*, 363 (1976).
(69) J. W. Petrozzi, K. M. Kaidbey, and A. M. Kligman, *Arch. Dermatol.*, *113*, 292 (1977).
(70) *Archives of Dermatology*, *112*, 35 (1976).
(71) T. Lakshmipathi, P. W. Gould, L. A. Machenzie, B. E. Johnson, and W. Frain-Bell, *Br. J. Dermatol.*, *96*, 587 (1977).
(72) K. W. Wolff, T. B. Fitzpatrick, J. A. Parrish, F. Gschnait, B. Gilchrest, H. Honigsmann, M. A. Pathak, and L. Tanenbaum, *Arch. Dermatol.*, *112*, 943 (1976).
(73) J. W. Melski, L. Tanenbaum, J. A. Parrish, T. B. Fitzpatrick, and H. L. Bleich, *J. Invest. Dermatol.*, *68*, 328 (1977).
(74) L. E. King, Jr., *Arch. Dermatol.*, *111*, 131 (1975).
(75) R. G. Bergstresser, S. H. Schreiber, and G. D. Weinstein, *Arch. Dermatol.*, *112*, 977 (1976).
(76) "Textbook of Dermatology," Vol. 2, 2nd ed., A. Rook, D. S. Wilkinson, and F. J. G. Ebling, Eds., Blackwell Scientific Publications, London, England, 1972, pp. 256-294.
(77) H. Baker, *Br. Med. J.*, *4*, 544 (1973).
(78) D. Munro-Ashman, *Br. J. Clin. Pract.*, *17*, 537 (1963).
(79) L. Fry, *Update Int.*, *1*, 113 (1974).
(80) D. G. C. Presbury, *Update Int.*, *1*, 334 (1974).
(81) R. B. Stoughton, *Arch. Dermatol.*, *92*, 281 (1965).
(82) I. Sarkany, *Nurs. Times*, *1211*, 1212 (1971).
(83) *Product Marketing*, July 1978.
(84) H. Goldschmidt and M. A. Thew, *Arch. Dermatol.*, *106*, 476 (1972).
(85) J. J. Leyden, K. J. McGinley, and A. M. Kligman, *Arch. Dermatol.*, *112*, 333 (1976).

Product (Manufacturer)	Application Form	Keratolytic	Cytostatic Agent	Other
Aeroseb-HC (Herbert)	spray	—	—	hydrocortisone, 0.5%; alcohol, 47.2%
Anti-Dandruff Brylcreem (Beecham)	shampoo	—	zinc pyrithione, 0.1%	mineral oil, propylene glycol, paraffin wax, water, excipients
Breck One (Breck)	cream lotion shampoo	—	zinc pyrithione, 1.0%	anionic surfactants, 15.6%
Cuticura Anti-Dandruff Shampoo (Purex)	shampoo	sulfur, 2% salicylic acid, 2%	—	protein, surfactants
Dalex (Herbert)	shampoo	—	zinc pyrithione, 1%	surfactants
Danex (Herbert)	shampoo	—	zinc pyrithione, 1.0%	sodium methyl cocoyl taurate, magnesium aluminum silicate, sodium cocoyl isethionate, citric acid, fragrance
Diasporal (Doak)	cream	colloidal sulfur, 3% salicylic acid, 2%	—	isopropyl alcohol, 95%
Duponol Shampoo with 10% LCD (C&M)	shampoo	—	—	sodium lauryl sulfate, 15% coal tar, 10%
Head & Shoulders Cream (Procter & Gamble)	shampoo	—	zinc pyrithione, 2%	anionic detergent
Head & Shoulders Lotion (Procter & Gamble)	shampoo	—	zinc pyrithione, 2%	lauryl sulfate, cocamide, ethanolamine, triethanolamine, magnesium aluminum silicate, hydroxypropyl methylcellulose
Ionil (Owen)	shampoo	salicylic acid, 2%	—	polyoxyethylene ethers (nonionic); benzalkonium chloride, 0.2%; alcohol, 12%
Klaron (Dermik)	lotion	colloidal sulfur, 5% salicylic acid, 2%	—	greaseless, hydroalcoholic vehicle; alcohol, 13.1%
Long Aid Sulphur (Keystone)	ointment	sulfur, 2% salicylic acid, 0.5%	—	—
Meted (Texas Pharmacal)	shampoo	sulfur, 3% salicylic acid, 2%	—	highly concentrated detergents
Meted 2 (Texas Pharmacal)	shampoo	colloidal sulfur, 2.3% salicylic acid, 1%	—	mild detergent blend
Neomark (C&M)	lotion	salicylic acid, 1.6% resorcinol monoacetate, 1%	—	coal tar solution, 2%; betanaphthol, 1%; castor oil; isopropyl alcohol, 68%; purified water
Ogilvie (Tussy)	shampoo	—	—	monoundecylenamido MEA-sulfosuccinate disodium
Pernox (Westwood)	shampoo	—	—	sodium laureth sulfate, lauramide DEA, quaternium 22, lanate 25, sodium chloride, lactic acid
pHisoDan (Winthrop)	shampoo	precipitated sulfur, 5% sodium salicylate, 0.5%	—	entsufon sodium, lanolin cholesterols, petrolatum
Resorcitate (Schieffelin)	lotion	salicylic acid, 1.5% resorcinol monoacetate, 1.5%	—	alcohol, 66%
Resorcitate with Oil (Schieffelin)	lotion	salicylic acid, 1.5% resorcinol monoacetate, 1.5%	—	castor oil, 1.5%; alcohol, 81%
Rezamid Tinted (Dermik)	shampoo lotion	microsize sulfur, 2% (shampoo) 5% (lotion) resorcinol, 2% (lotion)	—	chloroxylenol, 0.5% (lotion); alcohol, 28.5% (lotion); salicylic acid, 2% (shampoo)
Rinse Away (Alberto Culver)	liquid	—	—	benzalkonium chloride, 0.05%; laurylisoquinolinium bromide, 0.05%
Sebaquin (Summers)	shampoo	—	—	diiodohydroxyquin, 3%
Sebaveen (Cooper)	shampoo	salicylic acid, 2% sulfur, 2%	—	colloidal oatmeal, 5%; emollients, 4%

Product (Manufacturer)	Application Form	Keratolytic	Cytostatic Agent	Other
Sebb (Max Factor)	shampoo	—	—	*N*-trichloromethylmercapto-4-cyclohexene-1,2-dicarboximide
Sebisol (C&M)	shampoo	salicylic acid, 2%	—	clorophene, 0.1%; betanaphthol, 1%; alkyl aryl surfactant base (biodegradable); aliphatic alcoholamide conditioner; purified water
Sebucare (Westwood)	lotion	salicylic acid, 1.8%	—	laureth-4, 4.5%; alcohol; water; butyl ether; dihydroabietyl alcohol
Sebulex (Westwood)	shampoo	sulfur, 2% salicylic acid, 2%	—	surfactants
Sebutone (Westwood)	shampoo	sulfur, 2% salicylic acid, 2%	—	tar, 0.5%; surfactants; cleansers; wetting agents
Selsun Blue (Abbott)	shampoo	—	selenium sulfide, 1%	surfactants
Soltex (C&M)	shampoo	—	—	clorophene, 0.1%; alkyl aryl surfactant base (biodegradable); aliphatic alcoholamide conditioner; purified water
Sul-Blue (Columbia Medical)	shampoo	—	selenium sulfide, 1%	—
Sulfoam (Alvin Last)	shampoo	sulfur	—	sodium lauryl sulfate, lauramide DEA, glycol stearate, lanolin, citric acid, fragrance, formaldehyde
Sulfur-8 Hair and Scalp Conditioner (Plough)	ointment	sulfur, 2%	—	menthol, triclosan
Sulfur-8 Shampoo (Plough)	shampoo	—	—	triclosan
Thilene (Quality)	lotion	allantoin, 0.25%	—	cleansers, wetting agents, emulsifiers, dispersants
Thylox PDC (Dent)	shampoo	—	—	zinc sulfide, salicylanilide
Vanseb (Herbert)	shampoo	sulfur, 2% salicylic acid, 1%	—	proteins, surfactants
Zincon (Lederle)	shampoo	—	zinc pyrithione, 1%	surfactants

Dry Skin Products

Product (Manufacturer)	Application Form	Keratin Softener	Humectant	Other
Acid Mantle (Dorsey)	cream lotion	—	glycerin	aluminum acetate, water, cetearyl alcohol, sodium lauryl sulfate, petrolatum, synthetic beeswax, mineral oil, methylparaben
Alpha Keri (Westwood)	bath oil	—	—	mineral oil, lanolin oil, polyethylene glycol-4-dilaurate, benzophenone-3, fragrance
Alpha Keri Soap (Westwood)	soap	—	—	nondetergent soap
Aquacare (Herbert)	cream lotion	urea, 2%	glycerin	oleth-3 phosphate, petrolatum, triethanolamine, synthetic spermaceti, carbomer 934P, mineral oil, lanolin alcohol, cetyl stearyl glycol, lanolin oil, benzyl alcohol, perfume
Aquacare/HP (Herbert)	cream lotion	urea, 10%	glycerin	oleth-3 phosphate, cetyl stearyl glycol, petrolatum, triethanolamine, synthetic spermaceti, carbomer 934P, mineral oil, lanolin alcohol, lanolin oil, benzyl alcohol, perfume
Carmol 20 (Ingram)	cream	urea, 20%	—	nonlipid base
Carmol 10 (Ingram)	cream	urea, 10%	—	nonlipid base
Clocream Ointment (Upjohn)	ointment	—	—	vitamins A and D, vanishing cream base
Corn Huskers Lotion (Warner-Lambert)	—	—	glycerin, 6.7%	alcohol, 5.7%; sodium alginate; galactomannan
Dermidol (C&M)	lotion	—	propylene glycol	water, mineral oil, polyethylene glycol 6-32 stearate, cellulose gum, fragrance

Product (Manufacturer)	Application Form	Keratin Softener	Humectant	Other
Emulave (Cooper)	soap	—	glycerin	vegetable oils and dewaxed lanolin, 25%; colloidal oatmeal, 30%
Extra Strength Vaseline Intensive Care (Chesebrough-Ponds)	lotion	—	glycerin	white petrolatum, zinc oxide
Jergens Direct Aid (Jergens)	lotion	allantoin	—	deionized water, sorbitol, stearic acid, glyceryl dilaurate, glyceryl stearate, lard glyceride, stearamide, hydrogenated vegetable oil, isopropyl palmitate, polyethylene glycol 100 stearate, dimethicone, petrolatum, sodium carbomer 941, fragrance, methylparaben, quaternium-15, propylparaben, simethicone, cetearyl alcohol
Jergens for Extra Dry Skin (Jergens)	lotion	allantoin	glycerin	deionized water, glyceryl dilaurate, palm oil glyceride, mineral oil, isopropyl palmitate, stearic acid, dimethicone, methylparaben, sodium carbomer 941, fragrance, propylparaben, cetearyl alcohol, petrolatum
Jergens Hand Cream (Jergens)	cream	allantoin salicylic acid	glycerin	deionized water, stearic acid, alcohol, potassium stearate, propylene glycol dipelargonate, fragrance, lanolin oil, tetrasodium dicarboxyethylstearyl sulfosuccinamate, potassium carbomer 934, methylparaben, polysorbate 81, simethicone, cellulose gum, propylparaben
Jeri-Bath (Dermik)	oil	—	—	dewaxed oil-soluble fraction of lanolin, mineral oil, nonionic emulsifier
Jeri-Lotion (Dermik)	lotion	—	—	dewaxed oil-soluble fraction of lanolin, mineral oil, nonionic emulsifier
Keri Cream (Westwood)	cream	—	—	water, mineral oil, talc, sorbitol, lanolin alcohol, magnesium stearate, glycerol oleate, methylparaben, propylparaben, fragrance
Keri Lotion (Westwood)	lotion	—	—	mineral oil, lanolin oil, water, propylene glycol, glyceryl stearate, polyethylene glycol 40 stearate, polyethylene glycol 100 stearate, polyethylene glycol 40 dilaurate, laureth-4, methylparaben, propylparaben, carbomer 934, triethanolamine, dioctyl sodium sulfosuccinate
Lacti Care (Stiefel)	lotion	—	lactic acid sodium PCA	—
Lowila Cake (Westwood)	cleanser bar	urea	lactic acid	dextrin, sodium lauryl sulfoacetate, boric acid, sorbitol, mineral oil, polyethylene glycol 14-M, cellulose gum, dioctyl sodium sulfosuccinate
Lubriderm (Texas Pharmacal)	cream	—	glycerin	lanolin derivatives, cetyl alcohol, petrolatum blend
Lubriderm Lotion (Texas Pharmacal)	lotion	—	—	lanolin derivatives, mineral oil, sorbitol, cetyl alcohol, triethanolamine stearate
Mammol (Abbott)	ointment	—	—	bismuth subnitrate, 40%
Moisture Cream (C&M)	cream	salicylic acid	glycerin	water, propylene glycol, oxtoxynol-9, fragrance, acid pH
Nutraderm (Owen)	lotion cream	—	—	mineral oil, aliphatic alcohols, balanced emulsifiers
Nutraplus (Owen)	cream lotion	urea, 10%	—	glyceryl stearate, acetylated lanolin, alcohol, isopropyl palmitate
Nutraspa (Owen)	liquid	—	—	dewaxed fraction of lanolin, mineral oil, soapless surfactant
Oilatum Soap (Stiefel)	soap	—	—	polyunsaturated vegetable oil, 7.5%
Saratoga Ointment (Blair)	ointment	—	—	zinc oxide, 14%; boric acid, 1.75%; eucalyptol, 1.1%; servum preparatum; white petrolatum
Sardo (Plough)	bath oil	—	—	mineral oil, isopropyl myristate, isopropyl palmitate
Sardoettes (Plough)	towelettes	—	—	mineral oil, isopropyl myristate, isopropyl palmitate
Sayman Salve (Carson)	ointment	—	propylene glycol	petrolatum, zinc oxide, camphor, lanolin
Shepard's (Dermik)	lotion	—	—	sesame oil
Siliderm (C&M)	lotion	—	glycerin	silicone, nonsensitizing lanolin, purified water, perfume, sorbic acid
Sofenol (C&M)	lotion	—	glycerin	peanut oil, lanolin, cetyl alcohol, stearyl alcohol, purified water, perfume, triethanolamine stearate, sorbic acid
Surfol (Stiefel)	bath oil	—	—	mineral oil, isopropyl myristate

Product (Manufacturer)	Application Form	Keratin Softener	Humectant	Other
Tega E (Ortega)	cream	—	—	vitamin E, 50 IU/g; cream base
Thilene 4-M (Quality Products)	lotion	allantoin, 0.25%	—	cleansers, wetting agents, emulsifiers, dispersants
Triapon (Spirt)	liquid	—	—	olive oil, vegetable oils, nonionic surfactant
Vaseline Pure Petroleum Jelly (Chesebrough-Pond)	gel	—	—	white petrolatum
Wibi (Owen)	lotion	—	—	emulsifying wax, polyglycols, alcohol, menthol, glycerol
Woodbury for Extra Dry Skin (Jergens)	lotion	allantoin	glycerin	deionized water, alcohol, mineral oil, triethanolamine stearate, stearyl alcohol, lanolin, hydrogenated vegetable oil, cetyl alcohol, sodium carbomer 941, methylparaben, propylparaben, fragrance

Eczema and Psoriasis Products

Product (Manufacturer)	Application Form	Keratolytic/ Keratin Softener	Tar Product	Other
Alma Tar (Schieffelin)	bath shampoo	—	juniper tar, 35% (bath) 4% (shampoo)	polyoxyethylene ether, edetate sodium, sulfonated castor oil, coconut oil, triethanolamine (all in shampoo only)
Alphosyl (Reed & Carnrick)	lotion cream	allantoin, 2%	coal tar extract, 5%	hydrophilic base
Balentar (Westwood)	bath	—	tar equiv. to 5% coal tar	mineral oil, lanolin oil
Denorex (Whitehall)	shampoo	—	coal tar solution	menthol; alcohol, 7.5%
DHS Tar (Person & Covey)	shampoo	—	coal tar, 0.5%	cleansing agents
Diasporal-Tar (Doak)	cream	colloidal sulfur, 3% salicylic acid, 2%	tar distillate, 5%	isopropyl alcohol, 90%
Estar (Westwood)	gel	—	tar equiv. to 5% coal tar	hydroalcoholic gel
Ichthyol (Stiefel)	ointment	—	ichthyol, 10%	—
Ionil T (Owen)	shampoo	salicylic acid, 2%	coal tar solution, 5% (equivalent)	polyoxyethylene ethers (nonionic); benzalkonium chloride, 0.2%; alcohol, 12%
Kay-San (Commerce)	cream	allantoin resorcinol	coal tar	sodium salicylate, chloroxylenol
Lavatar (Doak)	bath oil	—	tar distillate, 25%	—
L.C.D. (Schieffelin)	cream	—	coal tar solution, 5.8% (cream)	—
Lipoderm (Spirt)	capsule	—	—	pancreas, 500 mg; pyridoxine hydrochloride, 3 mg
Mazon Cream (Norcliff Thayer)	cream	salicylic acid, 1% resorcinol, 1%	coal tar, 0.18%	benzoic acid, 0.5%
Mazon Shampoo (Norcliff Thayer)	shampoo	sulfur, 1% salicylic acid, 0.5%	coal tar, 0.05%	—
Oxipor VHC (Whitehall)	lotion	salicylic acid	coal tar solution	benzocaine; alcohol, 81%
Packer's Pine Tar (Cooper)	soap	—	pine tar, 6%	soap chips, 93%
Packer's Pine Tar Shampoo (Cooper)	shampoo	—	pine tar, 0.82%	isopropyl alcohol, 2.175%
Pentrax (Texas Pharmacal)	shampoo	—	coal tar, 8.75%	highly concentrated detergents

Product (Manufacturer)	Application Form	Keratolytic/ Keratin Softener	Tar Product	Other
Polytar (Stiefel)	soap bath oil shampoo	—	juniper, pine, and coal tars, 1% (soap, shampoo) 25% (bath oil)	surfactant base (soap, shampoo)
Poslam (Royal)	ointment	sulfur salicylic acid	tar distillate	phenol, 0.035%; zinc oxide; menthol; lanolin
Pragmatar (Smith Kline & French)	cream	salicylic acid, 3% colloidal sulfur, 3%	cetyl alcohol–coal tar, 4%	emulsion base
Psorelief (Columbia Medical)	cream	allantoin salicylic acid	coal tar solution	isopropyl myristate, psoralen
Psorex (Jeffrey Martin)	shampoo	allantoin, 0.2%	coal tar, 2%	surfactants
Psorex Medicated (Jeffrey Martin)	cream shampoo	allantoin, 0.25% (cream) 0.20% (shampoo)	coal tar, 0.50%	silicone base (cream), lanolin and protein base (shampoo), surfactants
Riasol (also known as Dermoil) (Blair)	lotion	—	—	phenol, 0.5%; mercury, 0.45% (as coconut oil soap); cresol, 0.75%
Supertah (Purdue Frederick)	ointment	—	coal tar fraction, 1.25%	zinc oxide, starch
Tarbonis (Reed & Carnrick)	cream	—	coal tar extract, 5%	hydrophilic base
Tar-Doak (Doak)	lotion	—	tar distillate	—
Tarpaste (Doak)	paste	—	tar distillate, 5%	zinc oxide
Tarsum (Summers)	shampoo	salicylic acid, 5%	coal tar solution, 10%	—
Tegrin (Block)	cream lotion shampoo	allantoin, 0.2%	coal tar extract, 5%	—
Tersa-Tar (Doak)	shampoo	—	tar distillate, 3%	—
Vanseb-T (Herbert)	shampoo	sulfur, 2% salicylic acid, 1%	coal tar, 5%	sodium lauryl sulfate, sodium stearate, fatty alkylolamide condensate, hydrolyzed animal protein, polyethylene glycol 75, lanolin, silicone–glycol copolymer, imidazolidinylurea, perfume
Vaseline Pure Petroleum Jelly (Chesebrough-Pond)	gel	—	—	petrolatum, 100%
Zetar (Dermik)	shampoo	—	crude colloidal coal tar, 1%	chloroxylenol, 0.5%

Poison Ivy and Poison Oak Products

Henry Wormser

Chapter 29

Questions to Ask the Patient

Have you been exposed to poisonous plants recently?

Have you had poison ivy/oak/sumac rash before?

How long have you had the rash?

Where is it located? How extensive is it?

Are the lesions weeping?

What treatments have you tried? Were they effective?

Poison ivy, poison oak, or poison sumac dermatitis is a common, seasonal, allergic contact dermatitis. It may be acute or chronic depending on the extent of exposure and the degree of sensitivity to the allergens. Symptoms range from transient redness to severe swelling and the formation of bullae; itching and vesiculation nearly always occur.

SKIN ANATOMY AND PHYSIOLOGY

The skin performs many essential functions, such as protection, temperature regulation, and sensation. It consists primarily of two layers which differ not only in structure but also in embryological origin: the outer and thinnest layer, called the epidermis (originating from the ectoderm), and the dense and thicker dermis (originating from embryonic mesoderm).

The thickness of the epidermis, or cuticle, varies in different areas, from up to 3–4 mm thick on the palms and soles to less than 0.5 mm on the eyelids. Composed of stratified squamous keratinizing epithelium, the epidermis is subdivided into five layers: the outermost horny layer, or stratum corneum; the thin and clear layer, or stratum lucidum; the granular cell layer, or stratum granulosum; the prickle cell layer, or stratum spinosum; and the innermost layer responsible for mitotic growth of the epidermis, the stratum basale, also called the stratum germinativum. Although the epidermis contains no blood vessels, it receives nourishment by way of the tissue fluid derived from the dermal capillaries. The epidermis not only provides mechanical protection of subcutaneous tissues, but also protects them from light by forming melanin and prevents dehydration and osmotic shock.

The dermis, or corium, contributes strength, distensibility, and elasticity to the skin. These features are evident in the swollen extremities of the edematous patient or in the abdominal skin of the obese or pregnant person. The uneven dermal surface is due to the presence of conelike elevations, or papillae, which serve to attach it to the epidermis. The lower portion is called the reticular layer. Both layers (papillary and reticular) contain bundles of collagen and elastic fibers.

In addition to its primary layers, the skin has several appendages: the cutaneous glands (sweat glands and sebaceous glands), the hair and hair follicles, and the nails (1).

ETIOLOGY

Causative Plants

Many chemical substances and products (e.g., nickel and chromium salts, halogenated aromatic chemicals, epoxy resins, and aniline derivatives) cause allergic contact dermatitis. Various plants and parts of plants—trees, grasses, flowers, vegetables, fruits, weeds, and airborne pollen—also may produce this type of allergy (3). Among the 60 or more plants that frequently cause contact dermatitis, those most commonly encountered and responsible for the more severe lesions are poison ivy *(Toxicodendron radicans),* western poison oak *(T. diversilobum),* eastern poison oak *(T. toxicarium),* and poison sumac, or thunderwood (*T. vernix*) (4). Formerly the species were assigned to genus *Rhus,* hence rhus dermatitis. These plants belong to the Anacardiaceae family, members of which are often both noxious and useful and are found in many parts of the world. Members include the Japanese lacquer tree (*Rhus verniciflua*), which grows in Japan, China, and Indochina and from which a rich furniture lacquer is obtained; the cashew nut tree *(Anacardium occidentale),* found in India and Pakistan, the East Indies, Africa, and Central and South America; and the mango tree *(Mangifera indica),* found in tropical areas. Cross-sensitivity may occur on contact of skin with tables painted with natural lacquer, cashew nut shells, and mango rinds.

Poison ivy and poison oak are the main causes of rhus dermatitis in the United States. Poison ivy is particularly abundant in the eastern United States and southeastern Canada. It may be either a shrub or a vine and is identified readily by its characteristic leaves with leaflets arranged in a cluster of three per stalk, by white berries produced in the fall, and by its usual climbing nature (when it is a vine) (Figure 1). Western poison oak is found along the Pacific coast area from New Mexico to Canada. It commonly grows as a bush without support, and the center leaf of the three-leaflet cluster resembles an oak leaf. Eastern poison oak is found from New Jersey to Florida and from central Texas to Kansas. Poison sumac, or poison dogwood, is a coarse, woody shrub or small tree commonly found in swamps of the southern and eastern United States. It differs from the other two plants by having 7–13 leaflets per leaf arranged in two stalks (5).

characteristics and distribution of causative plants

In England and western Europe, primrose dermatitis, due to the sensitizing agent primulin, is more common than poison ivy dermatitis (6). Dark-skinned people seem somewhat less susceptible to these dermatitides than others. Young people are more susceptible than the elderly, and newborns may be sensitized readily by applying the sap of the plant to the body (7). It is estimated that at least 70% of the American population would acquire the poison ivy dermatitis if casually exposed to the plants. However, most estimates show about 40% incidence of the allergy.

toxicodendrol and urushiol

phases of contact dermatitis

Allergenic Constituents

A phenolic oily resin, toxicodendrol, is present in all of the poisonous species and contains a complex active principle, urushiol. Urushiol is distributed widely in the roots, stems, leaves, and fruit of the plant, but not in the flower, pollen, or epidermis (8). Therefore contact with the intact epidermis of the plant is harmless; dermatitis occurs only if contact is made with a bruised or injured plant or its juice. The dermatitis cannot be contracted by emanation per se because neither toxicodendrol nor urushiol is volatile. However, smoke from burning plants carries a substantial amount of the oleoresin and may cause serious reactions in susceptible individuals.

The identification and structure elucidation of poison ivy's allergenic constituents are credited mainly to research (9–11) at Columbia University. Investigators found four antigens, all possessing a 1,2-dihydroxybenzene or catechol nucleus with a 15-carbon atom side chain at position 3. The only difference among the antigens is the degree of unsaturation of the side chain. There is a saturated component (3-pentadecylcatechol, or 3-PDC), a mono-olefin (unsaturated at C-8), a diolefin (unsaturated at C-8 and C-11), and a triolefin (unsaturated at C-8, C-11, and C-14). Certain individuals hypersensitive to 3-pentadecylcatechol show cross-reactivity with other compounds such as resorcinol, hexylresorcinol, and the hydroquinones, but not with phenol itself (12).

It has been reported that as little as 1 μg of crude urushiol causes dermatitis in sensitive individuals (13). Direct contact with the plant is not necessary in a sensitive person; contact with the antigens may be made from an article that injured the plant or from soot particles that contain antigenic material from the plant. Stroking a dog whose hair is contaminated is also a common source of antigens. Contaminated clothing, a frequent source of antigens, is rendered harmless by machine laundering with an effective commercial detergent.

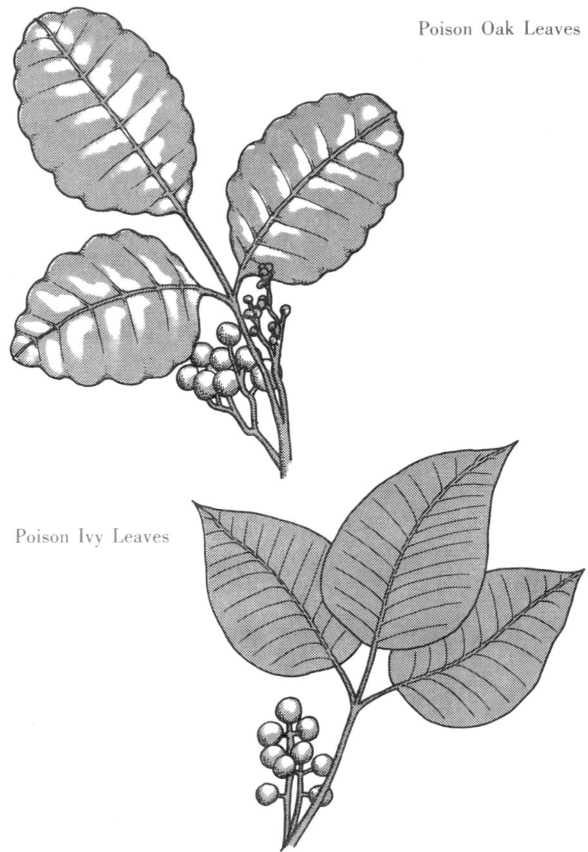

Figure 1. Poison ivy and poison oak leaves.

Although the highest incidence of the dermatitis occurs in the spring and summer months when the leaves are young, soft, and easily bruised, it also may occur in the fall and winter. Fall's yellow leaves still have antigenic properties, but they are more resistant to injury than they were earlier in the season. Once they wither and fall, the leaves are much less antigenic. Winter dermatitis, which occurs most often around Christmas in tree nursery employees and in those who cut their own trees, is due to contact with the plant's roots.

Mechanism of Contact Dermatitis

The natural course of contact dermatitis is divided into two phases: a sensitization phase, during which a specific hypersensitivity to the allergen is acquired, and an elicitation phase, during which subsequent contact with the allergen elicits a visual dermatological response (2). In the sensitization phase, urushiol components combine readily with epidermal proteins to form complete antigens on conjugated proteins. Each conjugate leaves the skin via the lymphatic system and is carried to the reticuloendothelial system, where special globulins and antibodies are synthesized and lymphocytes are sensitized in response to the antigenic stimulus of the conjugate. In the elicitation phase, repeated contact with the allergen again produces the antigenic conjugate, this time causing a noticeable reaction. The reaction appears to be triggered by the association of specific immunological elements carried by the blood to the skin in very low concentration with antigenic conjugates in the papillary dermal layer.

The interval between contact with the antigen and the appearance of the rash varies with the degree of sensitivity and the amount of antigen contacted. Reaction time, the time between contact of sensitized skin with the allergen and the first sign of reaction, is usually not less than 12 hours. This interval is characteristic of delayed hypersensitivity reactions involving cell-mediated immunity.

Lesions vary from simple macules to vesicles and bullae. Contrary to popular belief, fluids in the vesicles and bullae are not antigenic, and patch tests with the fluids give negative reactions. Histologically, nonspecific inflammatory changes occur in the dermis, and spongiosis followed by intraepidermal vesicles is seen in the epidermis in the acute state of the disease. Bursting of the vesicles is a problem, because it may lead to secondary infection.

SIGNS AND SYMPTOMS

Although the limbs, face, and neck are common sites of the dermatitis, all skin areas that come in contact with the sensitizing substance may be affected. Sometimes, distribution of the lesions is bizarre, especially if the antigenic agent is in the clothes or is transferred to various parts of the body by the fingers. Different parts of the body may not have the same sensitivity. Thus the dermatitis may appear first in one area and later in another. The phenomenon is often called "spreading," but this description is inaccurate. Often, parts of the body that may sustain a heavy concentration of the allergen and exhibit more severe reactions remain "hypersensitive" for several years.

The initial reaction following exposure to the antigen is erythema or rash. The development of raised lesions (erythematous macules and papules) follows, and finally, vesicle formation, caused by fluid accumulation in the epidermis. The initial lesions usually are marked by mild to intensive itching and burning. The affected area, often hot and swollen, oozes and eventually dries and crusts (14). Secondary bacterial infections may occur. Very rare complications include eosinophilia, kidney damage, urticaria, dyshidrosis, marked pigmentation, and leukoderma. The majority of cases of the dermatitis are self-limiting and disappear in 14–20 days. Again, disappearance depends on the degree of sensitization and frequency of re-exposure to the allergen.

Rhus dermatitis may be diagnosed not only from the morphological appearance of the lesions but also from their distribution—linear streaking is common and occurs naturally as the result of "brushing" the skin against the poison plant. A history of exposure facilitates the diagnosis. *Toxicodendron* plants are not photosensitizers. The dermatitis occurs on covered and uncovered parts of the body and does not require sunlight to develop.

Diagnostic patch testing is a valuable tool in investigating allergic contact dermatitis (15). However, it should be employed only by individuals thoroughly familiar with accepted techniques. Patch testing should not be done during the acute phase of any dermatitis. It must be understood that substances used for patch testing may sensitize the patient during testing. Positive and negative results of patch testing are not diagnostic in themselves but are interpreted properly in light of the history, the physical findings, and the practitioner's clinical experience.

TREATMENT

The best treatment of poison ivy or poison oak dermatitis is prevention of the condition. Cases of contact dermatitis may be treated either topically or systemically.

Prophylaxis

Topical prophylactic measures used for poison ivy and poison oak dermatitis include removal of the antigen by washing with soap and water or organic solvents, prior use of barrier creams, and/or use of detoxicants (oxidizing and complexing agents that chemically inactivate the antigen) (12). However, many investigators have shown that the benefits derived from these measures are questionable (16–18). Removing the antigen by washing has been largely ineffective, probably because alkyl and alkenyl catechols of the sap, in contact with the skin, readily form a tightly bound complex with one or more specific skin proteins.

A test was made of 34 barrier preparations over a 2-year period on a group of highly sensitive people (12). The preparations were detoxicants that contained substances such as potassium permanganate, hydrogen peroxide, sodium perborate, iodine, and iron and silver salts. The investigator concluded that all the preparations were incapable of preventing the dermatitis. It is inferred by this conclusion that the antigen reacts rapidly and quite selectively with the skin and that irreversible damage occurs before preventive action can be taken. Enthusiastic claims have been made for zirconium oxide, an agent used in many OTC products. However, tests found it completely ineffective (12). In addition, several researchers found extensive, sarcoidlike granulomas of glabrous skin that develop because of allergic hypersensitivity to insoluble zirconium oxide (19–21).

Specific hyposensitization may be tried by administering repeated doses of rhus toxicodendron antigens, but such prophylaxis is neither complete nor permanent; the original sensitivity returns about 6 months after the treatment is stopped (22, 23). Various forms of the plant antigens and several routes of administration have been used. Prophylaxis may be accomplished intramuscularly or orally. For equivalent effects, larger amounts of the oleoresin are required orally than parenterally. Sustained release is probably the major factor in the superior efficacy of the intramuscular route. Orally, there may be inactivation and imperfect absorption. Maximum hyposensitization is obtained with approximately 2–2.5 g im or 2.5–3 g orally of the poison ivy oleoresin antigen. If available, pure (less potent) pentadecylcatechol may

contact dermatitis mechanisms and symptoms

patch testing in diagnosis

prevention—the best treatment

topical prophylactic measures

zirconium oxide effectiveness

hyposensitization

be administered in doses of 2.5–3 g im or 3.5–4 g orally.

Hyposensitization by administering crude extracts or oleoresins from plants usually has been ineffective because extract potency varies and recommended dosages are usually far below those required. Three or four injections cannot provide clinical protection for moderately or extremely sensitive people. An alum-precipitated pyridine extract has been used with a weak to moderate degree of success. The outlook for successful hyposensitization has been improved by the availability of intramuscularly administered 3-pentadecylcatechol. Large amounts (1–3 g) may be needed in a course of 8–20 injections to provide clinical protection. The greater the sensitivity, the larger the amount needed. Administering an antigenic substance to sensitive individuals involves a certain degree of risk. The exact course of treatment must be individualized and geared to the particular sensitivity level and the person's capacity to tolerate the antigen without serious allergic reactions. If the dermatitis appears during prophylactic treatment, the treatment should be stopped for the duration of the eruption. Chewing poison ivy leaves may result in edematous swelling and pain of the tongue, cheeks, palate, pharynx, and anal region (24).

hyposensitization drawbacks

avoiding the allergen

simplicity and safety—keynotes of treatment

treatment objectives

Hyposensitization is temporary, and maintenance doses of the antigen should be administered at predetermined intervals. Hyposensitization generally results in milder and shorter reactions and lessens the reaction's tendency to "spread" to other parts of the body. It is important that the dermatitis be diagnosed properly by a qualified dermatologist before hyposensitization because prophylactic administration of *Toxicodendron* antigens has no effect on contact dermatitis due to other causes. The only objective proof of successful hyposensitization is a negative or weakly positive patch test reaction to the antigens at a previous strongly positive reaction site.

The best prophylaxis for allergic contact dermatitis is complete avoidance of the allergen. People should be taught to recognize and avoid poison ivy and related plants and to observe and search surrounding terrain carefully before choosing a picnic area or campsite. When a poisonous plant is in a garden or cannot be avoided, it should be removed physically or destroyed chemically. The latter method is easier and less dangerous, but there are places where chemicals cannot be used, such as hedges and shrubbery, where the poison ivy is mixed closely with the valuable plants. In such situations, digging and pulling (use gloves!) are the only satisfactory methods. The chemicals most effective against poison ivy include amitrole (aminotriazole), ammonium sulfamate, (2,4-dichlorophenoxy)acetic acid (2,4-D), (2,4,5-trichlorophenoxy)acetic acid (2,4,5-T), ammonium thiocyanate, borax, carbon disulfide, coal tar creosote oils, fuel oil and similar petroleum distillates, sodium chlorate, and sodium arsenite. Chemical sprays may be used at any time when poison ivy is in full leaf, June and July being perhaps the best months. Ordinarily, treatments should begin no later than August 15, since poison ivy then begins to go dormant and sprays are ineffective. At least three to four treatments at an interval of 2–8 weeks are necessary before all plants are dead (25).

Topical and Systemic Therapy

No treatment is effective unless the offending agent is removed so that continued contact is avoided. The most prevalent method of treatment for localized inflammatory reactions is topical. When the reaction is spread over the body and/or is associated with major swelling, systemic treatment is necessary. Systemic treatment always involves prescription drugs such as anti-inflammatory steroids. Prednisone commonly is administered orally over about 7–10 days in a gradually descending dosage schedule. This type of treatment is relatively safe, since it does not lead to hypercorticism or depress adrenal cortical function significantly, as is inevitably the case in more chronic conditions. Corticosteroids in topical forms do not appear very effective in severe cases of poison ivy dermatitis, since these agents cannot penetrate the epithelium of vesicles and bullae, and when such blisters break, the fluid flow simply washes away the drug. Oral antihistamines, which theoretically should be of value, have proven ineffective (2). One of the first precepts of local treatment is to avoid unnecessary local skin irritation; the pharmacist should caution against bathing and scrubbing the lesions frequently and using irritating chemicals, cosmetics, greases, and soaps.

The initial signs and symptoms of the reaction may be alarming, and the temptation to meddle therapeutically is strong. Simplicity and safety are keynotes of treatment. Many claims for products used for self-medication take credit for the body's own natural reparative processes; in most cases, contact dermatitis is self-resolving. The major treatment objectives are:

- To provide protection to the damaged tissue until the acute reaction has subsided;
- To prevent excessive accumulation of debris resulting from oozing, scaling, and crusting, without disturbing normal tissue;
- To relieve itching and prevent excoriation.

Generally, the local treatment should be adapted to the stage or severity of the lesions. During the acute weeping and oozing stage, aluminum acetate, saline, or sodium bicarbonate solution should be used as either soothing or astringent soaks, baths, or wet dressings for 30 minutes, three or four times per day. Shake lotions (e.g., calamine, zinc oxide, and starch) are used at night or when wet dressings are not desirable. Greasy ointments should not be used during active vesiculation and oozing. Creams and ointments should be reserved for subacute and chronic dermatitis.

Large bullae may be drained to reduce discomfort. Aseptic techniques should be used, and the blister punctured at the edge. The tops of the lesions should be kept intact because they protect the underlying, denuded epidermis of the lesions as they dry. The patient should be reassured that the fluid from the lesions will not lead to spreading of the dermatitis, nor will touching someone with the dermatitis transmit the dermatitis. During the healing phase, application of a neutral soothing cream, e.g., cold cream, helps prevent crusting, scaling, and lichenification of the lesions.

Ingredients in OTC Products

Four major types of pharmacological agents—local anesthetics, antipruritics, antiseptics, and astringents—are used in topical OTC products for poison ivy and poison oak dermatitides.

Local Anesthetics

Local anesthetics affect sensation by interfering with the transmission of the action potential along the sensory nerve fiber. Many nerve fibers, specialized endings or receptors, and free nerve endings are in the epidermis. The superficially applied anesthetic acts very near the application site. However, it is questionable whether the agent can reach the nerve endings when applied to unbroken skin. The most commonly used anesthetic in poison ivy/poison oak products is benzocaine. Other products contain diperodon hydrochloride, pramoxine hydrochloride, and tetracaine. Systemic toxic effects attributed to local anesthetics occur at relatively high serum concentrations. Fortunately, these high levels are difficult to obtain by applying topical products now available. A more likely undesirable effect is an allergic one characterized by cutaneous lesions, urticaria, edema, and anaphylactoid reactions. Topically applied "caine" anesthetics are strong sensitizers in susceptible individuals.

Antipruritics

Topically applied antipruritics, which include antihistamines and counterirritants, are agents that alleviate itching. Antihistamines (diphenhydramine, pyrilamine, and methapyrilene) are used essentially as local anesthetics, but like the "caine" anesthetics, they also may be sensitizers. Counterirritants, such as menthol, phenol, and camphor, produce a feeling of coolness and reduce the irritation of the dermatitis. The sensation is difficult to explain because these chemicals produce local hyperemia. However, the counterirritants have a local anesthetic effect.

Antiseptics

Antiseptics used in poison ivy and poison oak products probably are intended for prophylaxis against secondary infections, but their effectiveness is questionable. Of the available antiseptics (phenols, alcohols, and oxidizing agents) and quaternary ammonium compounds such as benzalkonium chloride, the quaternary ammoni-

components of topical products

benzocaine, diperodon, pramoxine, and tetracaine

antihistamines and counterirritants

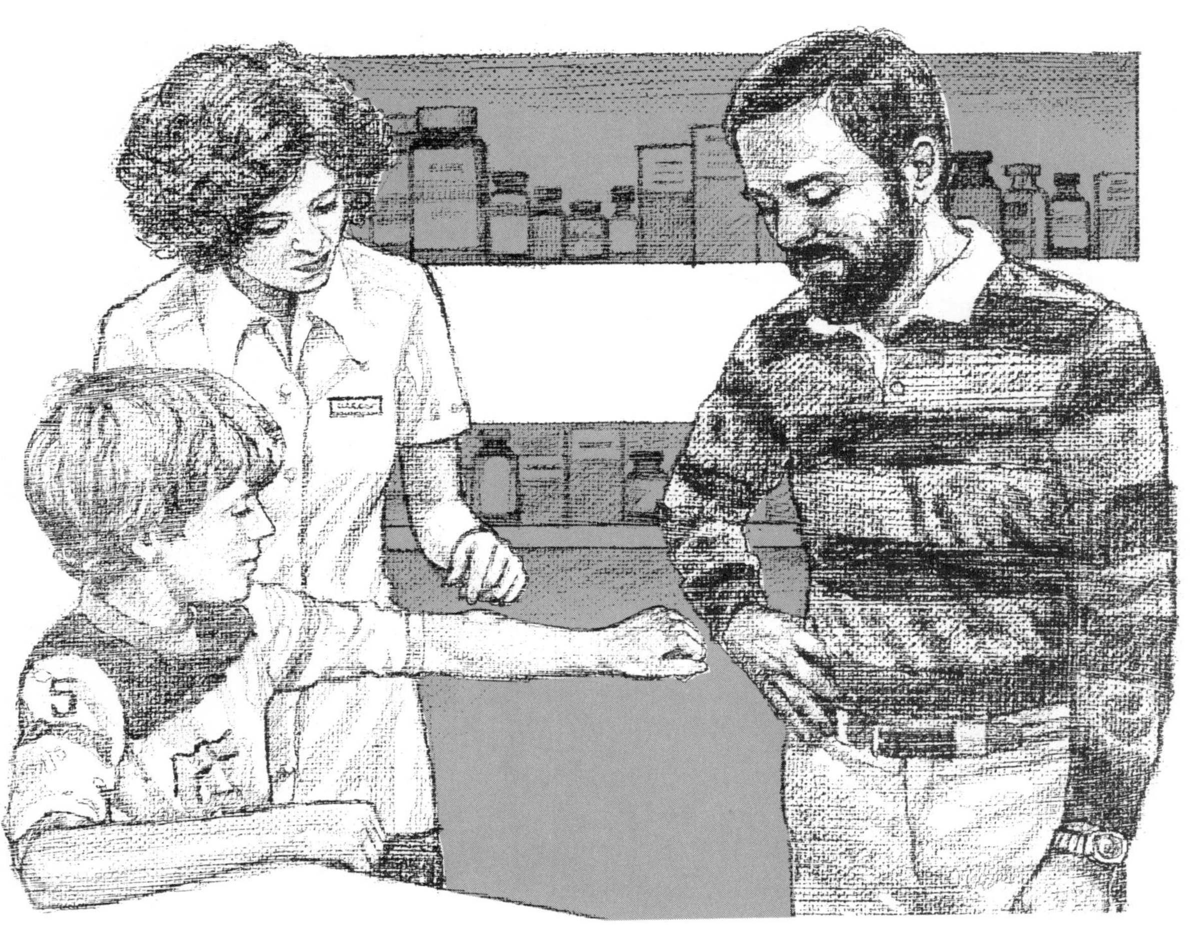

um agents seem more effective. Unfortunately, their action is antagonized by anionic compounds such as soap.

Astringents

Astringents are mild protein precipitants that form a thick coagulum on the surface of lesions or coagulate and remove overlying debris. These substances, which include aluminum acetate, tannic acid, zinc, iron and zirconium oxides, and potassium permanganate, are used to stop oozing, reduce inflammation, and promote healing. Astringents also are antiseptic. Potassium permanganate may not be desirable because it leaves an objectionable stain.

PRODUCT SELECTION GUIDELINES

other agents in topical products

advice to the patient

Selection of products depends on the severity of the dermatitis. Mild to moderately severe cases of poison ivy or poison oak dermatitis usually can be treated with local or topical products. Preparations that contain benzocaine or other local anesthetics or zirconium oxide should be avoided because they may act as sensitizers. Products containing iron salts also should be avoided because they may leave a permanent tattoo. A physician should be consulted in severe cases of poison ivy dermatitis.

Individuals sensitive to *Toxicodendron* plants should be informed of certain cosmetics, hair dyes, bleaches, and other commercial products that contain compounds related to 3-pentadecylcatechol which could exhibit cross-allergenicity. Shake lotions (which may contain phenol or menthol) provide immediate relief due to the cooling effect of water evaporation. Phenol and menthol lengthen the antipruritic activity. However, consultation should include cautioning against the frequent use of shake lotions, which pile masses of plasterlike material on the skin that are difficult and painful to remove. Men with facial dermatitis should shave, because shaving is less uncomfortable and irritating than accumulating crust and debris in the beard. In more severe cases, potassium permanganate baths (1 tsp potassium permanganate crystals per tub of lukewarm water, for 15–20 minutes) should be recommended for their drying effect and the prevention of secondary infection after the vesicles and bullae are open. Colloid baths (oatmeal colloid or a protein complex) also clean and soothe, but they make the tub slippery. If a soap is used, it should be bland.

SUMMARY

Poison ivy, poison oak, and poison sumac cause a contact dermatitis in many people every year. Prophylaxis and therapy of this allergy are still in the early stages of study, although much research is being done and progress is being made. Better understanding of the mechanism of the allergic reaction, of cross-sensitivity, and of hyposensitization will help in designing better products to alleviate and possibly eradicate this annoying and often serious disorder.

REFERENCES

(1) W. Montagna, "The Structure and Function of the Skin," 2nd ed., Academic, New York, N.Y., 1962.

(2) A. L. de Weck, in "Dermatology in General Medicine," T. B. Fitzpatrick, K. A. Arndt, W. H. Clark, Jr., A. Z. Isen, E. J. Van Scott, and J. J. Vaughan, Eds., McGraw-Hill, New York, N.Y., 1971, p. 669.

(3) A. A. Fisher, "Contact Dermatitis," 2nd ed., Lea and Febiger, Philadelphia, Pa., 1973, p. 1.

(4) M. A. Lesser, *Drug Cosmet. Ind.*, *70*, 610 (1952).

(5) C. R. Dawson, *Trans. N.Y. Acad. Sci. Sect. Phys. Chem.*, *18*, 427 (1956).

(6) A. Rook and H. T. H. Wilson, *Br. Med. J.*, *1*, 220 (1965).

(7) A. A. Fisher, "Contact Dermatitis," 2nd ed., Lea and Febiger, Philadelphia, Pa., 1973, p. 260.

(8) J. H. Doyle, *Pediatr. Clin. North Am.*, *8*, 259 (1961).

(9) S. V. Sunthankar and C. R. Dawson, *J. Am. Chem. Soc.*, *76*, 5070 (1954).

(10) W. E. Symes and C. R. Dawson, *J. Am. Chem. Soc.*, *76*, 2959 (1954).

(11) B. Loev and C. R. Dawson, *J. Am. Chem. Soc.*, *78*, 1180 (1956).

(12) A. M. Kligman, *Arch. Dermatol.*, *77*, 149 (1958).

(13) F. A. Stevens, *J. Am. Med. Assoc.*, *127*, 912 (1945).

(14) P. M. Selfon, *Mil. Med.*, *128*, 895 (1963).

(15) A. M. Kligman, *J. Invest. Dermatol.*, *47*, 369, 375, 393 (1966).

(16) B. Shelmire, *J. Am. Med. Assoc.*, *113*, 1085 (1939).

(17) O. Gisvold, *J. Am. Pharm. Assoc. Sci. Ed.*, *30*, 17 (1941).

(18) J. B. Howell, *Arch. Dermatol. Syphitol.*, *48*, 373 (1943).

(19) P. J. LoPresti and G. W. Hambrick, Jr., *Arch. Dermatol.*, *92*, 188 (1965).

(20) W. L. Epstein and J. R. Allen, *J. Am. Med. Assoc.*, *190*, 940 (1964).

(21) N. A. Hall, *J. Am. Pharm. Assoc.*, *NS12*, 576 (1972).

(22) A. M. Kligman, *Arch. Dermatol.*, *78*, 47 (1958).

(23) *Ibid.*, p. 359.

(24) S. H. Silvers, *J. Am. Med. Assoc.*, *116*, 2257 (1941).

(25) D. M. Crooks and L. W. Kephart, "Farmers' Bulletin," No. 1972, U.S. Department of Agriculture, Washington, D.C., 1951, 30 pp.

Product (Manufacturer)	Application Form	Anesthetic	Antipruritic/ Antihistamine	Antiseptic	Astringent	Other
Albitox (Pfeiffer)	lotion spray	benzocaine, 3%	—	benzalkonium chloride, 1:750 (lotion) chloroxylenol, 0.5% (spray)	—	alcohol
Americaine (Arnar-Stone)	spray	benzocaine, 10%	—	benzethonium chloride, 0.1%	—	alcohol
Caladryl (Parke-Davis)	cream lotion	—	diphenhydramine hydrochloride, 1% camphor, 0.1%	—	calamine	alcohol, 2% (lotion)
Calamatum (Blair)	ointment lotion spray	benzocaine, 3%	camphor	phenol	zinc oxide calamine	—
Calamox (Mallard)	ointment	—	camphor, 0.5%	phenol, 0.5%	calamine, 20% zinc oxide, 10%	pyrilamine maleate, 1%
Caleate (Elder)	ointment	—	—	—	neocalamine, 4.4% zinc oxide, 4.4%	pyrilamine maleate, 0.125%
CZO (Elder)	lotion	—	—	—	calamine, 65 mg/ml zinc oxide, 65 mg/ml	glycerin aromatics
Dalicote (Dalin)	lotion	diperodon hydrochloride, 0.25%	pyrilamine maleate camphor	—	zinc oxide	dimethyl poly-siloxane silicone greaseless base
Dermapax (Recsei)	lotion	—	pyrilamine maleate, 0.22% methapyrilene hydrochloride, 0.22% chlorpheniramine maleate, 0.06%	chlorobutanol, 1% benzyl alcohol, 1%	—	isopropyl alcohol, 40%
Didelamine (Commerce)	gel	—	tripelennamine hydrochloride methapyrilene hydrochloride menthol	benzalkonium chloride	—	clear gel
Dri Toxen (Walker Corp)	cream	—	methapyrilene hydrochloride, 1% menthol, 0.5%	phenol, 1%	zinc oxide, 10% zinc sulfate, 0.5%	washable grease-less base
Hist-A-Balm Medicated Lotion (Columbia Medical)	lotion	diperodon hydrochloride, 0.25%	phenyltoloxamine dihydrogen citrate, 0.75% menthol camphor	benzalkonium chloride, 0.1%	—	—
Hista-Calma Lotion (Rexall)	lotion	benzocaine, 1%	phenyltoloxamine dihydrogen citrate, 1%	—	calamine	—
Ivarest (Carbisulphoil-Blistex)	cream lotion	benzocaine, 1%	pyrilamine maleate, 1.5% menthol, 0.7% camphor, 0.3%	—	calamine, 10% zirconium oxide, 4%	—
Ivy-Chex (Bowman)	aerosol	—	—	benzalkonium chloride, 1:1000	—	alcohol acetone polyvinylpyrrolidone-vinyl acetate copolymers

Product (Manufacturer)	Application Form	Anesthetic	Antipruritic/ Antihistamine	Antiseptic	Astringent	Other
Ivy Dry Cream (Ivy)	cream	benzocaine	menthol camphor	—	tannic acid, 8%	methylparaben propylparaben isopropyl alcohol, 7.5%
Ivy Dry Liquid (Ivy)	liquid	—	—	—	tannic acid	isopropyl alcohol, 12.5%
Ivy-Rid (Mallard)	aerosol	—	—	benzalkonium chloride	—	alcohol acetone isobutane methylene chloride polyvinylpyrrolidone-vinyl acetate copolymers
Ivy Supra Dry (Ivy)	liquid	benzocaine	menthol camphor	—	tannic acid	isopropyl alcohol, 35% methylparaben propylparaben
Neoxyn (Rorer)	solution	—	—	hydrogen peroxide, 2.85% benzethonium chloride, 0.26%	—	acetic acid, 1.15% propylparaben, 0.02% acetanilide, 0.0169%
Nupercainal Cream (Ciba)	cream	dibucaine, 0.5%	—	—	—	acetone sodium bisulfite, 0.37% water-washable base
Nupercainal Ointment (Ciba)	ointment	dibucaine, 1%	—	—	—	acetone sodium bisulfite, 0.5%
Obtundia Calamine Cream (Otis Clapp)	cream	—	—	cresol–camphor complex	calamine zinc oxide	—
Peterson's Ointment (Peterson's Ointment Co.)	ointment	—	camphor, 3.88%	phenol, 2.50%	zinc oxide, 6.60% tannic acid, 2.20%	beeswax, 4% lavender oil petrolatum
Poison Ivy Cream (McKesson)	cream	benzocaine, 2.5%	pyrilamine maleate	povidone	zirconium oxide, 4% (as carbonated hydrous zirconia)	—
Poison Ivy Spray (McKesson)	aerosol	benzocaine, 0.5%	menthol camphor	—	calamine, 2% zinc oxide, 1%	isopropyl alcohol, 9.44%
Pontocaine (Breon)	cream ointment	tetracaine hydrochloride, (equivalent to 1% base) (cream) base, 0.5% (ointment)	menthol, 0.5% (ointment)	—	—	methylparaben (cream) sodium bisulfite (cream) white petrolatum (ointment) white wax (ointment)
Pyribenzamine (Ciba)	cream ointment	—	tripelennamine, 2%	—	—	water-washable base (cream) petrolatum base (ointment)
Rhuli Cream (Lederle)	cream	benzocaine, 1%	menthol, 0.7% camphor, 0.3%	—	zirconium oxide, 1%	isopropyl alcohol, 8.8%
Rhuligel (Lederle)	gel	—	menthol, 0.3% camphor, 0.3%	benzyl alcohol, 2%	—	alcohol, 31%
Rhulihist (Lederle)	lotion	benzocaine, 1.153%	camphor, 0.253% menthol, 0.025%	benzyl alcohol, 0.674%	calamine, 4.710%	alcohol, 28.76%
Rhuli Spray (Lederle)	spray	benzocaine, 0.98%	camphor, 0.098% menthol, 0.009%	—	zirconium oxide, 1% calamine, 0.98%	isopropyl alcohol, 9.5%

Product (Manufacturer)	Application Form	Anesthetic	Antipruritic/ Antihistamine	Antiseptic	Astringent	Other
Surfadil (Lilly)	cream lotion	cyclomethycaine, 0.5%	methapyrilene hydrochloride, 2%	—	—	titanium dioxide, 5% (lotion)
Topic (Ingram)	gel	benzyl alcohol, 5%	camphor menthol	—	—	isopropyl alcohol, 30% greaseless base
Tronothane Hydrochloride (Abbott)	cream jelly	pramoxine hydrochloride, 1%	—	—	—	water-miscible base
Tyrohist Cream (Columbia Medical)	cream	benzocaine	pyrilamine maleate camphor menthol	benzalkonium chloride	neocalamine	—
Ziradryl (Parke-Davis)	lotion	—	diphenhydramine hydrochloride, 2% camphor, 0.1%	—	zinc oxide, 2%	alcohol, 2%
Zotox (Commerce)	spray	benzocaine	menthol camphor	—	calamine zinc oxide	isopropyl alcohol

Diaper Rash and Prickly Heat Products

Gary H. Smith

Chapter 30

Questions to Ask the Patient

Diaper Rash	*Prickly Heat*
How often do you change the diaper?	*What is the temperature of the infant's room?*
Do you use disposable or cloth diapers?	*Is the rash associated with increased temperature?*
Do you use a diaper service?	*Where is the rash located?*
What type of lesion is present?	*How long has the rash been present?*
What products have you tried?	*Is any treatment being used now? If so, what?*

Diaper rash and prickly heat (miliaria rubra) are acute, transient, inflammatory skin conditions that occur in nearly all infants and young children. Both conditions are unpleasant to the child. They cause burning and itching which result in restlessness, irritability, and sleep interruption. Prevention is the best treatment, but most cases are reversed easily by simple home remedies.

The skin of most adults is about 2 mm thick, but infant skin is considerably thinner, i.e., about 1 mm. The epidermis (the outermost skin layer) represents about 5% of the total skin thickness; therefore the external barrier that protects the infant from the environment is very thin (1). (See Chapter 26 for a discussion of skin anatomy.) The main functions of the skin are:

- To retard the loss of body fluids to the external environment;
- To retard the exchange of fluids between the body and the environment;
- To protect the body from external factors, such as heat, bacteria, fungi, and chemical toxins.

For the skin to function most efficiently, it should remain dry, smooth, and at a low pH.

DIAPER RASH

Diaper rash, or diaper dermatitis, is one of the most common dermatitides in infants. It is an acute, inflammatory reaction of the skin in the diaper area caused by one or more factors. One report indicated a 17% incidence in week-old infants (2).

Etiology

The histopathological changes vary with the causative factors and the severity of the dermatitis. Several predisposing factors that should be considered include inherited skin anomalies (e.g., hypersensitive skin and seborrheic diathesis) and systemic diseases (e.g., syphilis), acrodermatitis, chronica enteropathica, Letterer–Siwe disease, and gastroenteritis causing frequent stools, all of which may lower skin resistance (3, 4).

Normal newborns begin urinating within 24 hours after birth. They urinate up to 20 times per day until 2 months of age and as many as 8 times per day from 2 months to 8 years of age. Defecation also occurs several times per day (5). Breast-fed infants tend to urinate less frequently and have a lower incidence of dermatitis than bottle-fed infants, because of the lower alkalinity of the urine and feces (6, 7).

Diaper rash begins between folds of skin, e.g., between the buttocks or between the scrotum and the thighs. It may spread to the entire diaper area, depending on when therapy begins and what caused the rash. The diaper area is vulnerable to inflammation because the skin is often warm and moist and is exposed to irritants and bacteria. Diaper rash may range from mild erythema with maceration and chafing to nodular, infiltrated lesions that may become vesicular, pustular, and bullous, depending on the primary cause of the dermatitis. The causative factors of diaper rash include ammonia, sweat retention, mechanical and chemical irritants, and secondary infections and complications.

Ammonia

The most widely accepted theory of the etiology of diaper rash is the presence of ammonia and other end products of the enzymatic breakdown of the urine. Ammoniacal dermatitis was described first in 1886 (8), and other reports followed in the early 1900's (9, 10). Later, it was determined that ammonia in the diaper area was produced by urea-splitting bacteria found in the stool (11). The causative organism, *Bacillus ammoniagenes*, was isolated from stool samples of 31 children with diaper rash. This aerobic, nonmotile, gram-positive bacillus is a saprophyte that can ferment urea to produce ammonia as follows:

$$CO(NH_2)_2 + 2H_2O \rightleftharpoons (NH_4)_2CO_3 \rightleftharpoons 2NH_3 + H_2O + CO_2$$

Ammonia causes diaper rash because it raises the pH and forms soaps with some constituents of the natural skin oils.

A later study found a close correlation between urine's odor and its ability to produce erythema, regardless of the urinary pH (12). This extensive study showed that malodorous putrescent materials, in the absence of ammonia and high pH, may cause erythema. These materials also are produced by enzymatic degradation in the urine. Urine causes diaper dermatitis characterized by the pungent odor of ammonia and erythematous papules on the buttocks, the inner surface of the thighs, and other sites in the diaper area.

role of ammonia in diaper rash

contributing factors

secondary bacterial and fungal infections

causative organisms

Sweat Retention

If a soiled diaper is not changed promptly, the stratum corneum in the diaper area becomes waterlogged. This saturation causes keratotic plugging of the sweat glands (plugging with loose protein material on the skin), which results in sweat retention and may cause erythematous papules (13).

Mechanical and Chemical Irritants

Tightly fitting diapers covered with plastic pants increase the humidity and temperature in the diaper area and keep air away from the skin, producing an environment conducive to irritation. If diapers are changed frequently, irritation may be prevented. Irritation results from the diaper's constant rubbing against the skin. Feces remaining in contact with the skin cause irritation, especially if the infant's diet promotes the elimination of irritating substances. Preparations commonly applied to the diaper area, such as proprietary antiseptic agents and harsh soaps containing mercury, phenol, tars, salicylic acid, or sulfur, also may cause diaper rash. Diapers rinsed inadequately after washing may irritate the diaper area or cause an allergic reaction. Improper rinsing of the diaper area after bathing may leave an irritating soapy residue. Therefore precautions should be taken to avoid exposing the sensitive skin of infants and young children to these irritating substances (4, 13).

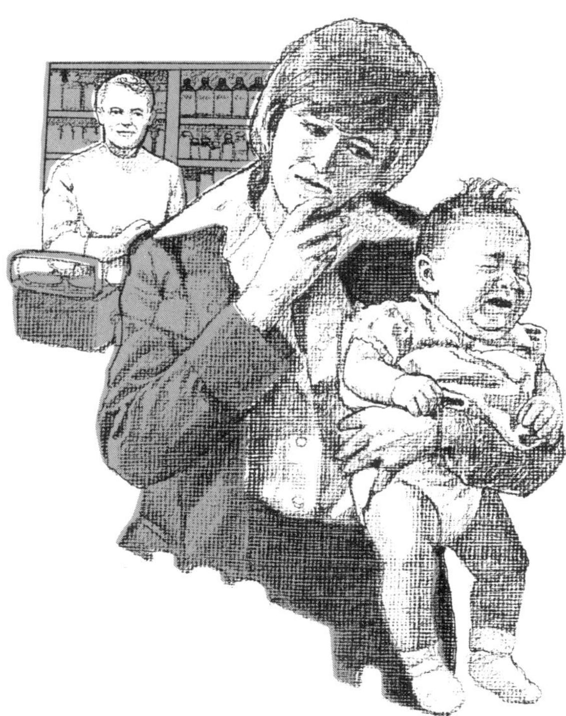

Complications

Fungal and bacterial infections are the most common complications of diaper rash. These cutaneous infections usually result from untreated or improperly treated diaper dermatitis. The moist, warm, alkaline environment created by unchanged diapers is conducive to the development and multiplication of many pathogenic bacteria and fungi (14). Most bacteria and fungi do not produce lesions on normal skin. However, if the skin is broken or macerated or the normal balance of the skin's bacterial flora is disturbed, these organisms may become pathogenic and cause a serious infection in the diaper area (6).

Fungal infections are caused most commonly by *Candida albicans*, an organism that is part of the normal colonic flora. The stool therefore is the most common source of this organism (14). Because monilial infections of the diaper area are usually a complication of ammoniacal diaper dermatitis, the clinical picture is often obscure, and the only precise method of diagnosis is finding *C. albicans* in scrapings and cultures from the skin lesions (15). In newborns less than 2 weeks old, monilial diaper dermatitis usually is accompanied by oral thrush. Both conditions probably result from the mother's having had a *Candida* vaginal infection before and during delivery. Monilial dermatitis is characterized by lesions in the groin, intergluteal fold, and lower abdomen. The lesions usually are eroded and weeping and are surrounded by satellite pustules. A physician should be consulted for appropriate treatment of this condition.

Bacterial infection of the diaper area is caused most commonly by *Staphylococcus* and is often a form of folliculitis. The lesions are pinhead-sized or slightly larger pustules surrounded by a narrow area of erythema. They may coalesce to form an area of infectious eczematoid dermatitis. Occasionally, bullous impetigo (also staphylococcal in origin) may occur. In some cases, Group A *Streptococcus* may be the pathogen, and glomerulonephritis may develop. As with monilia, if a bacterial infection in the diaper area is suspected, a physician should be consulted for appropriate diagnosis and therapy (16).

Ulceration of the penile meatus may be a painful complication of diaper rash in circumcized babies. The pain associated with this condition leads to reflex inhibition of micturition and secondary distention of the bladder (17, 18).

Diaper rash also may accompany other dermatological conditions, such as eczema, seborrheic dermatitis, or systemic disease.

PRICKLY HEAT

The lesions associated with this acute dermatitis result from obstruction of the sweat gland ducts. Sweat retained behind the obstruction causes the dilation and rupture of the epidermal sweat duct, which produces swelling and inflammation. The term "prickly heat" was coined because the lesions usually produce itching and stinging. Prickly heat occurs primarily during hot, humid weather or during a febrile illness with heavy sweating. It also may occur as a result of overclothing and overcovering at night in warm rooms.

The lesions appear in areas of maceration and under plastic pants, diapers, adhesive tape, or anything that occludes the sweat gland duct. The lesions, which are erythematous and papulovesicular, occur most frequently on the cheeks, neck, trunk, and skin folds and in the diaper area (3, 19, 20).

DIAPER RASH VS. PRICKLY HEAT

In general, if the diaper dermatitis is confined to the diaper area and does not present signs or symptoms of fungal or bacterial infection, the pharmacist may recommend OTC therapy. If the infant has had diaper rash for only a few days, the diapers smell of ammonia, and the diapers have not been changed frequently, self-treatment may be recommended. The pharmacist should determine whether laundry detergents that contain irritants are being used. If diaper rash persists 1 week or more after the infant has been treated with protectants and has been changed frequently, the rash may be caused by a problem other than the diaper, and a physician should be consulted. If the infant has had consistent diarrhea, has awakened frequently, and is resistant to OTC treatment, a physician should be consulted because the problem may be more serious than simple diaper rash.

If the rash is more widespread than the diaper area (groin, intergluteal fold, or lower abdomen), the infant may be hypersensitive to food in the diet, and the cause of the allergy should be ascertained by a physician. Eroded, weeping lesions surrounded by satellite pustules may be secondary to *Candida* infection; a definitive diagnosis should be made by a physician. If the lesions are of the pinhead kind and bullous or look like impetigo, a bacterial infection may be the cause.

The pharmacist may be able to recognize the cause of many conditions by questioning the parents. In addition to explaining the steps that must be taken to prevent diaper rash and prickly heat, the pharmacist may recommend several products suited to the child's condition. If the pharmacist ascertains that the dermatitis has persisted and appears to be complicated by infection or another process, it should be suggested that the child be taken to a physician.

TREATMENT

The treatments for diaper rash and prickly heat may be considered together. The active treatment of diaper rash involves removing the source of irritation, reducing the immediate skin reaction, relieving discomfort, and preventing secondary infection and other complications. The treatment plan should be individualized for both diaper rash and prickly heat. Products helpful in treatment include protectants, agents to promote healing, antiseptics, and antifungal and anti-inflammatory agents. The pharmacist is in a good position to advise parents which products should be used for a particular kind of dermatitis. As with most forms of therapy, the simplest regimen is the one most likely to be followed by parents. A baby's skin is sensitive, and many babies may be allergic to some available products.

In treating mild forms of diaper rash the best remedy is changing diapers frequently and leaving diapers off during naps, so that the buttocks are exposed to the air. An incandescent lamp also was recommended as a heat source that may speed healing (21, 22). A lamp with a 25-W bulb should be placed about 30 cm from the buttocks. The condition of infants with ammoniacal dermatitis improved when they were exposed to air as often as possible. Parents should be warned not to hold the bulb too close to the buttocks because of the danger of burning the skin. In other respects, treatment is the same as for mild cases and includes the use of a good protective agent such as zinc oxide paste (Lassar's paste) or white petrolatum.

characteristics of prickly heat

differentiating diaper rash and prickly heat

treatment plan

Prescription-only corticosteroid creams and ointments also are used in treating severe diaper dermatitis and prickly heat. However, several studies showed systemic effects resulting from percutaneous absorption of steroids after topical application (23–25). Occlusive dressings facilitate the absorption of topically applied steroids through normal (not inflamed) skin (23). When steroid creams are applied topically to inflamed or abraded skin, systemic levels may be higher than when they are applied to normal skin (24). Because of the large absorptive area of diaper rash and the covering of the area with a diaper, infants treated with topical steroids may experience systemic steroid effects resulting from adrenal suppression. Using topical steroids to treat diaper dermatitis should be discouraged. These products should be used only for the most severe cases, and then only for short periods.

Removal of Irritants

When irritants cause diaper rash, they should be avoided if possible. The theory that various foods cause a higher incidence of diaper rash has not been substantiated. In a study of 1184 infants there was no significant difference in diaper rash between infants fed an iron-fortified formula and those fed formulas without iron (26). If an infant displays hypersensitivity to a particular food, a rash may appear, but it is not confined to the diaper area.

Treatment of Secondary Complications

Secondary infections caused by bacteria or fungi should be diagnosed and treated by a physician. Various antiseptic agents have been used to treat *Staphylococcus*- and *Streptococcus*-induced infections. These infections usually respond to local treatment with neomycin, bacitracin, and polymyxin B sulfate. Quaternary ammonium chloride compounds often are included in commercial products. However, their antibacterial action has been questioned, and they may not be effective. In addition, these compounds may act as irritants in some cases, exacerbating the inflammation (27). Aluminum acetate (Burow's) solution also is used for its astringent action. All of these agents may be irritating to an infant's skin, causing discomfort when applied. Antibiotic ointments, especially neomycin, should be used only when clearly indicated because they may cause hypersensitivity reactions (28).

In *Candida*-induced diaper rash the use of antifungal agents may be necessary. Aluminum acetate solution soaks may be used for severe dermatitis followed by the application of nystatin dusting powder or ointment at a concentration of 100,000 units/g (15, 29). A 2% amphotericin B ointment also is effective (30). Hydroxyquinoline is applied topically for its antibacterial and antifungal activity. Calcium undecylenate is used for its antifungal activity. Nystatin, amphotericin B, and hydroxyquinoline are prescription-only products (except for Bagbalm); aluminum acetate solution and calcium undecylenate are available over the counter.

treating secondary bacterial and fungal infections

components of OTC products

petroleum jelly and zinc oxide paste

talc and magnesium stearate

boric acid and other antiseptics

Ingredients in OTC Products

OTC products for diaper rash and prickly heat treatment include protectants, powders, and antiseptics.

Protectants

Before a dry diaper is put on, a thin layer of petroleum jelly, zinc oxide paste (Lassar's paste), or some other similar preparation should be applied as a protectant. Zinc oxide, an excellent protectant found in many products used to treat diaper rash and prickly heat, is a mild astringent with weak antiseptic properties. Plain white petrolatum serves the same purpose and is less expensive and easier to remove from the diaper and skin. Many products contain various concentrations of zinc oxide and petrolatum. Zinc oxide paste USP, the simplest of these formulations, contains 25% zinc oxide, 25% corn starch, and 50% white petrolatum. This combination serves as a highly water immiscible base. Many commercial preparations contain zinc oxide, in some cases at a higher concentration than Lassar's paste (Desitin contains 40% zinc oxide), but most of these preparations also contain one or more of various other medicaments such as cod liver oil, vitamins A and D, lanolin, peruvian balsam, and silicone.

In general, these various products are popular and are promoted primarily for the treatment of diaper rash and prickly heat. Only recently have there been controlled studies with these products (31–33). Recent reports from Leeming/Pacquin (32, 33) showed Desitin Ointment to be superior to bland soap and unmedicated talcum powder in the treatment of diaper rash. Only one report has been published that compares one product with the other (33). In this report, Lantiseptic Ointment (Corona) in a controlled study was shown to be equal or superior to vitamin A and D ointment in the treatment of diaper rash. While several anecdotal reports indicate that vitamin A and D ointment or cod liver oil containing ointments may be beneficial in preventing and treating diaper rash (34–37), no evidence exists that indicates any of these products to be superior to zinc oxide paste or white petrolatum. Therefore zinc oxide paste or white petrolatum should be recommended as a protectant and as initial treatment for diaper rash. Use of these products avoids subjecting the infant to compounds that may cause skin sensitization.

Powders

The powdered agents used in treating diaper rash and prickly heat are talc and magnesium stearate. Talc is a natural hydrous magnesium silicate that allays irritation, prevents chafing, and absorbs sweat. Talc is similar to ointments and creams in that it adheres well to the skin. Magnesium stearate is included in some dusting powders promoted for infant use because of its ability to adhere to the skin and to serve as a mechanical barrier to irritants. When applied after each changing, these products serve primarily to keep the diaper area dry. They should be used cautiously because inhalation of the dust by the infant may be harmful and could lead to chemical pneumonia.

Antiseptics

Boric acid has been used extensively in the past for its bacteriostatic and fungistatic activity in diaper dermatitis and prickly heat treatment. It has been incorporated into ointments in concentrations of as much as 3% and into dusting powders. However, there have been reports of toxicity and, in two instances, death associated with boric acid use (38, 39). In one quantitative study of 16 infants, boron levels were significantly high in infants treated with 3% boric acid/borate ointments (40). Concern about boron toxicity has prompted the American Academy of Pediatrics Committee on Drugs to recommend to the FDA that products containing boric acid be reformulated, eliminating boric acid as an ingredient.

Most recently, Lantiseptic Ointment has been investigated for the treatment of diaper rash (33). Lantiseptic contains an organic compound. *p*-chloromercuriphenol (1:1500), in a lanolin and petrolatum base that appears to reduce or eliminate most fungus and bacteria from the diaper area. In a controlled study of 39 cases of diaper rash in which Lantiseptic was compared to vitamin A and D ointment, Lantiseptic, in all cases, was equal or superior to the vitamin A and D ointment in improving the diaper rash (31). This product, which has been used for more than 70 years in veterinary medicine, only recently has been used in the treatment of human skin irritations. Another veterinary product recently used in diaper rash is Bagbalm, which contains 8-hydroxyquinoline sulfate in a petrolatum and lanolin base.

Methods of Prevention

Diaper rash and prickly heat exemplify well the old saying, "An ounce of prevention is worth a pound of cure." Good prophylactic practices depend on parental cooperation and responsibility. Common sense is perhaps the best guide for preventive therapy.

A diaper should be changed as soon as it is soiled; leaving a wet diaper on for several hours increases the chances of diaper rash. Diapers should be made of soft material and fastened loosely to prevent rubbing. Plastic pants should be used as seldom as possible, since they impede the passage of air through the diaper, and their use at night should be discouraged.

Diapers cleaned by a diaper service were associated with the lowest incidence of diaper rash (24.4%), disposable diapers showed a similar low incidence (25%), and home-laundered diapers were associated with the greatest incidence (35.6%) (41). The home-laundered diapers were not rinsed with a bacteriostatic agent. These reports show the necessity of using a bacteriostatic agent either in the rinse water or in the diaper pail. Diapers containing fecal material should be rinsed well in the toilet before they are placed in the diaper pail. Commercial diaper services provide essentially sterile diapers. Although disposable diapers were comparable in this study, their routine use should be discouraged because they have a plastic covering that reduces the amount of air available to the skin under the diaper.

The prevention of prickly heat consists of eliminating the cause—overheating. Overclothing and overcovering of infants should be avoided. Light clothing and covering are recommended to allow air to reach the skin. In hot weather, frequent removal of clothes for relatively short periods helps to keep the skin dry. Air conditioning the environment helps lower humidity and temperature. Perspiration may be reduced by frequent bathing or sponge baths and the use of bland dusting powder. Oatmeal (1 cup of Aveeno Colloidal Oatmeal in a tub of warm water) and soy protein (1 packet of protein colloidal bath powder in a tub of warm water) also may help in treating prickly heat.

Infants often urinate soon after they are put to bed for the night. Parents can reduce the time a child is exposed to a wet diaper and the amount of urine accumulated at night by changing the diaper within several hours after putting the child to bed.

The diaper area should be cleaned at each diaper change. A mild ointment or dusting powder (such as white petrolatum or talcum powder) may be recommended after washing. Mild soap (Oilatum or a commercial baby soap) should be used for cleaning the diaper area and for bathing. It is important that skin folds that entrap sweat and feces be cleaned thoroughly and rinsed well with clean water. The diaper area should be completely dry before a clean diaper is put on. Exposing the diaper area to warm, dry air for a few minutes between changes helps to keep the skin dry.

To prevent ammoniacal diaper rash, it is important to keep urea-splitting bacteria at a minimum. Several reports dealt with the use of antibacterial compounds in laundering diapers. If home-laundered diapers are used, they should be soaked in a solution of Borax (½ cup Borax per gallon of water) before washing (21). Other antibacterial compounds that can be used for presoaking, to reduce odor, and to disinfect diapers are quaternary ammonium compounds or a diluted sodium hypochlorite solution. Diapers should be washed with mild soap. The use of harsh detergents and water softeners should be avoided. After they are washed, the diapers should be rinsed thoroughly and, if possible, dried outside in the sun.

If an antibacterial presoak is not used, a disinfectant should be used during the washing process. A 5.25% sodium hypochlorite bleach (Clorox) properly diluted reduced the number of organisms from 277/in^2 to 2/in^2 (42). The use of clorophene [(*o*-benzyl-*p*-chloro)phenol] in the first rinse of diapers in a concentration of 1 part chlorophene to 2500 parts water also is effective in treating and preventing ammoniacal diaper dermatitis (43).

PRODUCT SELECTION GUIDELINES

recommendations for prevention

advice to parents

Pharmacists should advise parents about the correct use of any product recommended. Some general precautions should be mentioned, such as expiration dates on antimicrobial ointments and the possibility of stinging and irritation when the ointment is applied. If powders are recommended, parents should be instructed to apply them carefully to prevent the infant from inhaling the powder, which could lead to chemical pneumonia. When soaks and solutions (such as aluminum acetate solution) are used, the unused portion should be discarded after each use; i.e., only fresh preparations should be used each time.

Above all, pharmacists should caution parents about the general use of any medication for a baby's skin. The best therapy for diaper dermatitis is keeping the skin clean and dry.

Few infants escape diaper rash. The pharmacist may help by teaching parents the proper procedures for preventing diaper rash and prickly heat. Parents should understand that using medications indiscriminately is not the proper way to treat either condition and is ill advised. Drugs alone cannot stop or prevent diaper rash or prickly heat. Many newborns, infants, and young children may be hypersensitive to various medicaments, and more harm than good can result from their use. Diaper dermatitis may be inadvertently induced by the overuse of medications (especially those containing sulfonamides, neomycin, and other sensitizing antibacterial agents). This condition has been referred to as "dermatitis medicamentosa" (44).

SUMMARY

Pharmacists should be prepared to offer sound advice on a good prophylactic program and to recommend therapy for uncomplicated, uninfected cases. They also should be prepared to assess severity of the rash and be able to recommend appropriate action, either referral to a physician or a treatment plan.

Diaper dermatitis and prickly heat are the two most common afflictions of newborns, infants, and young children, but the incidence and severity may be reduced by following the proper procedures. If the dermatitis does not respond to frequent diaper changes, frequent exposure to air, and application of a good protectant, e.g., zinc oxide paste, within 1 week, a physician should be consulted.

REFERENCES

(1) M. Kieder, "Practical Pediatric Dermatology," Mosby, St. Louis, Mo., 1961, p. 220.
(2) G. Weipole, *Klin. Paediatr.*, *186*, 259 (1974).
(3) W. E. Nelson, V. C. Vaughan, and R. J. McKay, "Textbook of Pediatrics," 9th ed., Saunders, Philadelphia, Pa., 1969, p. 1398.
(4) M. D. Lewis, *Med. J. Aust.*, *2*, 83 (1976).
(5) K. S. Shepard, "Care of the Well Baby," Lippincott, Philadelphia, Pa., 1968, p. 2310.
(6) D. R. Marlow, "Textbook of Pediatric Nursing," Saunders, Philadelphia, Pa., 1973, pp. 136–137.
(7) P. J. Koblenzer, *Clin. Pediatr.*, *12*, 386 (1973).
(8) L. Jacquet, *Rev. Mens. Mal Enf.*, *4*, 208 (1886).
(9) T. S. Southworth, *Arch. Pediatr.*, *30*, 730 (1913).
(10) J. Zahorsky, *Am. J. Dis. Child.*, *10*, 436 (1915).
(11) J. V. Cooke, *Am. J. Dis. Child.*, *22*, 481 (1921).
(12) G. W. Rapp, *Arch. Pediatr.*, *72*, 113 (1955).
(13) L. M. Solomon and N. E. Easterly, "Neonatal Dermatology: Major Problems in Clinical Pediatrics," Vol. 9, Saunders, Philadelphia, Pa., 1973.
(14) R. F. Pittillo, *J. Dermatol.*, *12*, 245 (1973).
(15) P. J. Kozinn, *Antibiot. Annu.*, 910 (1958–1959).
(16) L. F. Montes, R. F. Pittillo, D. Hunt, A. J. Narketes, and M. D. Dillon, *Arch. Dermatol.*, *103*, 400 (1971).
(17) S. Swift, *Pediatr. Clin. North Am.*, *3*, 759 (1956).
(18) J. Brennemann, *Am. J. Dis. Child.*, *21*, 38 (1921).
(19) H. L. Barnett, "Pediatrics," Appleton-Century-Crofts, New York, N.Y., 1968, pp. 1808–1809.
(20) K. J. Collins, *Practitioner*, *219*, 193 (1977).
(21) M. M. Alexander and M. S. Brown, "Pediatric Physical Diagnosis for Nurses," McGraw-Hill, New York, N.Y., 1974, pp. 22–23.
(22) D. A. Humphries, Master of Nursing Thesis, University of Washington, Seattle, Wash., 1966.
(23) R. B. Scoggins and B. Kliman, *N. Engl. J. Med.*, *273*, 831 (1965).
(24) R. J. Feldman and H. I. Maibach, *Arch. Dermatol.*, *91*, 661 (1965).
(25) R. D. Carr and W. M. Tarnowski, *Acta Derm. Venereol.*, *48*, 417 (1968).
(26) W. W. Grant, L. Street, and R. G. Fearnow, *J. Pediatr.*, *81*, 973 (1972).
(27) E. Shmunes and E. J. Levy, *Arch. Dermatol.*, *105*, 91 (1972).
(28) J. Patrick, J. D. Panzer, and V. J. Darbes, *Arch. Dermatol.*, *102*, 532 (1970).
(29) P. J. Kozinn, *J. Pediatr.*, *59*, 76 (1961).
(30) P. J. Kozinn, *Antibiot. Annu.*, 128 (1956–1957).
(31) Leeming/Pacquin Pharmaceutical Co., research report, 1972.
(32) *Ibid.*, 1974.
(33) W. S. James, *J. Med. Assoc. Ga.*, *64*, 133 (1975).
(34) H. T. Behram, F. C. Combes, A. Bobroff, and R. Leviticus, *Ind. Med. Surg.*, *18*, 512 (1949).
(35) C. B. Heimer, H. G. Grayzel, and B. Kramer, *Arch. Pediatr.*, *68*, 382 (1951).
(36) O. M. Kurschner, H. F. Cohen, H. R. Moskow, and A. Snyder, *J. Am. Osteopath. Assoc.*, *53*, 215 (1953).
(37) H. G. Grayzel, C. B. Heimer, and R. B. Grayzel, *N.Y. State J. Med.*, *53*, 2233 (1953).
(38) W. T. Maxon, *J. Ky. Med. Assoc.*, *52*, 423 (1954).
(39) *British Medical Journal*, *2*, 603 (1970).
(40) P. Jensen, *Nord. Med.*, *86*, 1425 (1971).
(41) W. W. Grant, L. Street, and R. G. Fearnow, *Clin. Pediatr.*, *12*, 714 (1973).
(42) H. S. Whitehouse and N. W. Ryan, *Am. J. Dis. Child.*, *112*, 225 (1967).
(43) W. Friend, *Calif. Med.*, *87*, 56 (1962).
(44) V. J. Fontana, *J. Med. Soc. N.J.*, *70*, 819 (1973).

Product (Manufacturer)	Application Form	Protectant	Powdered Agent	Antimicrobial	Other
A and D Ointment (Schering)	ointment	—	—	—	petrolatum anhydrous lanolin base
Ammens Medicated Powder (Bristol-Myers)	powder	zinc oxide, 9.10%	talc, 45.06% starch, 41%	boric acid, 4.55% 8-hydroxyquinoline, 0.1% 8-hydroxyquinoline sulfate, 0.05%	aromatic oils, 0.14%
Ammorid Dermatologic Ointment (Kinney)	ointment	zinc oxide	—	benzethonium chloride	lanolin
Ammorid Diaper Rinse (Kinney)	powder	—	—	methylbenzethonium chloride	edetate disodium
Aveeno Bar (Cooper)	cleanser	—	—	—	colloidal oatmeal, 50% mild sudsing agent (soap free) lanolin
Aveeno Colloidal Oatmeal (Cooper)	powder	—	—	—	oatmeal derivatives
Aveeno Lotion (Cooper)	lotion	—	—	—	colloidal oatmeal, 10% nonionic surfactants emollients
Aveeno Oilated (Cooper)	liquid	—	—	—	colloidal oatmeal, 43% lanolin fraction liquid petrolatum
Bab-Eze Diaper Rash Cream (A.V.P.)	cream	zinc oxide	starch	—	cod liver oil diperodon hydrochloride, 0.25% aluminum acetate peruvian balsam
Baby Magic Lotion (Mennen)	lotion	—	—	benzalkonium chloride	lanolin refined sterols
Baby Magic Oil (Mennen)	oil	—	—	—	mineral oil lanolin
Baby Magic Powder (Mennen)	powder	—	—	methylbenzethonium chloride	—
Baby Ointment (Beecham Labs)	ointment	zinc oxide benzoin	—	boric acid	aluminum hydroxide balsam tolu phenol lanolin–petrolatum base
Bagbalm (Dairy Associates)	ointment	—	—	8-hydroxyquinoline sulfate, 0.5%	petrolatum and lanolin base
Balmex Baby Powder (Macsil)	powder	zinc oxide	talc starch purified calcium carbonate	—	peruvian balsam
Balmex Emollient Lotion (Macsil)	lotion	—	—	—	peruvian balsam, purified silicone lanolin fraction
Balmex Ointment (Macsil)	ointment	zinc oxide bismuth subnitrate	—	—	vitamins A and D peruvian balsam, base containing silicone
B-Balm Baby Ointment (North American)	ointment	zinc oxide, 10% compound benzoin tincture, 0.005 ml/g	—	—	phenol, 2.17 mg/g methyl salicylate, 0.67 mg/g
Biotres (Central)	ointment	—	—	polymyxin B sulfate, 10,000 units/g bacitracin zinc, 500 units/g	—
Borofax (Burroughs Wellcome)	ointment	—	—	boric acid, 5%	lanolin

Product (Manufacturer)	Application Form	Protectant	Powdered Agent	Antimicrobial	Other
Caldesene Medicated Ointment (Pharmacraft)	ointment	zinc oxide	talc	—	cod liver oil lanolin petrolatum
Caldesene Medicated Powder (Pharmacraft)	powder	—	talc	calcium undecylenate, 10%	—
Codanol A & D (Amer. Pharm.)	ointment	—	—	—	vitamin A, 1500 units/g vitamin D, 200 units/g white petrolatum lanolin
Comfortine (Dermik)	ointment	zinc oxide, 12%	—	—	lanolin vitamins A and D
Cruex (Pharmacraft)	aerosol powder powder cream	—	talc	calcium undecylenate, 10% zinc undecylenate, 20% chloroxylenol, 3%	—
Dalicreme (Dalin)	cream	—	—	methylbenzethonium chloride, 0.1%	vitamins A and D diperodon hydrochloride, 0.25% scented greaseless base
Dalisept (Dalin)	ointment	—	—	methylbenzethonium chloride, 0.1% hexachlorophene, 1%	vitamin A, 750 units/g vitamin D, 75 units/g diperodon hydrochloride, 1% petrolatum–lanolin base
Desitin Ointment (Leeming)	ointment	zinc oxide	talc	—	cod liver oil petrolatum lanolin
Diapa-Care Baby Powder (Paddock)	powder	—	corn starch	benzethonium chloride	sodium bicarbonate
Diaparene Baby Powder (Glenbrook)	powder	magnesium carbonate	corn starch	methylbenzethonium chloride, 1:1800	—
Diaparene Ointment (Glenbrook)	ointment	—	—	methylbenzethonium chloride, 1:1000	petrolatum glycerin
Diaparene Peri-Anal Creme (Glenbrook)	cream	—	—	methylbenzethonium chloride, 1:1000	cod liver oil water-repellent base
Diaprex (Moss, Belle)	ointment	zinc oxide	zinc stearate	boric acid	peruvian balsam water-resistant base
Johnson & Johnson Medicated Powder (Johnson & Johnson)	powder	zinc oxide	talc	—	menthol fragrance
Johnson's Baby Cream (Johnson & Johnson)	cream	—	—	—	mineral oil water paraffin sodium borate lanolin white beeswax ceresin glyceryl stearate
Johnson's Baby Powder (Johnson & Johnson)	powder	—	talc	—	fragrance
Mediconet (Medicone)	cloth wipe	—	—	benzalkonium chloride, 0.02%	hamamelis water, 50% glycerin, 10% ethoxylated lanolin, 0.5% methylparaben, 0.15% perfume
Methakote Pediatric Cream (Syntex)	cream	—	talc	benzethonium chloride	protein hydrolysate
Mexsana Medicated Powder (Plough)	powder	zinc oxide	corn starch kaolin	triclosan	camphor eucalyptus oil
Moruguent (Beecham Labs)	ointment	—	—	—	cod liver oil concentrate lanolin–petrolatum base
Oilatum Soap (Stiefel)	cleanser	—	—	—	polyunsaturated vegetable oil, 7.5%

Product (Manufacturer)	Application Form	Protectant	Powdered Agent	Antimicrobial	Other
Panthoderm (USV)	lotion	—	—	—	dexpanthenol, 2% water-miscible base
Rexall Baby Powder (Rexall)	powder	—	talc	—	fragrance
Silicote (Arnar-Stone)	cream ointment	dimethicone, 30% (cream) 33.3% (ointment) titanium dioxide, 1% (cream)	—	—	—
Spectro-Jel (Recsei)	gel	—	—	cetylpyridinium chloride, 0.1%	glycol–polysiloxane, 1% isopropyl alcohol, 15% methylcellulose, 1.5%
Taloin (Warren-Teed)	ointment	calamine	—	methylbenzethonium chloride	eucalyptol silicone base
Vaseline Pure Petroleum Jelly (Chesebrough-Pond)	gel	—	—	—	white petrolatum, 100%
Zea Sorb (Stiefel)	powder	—	microporous cellulose	—	—
Zincofax Cream (Burroughs Wellcome)	cream	zinc oxide, 15%	—	—	petrolatum–lanolin base

Foot Care Products

Nicholas G. Popovich

Chapter 31

Questions to Ask the Patient

What is the problem—inflammation, itching, blisters, oozing lesions (sores), scaling, or bleeding?

Did you see your physician about this problem? If so, what did he or she tell you to do? What have you done? Did it help?

Where is the lesion located—on or between the toes or on the bottom of the foot?

How long have you had the problem?

What have you done about it? Have you put any medication on the foot?

Did the problem begin with the use of new shoes, socks, or soaps?

Do you have any allergies?

Do your feet sweat a lot? Too much?

Do other members of your family have this problem?

Is a doctor treating you for any other condition, such as diabetes, heart trouble, or circulatory disorders?

Do you take insulin? What other medicines do you take?

Although foot conditions generally are not life-threatening, except perhaps in diabetes, they may cause some measure of discomfort and impaired mobility—from a limitation of activity to a serious disease condition (1). Corns and calluses, for example, are common and widespread and may contribute to impairment.

Pain usually is associated with corns and warts. In corns, pain may be severe and sharp (when downward pressure is applied) or dull and discomforting. Calluses usually are asymptomatic, causing pain only when pressure is applied (2). Individuals who suffer from calluses on the sole of the foot frequently draw a parallel of their discomfort to that of a person walking with a pebble in the shoe. Another important sign with foot problems is the hardening of the skin, which signals a biochemical problem causing abnormal weight distribution in that particular area of the foot. This hardening, which can be identified physically by the physician and the patient, is an objective sign, as opposed to pain, which is subjective. A podiatric examination is warranted to determine whether an imbalance is present.

Human mycotic (fungus) infections that have cutaneous manifestation may be conveniently subdivided into five categories based on site of invasion (3). Usually, the superficial and cutaneous types are those that warrant the pharmacist's advice.

The primary lesions of athlete's foot often consist of macerated tissues, slight scaling, occasional vesiculation, and fissuring between and under the toes. Any or all of the interdigital webs of the foot may be affected, although usually the skin beneath the fourth and fifth toes of each foot is involved. A relapse of the disease is inevitable if there is nail involvement or if the infection is present on the soles of the feet (4, 5).

CORNS, CALLUSES, BUNIONS, WARTS

Pressure (tightly fitting shoes) is the most frequent cause of the pain of corns. Friction (loosely fitting shoes), walking barefooted, and orthopedic problems contribute to the development of calluses. Orthopedic problems include improper weight distribution, pressure, and the development of bunions with age (6). Improperly fitting hosiery and nonlubricated friction in hosiery may cause blisters, calluses, and corns.

A corn and callus are strikingly similar in one respect: each has a marked hyperkeratosis of the stratum corneum. (See Chapter 26 for a discussion of skin anatomy.) Beyond this feature, however, there are marked differences.

A corn (clavus) is a small, sharply demarcated, hyperkeratotic lesion having a central core (Figure 1) (7). It is raised and yellowish gray and ranges from a few millimeters to 1 cm or more in diameter. The base of the corn is on the skin surface; the apex points inward and presses nerve endings in the dermis, causing pain.

Corns are hard or soft. Hard corns occur on the surfaces of the toes and are shiny and polished. Soft corns are whitish thickenings of the skin usually found on the webs between the fourth and fifth toes. They are continually macerated by accumulated sweat (8).

Soft and hard corns usually are caused by underlying bony prominences. A bony spur, or exostosis (a bony tumor in the form of an ossified muscular attachment to the bone surface), nearly always exists beneath long-last-

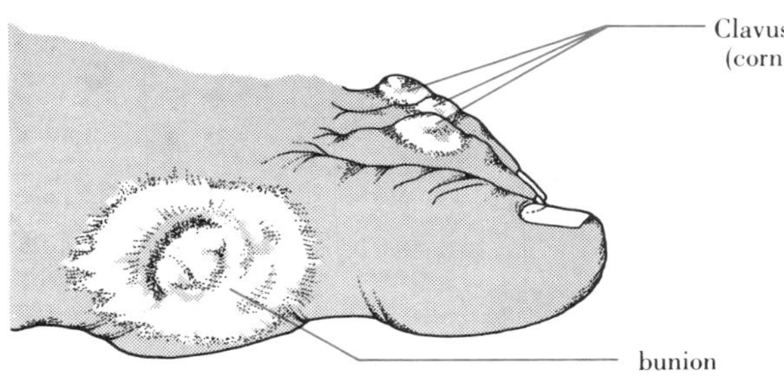

Figure 1. Conditions affecting the top of the foot.

characteristics of corn, callus, and bunion development

warts/verrucae—a common viral skin infection

patient susceptibility

plantar warts

acquired immunity

ing hard and soft corns. A lesion located over non-weight-bearing bony prominences or joints, such as metatarsal heads, the bulb of the large toe, the dorsum of the fifth toe, or the tips of the middle toes, is usually a corn (8).

A callus differs from a corn in that it has no central core and has more diffuse thickening of the skin (Figure 1) (6, 7). It has indefinite borders and ranges from a few millimeters to several centimeters in diameter. It is usually raised, yellow, and has a normal pattern of skin ridges on its surface. Calluses form on weight-bearing areas other than joints (e.g., on the palms of the hands and the sides and soles of the feet).

During corn or callus development, the cells in the basal cell skin layer undergo mitotic division, which leads to the migration of maturing cells through the prickle cell (stratum spinosum) and the granular (stratum granulosum) skin layer. The rate is equal to the continual surface cellular desquamation. Normal mitotic activity and subsequent desquamation lead to complete replacement of the epidermis in about 1 month (9). In the case of a callus, friction and pressure cause faster mitotic activity of the basal cell layer (9). This activity produces a thicker stratum corneum as more cells reach the outer skin surface. When the friction or pressure is relieved, mitotic activity returns to normal, causing remission and disappearance of the callus.

Bunions are swellings of the bursae caused by various conditions. Pressure from a tightly fitting shoe generally causes this condition, but pressure may result from the way a person sits, walks, or stands. Friction on the toes from malformations of the bones of the toes (e.g., wide heads or lateral bending) also causes bunions.

The hallux, or great toe, along with the inner side of the foot provides the elasticity and mobility needed to propel oneself. The hallux is therefore a dynamic organ (10). However, this mobility causes a number of anatomical disorders associated with the foot, e.g., hallux valgus, the deviation of the great toe toward the lateral (outer) side of the foot (11). Prolonged pressure caused by hallux valgus may result in pressure over the angulation of the metatarsophalangeal joint of the great toe, causing inflammatory swelling of the bursa over the metatarsophalangeal joint and resultant bunion formation (Figure 1) (12).

Warts (verrucae), or intraepidermal tumors of the skin, are the most common viral skin infection; they are caused by a human wart virus (human papilloma virus) (13). Although there are several kinds of warts, it is presumed that the human papilloma virus is responsible for a majority of them. Human papilloma virus belongs biologically to the papovavirus group (papilloma, polyoma, vacuolating viruses) (14). Because this virus has not been grown in tissue culture or laboratory animals, little information is known about its growth pattern, immunology, or metabolism. Information is based on various observations of infections in humans.

Warts begin as minute, smooth-surfaced, skin-colored lesions that enlarge over time. Repeated irritation causes the wart to continue enlarging. Plantar warts (on the soles of the feet) usually are asymptomatic and may not be noticed. However, if the plantar warts are large or occur in certain areas, the limitation of function and the discomfort may be bothersome to the point where professional advice is sought.

Three criteria must be met for an individual to develop a wart. The papovavirus must be in the area, there must be an open avenue for the virus to enter through the skin (i.e., abraded skin), and the patient must be susceptible to the virus (probably the key reason certain individuals develop warts and others do not).

Warts are most common in children and young adults and usually appear on exposed areas of the fingers, hands, face, and soles of the feet. They may spread by contact or autoinoculation. The incubation period after inoculation is 1–20 months, with an average of 4 months. An increase in plantar warts in England may have been due to an increase in the number and use of swimming pools (15). The hypothesis was that swimming, especially in warm water with a pH greater than 5, produced swelling and softening of the horny skin layer cells on the sole of the foot. The surrounding surface area of the pool and diving board is abrasive enough to contribute to tissue debridement, and inoculation in the area of heavy foot traffic around the pool (e.g., the diving board) is likely, especially when running and springing contribute to stress on the soles of the feet. Scrapings of the horny layer of plantar warts contain virus particles, and therefore it is conceivable that an area of heavy traffic of a pool can be contaminated easily by one person with a plantar wart.

Warts are not necessarily permanent—30% clear spontaneously in 6 months, 65% in 2 years, and most warts in 5 years (16, 17). The mechanism of spontaneous resolution is not fully understood. Acquired immunity may account for the remission (18). The wart virus stimulates the production of two immunoglobulins, IgM and IgG (19). The cure of warts in one population sample seemed to be correlated with the presence of complement fixation antibodies (IgG) (20). The rapid occurrence of complement fixation antibodies was associated with rapid healing; 75% of these patients were cured during the first 2 months of the observation period. In contrast, in patients with antibodies measurable only by immunodiffusion technique (i.e., IgM and/or low titers of IgG), only

16% were cured during the first month.

The development of immunity is directly related to the amount of virus present. This amount may vary among the different types of warts and their duration (20). Plane and mosaic warts and those of long duration, which are all known to be clinically difficult to cure, are those in which little virus is found. In a prior study, 65% of patients treated topically for plantar warts and cured in a 12-week treatment period had wart antibody (21). These results demonstrate that topical therapy will not prevent the formation of protective antibodies, as would be the case if the antigenic stimulus was removed by early curettage of the wart. Destroying a wart too early by curettage may lead to reinfection, because protective immunity seems to develop in about 6 months. Immunity may be correlated with the "not exceptionally high" rate of cure of electrodestruction and curettage (16). Electron microscopic counting procedures demonstrate that warts contain their highest concentration of virus particles when they are about 6 months old. It is in the period 6–12 months after inoculation that peak antibody titers in the body are reached (14).

wart immunity

should warts be treated

common virogenic warts

plantar warts

In light of this finding, it is questionable whether warts should be treated at all. The determination can be made only after making appropriate differential diagnosis and weighing the advantages and disadvantages of therapy predicated on patient circumstance. Indeed, when tests for wart antibody become routine, it will be possible to predict which patients will be likely to enjoy early spontaneous remission. Many practitioners believe that because of the contagious nature of plantar warts, early and vigorous treatment provides the best results. Prolonged treatment with OTC products may make the lesions more resistive to future treatment and increase the chance of autoinoculation.

Common virogenic warts are defined according to their location. Common warts (verruca vulgaris) are located on the hands and fingers, although they may occur on the face. Periungual and subungual verrucae occur around and underneath the nail beds. Juvenile, or flat, warts (verruca plana) usually occur in groups on the face, neck, and dorsa of the hands, wrists, and knees. Venereal warts (condyloma latum) occur near the genitalia and anus. Plantar warts (verruca plantaris) are common on the soles of the feet (22).

Plantar warts, hyperkeratotic lesions resulting from pressure, are more common in older children and adolescents but also occur in adults (23). They may be confined to the weight-bearing areas of the foot (the sole of the heel, the big toe, the areas below the heads of the metatarsal bones, and the ball), or they may occur in non-weight-bearing areas of the sole of the foot (Figure 2A). Because calluses also are more commonly found under weight-bearing areas of the foot, a differential diagnosis must be made by a podiatrist.

Plantar warts demonstrate marked hypertrophy of the horny skin layer, thickening of the prickle cell layer (acanthosis), formation of minute spaces (vacuolization) in the granular layer, and development of many papillomas (circumscribed overgrowth of a small nipplelike process) (18). The causative virus stimulates mitosis in

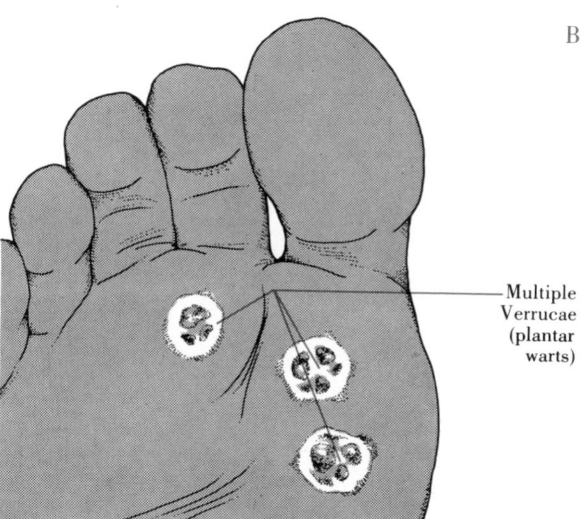

Figure 2. Conditions affecting the sole of the foot.

the prickle cell layer, resulting in the formation of the warty lesion (24). The warts are circumscribed lesions under constant pressure and are usually not raised above the skin surface unless they are on non-weight-bearing surfaces. In the center of the lesion is the wart itself. It is roughly circular with a diameter of 0.5–1 cm. The surface is grayish and friable, and the surrounding skin is thick and heaped. The entire area forms a uniform, slight swelling (23, 25). The surface of the planter wart may contain small black points which are the result of hypertrophied papillae that contain highly distended blood vessels. Rupture of the vessels allows coagulated blood into the epidermis which is eventually carried to the outer surface of the epidermis (13).

Plantar warts occur in clusters (Figure 2B), or several contiguous warts are fused, giving the appearance of one wart (mosaic wart) (12). They are often confused with corns and calluses, which are mainly thickened areas of the corneous layer (23). Plantar warts can grow under a callus (13).

Evaluation

Many foot conditions require a physician's attention, especially those accompanying chronic, debilitating diseases (e.g., diabetes mellitus or arteriosclerosis). Without proper supervision, OTC products may induce more ulceration and possibly gangrene, particularly in cases of vascular insufficiency in the foot (1). In addition, simple lesions may mask more serious abscesses or ulcerations. If exostoses associated with corns are not excised by a physician, the corns will persist. Sites with many corns and calluses and lesions that ooze purulent material (a sign of secondary infection) should be examined by a physician.

when physician referral is indicated

when self-treatment is appropriate

corn and callus treatment—eliminating pressure and friction

bunion and wart treatment

A physician (either a doctor of medicine or podiatrist) should be consulted if:

- A peripheral circulatory disease, diabetes, or a condition already under a physician's care exists;
- Hemorrhaging or oozing of purulent material occurs;
- Corns and calluses indicate an anatomical defect or faulty weight distribution;
- Corns or calluses are extensive on the foot and are painful and debilitating;
- Warts are not confined to the foot, are extensive on one site, or are in the perianal and genital areas;
- Proper self-medication for warts has been tried for an adequate period with no beneficial results.

Self-treatment is appropriate if:

- The directions for use of the products can be followed with no difficulty;
- Chronic, debilitating diseases do not contraindicate the use of these products;
- Predisposing factors (ill-fitting footwear and hosiery) of corns and calluses are removed;
- Corns and calluses are minor;
- Neither an anatomical defect nor faulty weight distribution is indicated by corns or calluses;
- Plantar warts are not spread extensively over the sole of the foot;
- No medication (e.g., immunosuppressives) is being taken for another condition that contraindicates the use of these products.

The medical history and medication profile are extremely valuable, particularly in cases where self-medication has been tried. Warts, calluses, and corns can mask more serious abscesses and ulcerations; if left medically unattended, they may lead to conditions that require hospitalization, such as osteomyelitis. Because circulation is impaired in these chronic, debilitating diseases, injury to normal skin treated with these OTC products may require a long time to heal. Diabetics and those not properly screened for ischemic changes are susceptible to disastrous gangrene (see Chapter 11).

The pharmacist must be cognizant that warts can occasionally be indicators for more serious conditions, such as squamous cell carcinoma and deep fungal infections (26). Squamous cell carcinomas may develop very rapidly, attaining a diameter of 1 cm within 2 weeks. The condition appears as a small, red, conical, hard nodule which quickly ulcerates (27). Subungual verrucae occur under the nail plate and may exist in conjunction with periungual verruca. The long-standing subungual verruca may be difficult to differentiate from a squamous cell carcinoma, especially in elderly patients (26). Condyloma acuminatum are moist and often cauliflowerlike in appearance. These warts must be differentiated from condyloma latuma (secondary syphilis), which have a smooth, whitish surface (28).

Most patients with rheumatoid arthritis eventually have foot involvement (29). Painful metatarsal heads, hallux valgus (deviation of the great toe toward the outer or lateral side of the foot), and clawtoes are the major forefoot deformities in patients with rheumatoid arthritis. Corrective surgical procedures often are indicated to reduce pain and improve function in these patients. There is little scientific evidence to support the effectiveness of conventional nonoperative therapy (e.g., orthopedic shoes, metatarsal inserts, conventional arch supports, or metatarsal bars) (29).

Medical history and medication profile should include characteristics (particularly oozing and bleeding of warts) and duration of the condition, whether similar problems have occurred in other family members, any medical treatment being given for the problem or other conditions (e.g., immunosuppressive therapy, diabetes, rheumatoid arthritis), and any drug allergies.

Treatment

The success of treatment of corns and calluses with OTC products depends on eliminating the causes: pressure and friction. This process entails the use of well-fitting, nonbinding footwear that distributes body weight evenly; for anatomical foot deformities, orthopedic corrections must be made. These measures relieve pressure and friction to allow for efficacious use of topical products used for corns and calluses, the resumption of normal mitosis of the basal cell layer, and the normalization of the stratum corneum after total desquamation of the hyperkeratotic tissue.

Corrective steps to alleviate bunions often depend on the degree of discomfort. Bunions may be asymptomatic but usually become quite painful, swollen, and tender. The bunion area itself usually is covered by an extensive keratinous overgrowth. Topical OTC drugs do not relieve this condition; palliative measures such as adhesive cushions provide some relief. Surgery may be indicated.

Warts are a result of viral infection. No specific effective medication is available, but topical agents and procedures help in their removal and relief of pain. Treatment is extremely difficult. Warts may reappear several months after they have been supposedly "cured."

Simple, not widespread warts may be helped by

self-medication depending on how the products are used and the use of ancillary procedures (e.g., foot baths and debridement with an emery board) that help make the treatment effective. When warts are widespread in a specific area, especially the perianal or genital area, medical attention and supervision are necessary.

Pharmacological Agents and Delivery

Drugs with enough keratolytic activity for use in products intended for the treatment of corns, calluses, and warts include ascorbic acid, calcium pantothenate, castor oil, glacial acetic acid, lactic acid, podophyllum resin, salicylic acid, and zinc chloride. Certain drugs, such as castor oil, are included in proprietary drug products for their emollient properties. Several topical products contain a local anesthetic, e.g., diperodon hydrochloride, to help alleviate the pain of corns or calluses. Salicylic acid is the most common ingredient in OTC drug products intended for corns, calluses, and warts. It usually appears in these products alone but may appear with other agents as well.

The pharmacist should be aware that there are several prescription products that might serve the patient better. At times, injection of a small amount of a corticosteroid beneath a painful corn results in a -amatic relief of symptoms (2).

Ascorbic Acid

Ascorbic acid is included in one topical product for wart therapy. Although ascorbic acid is essential to the development of supporting tissue (collagen and intracellular ground substance) and healing, there are no clinical reports to substantiate or refute its efficacy in topical wart therapy (30).

Cantharidin

Cantharidin is a potent vesicant available by prescription only as an ingredient of Cantharone. For wart therapy this liquid is applied lightly with a stick or swab, allowed to dry, and then covered by a piece of waterproof adhesive tape slightly larger than the wart (26). Depending on the physician's directions, the bandage is left in place between 24 hours and 1 week and then removed. In approximately 10 days the blister formed dries and peels off, taking with it the wart and leaving no scar. If the dressing is allowed to remain in place for 1 week, the skin under the tape becomes soggy and separates from underlying tissue. The physician debrides the dead material with a fine-curved iris scissors (31).

A disadvantage of cantharidin is that on occasion, annular warts develop at the periphery of the blister (32). In addition, since this method is considered dangerous, it is suggested that it should be performed only by the physician, and never by the patient at home (31). However, a successful trial of cantharidin treatment of warts at home was reported (33). Application of the occlusive tape was omitted from the instruction to simplify the process and produce fewer reactions. This mode demonstrated an easy, safe, and reasonably effective means of treating warts.

Castor Oil

Castor oil is included in several commercial products for corns and calluses for its emollient properties; it also may be used by itself. It keeps the keratinous tissue soft by forming an occlusive film, which prevents water loss and sweat evaporation from the surface of the corn or callus and allows the tissue to remain soft and pliable.

The oil usually is applied at bedtime, and the foot is covered by a sock. The sock serves a dual purpose in that it prevents oil stains on bed linens and helps occlude the affected area for better penetration of the medication.

Collodions

components of OTC products for corns, calluses, and warts

types of delivery systems used

Topical keratolytics used in treating corns, calluses, and warts generally are formulated in flexible collodion drug delivery systems containing pyroxylin, volatile solvents such as ether or alcohol, and a plasticizer, usually castor oil. Pyroxylin is a nitrocellulose derivative that, after evaporation of the volatile solvents, remains on the skin as a water-repellent film (34). Collodion drug delivery systems are advantageous because they form an adherent flexible or rigid film (35). They also prevent moisture evaporation and thus facilitate penetration of the active ingredient into the affected tissue, resulting in sustained local action of the drug. The systems are water insoluble, as are most of their active ingredients, e.g., salicylic acid. They are less apt to run than aqueous solutions.

The disadvantages of collodions are that they are extremely flammable and volatile and they may be mechanically irritating by occluding normal water transport through the skin. In addition, the collodions favor systemic absorption of some drugs by their occlusive nature, and their aromatic odors make them vehicles that children or adults might abuse by sniffing their contents (36).

Glacial Acetic Acid and Lactic Acid

Glacial acetic acid and lactic acid are organic acids included in OTC formulations for corns, calluses, and warts because of their corrosive properties. They should be applied only on the affected area, not on surrounding healthy skin. Either of these acids is usually included in low concentration (less than 10%) in formulations that also contain salicylic acid.

These acids are contraindicated in cases involving debilitating diseases. Overuse may cause skin irritation and ulceration. Used appropriately, these agents are safe for adults and children.

Local Anesthetics

To ease the pain of a corn or callus, several topical products contain a local anesthetic used with the keratolytic agents. Diperodon hydrochloride, usually incorporated into preparations at a concentration of 1%, is as potent as cocaine and has a longer duration of action. It should not be applied to abraded or denuded areas where systemic absorption is possible. Diperodon hydrochloride is contraindicated in patients who are hypersensitive to other local anesthetic agents, e.g., benzocaine. Menthol or camphor is included in several OTC products for wart removal as a counterirritant and mild, local anesthetic.

Pantothenic Acid and Derivatives

Calcium pantothenate is used for warts. Application of the alcohol derivative pantothenol in various ulcerative and pyogenic dermatoses stimulates epithelialization and allays itching. There have been no reports of sensitization or allergic reaction to topical therapy with pantothenic acid or its derivatives (30). The use of these drugs in adults and children seems safe. Topical formulations have a 2–5% concentration of the active pantothenic acid derivative.

Podophyllum

components of OTC products for corns, calluses, and warts

mechanisms, cautions, and possible toxicity

Podophyllum resin (20%) dispensed in compound benzoin tincture or as a solution in alcohol is effective in the treatment of condyloma acuminatum (genital warts). This caustic and powerful skin irritant is available by prescription only for short-term use. In 24–48 hours after application, lesions become necrotic and in the following days begin to slough off and gradually disappear.

The primary toxicological problem associated with the use of podophyllum resin, aside from its topical irritant qualities, is peripheral neuropathy when it is absorbed percutaneously into the systemic circulation (35–37). Podophyllum should be applied only in small amounts by the physician. The patient should be instructed to wash off the podophyllum preparation with soap and water within 8–12 hours from the time of application. Because the usual delivery system is a low-viscosity suspension (compound tincture of benzoin) or tincture (alcohol), the solution tends to run onto adjacent tissue and cause damage. This risk may be minimized if white petrolatum is applied to healthy surrounding skin before the podophyllum preparation is applied to the wart (28).

Podophyllum resin for vulvar warts in pregnant women should be used cautiously, if at all, and should not be used where hemorrhaging or an extensive skin surface area is involved. These conditions increase the possibility of percutaneous absorption. Because podophyllum is such a potent corrosive, it should not be used in conjunction with other keratolytic agents (e.g., salicylic acid).

Salicylic Acid

Salicylic acid, in concentrations of 5–10% and higher, softens and destroys the stratum corneum by increasing endogenous hydration, probably the result of lowering the pH, which causes the cornified epithelium to swell, soften, macerate, and then desquamate (38). This concentration is advantageous in hyperkeratotic conditions such as corns and calluses. However, on normal skin tissue, damage and necrosis are associated with the overuse (six times per day) or long-term use of salicylic acid in concentrations as low as 3–6% (39, 40).

The presence of moisture is important for therapeutic efficacy of salicylic acid in corn and callus therapy. If there is no moisture, tolerable amounts of salicylic acid will not soften cornified epithelium. Thus salicylic acid usually is incorporated in dosage forms (e.g., plasters, flexible collodions, and occlusive ointments) that occlude the area and promote moisture buildup, causing maceration and sloughing of tissues (41). These occlusive dosage forms may cause percutaneous absorption of salicylic acid (40). If enough salicylic acid is absorbed, salicylism may result. However, this condition may develop only when the salicylic acid preparation is used over an extensive area of the foot. Absorbed salicylic acid is metabolized to a degree and excreted in urine; patients with impaired liver and/or kidney function are predisposed to systemic salicylate buildup. These patients cannot tolerate absorbed salicylate because toxic serum levels may develop (39, 42).

In concentrations of 3–6%, salicylic acid is keratolytic. However, salicylic acid preparations of 10–40%, in appropriate dosage forms applied only to the affected area, are needed to soften hyperkeratotic tissue. Thus large amounts of salicylic acid preparations should be applied carefully to avoid destruction of skin, particularly adjacent healthy skin. Patients with diabetes mellitus or peripheral vascular disease, where acute inflammation or ulcer formation from topical salicylic acid would be difficult to treat, should not use products containing salicylic acid except under direct physician supervision.

A plaster provides direct and prolonged contact of drugs with corns, calluses, and warts. Salicylic acid plaster (USP XIX) is a uniform solid or semisolid adhesive mixture of salicylic acid in a suitable base, spread on appropriate backing material (felt, moleskin, cotton, or plastic) and applied to the affected area. The usual concentration of salicylic acid in the base is 40%. A small piece of the 40% plaster may be cut to the size of the wart and held in place by a larger piece of waterproof tape (31), then replaced every 3 days until the warty tissue turns white. This material is preferably pared away with a sharp blade every week under the physician's direction. Plasters are occlusive and prevent the dissipation of moisture (37).

Salicylic acid is used most often in conjunction with lactic acid or glacial acetic acid in the following classic prescription for corns and warts (6): one part each of salicylic and lactic acids to up to 10 parts with flexible collodion. Apply every day to the corn or twice per day to the wart without occlusion. Although this combination is favored by dermatologists for common warts, especially in pediatric patients, a case of permanent scarring with inappropriate use of the product has been reported (43). Seemingly appropriate instructions resulted in a misinterpretation of the instructions and overapplication of the material.

There are no clear-cut guidelines of how much salicylic acid or other keratolytic in an appropriate vehicle is needed before the product is considered a prescription-only item.

Zinc Chloride

Zinc chloride is included in several formulations of topical OTC products for corns and calluses. Because it is irritating and caustic, its concentration is low, usually less than 3%. Zinc chloride is very water soluble and ether soluble and may be used in either drug delivery system. It owes its activity to zinc ion, which precipitates protein. Because zinc chloride is extremely corrosive and irritating, it should not come into contact with mucous membranes or healthy skin (44) and should not be used for long periods.

Miscellaneous Prescription Drugs

Other prescription drugs used fairly successfully in treating warts are the antibiotic bleomycin sulfate (Blenoxane) for recurrent or recalcitrant plantar warts (31), tretinoin (retinoic acid) for flat warts and plantar warts (31, 45, 46), and fluorouracil (47). Bleomycin has not been approved by the FDA for wart treatment. Theoretical objection to the local use of this drug is that the drug may interfere with DNA metabolism and induce skin cancer (48). Results with tretinoin and fluorouracil therapy are variable, and in those cases that do respond it has not been determined whether the disease is simply taking its natural course (26).

Experiments have been made to treat corns by injecting fluid silicone subdermally (49). The injected silicone seems to augment digital and plantar tissues, causing a cushioning effect that enhances pain reduction and decreases the need for regular palliation.

Therapy for Bunions

Bunions are not amenable to topical drug therapy. The patient should correct the condition by wearing properly fitting shoes or by seeing a podiatrist or orthopedist. If the condition is not severe, shielding the bunion with protective pads (e.g., moleskin) may be all that is necessary. However, if the manifestation is severe or particularly unsightly, surgical correction is usually indicated.

Larger footwear may be necessary to compensate for the space taken up by the pad; not increasing shoe size may cause pressure in other areas. Also, protective pads should not be used on bunions when the skin is broken or blistered. In these cases, palliative treatment should first involve treatment of the abraded skin before pads are applied. If these conditions persist (e.g., in diabetic patients), the pharmacist should recommend that the patient see a podiatrist or orthopedist. Surgical treatment may be necessary to save the patient from further suffering and expense.

Adjunctive Therapy

In addition to OTC products, self-therapy measures include daily soaking of the affected area throughout the treatment period for at least 5 minutes in very warm (not hot) water to remove dead tissue (32). Dead tissue should be removed gently after normal washing. Skin should not be removed forcibly because further damage could result. Sharp knives or razor blades should not be used to cut dead tissue because they are not sterile and may cause bacterial infection. A rough towel, callus file, or pumice stone effectively removes dead tissue of corns and calluses. Petroleum jelly should be applied on the healthy skin surrounding the affected area to avoid accidental application of corrosive products. This precaution is especially important in cases where poor eyesight increases the chances of misapplication.

To relieve painful pressure emanating from inflamed underlying tissue and irritated or hypertrophied bones directly underneath the corn or callus, patients may use a pad (e.g., Dr. Scholl's) with an aperture for the corn or callus. If the skin can tolerate the pads, they may be used up to 1 week (50) or even for several weeks. To prevent the pads from adhering to hosiery, patients may wax the pads with paraffin or a candle and powder them daily with a hygienic foot powder. If, despite these measures, friction causes the pads to peel up at the edge and stick to hosiery, the pharmacist may recommend that patients cover their toes with the forefoot of an old stocking or pantyhose before putting on hosiery (50).

Patients should be advised that if at any time the pad begins to cause itching, burning, or pain, it should be removed, and a podiatrist consulted. The pharmacist also should advise the patient that these pads will provide only temporary help and rarely effect a cure for a corn or a callus.

bunion therapy

nondrug measures

preferred therapy for corns, calluses, and warts

To avoid the spread of warts, which are contagious, patients should wash their hands before and after treating or touching wart tissue, and a specific towel should be used only for drying the affected area after cleaning. Patients should not pick at the wart. Footwear should be worn in the case of plantar warts. If warts are on the sole of the foot, patients should be advised not to walk around in bare feet unless the wart is covered securely.

Product Selection Guidelines

There are no clinical studies to indicate whether prescription-only products are superior to OTC products. Conclusions are based only on subjective physician evaluation reports (2, 8). Salicylic acid in a plaster or collodion dosage form appears to be the most effective treatment for corns and calluses. Some studies advocate the use of a 50% solution of silver nitrate, applied by the physician, followed by weekly applications of 40% salicylic acid plasters for corns (6, 8).

If the pharmacist recommends the use of topical adhesive cushioning to alleviate the pressure on a bunion, instructions should be given on proper use. Before the protective pad is applied, the foot should be bathed and dried thoroughly. The pad is then cut into a shape that conforms to the bunion. If the intent is to relieve the pressure from the center of the bunion area, the pad can be cut such that it surrounds the bunion. The pressure is then transferred to the surrounding pad instead of to the bunion. Precut pads are available for immediate patient use.

Opinions about the best treatment for warts vary from recommendations to use nitric acid for plantar warts (51) to recommendations of cantharidin preparations for common warts (18, 26, 52).

In an evaluation of four plantar wart products, a benzyldimethylammonium dibromide solution (Callusolve paint) was less effective than either a 50% podophyllum resin/liquid paraffin preparation or an established salicylic acid/lactic acid/collodion preparation of 1 part:1 part:4

parts (21). A flexible collodion was used as the control preparation. The study also showed that the basic treatment time for simple plantar warts was about 6 weeks and that the cure rate was fastest with salicylic acid paint. The conclusion stated that the treatment of plantar warts with salicylic acid/lactic acid/flexible collodion mixture was enhanced when the method of application of the product was understood and was carried out under a physician's supervision.

The salicylic acid/lactic acid/flexible collodion preparation used in this study was safe and effective in children and adults; no incidences of hypersensitivity or systemic involvement were reported. Podophyllum also was used with no acute reactions, but it was used under the direct supervision of a physician, and the therapy was for plantar, not genital, warts. Podophyllum toxicity is associated with genital warts (53, 54).

advice for the patient with corns, calluses, or warts

tinea pedis

causative organisms in athlete's foot

predisposing factors in athlete's foot

Patient Consultation

Remission of corns, calluses, and warts does not happen quickly; it can take several days to several months (in cases of persistent warts). Usually, OTC treatment lasts 3–7 days for corns and calluses and 6–7 days for warts and is repeated if necessary. (If the wart remains, a physician should be consulted.) Adherence to the dosage regimen and selection of a convenient time to apply the product are important. The pain and lack of mobility associated with corns, calluses, or warts usually is a strict reminder to adhere to the medication. Topical products should be applied daily—in the morning and at bedtime generally are the most convenient times for the majority of patients.

The pharmacist should explain clearly how to use the medication. Because many products contain corrosive materials, it should be understood that the product is applied only to the corn, callus, or wart. If a plaster or pad is used, the process of trimming it to follow the contours of the corn or callus should be explained.

If a solution is used, it is applied, one drop at a time, directly to the corn, callus, or wart and is allowed to dry and harden to avoid running; the procedure continues until the entire area is covered. Adjacent areas of normal healthy skin should not come into contact with the product. If the solution does touch healthy skin, it should be washed off immediately with soap and water. If the solution is intended for a soft corn between the toes, the toes should be held apart comfortably until the solution is applied and is allowed to dry. This procedure should be followed for 3–6 days. The solution should solidify before a dressing is applied.

A plaster should be cut to the size of the lesion, applied to the skin, and covered with adhesive, occlusive tape. The next day the dressing is removed, and the foot is soaked in warm water. The macerated, soft white skin of the corn or callus is then removed by scrubbing gently with a rough towel, pumice stone, or callus file, and the plaster is reapplied. Patients must be careful not to debride "healthy" skin when using a pumice stone or callus file.

Creams should be applied after the wart has been washed with soap and water. Then an occlusive dressing generally is placed over the wart.

Because OTC preparations contain volatile and irritating ingredients, precautions should be taken in using them. After use, the container should be tightly capped, avoiding evaporation and preventing the active ingredients from assuming a greater concentration. The volatile delivery systems are quite flammable, and the product should be stored away from direct sunlight or heat in amber or light-resistant containers.

The products that contain collodions are poisonous when they are taken orally, and they should be stored out of children's reach. They have an odor similar to that of airplane glue and may be subject to abuse by inhaling the vapors (37).

Nonprescription products are not recommended for patients with diabetes or circulatory problems. Contraindications should be pointed out to all patients to avoid the possibility of inadvertent use of these products by other family members who have such conditions. These products are keratolytic and cause skin tissue to slough off, leaving an unsightly, slightly pinkish tinge to the skin; nevertheless, they should continue being used. They should be discontinued only when a severe inflammatory response (swelling or reddening) or irritation occurs.

ATHLETE'S FOOT

The most prevalent cutaneous fungal infection in humans is athlete's foot (dermatophytosis of the foot, or tinea pedis), the itchy, scaling lesions between the toes. Since ringworm fungi (dermatophytes) generally are the causative or initiating organisms responsible, athlete's foot is often synonymous with a ringworm infection (3).

The clinical spectrum of athlete's foot ranges from a mild scaling to a severe, exudative inflammatory process characterized by fissuring and denudation. The prevalent type of athlete's foot, midway between these two extremes, is characterized by maceration, hyperkeratosis, pruritis, malodor, and a stinging sensation of the feet.

Etiology

Species of the genera *Trichophyton*, *Microsporum*, and *Epidermophyton* are common fungal pathogens found in cutaneous infections of the skin, nails, and hair. The most commonly implicated pathogens of tinea pedis are the *Trichophyton sp.*, specifically, *T. mentagrophytes* and *T. rubrum* (55). It is perplexing, however, to note that the rates of recovery of fungi have been low in cases clinically diagnosed as athlete's foot (56, 57) especially of the symptomatic, macerated hyperkeratotic type. Recent evidence supports the theory that normal resident skin aerobic diphtheroids and gram-negative organisms, such as *Pseudomonas sp.*, also may play a role in the manifestations of the disease process (3, 4).

In addition to microorganisms, other predisposing factors contribute to the disease's development. Overhydration of the foot's skin may be due to exercise, emotional hyperhidrosis, tightly fitting occlusive footwear, and/or hot, humid weather (4). These conditions may be accentuated by debilitating diseases (e.g., diabetes), poor nutrition, and/or poor body hygiene.

Although tinea pedis may occur at all ages, it is more common in adults. However, it should not be ignored as a diagnostic possibility in children just because of infrequent occurrence (58). This infection is acquired most often by walking barefoot on infected floors, such as those in hotel bathrooms and locker rooms of clubs, schools, and camps. Tinea pedis may be present among several members of a family, presumably due to the spread of the fungi via the bathroom floor, floor mats, or rugs. Pathogenic fungi and bacteria also may be found in contaminated shoes and socks.

Tinea pedis is not thought to be transmitted simply by exposure to the fungal infection. Trauma to the skin, especially blister-producing trauma (e.g., wearing ill-fitting footwear), may contribute significantly to the occurrence of human fungal infections (59).

Susceptibility

Although there are many pathogenic fungi in the environment, the overall incidence of actual superficial fungal infections is remarkably low. Many degrees of susceptibility produce a clinical infection—from instantaneous "takes" by as few as one spore to severe trauma by massive exposure (60). One of the most important determinants of susceptibility to clinical fungal infection may be undefined, host-resistant factors (61). Acquired protective immunity occurs in the majority of infected patients. Reinfection in such patients requires a greater exposure to fungi, and lesions appear to heal more rapidly. About 20% of those afflicted with an acute superficial fungal infection develop a chronic fungal infection. An adequate immune response is not acquired by these patients (62). They seem to have a fungus infection "which comes and goes and which no one can cure" (63).

Pathophysiology

Superficial fungi, such as dermatophytes, attach to, proliferate, and live in the horny skin layer. These fungi produce keratinase, an enzyme that enables them to digest keratin, causing the outermost skin layer to disintegrate and scale (64, 65). The more severe reactions characterized by vesicles, erythema, and infiltration are presumably due to the fungi releasing an exotoxin or metabolic product (66). Dermatophytic fungi grow only in keratinous tissue because a potent antifungal factor protects living tissue from deep penetration by fungal elements (67). However, after the initial invasion of the horny layer by dermatophytes, enough moisture may accumulate to trigger a bacterial overgrowth (3). Large numbers of normally resident aerobic diphtheroids may become involved. Increased moisture and temperature then lead to bacterial proliferation and release of products that diffuse easily through the underlying horny layer already damaged by fungal invasion.

Experimental manipulation of the microflora supports the concept that bacterial overgrowth in an interspace already damaged by dermatophyte invasion results in the symptomatic types of athlete's foot (67). When occlusive dressings were applied to feet harboring the dermatophytes, the interdigital spaces became macerated and symptomatic within 7–10 days. These changes, however, did not occur when antibiotics (gentamicin sulfate, 0.1% cream) were added daily to the dressings to prevent the overgrowth of bacteria (3). A combination of an antibiotic and an antifungal (either two separate agents or one of the newer broad-spectrum agents, such as miconazole nitrate or clotrimazole) produced faster and more complete resolution of symptoms (3).

acquired immunity to fungal infections

development of athlete's foot

There are two main clinical types of tinea pedis: vesicular and intertriginous. Vesicular tinea pedis is an acute, inflammatory condition, caused predominantly by *T. mentagrophytes* (55). Vesicles 2–3 mm wide appear on the soles or sides of the feet or between the toes. They may be sparse or closely grouped into areas 2.5–5 cm wide. Erythema may be extensive or absent altogether. Burning and itching usually are present, along with hyperhidrosis (excessive sweating). After a few days, vesicles may become yellowish and purulent; they may rupture, causing a weeping surface open to infection by pyrogenic cocci, or they may simply dry up as the acute stage subsides, leaving yellowish-brown crusts.

vesicular and intertriginous tinea pedis

characteristics of athlete's foot

Intertriginous tinea pedia, a chronic dermatophytosis, is caused primarily by *T. rubrum*. This type is divided into two subclassifications (3). Dermatophytosis simplex, characterized by dry, scaly lesions, is relatively asymptomatic except for periodic low-grade pruritis. Dermatophytosis complex, characterized by soggy, macerated skin, has symptoms of itching, malodor, and discomfort between the toes. Manifestations of this condition may range from hyperkeratotic, leukokeratotic plaques to erosions and fissures. The horny skin layer becomes white and macerated and usually peels off in large friable scales. Beneath the scales the epidermis appears dull and red. The pain and discomfort seem to be a consequence of the progression of bacterial proliferation in the fungus-infected interspace (3).

Intertriginous tinea pedis may be restricted to a small patch adjacent to a fungus-infected toenail (usually caused by *T. rubrum*) or to a patch between or under the toes (67). The absence of vesiculation is characteristic.

Evaluation

The most common complaint of patients suffering from tinea pedis is pruritus. However, if fissures are present, particularly between the toes, the patient also may complain of painful burning and stinging. If the foot area is abraded, denuded, or inflamed, weeping or oozing may occur in addition to frank pain. Some patients may merely remark on the bothersome scaling of dry skin, particularly if it has progressed to the soles of the feet. Small vesicular lesions may combine to form a larger bullous eruption marked by pain and irritation. The only symptoms may be brittleness and discoloration of a hypertrophied toenail.

The only true determinant of a fungal foot infection is clinical laboratory evaluation of tissue scrapings from the foot. This process involves a potassium hydroxide mount preparation of the scrapings and cuttings on special growth media to show the actual presence of fungi and the specific type (68). The procedure can be ordered and performed only at the direction of a physician. It must be noted, however, that the microscopic confirmation probably will be possible only in the dry, scaly type. In typical cases of dermatophytosis complex, fungus recovery rates are only about 25–50% (4).

The pharmacist should question the patient thoroughly as to the condition and its characteristics so as to obtain a description of the condition and determine the extent of the disease process, any mitigating circumstances (e.g., diabetes or obesity) that would render the patient susceptible, and previous patient compliance with medications.

other similar foot infections

when to recommend physician referral

components of OTC products for athlete's foot

The pharmacist should seek to distinguish tinea pedis from other diseases with similar symptoms. Dermatitis, allergic contact dermatitis, and atopic dermatitis may occur on the feet, and these conditions should be treated by a physician. In addition, hyperhidrosis of the sole of the foot and infection of toe webs by gram-negative bacteria are common. In hyperhidrosis, tender vesicles cover the sole of the foot and toes and may be quite painful. The skin generally turns white, erodes, and becomes macerated. This condition is accompanied by a foul foot odor.

Infection by gram-negative bacteria is characterized by a soggy wetness of the toe webs and immediately adjacent skin (69). The affected tissue is damp, softened, and boggy. The last or next to last (adjacent to the little toe) toe webs are the most common types of primary or initial involvement (69). Severe forms of this disease may progress to disintegration and denudation of the affected skin and profuse, serous, or purulent discharge. Denudation may involve all of the toe webs, the dorsal and plantar surfaces of the toes, and an area about 1 cm wide beyond the base of the toes on the plantar surface of the foot. When the disease is out of control, its progression is observed on the dorsum of the foot and the calf in the form of tiny red follicular crusts. This condition paradoxically may be caused by use of reputed germicidal soaps (e.g., pHisoHex, Dial, and Safeguard) (69). It was hypothesized that these soaps reduce harmless saprophytes and thus promote resistant pathogens (e.g., *Pseudomonas aeruginosa* and *Proteus mirabilis*) by removing their competitors.

If the patient has used an OTC antifungal product appropriately for several weeks without relief, a disease other than tinea pedis may be involved. Patients suffering from hyperhidrosis, allergic contact dermatitis, or atopic dermatitis or from a possible gram-negative infection of the toe should see a physician for treatment.

Treatment

Before self-medication can be effective, the correct type of tinea pedis as well as correct treatment must be evaluated. Treatment of an acute superficial tinea foot infection may be effective if certain conditions are met. In acute, inflammatory tinea pedis, characterized by reddened, oozing, vesicular eruptions, the inflammation must be counteracted before antifungal therapy can be instituted. This step is especially important if the eruptions are caused by a secondary bacterial infection (60).

Self-treatment is effective only if the patient understands the importance of compliance with all facets of the treatment plan. Specific antifungal products must be used appropriately in conjunction with other treatment objectives (e.g., general hygienic measures and local drying).

The pharmacist should recommend that the patient consult a physician in the following circumstances:

- If the toenail is involved, topical treatment is ineffective and does not allay the condition until the disease's primary focus is treated with oral griseofulvin or until other preventive measures are instituted (e.g., surgical avulsion, or tearing away of the nail).
- If vesicular eruptions are oozing, including purulent material that could indicate a secondary bacterial infection, topical astringent therapy and/or antibiotic therapy may be appropriate.
- If the foot is seriously inflamed and/or swollen and a major portion is involved, supportive therapy must be instituted before an antifungal agent may be applied.
- If the patient is under a physician's supervision for a disease (e.g., diabetes or asthma) where the normal defense mechanism may be deficient, OTC products should not be used.

Ingredients in OTC Products

Carbol–Fuchsin Solution

Basic fuchsin (NF XIII) dye is a mixture of rosaniline and pararosaniline hydrochlorides. It is used only in superficial fungal foot infections in the form of carbol–fuchsin solution (NF XIII) or Castellani's paint. The solution is dark purple but appears red when painted onto the affected area in a fine film. It has local anesthetic, drying, and antimicrobial properties.

The use of carbol–fuchsin solution in tinea pedis is indicated in the subacute or chronic stages of infection when there is little or no inflammation. The solution should not be applied to inflamed or denuded skin.

In one study, carbol–fuchsin solution demonstrated equivalent efficacy to a 30% aluminum chloride solution for interdigital dermatophytosis (4). The drying and antimicrobial properties of carbol–fuchsin are well suited for the ultrasoggy, steaming athlete's foot. However, the staining properties of the dye and the poisonous nature of the solution limit this medication's usefulness.

Before the solution is applied, the affected area should be cleaned thoroughly with soap and water and dried. The solution is then applied to the area with an applicator and reapplied once or twice per day for 1 week. After this time, if the condition has not improved, choice of medication as well as assessment of the actual condition should be re-evaluated.

The efficacy of carbol–fuchsin solution must be questioned especially if an infected toenail is involved. Because the preparation contains several volatile components, the patient should tighten the cap securely to avoid evaporation. Otherwise, volatile ingredients escape, causing other, nonvolatile components (e.g., resorcinol) to become more concentrated, and irritation may result with subsequent applications.

The effectiveness of the product is limited because it can be applied to only 10% of the foot. This limitation, its staining properties, and possible patient sensitivity to ingredients in the product limit the usefulness of carbol–fuchsin solution for tinea pedis. This is indeed unfortunate, since carbol–fuchsin solution possesses all facets necessary for effective athlete's foot therapy. The solution suppresses fungi and bacteria and simultaneously produces a local drying or astringent effect.

Naphthol Derivatives

The most notable naphthol derivative synthesized for antifungal activity is tolnaftate (70). Its spectrum of action encompasses typical fungi responsible for tinea pedis, including *T. mentagrophytes* and *T. rubrum.* In addition, it is effective against *E. floccosum* and *Microsporum sp.* Although the exact mechanism of action of tolnaftate has not been reported, it is believed that it distorts the hyphae and stunts the mycelial growth of the fungi species. Tolnaftate is more effective in tinea pedis than in onychomycosis or tinea capitis. For onychomycosis and tinea capitis, concomitant administration of oral griseofulvin is necessary, unless the condition is superficial.

Tolnaftate is tolerated well when applied to intact or broken skin in either exposed or intertriginous areas. Tolnaftate usually causes a slight stinging sensation when applied. Although there has been one report of a developed delayed hypersensitivity reaction to tolnaftate, there have been no references to hypersensitivity associated with its use (71). As with all topical medicaments, irritation, sensitization, or worsening of the skin condition warrants discontinuance of the product.

Tolnaftate (1% solution or 1% cream) is applied sparingly twice per day after the affected area is cleansed thoroughly. The usual period for effective therapy is 2–4 weeks, although treatment of 4–6 weeks may be necessary for some individuals, e.g., patients with lesions between the toes or on pressure areas of the foot. When medication is applied to pressure areas of the foot, where the horny skin layer is thicker than normal, concomitant use of a keratolytic agent may be advisable. Neither keratolytic agents nor wet compresses, such as aluminum acetate (Burow's) solution, which promote the healing of oozing lesions, interfere with the efficacy of tolnaftate. If weeping lesions are present, the inflammation should be treated before tolnaftate is applied.

The cream dosage form of tolnaftate is formulated in a polyethylene glycol 400/propylene glycol vehicle, the solution in polyethylene glycol 400. The solution may be more effective than the cream. These vehicles are particularly advantageous in superficial antifungal therapy because they are nonocclusive, nontoxic, nonsensitizing, water miscible, anhydrous, easy to apply, and efficient in delivering the drug to the affected area.

High molecular weight polyethylene glycol bases have been reported to form associated complexes with some medicaments, e.g., benzoic and salicylic acids. Although diffusion of the medicament to the skin is adequate with polyethylene glycol bases, little percutaneous absorption occurs (72, 73). In regard to topical antifungal therapy, however, complex formation seems inconsequential because the role of the vehicle in this instance is to supply drug to the horny layer of the skin.

Tolnaftate solution solidifies when exposed to cold. However, if the preparation is allowed to warm, it will liquefy with no loss in potency.

The topical powder formulation of tolnaftate uses corn starch–talc as its vehicle. This vehicle not only is an effective drug delivery system but also offers therapeutic advantage due to the water-retaining nature of the two agents. Tolnaftate powder was more effective than its vehicle in reducing the incidence of tinea pedis in patients who, on initial examination, demonstrated laboratory-confirmed dermatophytosis of the foot (74). The topical aerosol formulation of tolnaftate includes talc in addition to the propellant vehicle.

tolnaftate—indications, dosage forms, and concentrations

Tolnaftate has demonstrated marked clinical efficacy since its commercial introduction into the United States in 1965, and it has become the standard topical antifungal medicament (75). In addition, there has been a consistent absence of signs of irritation or hypersensitivity to tolnaftate in cream, solution, or powder form, thus enabling its approval for OTC use as well.

Tolnaftate is valuable primarily in the dry, scaly type of athlete's foot. Superficial fungal infection relapse has occurred after tolnaftate therapy was discontinued (76). However, the relapse may have been caused by an inadequate treatment time, patient noncompliance with the medication, or the use of tolnaftate where oral griseofulvin should have been instituted. Since tolnaftate does not possess antibacterial properties, its value in the soggy, macerated type of athlete's foot must be viewed with skepticism, if indeed bacteria are at the root of the problem (3).

Organic Fatty Acids

fatty acid use

Studies of the antifungal effect of various fatty acids and their salts on dermatophytes reported encouraging clinical results with sodium propionate, a constituent of sweat (77). The sodium salt of caprylic acid (C_8 fatty acid) was more effective than sodium undecylenate in treating dermatophytosis of the foot (78). However, both propionic and undecylenic acids are weakly fungistatic (79).

Whether organic fatty acids are more effective than sulfur and/or iodine preparations in treating superficial fungal infections is questionable. Organic acid preparations should be used, if at all, only for very mild or chronic forms of tinea pedis.

These organic fatty acids and/or their salts are available in various dosage forms. The cream or ointment form is usually used at bedtime, and solutions should be used for their soothing effects after a footbath. The powder is usually sprinkled into the socks and shoes in the morning.

triacetin

Acetic acid. Acetic acid is delivered to the infected area as triacetin. The fungistatic activity of triacetin is based on the fact that at the neutral or alkaline pH of infected skin, fungal esterase enzymes cleave triacetin into acetic acid and glycerin (80). The acetic acid then effects antifungal activity by lowering the pH at the infection site. As the pH increases after the initial release of acetic acid, more acetic acid is generated by the enzymes, and the process is repeated. The efficacy of products containing triacetin has not been proven by controlled clinical trials (76).

Used topically, triacetin is relatively colorless and odorless. In the concentrations used, the small amount of acetic acid liberated is probably nonirritating to the skin in most cases. The corresponding incidence of sensitization also is low. However, the acetic acid formed may damage rayon fabrics, so the treated areas should be covered with a clean bandage to prevent contact. Triacetin must not come into contact with the eyes.

Triacetin as a topical aerosol (15%), cream (25%), or powder pack (33.3%) should be applied every evening after thorough cleansing. The aerosol and powder may be used adjunctively to the cream form. The product should be used until the infection has cleared entirely, then once per week as a preventive measure.

mechanism of action of undecylenic acid and zinc undecylenate

phenol, resorcinol, and chloroxylenol

Undecylenic acid–zinc undecylenate. This combination is widely used for various superficial fungal infections excluding those involving nails and/or hairy parts of the body. It is fungistatic and is effective in mild, chronic cases of tinea pedis. Compound undecylenic acid ointment (USP XIX) contains undecylenic acid and 20% zinc undecylenate in a polyethylene glycol vehicle. It is believed that zinc undecylenate liberates undecylenic acid (the active antifungal entity) on contact with moisture (e.g., perspiration). In addition, zinc undecylenate has astringent properties due to the presence of zinc ion (66). This astringent activity decreases the irritation and inflammation of the infection.

Applied to the skin as an ointment, diluted solution, or dusting powder, the combination (undecylenic acid–zinc undecylenate) is relatively nonirritating, and hypersensitivity reactions associated with its use are uncommon. The undiluted solution, however, may cause transient stinging when applied to broken skin, due to its alcohol content. Caution must be exercised to ensure that these ingredients do not come into contact with the eye or that the powder is not inhaled.

The vehicle in compound undecylenic acid ointment has a water-miscible base, making it nonocclusive, water removable, and easy to apply. The powder uses talc as its vehicle and adsorbent. The aerosol contains menthol, which serves as a counterirritant and antipruritic. The solution contains 10% undecylenic acid in a vehicle solution of propanol, propylene glycol, and water. The product is applied twice daily after the affected area is cleansed. The usual period for therapeutic results depends on the patient. However, improvement should occur in 2–4 weeks, after which time the condition should be re-evaluated and an alternative medication tried.

To avoid contamination of the product, a small amount of solution is poured from the stock solution into a smaller glass container. With an applicator or cotton swab, the solution is then applied from the smaller container. Another precaution is to allow the solution to air-dry after it has been applied. Otherwise the water accumulates, resulting in further tissue maceration. Undecylenic acid's rancid odor may be objectionable to some patients and may promote ultimate patient noncompliance.

Undecylenic acid–zinc undecylenate combinations are useless when the condition is complicated by an infected toenail, since they cannot eradicate the disease's primary foci. The combination may be beneficial to patients with mild, chronic forms of tinea pedis.

A comparison study of two 20% zinc undecylenate–2% undecylenic acid powder formulations used in the treatment of tinea pedis found no difference in clinical efficacy between a product with a new formulation and an OTC antifungal preparation available for a number of years (81). However, these formulations collectively effected clinical and mycological cures in 53% of the patients treated as compared with 7% of those treated with the talc vehicle or left untreated (using daily foot washings or changes of socks). There was no indication whether patients failing to respond to either formulation possessed the more severe forms of tinea pedis.

Other preparations, e.g., ointments, powders, and tinctures, incorporate undecylenic acid (10%) by itself in the vehicle. This concentration has minor irritant effects on the skin. However, undecylenic acid should not be applied directly to mucous membranes in concentrations of more than 1%.

Phenolic Compounds and Derivatives

These aromatic compounds are included in topical OTC athlete's foot products for their keratolytic or fungicidal effects.

Phenol and substituted phenols. Phenol and substituted phenols (e.g., resorcinol) are included in many topical antifungal products. Phenol is fungicidal at a concentration of 1.3%. Resorcinol is also fungicidal, but its potency is about one-third that of phenol. Phenol is reported to be more effective in aqueous solutions than in glycerin or fats; it is relatively ineffective when incorporated into fats (82).

Applied to unabraded skin in low concentrations, phenol causes warmth and a tingling sensation. Its irritant qualities usually restrict its effectiveness in athlete's foot remedies. To be fungicidal in these preparations, concentrations irritating to human skin generally must be used.

Resorcinol, in concentrations usually applied topically (<10%), is nonirritating; higher concentrations may be irritating. Although resorcinol may produce allergic reactions, they rarely occur.

Phenol and resorcinol resemble each other with regard to systemic action, particularly on the CNS. Thus preparations containing either of these agents should never be applied to large areas or to irritated or denuded skin because of possible absorption and systemic toxicity.

Chloroxylenol, a substituted phenol, is a nonirritating antiseptic agent. Chloroxylenol (0.5% solution) was reported to be effective in treating and preventing athlete's foot (83). It is included in some topical preparations in liquid, cream, and powder forms. Chloroxylenol's limited water solubility makes its efficacy in powder drug delivery systems questionable. If the inert agents of the vehicle are effective in adsorbing moisture, the effect of the chloroxylenol may be diminished. Chloroxylenol causes no cutaneous irritation at a concentration of 5% (84). It is less toxic than phenol, but eczematous reactions have followed its use (85).

Salicylic acid. In high concentrations, salicylic acid is a keratolytic agent, causing a shedding of the keratin layer of the skin and facilitating penetration of other drugs. Lower concentrations (<2%) are keratoplastic; they aid normal keratinization. Salicylic acid (5–10%) softens the stratum corneum by increasing the endogenous hydration of this layer. This effect probably results from lowering the pH, which causes the cornified epithelium to swell, soften, macerate, and then desquamate (86). If no moisture is present, cornified epithelium is not softened significantly by tolerable amounts of salicylic acid. Because salicylic acid accelerates exfoliation of the infected keratin tissue, its use in conjunction with topical antifungals in appropriate conditions may be very beneficial (76).

Salicylic acid alone has little or no antifungal activity. It usually is applied to the skin as a combination of 3% salicylic acid and 6% benzoic acid in a polyethylene glycol base (Whitfield's ointment). Benzoic acid alone is alleged to have some fungistatic activity, but this claim is debatable at best. This ointment is available in double strength and half strength. The half-strength formula (1.5% salicylic acid) does not have the keratolytic properties of the regular or double strength and therefore should never be used when keratolytic activity is necessary. The basic criterion for evaluating the efficacy of salicylic acid products as keratolytic agents is the concentration of salicylic acid. Thus on the basis of current literature, these products should contain concentrations of more than 2% salicylic acid.

The pharmacist should be aware of the irritant properties of topically applied salicylic acid. Many skin irritations have been reported following unsupervised self-medication.

Quaternary Ammonium Compounds

Quaternary ammonium compounds (e.g., benzethonium chloride and methylbenzethonium chloride) are used in several antifungal aids for their skin antiseptic and detergent properties. Solutions of these agents have emulsifying properties that favor wetting and penetration of surfaces to which they are applied. These compounds are germicidal to most pathogenic fungi.

The disinfectant action of these compounds may not be as great as expected. They are cationic and have a chemical incompatibility with anionic compounds such as soaps. Thus any residual soap or soap film on the skin may inactivate them (87). In athlete's foot, where patients are told to clean their feet thoroughly on a daily basis, patients also must be instructed to rinse the affected area thoroughly before drying it. Otherwise, if the OTC product used contains a quaternary ammonium compound, any beneficial effects may be negated. A tincture delivery system of these cationic compounds is more effective as a skin disinfectant and is less affected by soap than an aqueous solution (88). Accordingly, tincture forms of these agents are used in more dilute concentrations than aqueous solutions.

Therefore in a liquid form, especially a tincture, quaternary compounds should be effective if appropriate concentrations are used. However, when applied topically in powder form with adsorbent agents included in the formulation, their efficacy may be in doubt. If all moisture is removed effectively by the adsorbing material, the quaternary compound may be unable to dissolve and exert its germicidal activity, but these compounds dissolve in a minimal amount of water.

Quaternary ammonium compounds generally are safe applied topically. However, each compound has its own sensitization index and its own ability to produce contact dermatitis as a result of widespread usage and multiple sources of patient exposure to these chemicals.

Quinoline Derivatives

salicylic acid as a keratolytic

benzethonium and methylbenzethonium chlorides

8-hydroxyquinoline/benzoxiquine

aluminum salt solutions/Burow's solution

Of 24 quinoline derivatives investigated in vitro, only benzoxiquine (8-hydroxyquinoline benzoate) was found to be active in fungistatic and fungicidal testing (89). It was postulated that the activity of 8-hydroxyquinoline was due to chemical inactivation via chelation of trace metals, essential for the growth of fungi, in either the nutritive media or the cell of the fungus (90). A 3% benzoxiquine preparation in a vanishing cream base was fungicidal in in vitro testing when compared to other antifungal ointments (79). Subsequently, an antifungal preparation containing 2.5% benzoxiquine was used successfully in the treatment of dermatophytosis (91).

Several proprietary powder antifungals use 8-hydroxyquinoline sulfate in their formulations. This compound is fungicidal. Because the sulfate salt is fairly water soluble and forms an acidic solution in the presence of moisture, it may lend more efficacy to the antifungal effect of the 8-hydroxyquinoline. However, there is no clinical evidence to confirm or refute this assumption.

Salts of Aluminum

Historically, the foremost astringent used for the acute, inflammatory stage of tinea pedis and the wet, soggy type of tinea pedis has been aluminum acetate (e.g., Burow's solution). Recent evidence, however, also has supported the use of aluminum chloride in treating the wet, soggy type (4).

The action and efficacy of these aluminum salts appear to be two-pronged. First, these compounds act as astringents. Their drying ability probably involves the complexing of the astringent agent with proteins, thereby altering the proteins' ability to swell and hold water (4). These astringents decrease edema, exudation, and inflammation by reducing the cell membrane permeability and hardening the cement substance of the capillary epithelium. Second, in concentrations greater than 20%, aluminum chloride, for instance, possesses antibacterial activity. Aluminum chloride may exhibit its antibacterial activity in two ways: by directly killing bacteria and by making the interspaces inhospitable through drying (4). Solutions of 20% aluminum acetate and 20% aluminum chloride demonstrated equal in vitro antibacterial efficacy (4).

Aluminum acetate solution for use in tinea pedis generally is diluted with about 10–40 parts of water. Depending on the situation, the patient either immerses the whole foot in the solution for 20 minutes up to three times per day or merely applies the solution to the area in the form of a wet dressing. In a recent trial, 10 subjects compared aluminum acetate solution (5%) to the recommended 1:20 dilution on the macerated, soggy type of athlete's foot (4). After 7 days the 5% solution produced moderate drying and symptomatic improvement in five subjects; the 1:20 dilution was ineffective.

When topical aluminum acetate solution dressings are indicated, an appropriate product can be selected depending on the involvement of the acute, inflammatory lesion. Convenient to use, these products are intended for external use, are not to be ingested, and should be kept away from contact with the eyes. Prolonged or continuous use of aluminum acetate solution for extended periods may produce necrosis (92). However, in the acute, inflammatory stage of tinea pedis, this solution should be used less than 1 week. The pharmacist should instruct the patient to discontinue use of the solution if extensive inflammatory lesions appear to worsen or if irritation becomes more apparent.

aluminum salt solutions
benzoyl peroxide
dosage forms
vehicle considerations

Concentrations of 20–30% aluminum chloride have been the most beneficial for the wet, soggy type of athlete's foot (4). Twice-daily applications of aluminum chloride generally are used until the signs and symptoms (e.g., odor, wetness, and whiteness) abate. Once-daily applications control the symptoms after that time (68). In hot, humid weather the original condition returns within 7–10 days after the application is stopped (68).

The application of aluminum salts does not cure athlete's foot entirely. This treatment modality merely shifts the disease process back to the simple dry type of athlete's foot, which then can be controlled with other agents (e.g., tolnaftate).

Since aluminum salts penetrate skin poorly, the toxicity of salts like aluminum chloride is rather low. However, one study demonstrated a few cases of irritation in patients where deep fissures were present (4), so that the aluminum salt was able to come into contact with living skin. Thus a contraindication to the use of concentrated solutions of aluminum salts would be severely eroded or deeply fissured skin. In these cases, dilution of the salts to a lower concentration (e.g., 10% aluminum chloride) is necessary for initial treatment.

Used appropriately, aluminum acetate solution or aluminum chloride solution is valuable in the wet, soggy, macerated form of athlete's foot and acute, inflammatory stages of athlete's foot. However, each solution has a potential for misuse (e.g., accidental childhood poisoning by ingesting the solutions or ingesting the solid tablets). The problem is real, and precautions must be taken to prevent this occurrence.

Miscellaneous

A 5% or 10% gel of benzoyl peroxide has been suggested for use in the symptomatic interdigital treatment of athlete's foot (93). The drying or astringent effect of this prescription formulation coupled with the antimicrobial activity of the benzoyl peroxide offers the advantage of rapid clinical improvement of this form of tinea pedis. However, this product must be used with caution, since it may be irritating, particularly to denuded areas or deep fissures. Prolonged use of benzoyl peroxide on inflamed or ulcerated skin should be avoided because of its strong sensitizing ability.

Other Ingredients and Dosage Forms

The primary drug delivery systems used for treatment of tinea pedis are creams, solutions, and powders. Powders, including those in aerosol dosage forms, generally are indicated for adjunctive use with solutions and creams. In very mild conditions, powders may suffice as the sole therapy.

The vehicle of the solution or cream forms should be:

- Nonocclusive (i.e., it should not retain moisture or sweat, which exacerbates the condition);
- Water miscible or water washable (i.e., removable with minimal cleansing efforts, since hard scrubbing of the affected area further abrades the skin);
- Anhydrous, since including water in the formulation introduces a variable that is one of the primary causes of the condition;
- Spreadable with minimal effort and without waste;
- Capable of efficient drug delivery (i.e., it must not interact with the active ingredient, but allow it to penetrate to the seat of the fungal infection);
- Nonsensitizing and nontoxic when applied to intact or denuded skin, especially if it is absorbed into the systemic circulation.

Most vehicles used to deliver topical solutions and creams are essentially polyethylene glycol and alcohols, which meet these criteria. Polyethylene glycol bases deliver water-insoluble drugs topically more efficiently than water-soluble agents. This feature is an added advantage because most topical antifungal drugs are basically water insoluble (e.g., tolnaftate).

The criteria for the powder dosage form (normal or under pressure) are basically the same as those for creams or solutions. Certain agents in powder forms are therapeutic and also serve as vehicles, e.g., talc and/or corn starch. Some OTC powder formulations state that the active ingredient is contained in a moisture-absorbent base (Enzactin). Powders inhibit the propagation of fungi by absorbing moisture and preventing skin maceration. Thus they actually alter the ecological conditions of the fungi, but the actual effective agent in these formulations is unknown (74). For example, the adsorbing material within the powder might be responsible for the remission of the disease instead of the intended active ingredient.

Many authorities consider corn starch superior to talc for these formulations, since it is virtually free of chemical contamination and it does not tend to produce granulomatous reactions in wounds as readily as talc (94). Moreover, a study comparing adsorbancy showed that corn starch adsorbed 25 times more mositure from moisture-saturated air than talc (95).

Product Selection Guidelines

Since the product chosen may influence patient compliance, the pharmacist should recommend an appropriate dosage form designed to cause the least interference with daily habits and activities without sacrificing efficacy. Product selection should be geared to the particular patient. For example, elderly patients may require a preparation that is easier than normal to use, and obese patients, in whom excessive sweating may contribute to the disease, should use topical talcum powders as adjunctive therapy.

Before recommending an OTC product, the pharmacist should review the patient's medical history. In patients with diabetes, for example, the glucose level, which as a normal constituent of sweat provides an excellent growth medium for fungi, must be under control (83). Patients with allergic dermatitides are extremely sensitive to most oral and topical agents. Such patients usually have a history of asthma, hay fever, or atopic dermatitis, which is indicated on the medication profile. Thus the pharmacist can distinguish a tinea infection from atopic dermatitis and avoid recommending a product that may cause skin irritation.

The concentration of organic fatty acids and/or their salt forms is usually too low to be irritating to the skin. Although these products are nonsensitizing, if irritation or sensitivity develops with their use, treatment should be discontinued.

The pharmacist should bear in mind that prescription-only drugs may be more beneficial in some cases than OTC products (96, 97). In the soggy, macerated athlete's foot complicated by bacteria the broad-spectrum antifungal agents miconazole nitrate (Mica-Tin) and clotrimazole (Lotrimin) are preferable to both tolnaftate and the prescription drug haloprogin (Halotex) (3). A recent study showed that clotrimazole was significantly more effective clinically and mycologically than haloprogin in treating tinea cruris (98).

Patient Consultation

The pharmacist should advise patients not to expect dramatic remission of the condition initially. The onset of symptomatic relief may take several days because healing generally is gradual. Patients should be advised that, depending on certain factors (e.g., extent of the affected area and patient variability to medication), the medication may have to be used a minimum of 2–4 weeks. The patient should be told of the necessity to adhere to the physician-prescribed dosage regimen or the suggested directions on the OTC product label. Although patient noncompliance is not documented, it probably contributes to the failure of topical products in treating tinea pedis. The pharmacist should ask the patient to continue the medication for a few days after the recommended time period to help prevent the possibility of a relapse of the infection.

All topical antifungal products may induce various hypersensitivity reactions. Although the incidence is small, patients should be advised to discontinue the product if itching, swelling, or further exacerbation of the disease occurs. In addition, patients should avoid contact of the product with the eyes. After applying the product, patients should wash their hands thoroughly with soap and water.

Before effective drug therapy for athlete's foot can be instituted, the pharmacist should emphasize the need for proper hygiene. The feet should be cleaned and dried thoroughly each day. Even though transmission of the disease to other individuals may be rare, patients should have their own washcloths and towels. The affected area should be patted dry thoroughly. After bathing, the feet should be dried last so as not to spread the infection with the towel to other sites.

General measures should be taken to eliminate the predisposing factors: heat and perspiration. Shoes and light cotton socks that allow ventilation should be worn. Wool and some newer synthetic fabrics interfere with foot moisture dissipation. Occlusive footwear, including canvas rubber-soled athletic shoes, should not be worn. Shoes should be alternated as often as possible so that the insides can dry adequately. Socks should be changed daily and washed thoroughly after use. Shoes should be dusted with drying powders.

product considerations

advice to the patient

proper hygiene

eliminating predisposing factors

Clothing and towels should be changed frequently and laundered well in hot water. The feet, particularly the area between the toes, should be dusted with a drying powder at every change of socks. Whenever possible, the feet should be aired to prevent moisture buildup. Nonocclusive protective footwear (e.g., rubber or wooden sandals) should be worn in areas of family or public use such as the home bathroom, community showers, or bathing areas.

The pharmacist should inform the patient of the need for protective measures that aid the topical antifungal product in eradicating the fungal infection. However, patients should be cautioned against overzealous cleansing with soap and water and vigorous drying between the toes; this practice may irritate the area further.

Dermatophytes enjoy living on moist warm wood. Public baths and shower areas should not be constructed with wooden grills for bathers to stand or walk on (63).

SUMMARY

The OTC drug of choice in the treatment of corns, calluses, and warts is salicylic acid in a flexible collodion (10%) or plaster (40%) form, whichever is more convenient. However, it is ineffective if predisposing factors responsible for corns and calluses are not corrected. (Surgical excision of corns associated with exostoses prevents development of corns only in that area.) The effectiveness of salicylic acid in warts is increased if the wart is pared to the point of bleeding or pain. This procedure should be performed only by a physician. Plantar warts should be treated with a higher concentration (20–40% of salicylic acid); warts on thin epidermis require a lower concentration (10–20%). Because warts are usually self-limiting, treatment should be conservative; vigorous therapy with salicylic acid may scar tissue.

The pharmacological OTC drug of choice in treating the dry, scaly type of athlete's foot is tolnaftate. However, other predisposing factors to tinea pedis must be eliminated by the patient for tolnaftate to be effective. Tolnaftate is effective in all its drug delivery systems, but the powder form should be reserved only for extremely mild conditions or as adjunctive therapy.

When it is recommended for suspected or actual dermatophytosis of the foot, tolnaftate should be used twice per day, morning and night. Because the vehicle forms of the solution and cream are spreadable, they should be used sparingly. Treatment should be continued 2–4 weeks, depending on the symptoms. After this time, effectiveness should be evaluated by the patient and pharmacist.

The value of any topical OTC product for the treatment of the soggy, macerated type of athlete's foot is dubious. The complex nature of the typical flora (i.e., resident aerobic diphtheroids) superimposed on the fungal infection dictates rigorous therapy with broader spectrum antifungals (miconazole nitrate or clotrimazole). Otherwise, soaks and compresses of astringent agents (aluminum chloride) may be indicated to dry the soggy, macerated tissue. Once this step is accomplished, tolnaftate therapy may be instituted.

Alleviation of the symptoms does not occur overnight. Patients should be made aware of this fact to avoid noncompliance associated with a product they believe to be ineffective.

REFERENCES

(1) S. Rosen, *J. Med. Assoc. State Ala.*, *43*, 617 (1974).
(2) K. A. Arndt, "Manual of Dermatological Therapeutics," Little, Brown, Boston, Mass., 1974, pp. 23–25.
(3) J. J. Leyden and A. M. Kligman, *Postgrad. Med.*, *61*, 113 (1977).
(4) J. J. Leyden and A. M. Kligman, *Arch. Dermatol.*, *111*, 1004 (1975).
(5) H. T. Behrmann, T. A. Labow, and J. H. Rozen, "Common Skin Diseases: Diagnosis and Treatment," 2nd ed., Grune and Stratton, New York, N.Y., 1971, p. 39.
(6) A. N. Domonkos, "Andrews' Diseases of the Skin," 6th ed., Saunders, Philadelphia, Pa., 1971, pp. 54–58.
(7) G. K. Potter, *J. Am. Podiat. Assoc.*, *63*, 57 (1973).
(8) "Current Dermatologic Management," S. Maddin and T. H. Brown, Eds., Mosby, St. Louis, Mo., 1970, pp. 114–116.
(9) W. D. Stewart, J. L. Danto, and S. Maddin, "Dermatology: Diagnosis and Treatment of Cutaneous Disorders," 3rd ed., Mosby, St. Louis, Mo., 1974, pp. 3–21.
(10) N. J. Giannestras, "Foot Disorders: Medical and Surgical Management," 2nd ed., Lea and Febiger, Philadelphia, Pa., 1973, pp. 24–26.
(11) I. Yale, "Podiatric Medicine," Williams and Wilkins, Baltimore, Md., 1974, pp. 244–246.
(12) "DuVries' Surgery of the Foot," 3rd ed., V. T. Inman, Ed., Mosby, St. Louis, Mo., 1973, pp. 206–223.
(13) A. N. Domonkos, "Andrews' Diseases of the Skin," 6th ed., Saunders, Philadelphia, Pa., 1971, pp. 548–553.
(14) E. Jawetz et al., "Review of Medical Microbiology," 11th ed., Lange Medical, Los Altos, Calif., 1974, pp. 449–450.
(15) J. S. Pegum, *Practitioner*, *209*, 453 (1972).
(16) F. A. Ive, *Br. Med. J.*, *4*, 475 (1973).
(17) K. A. Arndt, "Manual of Dermatological Therapeutics," Little, Brown, Boston, Mass., 1974, pp. 167–173.
(18) W. D. Stewart, J. L. Danto, and S. Maddin, "Dermatology: Diagnosis and Treatment of Cutaneous Disorders," 3rd ed., Mosby, St. Louis, Mo., 1974, pp. 281–285.
(19) A. P. Goffe, J. D. Almeida, and F. Brown, *Lancet*, *2*, 607 (1966).
(20) S. Pyrhonen and E. Johansson, *Lancet*, *1*, 592 (1975).
(21) M. H. Bunney, J. A. A. Hunter, M. M. Ogilvie, and M. A. Williams, *Practitioner*, *207*, 197 (1971).
(22) "Dermal Pathology," J. H. Graham, W. C. Johnson, and E. B. Helwig, Eds., Harper and Row, Hagerstown, Md., 1972, pp. 533–535.
(23) F. R. Bettley, "Skin Diseases in General Practice," Charles C Thomas, Springfield, Ill., 1965, pp. 243–253.
(24) N. Tobias, "Essentials of Dermatology," 6th ed., Lippincott, Philadelphia, Pa., 1963, p. 210.
(25) H. T. Behrman, T. A. Labow, and J. H. Rozen, "Common Skin Diseases: Diagnosis and Treatment," 2nd ed., Grune and Stratton, New York, N.Y., 1971, pp. 139–142.
(26) B. B. Sanders, Jr., and G. S. Stretcher, *J. Am. Med. Assoc.*, *235*, 2859 (1976).
(27) R. B. Rees, Jr., in "Current Diagnosis and Treatment," M. A. Krupp and M. J. Chatton, Eds., Lange Medical, Los Altos, Calif., 1976, p. 65.
(28) A. S. Wigfield, *Br. Med. J.*, *3*, 585 (1972).
(29) J. P. Barrett, Jr., *J. Am. Med. Assoc.*, *235*, 1138 (1976).
(30) "AMA Drug Evaluations," 3rd ed., Publishing Sciences Group, Littleton, Mass., 1977, pp. 188–189.
(31) A. L. Norins, in "Current Therapy, 1976," H. F. Conn, Ed., Saunders, Philadelphia, Pa., 1976, pp. 667–670.
(32) M. H. Bunney, *Drugs*, *13*, 445 (1977).
(33) E. W. Rosenberg, R. A. Amonette, and J. H. Gardner, *Arch. Dermatol.*, *113*, 1134 (1977).
(34) "Sprowls' American Pharmacy," 7th ed., L. W. Dittert, Ed., Lippincott, Philadelphia, Pa., 1974, p. 167.
(35) H. C. Ansel. "Introduction to Pharmaceutical Dosage Forms," Lea and Febiger, Philadelphia, Pa., 1969, p. 260.
(36) E. M. Brecher and Editors of Consumer Reports, "Licit and Illicit Drugs," Little, Brown, Boston, Mass., 1972, pp. 309–320.
(37) H. C. Ansel, "Introduction to Pharmaceutical Dosage Forms," Lea and Febiger, Philadelphia, Pa., 1969, p. 339.
(38) "Drug Design," Vol. 4, E. J. Ariens, Ed., Academic, New York, N.Y., 1973, p. 134.
(39) J. F. vonWeiss and W. F. Lever, *Arch. Dermatol.*, *90*, 614 (1964).
(40) M. E. Stolar, G. V. Rossi, and M. Barr, *J. Am. Pharm. Assoc. Sci. Ed.*, *49*, 144 (1960).
(41) "Drug Design," Vol. 4, E. J. Ariens, Ed., Academic, New York, N.Y., 1973, p. 178.
(42) J. A. Mills, *N. Engl. J. Med.*, *290*, 781 (1974).
(43) A. Gaisin, *Arch. Dermatol.*, *112*, 1791 (1976).
(44) M. N. Gleason, R. E. Gosselin, H. C. Hodge, and K. P. Smith, "Clinical Toxicology of Commercial Products, Acute Poisoning," 3rd ed., Williams and Wilkins, Baltimore, Md., 1969, Section 2, p. 154.
(45) R. R. M. McLaughlin, *Arch. Dermatol.*, *106*, 129 (1972).
(46) R. Lester and D. Rosenthal, *Arch. Dermatol.*, *104*, 330 (1971).
(47) M. W. Hursthouse, *Br. J. Dermatol.*, *92*, 93 (1975).
(48) Medical News, *J. Am. Med. Assoc.*, *237*, 940 (1977).
(49) S. W. Balkin, *Arch. Dermatol.*, *111*, 1143 (1975).
(50) L. Hymes and G. S. Hymes, *Am. Podiatry Assoc. J.*, *65*, 1023 (1975).
(51) D. F. Tutunji, *Br. Med. J.*, *4*, 241 (1972).
(52) W. L. Epstein and A. M. Kligman, *Arch. Dermatol.*, *77*, 508 (1958).
(53) A. N. G. Clark and M. J. Parsonage, *Br. Med. J.*, *2*, 1155 (1957).
(54) C. G. Schirren, *Hautarzt*, *17*, 321 (1966).
(55) G. C. Sauer, "Manual of Skin Diseases," 3rd ed., Lippincott, Philadelphia, Pa., 1973, pp. 159–181.
(56) L. Ajello, E. L. Keeney, and E. N. Broyles, *Johns Hopkins Med. J.*, *77*, 440 (1945).
(57) C. M. Davis, R. L. Garcia, J. P. Riordan, and D. Taplan, *Arch. Dermatol.*, *105*, 558 (1972).
(58) C. M. Caravati, Jr., E. M. Hudgins, and L. W. Kelly, Jr., *Cutis*, *17*, 313 (1976).
(59) R. L. Baer and S. A. Rosenthal, *J. Am. Med. Assoc.*, *197*, 187 (1966).
(60) W. D. Stewart, J. L. Danto, and S. Maddin, "Dermatology: Diagnosis and Treatment of Cutaneous Disorders," 3rd ed., Mosby, St. Louis, Mo., 1974, pp. 234–259.
(61) "An Introduction to the Biology of the Skin," R. H. Champion, T. Gillman, A. J. Rook, and R. T. Sims, Eds., Davis, Philadephia, Pa., 1970, pp. 206–221.
(62) K. A. Arndt, "Manual of Dermatologic Therapeutics," Little, Brown, Boston, Mass., 1974, pp. 61–77.
(63) J. H. S. Pettit, *Drugs*, *10*, 130 (1975).
(64) A. Jarrett, "The Physiology and Pathophysiology of the Skin: The Epidermis," Vol. 1, Academic, New York, N.Y., 1973, p. 155.
(65) R. J. Yu, S. R. Harmon, and F. Blank, *J. Bacteriol.*, *96*, 1435 (1968).
(66) F. Sadik, *PharmIndex*, *15*(7A), (1973).
(67) "Dermal Pathology," J. H. Graham, W. C. Johnson, and E. B. Helwig, Eds., Harper and Row, Hagerstown, Md., 1972, pp. 137–253.
(68) L. Goldman, in "Current Therapy, 1972," H. F. Conn, Ed., Saunders, Philadelphia, Pa., 1972, p. 585.
(69) R. A. Amonette and E. W. Rosenberg, *Arch. Dermatol.*, *107*, 71 (1973).
(70) T. Noguchi, A. Kaji, Y. Igarashi, A. Shigematsu, and K. Taniguchi, "Antitrichophyton Activity of Naphthiomates in Antimicrobial Agents and Chemotherapy," American Society for Microbiology, Ann Arbor, Mich., 1962, p. 259.
(71) G. A. Gellin, H. I. Maibach, and G. N. Wachs, *Arch. Dermatol.*, *106*, 715 (1972).
(72) J. B. Shelmire, Jr., *J. Invest. Dermatol.*, *26*, 105 (1956).
(73) K. H. Kaidbey and A. M. Kligman, *Arch. Dermatol.*, *110*, 868 (1974).
(74) E. B. Smith, J. E. Dickson, and J. M. Know, *South. Med. J.*, *67*, 776 (1974).
(75) A. H. Gould, *Dermatol. Trop. Ecol. Georg.*, *3*, 255 (1964).

(76) "AMA Drug Evaluations," 3rd ed., Publishing Sciences Group, Littleton Mass., 1977, pp. 821–838.
(77) S. M. Peck and H. Rosenfeld, *J. Invest. Dermatol.*, *1*, 237 (1938).
(78) E. L. Keeney, L. Ajello, E. Lankford, and L. Mary, *Bull. Johns Hopkins Hosp.*, *77*, 422 (1945).
(79) M. J. Golden and K. A. Oster, *J. Am. Pharm. Assoc. Sci. Ed.*, *39*, 47 (1950).
(80) W. C. Cutting, "Handbook of Pharmacology," 5th ed., Meredith, New York, N.Y., 1972, p. 56.
(81) E. B. Smith, R. F. Powell, and J. A. Ulrich, *Int. J. Dermatol.*, *16*, 52 (1977).
(82) "The Pharmacological Basis of Therapeutics," 5th ed., L. S. Goodman and A. Gilman, Eds., Macmillan, New York, N.Y., 1975, p. 990.
(83) M. H. Walker, *J. Am. Podiatr. Assoc.*, *52*, 737 (1962).
(84) M. N. Gleason, R. E. Gosselin, H. C. Hodge, and R. P. Smith, "Clinical Toxicology of Commercial Products, Acute Poisoning," 3rd ed., Williams and Wilkins, Baltimore, Md., 1969, p. 37.
(85) J. K. Morgan, *Br. J. Clin. Prac.*, *22*, 261 (1968).
(86) "The United States Dispensatory and Physician's Pharmacology," 26th ed., A. Osol et al., Eds., Lippincott, Philadelphia, Pa., 1967, p. 1024.
(87) "Sprowls' American Pharmacy," 7th ed., L. W. Dittert, Ed., Lippincott, Philadelphia, Pa., 1974, p. 49.
(88) P. B. Price, *Arch. Surg.*, *61*, 23 (1950).
(89) K. A. Oster and M. J. Golden, *J. Am. Pharm. Assoc. Sci. Ed.*, *37*, 429 (1948).
(90) G. A. Zentmyer, *Science*, *100*, 294 (1944).
(91) K. A. Oster and M. J. Golden, *Exp. Med. Surg.*, *1*, 37 (1949).
(92) M. N. Gleason, R. E. Gosselin, H. C. Hodge, and R. P. Smith, "Clinical Toxicology of Commercial Products, Acute Poisoning," 3rd ed., Williams and Wilkins, Baltimore, Md., 1969, p. 27.
(93) A. M. Kligman, J. J. Leyden, and R. Stewart, *Int. J. Dermatol.*, *16*, 413 (1977).
(94) H. Myllarniemi, M. Frilauder, M. Turunen, and L. Saxen, *Acta Chir. Scand.*, *131*, 312 (1966).
(95) *Federal Register*, *43*, 34636 (1978).
(96) L. E. Millikan, *Postgrad. Med.*, *60*, 52 (1976).
(97) E. B. Smith, J. L. Graham, and J. A. Ulrich, *South. Med. J.*, *70*, 47 (1977).
(98) J. V. VanDersarl and R. H. Sheppard, *Arch. Dermatol.*, *113*, 1233 (1977).

Product (Manufacturer)	Application Form	Antifungal	Keratolytic	Other
Aftate (Plough)	spray liquid spray powder powder gel	tolnaftate, 1%	—	—
Bevill's Lotion (Bevill)	lotion	—	salicylic acid	alcohol, 68% ether, 8% methyl salicylate, 1%
Blis-To-Sol (Chattem)	liquid aerosol powder powder	undecylenic acid, 5% (gel) 50 mg/g (liquid) zinc stearate, 10 mg/g (aerosol, powder) benzoic acid, 10 mg/g (aerosol) 19 mg/g (powder)	salicylic acid, 90 mg/g (liquid) 10 mg/g (aerosol) 19 mg/g (powder)	—
Bluboro (Herbert Labs)	liquid[a]	—	—	aluminum sulfate calcium acetate boric acid
Buro-Sol (Doak)	powder cream	—	—	aluminum acetate
Campho-Phenique (Winthrop)	liquid powder	phenol, 4.7% (liquid) 2% (powder)	—	camphor, 10.86% (liquid) 4.4% (powder)
Daliderm (Dalin)	powder	zinc undecylenate sodium propionate	salicylic acid	methylbenzethonium chloride corn starch magnesium carbonate boric acid bentonite zinc oxide talc aromatic oils
Desenex (Pharmacraft)	ointment powder aerosol powder soap	zinc undecylenate, 20% (not in soap) undecylenic acid, 5% (ointment) 2% (powder, soap)	—	—
Desenex Liquid (Pharmacraft)	solution	undecylenic acid, 10%	—	isopropyl alcohol, 40% propylene glycol triethanolamine
Deso-Creme (Columbia Medical)	cream	zinc undecylenate, 20% caprylic acid, 5% sodium propionate, 2%	—	—
Domeboro (Dome)	liquid[a]	—	—	aluminum sulfate calcium acetate
Enzactin (Ayerst)	cream	triacetin, 250 mg/g	—	—
Fungacetin (Blair)	liquid ointment powder	triacetin, 30% (liquid) 25% (ointment) 33.3% (powder)	—	—
Jim Wade Deodorant Foot Powder (Wade)	powder	8-hydroxyquinoline, 0.01%	—	aluminum sulfate, 15% menthol, 1% corn starch boric acid talc
Jim Wade Foot Medicine (Wade)	liquid	—	salicylic acid	sucrose octaacetate acetone
Medicated Foot Powder (Upjohn)	powder	benzoic acid, 2.5% chlorothymol, 0.04%	salicylic acid, 2.5%	boric acid, 10% zinc oxide, 2% camphor oil cinnamaldehyde, 0.08%
NP 27 Cream (Norwich)	cream	8-hydroxyquinoline benzoic acid	salicylic acid	propylparaben methylparaben

Product (Manufacturer)	Application Form	Antifungal	Keratolytic	Other
NP 27 Liquid (Norwich)	liquid	benzoic acid chlorothymol	salicylic acid	isopropyl alcohol, 50% propylparaben benzyl alcohol
NP 27 Powder (Norwich)	powder	benzoic acid	salicylic acid	eucalyptol menthol
Podiaspray (Dalin)	spray	undecylenic acid chloroxylenol	salicylic acid	cetyltrimethylammonium bromide aromatic base
Quin III (Pfeiffer)	cream	iodochlorhydroxyquin, 3%	—	—
Quinsana Plus (Mennen)	powder	zinc undecylenate, 20% undecylenic acid, 2%	—	talc silica fragrance
Rid-Itch Cream (Thomas & Thompson)	cream	zinc undecylenate, 20% undecylenic acid, 5%	—	emulsion base 2-(2-ethoxyethoxy)ethanol
Rid-Itch Liquid (Thomas & Thompson)	liquid	resorcinol, 1% benzoic acid, 2% chlorothymol, 1%	salicylic acid, 7%	boric acid, 5% alcohol glycerin
Salicresen (Upjohn)	liquid	secondary amyltricresols, 0.1% *o*-hydroxyphenylmercuric chloride, 0.1%	salicylic acid, 2%	acetone, 10% benzoic acid, 2% alcohol, 50%
Solvex Athlete's Foot Spray (Scholl)	spray	undecylenic acid chlorothymol triclosan	—	dichlorophene benzocaine propylene glycol alcohol
Solvex Ointment (Scholl)	ointment	benzoic acid	salicylic acid	thymol
Solvex Powder (Scholl)	powder	8-hydroxyquinoline sulfate chlorothymol	colloidal sulfur salicylic acid	—
Sopronol (Wyeth)	liquid ointment powder	sodium propionate, 12.3% (liquid, ointment) 5% (powder) sodium caprylate, 10% zinc caprylate, 5% (ointment) zinc propionate, 5% (powder)	—	—
T-4-L (Sorbol)	solution	—	salicylic acid benzoic acid	camphor alcohol, 79.9%
Tinactin Cream and Solution (Schering)	cream solution	tolnaftate, 1%	—	polyethylene glycol 400 propylene glycol (cream) butylated hydroxytoluene titanium dioxide (cream)
Tinactin Powder (Schering)	powder aerosol powder	tolnaftate, 1%	—	corn starch (powder) talc propellants (aerosol) butylated hydroxytoluene (aerosol)
Ting (Pharmacraft)	cream powder	zinc stearate benzoic acid	—	boric acid zinc oxide alcohol, 16% (cream)
Verdefam Cream (Texas Pharmacal)	cream	propionic acid, 3% undecylenic acid, 2% sodium propionate, 1% sodium caprylate, 1% copper undecylenate, 0.5%	salicylic acid, 3%	—

Athlete's Foot Products

Product (Manufacturer)	Application Form	Antifungal	Keratolytic	Other
Verdefam Solution (Texas Pharmacal)	solution	undecylenic acid, 5% propionic acid, 3% sodium propionate, 2% sodium caprylate, 2% copper undecylenate, 0.5%	salicylic acid, 5%	—

[a] Product is diluted or reconstituted and then applied to the skin.

Callus/Corn/Wart Products

Product (Manufacturer)	Application Form	Active Ingredients	Other
Bevill's Corn Remedy (Bevill)	lotion	salicylic acid ferric chloride tincture	alcohol, 70% ether methyl salicylate
Compound W Wart Remover (Whitehall)	liquid	salicylic acid, 14% glacial acetic acid, 11%	alcohol ether acetone menthol camphor
Corn Fix (Alvin Last)	liquid	phenol	soap turpentine oil
Derma-Soft Creme (Creighton)	cream	salicylic acid, 2.5%	cream base
Dr. Scholl's Corn/Callus Salve (Scholl)	ointment	salicylic acid	eucalyptus oil petrolatum lanolin mineral oil
Dr. Scholl's "2" Drop Corn-Callus Remover (Scholl)	liquid	salicylic acid	alcohol, 15% ether, 0.321 g/ml
Dr. Scholl's Fixo Corn Plaster (Scholl)	unmedicated pads medicated discs	salicylic acid	—
Dr. Scholl's Waterproof Corn Pads (Scholl)	unmedicated pads medicated discs	salicylic acid	—
Dr. Scholl's Zino-Pads (Scholl)	unmedicated pads medicated discs	salicylic acid	—
Freezone Corn and Callus Remover (Whitehall)	liquid	salicylic acid zinc chloride	alcohol Oregon balsam fir collodion hypophosphorous acid
Gets-It Liquid (Oakhurst)	liquid	salicylic acid, 13.9% zinc chloride, 2.7%	ether alcohol collodion
Johnson's Foot Soap (Combe)	liquid[a]	—	borax iodide bran
Mediplast (Beiersdorf)	plaster	salicylic acid, 40%	—
Mosco (Moss)	ointment	salicylic acid	methyl salicylate
Vergo (Daywell)	ointment	calcium pantothenate ascorbic acid	starch
Wart Fix (Alvin Last)	liquid	castor oil	—

[a] Product is diluted or reconstituted and then applied to the skin.

Hemorrhoidal Products

Benjamin Hodes

Chapter 32

Questions to Ask the Patient

What is the nature of the symptoms? How long have they been present?

Have you noticed any bleeding? Describe the bleeding.

Have you treated the symptoms without the use of medicine?

Have you previously used any OTC or prescription drugs for these symptoms?

Anorectal disease, including hemorrhoids, is one of the most annoying and uncomfortable disorders suffered by Americans. A number of diseases affecting the anorectal area are not amenable to self-treatment. However, many symptoms of hemorrhoids, the most prevalent anorectal disease, may be self-treated. Numerous OTC products are available for relief of the burning, pain, itching, and bleeding of hemorrhoids.

CLINICAL CONSIDERATIONS

In addition to hemorrhoids, anorectal disease encompasses other disorders, some of which may be serious. The pharmacist should evaluate patient symptom complaints carefully before recommending a product for self-medication. Some anorectal disorders require immediate physician referral.

Anatomy and Physiology

Three parts of the body are of concern with respect to anorectal disease. These are the perianal area, the anal canal, and the lower portion of the rectum (Figure 1).

Perianal Area

The perianal area (~7 cm in diameter) is the portion of the skin and buttocks immediately surrounding the anus. The skin is somewhat more likely to be moist than exposed skin in other areas of the body. The presence of sensory nerve endings makes the perianal area very sensitive to pain.

Anal Canal

The anal canal (~3 cm long) is the channel connecting the end of the GI tract (rectum) with the outside of the body. The lower two-thirds is covered by modified anal skin similar to normal skin.

Although no sensory nerve endings are present in the anal canal, "pressure receptors" do cause distention discomfort.

The point at which the skin lining changes to mucous membrane is the anorectal or pectinate line and delineates the upper margin of the anal canal.

Two sphincters encircling the anal canal control passage of fecal material. The external (anal) sphincter, located at the bottom of the anal canal, is a voluntary muscle. The internal sphincter, which allows passage into the anal canal, is an involuntary muscle. Both sphincters lie under the tissues of the anal canal and extend downward. Under normal conditions the external sphincter is closed and prevents the involuntary passage of feces and/or other discharges.

The skin covering the anal canal in healthy individuals serves as a barrier which severely limits absorption of substances into the body. Therefore treatment applied to the area of the anal canal can be expected to manifest only local effects. If disease is present, the character of the skin may be altered due to the loss of protective oils, and the ability to serve as a protective barrier is lost.

Anal crypts are pocketlike mucosal formations at the internal side of the anorectal line. They face upward and because of their position can retain small amounts of fecal material which can cause irritation. This irritation is believed by many to be the cause of subsequent infections and the development of some forms of hemorrhoidal disease. Some authors distinguish between rectal mucosa and anal mucosa and consider the anorectal ring to be the end of the anal canal (1). For the purposes of this discussion, the appearance of the mucosal region will mark the beginning of the rectal area.

Rectum

The rectum (~12–15 cm long) is the lower end of the GI tract that extends from the anorectal line up to the sigmoid colon. It is lined with semipermeable mucous membranes and is highly vascularized. Like the anal canal, it contains pressure receptors. The skin of the anal canal and mucous membrane in the rectum in individuals without anorectal disease protect the body from invasion by the bacteria present in the feces and from injury due to unabsorbed roughage.

Substances absorbed through the mucous membrane may exert systemic effects due to the plexus of hemorrhoidal vessels beneath the mucosa and the paths followed

sites of anorectal diseases

predisposing factors and causes of hemorrhoids

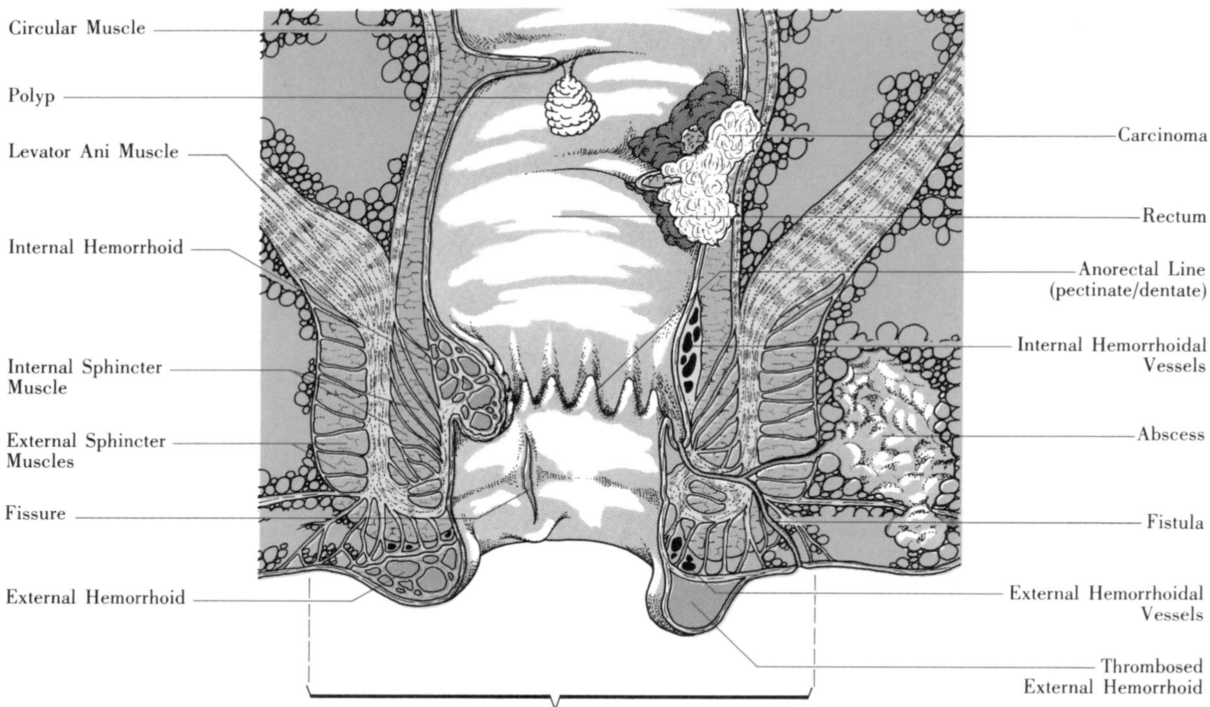

Figure 1. Selected disease states in anorectal region.

by the blood returning to the heart via the hemorrhoidal veins. This process allows substances to enter the systemic circulation without passing through the liver. This effect is important in evaluating the potential systemic toxicity of locally applied drugs. The rectal pH, ranging from neutral to decidedly basic, is important in determining the extent to which substances in the rectum are absorbed.

The most prominent parts of the vasculature in the region above and below the pectinate line are the three hemorrhoidal arteries along with the accompanying veins. Veins and arteries above the pectinate line are referred to as internal, and those below as external.

Etiology

Numerous etiological factors give rise to the considerable confusion regarding the cause or causes of hemorrhoidal disease. Etiological factors may be divided into predisposing and exciting causes (2).

Predisposing Causes

The main predisposing causes are the human upright position, heredity, and occupational status. The human upright position causes increased hydrostatic pressure within the hemorrhoidal veins. Because these veins contain no valves, they are unable to counteract the weight of the blood column impinging upon them and therefore produce continuous anorectal pressure. Heredity also is considered important to hemorrhoid formation, although there is far from universal agreement on this issue (3). Occupations involving severe muscular strain, prolonged sitting, or prolonged standing also are believed to be predisposing factors.

Dietary and cultural patterns also may predispose to hemorrhoids (4). Low-fiber diets contribute to hard and stiff stools, which in turn lead to constipation, an important exciting cause of hemorrhoids due to excessive straining for defecation.

Exciting Causes

Exciting causes of hemorrhoids are constipation and diarrhea, heart failure, portal hypertension, coughing, sneezing, vomiting, pregnancy, pelvic tumors, carcinoma of the rectum, physical exertion, and anal infection. Constipation leads to forcing defecation by straining, which in turn leads to greatly increased pressure within the hemorrhoidal venous plexuses. Diarrhea, coughing, sneezing, vomiting, heart failure, portal hypertension, and physical exertion all increase the pressure within the hemorrhoidal venous plexuses and thereby may precipitate hemorrhoids.

Pregnancy is by far the most common cause of hemorrhoids in young women. The enlarged and gravid uterus causes increased pressure in the middle and inferior hemorrhoidal plexuses. Labor also may intensify the hemorrhoidal condition and produce intense symptoms after delivery. Pelvic tumors may give rise to hemorrhoids by a similar process.

It is hypothetically possible that hemorrhoids may result from the alternating constipation and diarrhea associated with carcinoma of the rectum.

Anal infection is considered by some to be the principal cause of hemorrhoids (5), but this view is not generally accepted. Infections from bacteria in the feces cause inflammation, which leads to an erosion of the supporting tissue of the hemorrhoidal plexuses. Thus the weakened tissue is not able to withstand the normal pressure in the veins, and varicosities develop. Another possible cause of anorectal disorders is an infection occurring initially in the anal crypts that spreads to the veins nearby and results in a thrombosed hemorrhoid.

Description

Hemorrhoids (also known as piles) are abnormally large or symptomatic conglomerates of vessels, supporting tissues, and overlying mucous membrane or skin of the anorectal area. They may be classified according to degree of severity (6) or location (Figure 1).

External Hemorrhoids

External hemorrhoids occur below the anorectal line.

Thrombotic

A thrombotic hemorrhoid is either a hemorrhoidal vein in the anal canal or adjacent to the anus in which a blood clot develops or an accumulation of blood beneath the skin caused by a rupture of a hemorrhoidal vessel. The clot may vary in size from a pea to a walnut.

Cutaneous (Skin Tags)

These consist of fibrous connective tissue covered by anal skin and are located outside the anal sphincter at any point on the circumference of the anus. They may result from a previous thrombosed external hemorrhoid in which the clot has become organized and replaced by connective tissue (7) or from uneven skin healing after hemorrhoidectomy.

Internal Hemorrhoids

Internal hemorrhoids occur above the anorectal line. Occasionally, because of its size and distention, an internal hemorrhoid descends below the anorectal line and outside the anal sphincter. It is then referred to as a prolapsed hemorrhoid.

Internal–External Hemorrhoids

Also known as mixed hemorrhoids, these are a combination of external and internal hemorrhoids in continuity with one another and appear as baggy swellings. The following varieties occur:

- Prolapsed: characterized by pain until the prolapse is reduced. Bleeding may or may not be present.
- Without prolapse: bleeding may be present, but no pain.
- Strangulated: hemorrhoid that has prolapsed to such a degree and for so long that its blood supply is occluded by the anal sphincter's constricting action; very painful; usually becomes thrombosed.

Other Anorectal Disorders

Other anorectal diseases with symptoms amenable to self-medication are anal fissures and anal fistulas. Some potentially serious disorders also may present hemorrhoidal symptoms but should not be self-medicated.

- Abscess: a painful swelling in the perianal or anal canal area due to a bacterial infection and resulting in the formation of pus. Usually, *Staphylococcus* is the primary organism involved.
- Anal fissure: a slitlike ulcer in the anal canal. This condition may exist simultaneously with hemorrhoids.
- Anal fistula: a chronic lesion near the anus characterized by a cavity with swelling, pain, and pruritus among the major symptoms. Anorectal abscess or cryptitis usually results in an anal fistula.
- Condyloma latumi: one of the secondary lesions of syphilis. Its symptoms could very easily be mistaken for those of external hemorrhoid.
- Cryptitis: inflammation and hypertrophy of the semilunar anal valve; main symptom is anal discomfort aggravated by walking and defecation; probably originates in an anal gland.
- Malignant neoplasm: often characterized by a progressively enlarging "lump" beside the anus. Symptoms such as bleeding and pain may be associated with malignant anal tumors, the most common of which is squamous cell carcinoma. The seriousness of this disease cannot be overestimated.
- Polyps: benign tumors of the large bowel often characterized by bleeding, protrusion of a mass through the anus, and a feeling of fullness or pressure in the rectum.

characterteristics and types of hemorrhoids

common symptoms of anorectal disease

pruritus/itching

Signs and Symptoms

Itching, burning, pain, inflammation, irritation, swelling, and discomfort are common symptoms of anorectal disease that can be relieved by self-medication. Bleeding, seepage, protrusion, prolapse, and thrombosis are more serious symptoms of anorectal disease. These symptoms should not be self-medicated, either because a more serious disorder may be masked or because there is no appropriate OTC product.

Itching

Itching, or pruritus, occurs as a manifestation of mild inflammation associated with many anorectal disorders. Pruritus ani refers to itching in the anal and perianal area that may occur even if good hygiene is practiced. The most common symptom of anorectal disease, itching may be secondary to swelling or moisture in the anal area.

Itching is not always symptomatic of hemorrhoidal disease. Sensitivity to fabrics, detergents, and fecal contents may precipitate an itching attack. Fungal infections, parasites, allergies, and associated anorectal pathological lesions also may cause itching, and an adverse drug reaction to antibiotic therapy may trigger it as well. Sometimes, itching may be attributed to some psychological cause or possibly to no cause at all.

symptoms of anorectal disorders

Burning

Burning represents a somewhat greater degree of irritation of the anorectal sensory nerves than itching. The burning sensation may span the range from a feeling of warmth to a feeling of intense heat. Burning is a fairly common symptom of anorectal disease.

Pain

Pain is experienced in acute external hemorrhoids or in the presence of some other acute anal lesion. It results from acute inflammation of the anal tissues and may be accentuated by physical activity such as walking. The pain has a steady and aching character and is not necessarily relieved by defecation. There is no pain generally associated with chronic external hemorrhoids, and minimal or no pain is experienced in most uncomplicated cases of internal hemorrhoids. Patients with severe and/or persistent pain should be referred to a physician.

Inflammation

Inflammation often is caused by trauma, allergy, or infection. The inflammation itself may be relieved by self-medication but not its underlying cause.

Irritation, Swelling, and Discomfort

Irritation is a response to stimulation of the nerve ending. Tissue irritation is recognized by the appearance of burning, itching, pain, or swelling. Swelling represents accumulation of excess fluid associated with engorged hemorrhoids or hemorrhoidal tissue. Discomfort, a vague and generalized uneasiness, may result from any or all of the described symptoms.

Bleeding

Bleeding is almost always associated with internal hemorrhoids and may occur before, during, or after defecation. The amount of bleeding experienced is often variable and is not proportional to the amount of hemorrhoidal tissue present. When bleeding occurs from an external hemorrhoid, it is due to an acute thrombosis accompanied by rupture. Pain often accompanies the bleeding in this case, although a patient may experience some relief of the pain with the onset of the bleeding. Blood from hemorrhoids is usually bright red and externally covers the fecal material. Bleeding is stimulated by defecation and also may occur as an "oozing" which will soil underclothes.

Bleeding hemorrhoids may produce severe anemias due to the chronic blood loss. Bleeding may indicate the presence of serious anorectal disease and therefore should not be self-medicated.

Seepage

Seepage is caused by an anal sphincter that cannot close completely and involves the involuntary passing of fecal material or mucus. This symptom cannot be self-medicated, and physician referral is indicated.

Protrusion

Protrusion is a symptom of uncomplicated hemorrhoids. The rectal protrusion may vary in size and usually appears after defecation, prolonged standing, or unusual physical exertion. It is painless except when thrombosis, infection, or ulceration is present. Strangulation of a protruding hemorrhoid by the sphincter may occur and may lead to thrombosis.

Prolapse

A prolapsed hemorrhoid is an internal hemorrhoid which, because of distention, is located below the anorectal line and outside the anal sphincter.

When the anal sphincter contraction interferes with blood flow from a prolapsed internal or mixed hemorrhoid and thrombosis results, a painful lump forms. If this prolapsed hemorrhoid is returned to above the anal sphincter before thrombosis occurs, the pain and lump disappear. However, when defecation occurs at some later time, both the lump and pain are likely to recur. An observed symptom of permanently prolapsed internal hemorrhoids is a mucoid discharge, which may in turn lead to perianal irritation.

Thrombosis

Thrombosis, or blood clotting, within a hemorrhoid is a common complication. An abrupt onset of severe, constant pain in the anal area is a sign that thrombosis of a mixed or external hemorrhoid may have occurred. If untreated, the burning pain is experienced ~5–7 days, diminishing in intensity after the first day. A hard, tender lump at the site of the pain also appears; after the second day this lump slowly lessens and eventually leaves a skin tag.

If the thrombosed hemorrhoid resides entirely above the anorectal line (pure internal hemorrhoid), there probably is no pain because of the lack of sensory nerve supply. Patients are likely to be unaware of the presence of this type of hemorrhoid.

If thrombosed hemorrhoids do not disappear, gangrene and ulcers may develop on the hemorrhoid surface. This condition may lead to an oozing of blood as well as hemorrhaging, particularly at the time of defecation or if the patient is standing. If the clot remains exposed, infection may occur, and an abscess or fistula may eventually result.

ASSESSMENT

Questioning the patient should enable the pharmacist to determine whether self-medication is desirable and, if so, which OTC product is suitable. The pharmacist should recommend an appropriate OTC product for treatment of minor symptoms (itching, pain, or discomfort) associated with anorectal disease. The patient should be referred to a physician if there is bleeding, seepage, prolapse, or severe and persistent pain or if symptoms do not improve after 7 days of self-treatment.

TREATMENT

OTC products for treatment of anorectal disease symptoms are available in many dosage forms. The pharmacist also should emphasize the importance of good anal hygiene in helping to prevent and ameliorate symptoms of anorectal disease.

Patient Consultation

Specific advice to the patient should include the following reminders:

- If seepage, bleeding, and/or protrusion occurs, a physician should be contacted as soon as possible.
- Products designed for external use should not be inserted into the rectum.
- If insertion of a product in the rectum causes pain, use of the product should be discontinued and a physician consulted.
- Products to be used externally should be applied sparingly.
- Pile pipes may be too long and may deliver medication well beyond the hemorrhoidal problem area.
- If possible, the anorectal area should be washed with mild soap and warm water and then rinsed completely before any product is applied.
- If symptoms do not improve after 7 days, a physician should be consulted.

The role of good anal hygiene in preventing and ameliorating the symptoms of uncomplicated anorectal disease should be emphasized. Cleansing the anorectal area with a moistened toilet tissue after defecation is recommended. Sitz baths (a bath in which the patient sits in the tub with hips and buttocks immersed) are an alternative nondrug therapy for symptoms of uncomplicated anorectal disease. Also, the importance of maintaining normal bowel function by eating properly and avoiding excessive laxative use should be emphasized as a means of preventing anorectal disease.

Modern methods of treating hemorrhoids surgically include injection of sclerosing agents, rubber band ligation, dilatation of anal canal and lower rectum, cryosurgery, and hemorrhoidectomy (8).

Pharmacological Agents

The main pharmacological agents used for relief of anorectal disease symptoms are anesthetics, vasoconstrictors, protectants, counterirritants, astringents, wound-healing agents, antiseptics, keratolytics, and anticholinergics. Products containing an excessive number of agents may not be optimally effective because of potential interaction among ingredients. A summary of these agents and their effectiveness (as determined by the FDA OTC Panel on Hemorrhoidal Drug Products) in treating the symptoms of anorectal disease is given in Table 1.

Local Anesthetics

Local anesthetics relieve pain, burning, itching, and irritation by preventing the transmission of nerve impulses. As their name implies, they are designed to be used topically. In anorectal disease they should be used in the perianal region or the lower anal canal. Symptoms within the rectum itself generally are not relieved by local anesthetics because there are no rectal sensory nerve fibers (9–11).

Since absorption of local anesthetics through the rectal mucous mucosa may be quite rapid (12) and cause potentially toxic systemic effects (13), their application should be limited to the area below the rectum. Absorption through the perianal skin, even if abraded, would not be particularly rapid.

Local anesthetics may produce allergic reactions, both locally and systemically (14, 15). Such reactions may cause burning and itching that are indistinguishable from symptoms of the anorectal disease being treated.

Recommended Anesthetics

Of the local anesthetics used in hemorrhoidal preparations, only benzocaine and pramoxine hydrochloride are recommended, if used in appropriate doses (see Table 2).

Benzocaine. In the base form, benzocaine is effective locally in concentrations of 5–20% (16–18). Since absorption through the skin is poor, the possible systemic effects are minimized, and the most common adverse reaction to benzocaine is sensitization (19, 20). Polyethylene ointment and polyethylene glycol (PEG) ointment provide the same release of benzocaine; other vehicles may not release benzocaine as well.

advice to the patient

agents used for relief of anorectal disease symptoms

Pramoxine hydrochloride. Pramoxine hydrochloride is effective in a water-miscible base at a 1% concentration. Adverse effects are rare, and pramoxine hydrochloride is less sensitizing than other local anesthetics (21).

Nonrecommended Anesthetics

Other local anesthetics used in hemorrhoidal preparations are not recommended, either because they are not effective or because their safety is questionable. Studies have shown that diperodon is not effective (22), and phenacaine is considered unsafe because of the possibility of absorption leading to systemic toxicity (23). Additional evidence is required to show that the following local anesthetics are effective either intrarectally or externally: benzyl alcohol, dibucaine, dyclonine hydrochloride, lidocaine, tetracaine, and tetracaine hydrochloride (22).

Vasoconstrictors

Vasoconstrictors are chemical agents structurally related to the naturally occurring catecholamines epinephrine and norepinephrine, which function as transmitters of messages from nerves to receptors. Applied locally in the anorectal area, they attach to the α-adrenergic receptors in the vascular beds. Stimulation of these receptors causes constriction. While there is no evidence to support this theory, a vasoconstrictor applied locally to the rectal mucosa may have effects on β-receptors in other parts of the body (e.g., heart and lungs) due to possible systemic absorption. It has been demonstrated that there is a prompt altering of the blood supply to the mucosa when vasoconstrictors are applied locally (24). Vasoconstrictors also relieve local itching because they produce a slight anesthetic effect by an unknown mechanism (25). Conclusive evidence that vasoconstrictors reduce swollen hemorrhoids is lacking, even though they constrict vascular beds in skin and mucous membranes in other parts of the body.

Adverse Effects

The potential for systemic absorption of vasoconstrictors exists. As a result, increased blood pressure, cardiac arrhythmia, nervousness, tremor, insomnia, and aggravation of hyperthyroidism symptoms may occur (26), although this effect has never been demonstrated with vasoconstrictors applied rectally.

Because of these possible adverse reactions, vasoconstrictors should be used with caution in patients who have diabetes, hyperthyroidism, hypertension, and cardiovascular disease and in those who are taking monoamine oxidase inhibitors.

Recommended Vasoconstrictors

Three vasoconstrictors are recommended for use: ephedrine sulfate, epinephrine hydrochloride, and phenylephrine hydrochloride (see Table 2). Other drugs used in hemorrhoidal preparations, such as epinephrine undecylenate, have not been proven safe and effective.

agents used to relieve anorectal disease symptoms

summary of classes of agents used in hemorrhoidal products and their effectiveness for various symptoms

Ephedrine sulfate. This drug has a more prolonged effect than epinephrine and acts on both α- and β-adrenergic receptors. Because ephedrine antagonizes the effects of phenothiazines, it is contraindicated in patients receiving such therapy (27). Its onset of action ranges from a few seconds to 1 minute, its duration of action is 2–3 hours, and it is effective for itching and swelling.

Epinephrine hydrochloride. This drug is effective in the relief of itching and swelling only when used externally because epinephrine is inactivated at the pH of the rectum (28). Epinephrine is absorbed from the mucous membrane and acts on both α- and β-adrenergic receptors.

Phenylephrine hydrochloride. This drug relieves itching due to histamine release (22) and reduces congestion in the anorectal area (24). It acts primarily on the α-adrenergic receptors and produces vasoconstriction by a direct effect on receptors rather than by norepinephrine displacement.

Protectants

Protectants act to prevent irritation of the anorectal area and water loss from the stratum corneum skin layer by forming a physical barrier on the skin. Little or no absorption of protectants is expected. Protection of the perianal area from irritants such as fecal matter and air leads to a reduction in irritation and concomitant itching.

Absorbents, adsorbents, demulcents, and emollients are included in the protectant classification. Many substances classified as protectants also have uses as vehicles, bases, and carriers of pharmacologically active substances.

Adverse reactions are minimal with protectants as a class. Wool alcohols may cause allergic reactions, although a low incidence of allergic dermatitis has been associated with lanolin (29).

Recommended Protectants

The protectants recommended for use are aluminum hydroxide gel (in moist conditions only), calamine, cocoa butter, cod liver oil, glycerin, kaolin, lanolin, mineral oil, petrolatum, shark liver oil, starch, wool alcohols, and zinc oxide. All of these protectants are recommended for external and internal use, with the exception of glycerin, which is recommended for external use only. Of the

Table 1. Pharmacological Categories and Their Effectiveness in Treating Symptoms of Anorectal Disease

Symptom	Local Anesthetics	Vasoconstrictors	Protectants	Counterirritants	Astringents	Wound Healers	Antiseptics	Keratolytics	Anticholinergics	Miscellaneous
Itching	yes	yes	yes	yes	yes	no	no	yes	no	no
Discomfort	yes	no	yes	yes	yes	no	no	yes	no	no
Irritation	yes	no	yes	no	yes	no	no	no	no	no
Burning	yes	no	no	no	no	no	no	no	no	no
Swelling	no	yes	yes	no	no	no	no	no	no	no
Pain	yes	no	no	yes	yes	no	no	no	no	no
Inflammation	no	no	no	no	no	no	no	no	no	no

Modified from a table given in the "Tentative Findings of the FDA OTC Panel on Hemorrhoidal Drug Products," Information Copy, 1977, p. 42(1).
"Yes" means recommended as effective; "no" means not recommended.

recommended protectants, petrolatum is probably the most effective (30).

If one protectant is used, it must comprise at least 50% of the formulation. If two, three, or four protectants are used, their total concentration must be 50%. If protectant concentration is less than 50%, another protectant must be used. These dosages were arrived at by determining the amount of protectant required to provide adequate thickness to prevent water loss from the epidermis (22). For more specific dosage requirements, see Table 2. In general, two to four protectants are recommended.

Nonrecommended Protectants

The bismuth salts found in some hemorrhoidal products are not recommended as protectants. Bismuth subnitrate is not considered safe because it may be absorbed, producing toxic symptoms from the bismuth ion as well as the nitrate ion (31). The effectiveness of bismuth oxide, bismuth subcarbonate, and bismuth subgallate as protectants in the anorectal area has not been established by the FDA OTC Panel on Hemorrhoidal Drug Products.

Counterirritants

Counterirritants distract from the perception of pain and itching by stimulating nerve impulses to evoke a feeling of comfort, warmth, cooling, or tingling. Because the rectal mucosa contains no sensory nerve endings, counterirritants exert no effect in this area and thus, in general, are not recommended for intrarectal use.

Recommended Counterirritant

Menthol is the only recommended counterirritant. It is effective in concentrations of 0.25–2.0%, used externally (32). The primary adverse effect of menthol is the possibility of sensitivity reactions (33).

agents used in hemorrhoidal products

summary of recommended ingredients for anorectal products

Table 2. Recommended Ingredients

Class	Compound	Use	Amount/2 g
Anesthetics	benzocaine	external	100–400 mg (5–20%)
	pramoxine hydrochloride	external	20 mg (1%)
Vasoconstrictors	ephedrine sulfate	external, internal	10–20 mg
	epinephrine hydrochloride	external	0.1–0.2 mg
	phenylephrine hydrochloride	external, internal	0.5 mg
Protectants[a]	aluminum hydroxide gel	external, internal	
	calamine	external, internal	5–25%
	cocoa butter	external, internal	
	glycerin	external	20–45% aqueous solution
	kaolin	external, internal	
	lanolin	external, internal	
	petrolatum	external, internal	
	shark liver oil	external, internal	
	starch	external, internal	
	wool alcohols	external, internal	
	zinc oxide	external, internal	5–25%
	cod liver oil	external, internal	
	mineral oil	external, internal	
Counterirritants	menthol	external	0.25–2.0%
Astringents	calamine	external, internal	
	zinc oxide	external, internal	
	hamamelis water	external	10–50%
Wound healers	none		
Antiseptics	none		
Keratolytics	aluminum chlorhydroxy allantoinate	external	0.2–2.0%
Anticholinergics	none		
Miscellaneous	none		

[a] The total protectant concentration recommended is 50%.

Nonrecommended Counterirritants

Camphor, hydrastis (golden seal), juniper tar, and oil of turpentine are not recommended for use as counterirritants in the anorectal area. Because of camphor's rapid absorption due to its high lipid solubility, toxic concentrations may be reached (34). Both hydrastis and oil of turpentine are not considered safe and lack demonstrated effectiveness (35, 36). Juniper tar has not been proven effective.

Astringents

Applied to the skin or mucous membranes for a local and limited effect, astringents coagulate the protein in the skin cells, thereby protecting the underlying tissue and producing a decrease in the cell volume. When appropriately used, astringents lessen mucus and other secretions and help relieve local anorectal irritation and inflammation (37).

components of anorectal products

dosage form considerations

Calamine and zinc oxide are recommended as astringents for both external and internal use. The heavy metal zinc in these compounds acts as a protein precipitant and provides an astringent effect. Hamamelis water is recommended as an astringent for external use in anorectal disorders; its effectiveness is probably due to its alcohol content.

Tannic acid is not safe for anorectal use because it is well absorbed and may cause liver damage (38).

Wound-Healing Agents

Several ingredients in OTC hemorrhoidal products are claimed to be effective in promoting wound healing or tissue repair in anorectal disease. In particular, considerable controversy surrounds the substance skin respiratory factor (SRF), a water-soluble extract of Brewer's yeast also referred to as live yeast cell derivative (LYCD). Although some tests have supported manufacturer claims (39), there is no conclusive evidence that products containing skin respiratory factor promote the healing of diseased anorectal tissue. The FDA OTC Panel on Hemorrhoidal Drug Products evaluated live yeast cell derivative as well as cod liver oil, peruvian balsam, shark liver oil, vitamin A, and vitamin D and found them lacking in demonstrated effectiveness as wound healers (22). Well-designed and controlled studies are needed to determine the efficacy of wound healers in anorectal disease.

Antiseptics

Antiseptics generally inhibit the growth of microorganisms. Some OTC anorectal products contain compounds intended for use as antiseptics. However, because of the large numbers of microorganisms in feces, it is unlikely that the use of antiseptics in the anorectal area will provide a degree of antisepsis greater than that achieved by washing with soap and water. Antiseptics also are not recommended for use in the anorectal area because they may alter the normal flora in the anorectal region, which can lead to adverse effects, and because there is no convincing evidence that using antiseptics prevents infection in the anorectal area.

Specific compounds for which antiseptic properties have been claimed are boric acid, boric acid glycerite, hydrastis, phenol, resorcinol, and sodium salicylic acid phenolate. Boric acid and boric acid glycerite are not considered safe because of boric acid toxicity (40). As was mentioned earlier in the counterirritant discussion, hydrastis is not safe or effective for use in the anorectal region. Phenol, resorcinol (because of its resemblance to phenol), and sodium salicylic acid phenolate are not considered safe for use in the anorectal area (41).

Keratolytics

Keratolytics cause desquamation and debridement or sloughing of the epidermal surface cells. By loosening surface cells, keratolytics may help to expose underlying skin tissue to therapeutic agents. Used externally, they are useful in reducing itching, although their mechanism of action is unknown. Since mucous membranes contain no keratin layer, the use of keratolytics intrarectally is not justified.

The principal keratolytic recommended for external use is aluminum chlorhydroxy allantoinate. The dosage range established for it by the Panel is up to six applications per day of 0.2–2.0% ointment per 2-g dosage. In this concentration range it appears to be safe. Resorcinol and sulfur are not recommended as keratolytics for use in the anorectal area.

Anticholinergics

Anticholinergics inhibit or prevent the action of acetylcholine, the transmitter of cholinergic nerve impulses. Since anticholinergics produce their action systemically, they are not effective in ameliorating the local symptoms of anorectal disease.

Atropine, which is included in some products designed for anorectal use, is not safe because systemic poisoning may result from the absorption of the alkaloid through diseased skin (42) and through the rectal mucosa if the product is applied that high.

Miscellaneous

Collinsonia (stoneroot), *Escherichia coli* vaccines, lappa (burdock), leptandra (culver's root), and mullein are ingredients in OTC hemorrhoidal products that do not fall within the pharmacological classifications used above. With the exception of *E. coli* vaccines, these compounds are remnants of herbal medicine. There is no evidence that they are effective in treating symptoms of anorectal disease. The safety and effectiveness of *E. coli* vaccines also are unproven (22).

Dosage Forms

Drugs for treatment of anorectal disease symptoms are available in many dosage forms. For intrarectal use, suppositories, creams, ointments, gels, and foams are used, along with applicators, one's finger, and pile pipes to facilitate their application. Creams, ointments, gels, pads, liquids, and foam are used externally.

Ointments

Although from the pharmaceutical point of view there are considerable differences among ointments, creams, pastes, and gels, the therapeutic differences are not significant enough to classify them separately. Therefore "ointment" will be used to refer to all semisolid preparations designed for external or intrarectal use in the anorectal area.

Ointments may serve as vehicles for drugs used in treating anorectal disease symptoms and also possess inherent protectant and emollient properties. The primary function of an ointment base is the efficient delivery of the active ingredient(s). Applying an ointment may have a beneficial psychological effect on patients with anorectal disorders (22). When used externally, ointments should be applied to the perianal area and the anal canal as a thin covering.

For intrarectal use, pile pipes and one's finger have been used to apply ointments. Pile pipes have the advantage over a finger in that the drug product may be introduced onto the rectal mucosa where a finger cannot reach. For most efficient use, the pile pipe should have lateral openings, as well as a hole in the end, to allow the drug product to cover the greatest area of rectal mucosa. As was mentioned previously, the potential for systemic absorption is greatest from the mucosa.

Suppositories

Suppositories have been used for many centuries as a dosage form. A suppository may ease straining at the stool by a lubricating effect. Also, the insertion of a suppository may provide a beneficial psychological effect. However, because of their many disadvantages, suppositories are not recommended as a dosage form in treating anorectal disease symptoms. In prone patients, suppositories may leave the affected region and ascend into the rectum and lower colon. If the patient remains prone after inserting a suppository, the active ingredients may not be evenly distributed over the rectal mucosa. Suppositories are relatively slow acting because they must melt in order to release the active ingredient.

Foams

Foam products present no proven advantages over ointments. Their disadvantages are that there is difficulty in establishing that the foam will remain in the affected area and that the size of the foam bubbles determines the concentration of active ingredient available (43).

PRODUCT SELECTION GUIDELINES

Patient Considerations

Knowledge of a patient's present condition, medical history, and medication profile obtained from a patient interview is necessary to determine how an individual patient may respond to self-medication. Of prime importance is to determine that the patient has symptoms amenable to self-medication.

Conditions such as diarrhea and/or constipation will complicate, if not render impossible, the self-treatment of anorectal disease symptoms. If a patient is confined to bed, a suppository dosage form is probably not appropriate. Patients suffering from cardiovascular disease, diabetes, hypertension, and hyperthyroidism should not use a product containing a vasoconstrictor. Patients experiencing difficulty in urination and/or taking monoamine oxidase inhibitors should also not use an anorectal product containing a vasoconstrictor. Patients taking phenothiazines should avoid anorectal products containing ephedrine. Individuals who tend toward skin allergies should avoid ingredients such as wool alcohols and benzocaine in anorectal products. For pregnant women, an anorectal product that contains only a protectant should be used intrarectally.

Product Considerations

OTC anorectal preparations are intended to provide symptomatic relief for the burning, itching, pain, swelling, irritation, and discomfort of anorectal disorders. The prescription-only products available for treating the symptoms of mild anorectal disease differ from the OTC products mainly in that they contain a steroid compound. The superiority of prescription-only over OTC products is not known.

dosage form considerations

patient assessment

selecting an appropriate product

factors in bioavailability and effectiveness

In recommending an appropriate OTC product, the pharmacist should consider ingredients and dosage form. A product containing recommended ingredients (Table 2) in appropriate combination should be offered. For intrarectal use the only recommended ingredients are vasoconstrictors, protectants, and astringents. A pile pipe of appropriate length, with holes on the sides, may be used to apply an "ointment" type of product. Suppositories are not recommended as an anorectal product dosage form.

As a general rule, the products containing the least number of recommended ingredients in combination are the ones that should be suggested to a patient. These products minimize undesirable interactions and maximize effectiveness.

Biopharmaceutical Considerations

The bioavailability of drugs from anorectal dosage forms is a result of complex interplay among physiochemical, physiological, manufacturing, dosage form, dosage, and application variables. Absorption from anorectal dosage forms involves release from the vehicle, dissolution into surrounding medium, diffusion to a membrane, and penetration of the membranes. For oleaginous bases, diffusion from the base is the rate-limiting step in the release of a drug from its vehicle (44). Most drugs used in hemorrhoidal products are basic amines (e.g., local anesthetics and vasoconstrictors). The un-ionized base is soluble in lipid ointment bases; the salt form is not. The un-ionized form penetrates the lipid tissue barriers such as nerve membranes. Salt forms are converted to the un-ionized base at tissue pH.

The solubility of the drug in a base determines to a large extent its release rate from that base.

If a drug has in general a greater affinity for the base than for the surrounding medium, a relatively slow release rate is expected. Conversely, if a drug has a greater affinity for the surrounding medium than for the base, a relatively rapid release rate will be encountered. For example, ephedrine sulfate dissolved in an oleaginous base such as cocoa butter is released relatively rapidly into a surrounding aqueous medium.

For a water-soluble or water-miscible base (e.g.,

polyethylene glycol) a water-soluble drug form is preferred to facilitate absorption, because the absorption rate appears to be controlled by the transfer of the drug through the mucosa.

In the case of oleaginous bases, the rate-limiting step in the absorption process appears to be the rate at which the drug leaves the base and dissolves in the surrounding fluid (45). The rate at which a drug diffuses from its base depends on a number of factors, including the base pH, the drug concentration, the dissociation constant of the drug, the presence of surfactants, and the drug's particle size (46, 47).

(See Chapter 26 for a more in depth discussion of release and absorption of drugs from locally applied bases.)

In ointments, creams, and suppositories, additives such as viscosity-increasing and/or surface-active agents are required to achieve a high-quality product. These additives may increase or decrease drug absorption (48).

The absorption characteristics of an anorectal product may be affected by the manufacturing process. For example, the release rates associated with cocoa butter may vary according to the temperature at which the cocoa butter was melted. This effect may be explained by the polymorphic nature of cocoa butter.

SUMMARY

For external use, an ideal formulation would contain, in addition to one or two protectants totaling 50% of the formulation composition, three recommended ingredients (see Table 2)—each from a separate pharmacological category chosen from the following: local anesthetics, counterirritants, astringents, vasoconstrictors, and keratolytics. A combination containing a suitable local anesthetic, protectant, and astringent should be effective in relieving the itching, irritation, burning, and pain associated with anorectal disease.

For internal/intrarectal use a model product would contain one or two protectants totaling 50% of the dose and an appropriate astringent. An "ointment" type dosage form applied with a suitable pile pipe is recommended. This product should relieve the itching, swelling, and pain of anorectal disease.

Products containing benzocaine (20%) in a polyethylene glycol base would be expected, when used externally, to be effective in treating itching, burning, and pain. For internal use, a product consisting of 100% petrolatum is appropriate to recommend for relief of itching and swelling. This product is safe for use by pregnant women.

The pharmacist should make clear to the patient that if symptoms do not improve after 7 days or if bleeding, protrusion, and/or seepage occurs, a physician should be consulted as soon as possible.

REFERENCES

(1) R. L. Holt, "A Cure and Preventative: Hemorrhoids," California Health, Laguna Beach, Calif., 1977, p. 22.

(2) R. T. Shackelford, in "Diseases of Colon and Anorectum," R. Turell, Ed., Saunders, Philadelphia, Pa., 1969, pp. 899–904.

(3) E. Granet, "Manual of Proctology," Yearbook, Chicago, Ill., 1954, p. 115.

(4) R. L. Holt, "A Cure and Preventative: Hemorrhoids," California Health, Laguna Beach, Calif., 1977, pp. 50–69.

(5) J. P. Nesselrod, "Clinical Proctology," 3rd ed., Saunders, Philadelphia, Pa., 1964, p. 73.

(6) H. Dodd, *Am. J. Surg.*, *79*, 55 (1950).

(7) R. T. Shackelford, "Surgery of the Alimentary Tract," Vol. III, Saunders, Philadelphia, Pa., 1955, p. 1637.

(8) *Medical Letter*, *17*, 5 (1975).

(9) J. Adriani, Statement to FDA OTC Panel on Hemorrhoidal Drug Products, May 1, 1976.

(10) L. Van Dam, Statement to FDA OTC Panel on Hemorrhoidal Drug Products, May 1, 1976.

(11) J. C. White, Statement to FDA OTC Panel on Hemorrhoidal Drug Products, May 1, 1976.

(12) J. Adriani, "The Chemistry and Physics of Anesthesia," 2nd ed., Charles C Thomas, Springfield, Ill., 1962, p. 420.

(13) J. Adriani and D. Campbell, *J. Am. Med. Assoc.*, *162*, 1527 (1956).

(14) E. Epstein, *J. Am. Med. Assoc.*, *198*, 517 (1966).

(15) C. G. Lange and R. Luifart, *J. Am. Med. Assoc.*, *146*, 717 (1951).

(16) H. Dalili and J. Adriani, *Clin. Pharmacol. Ther.*, *12*, 913 (1971).

(17) J. Adriani and P. Zipernich, *J. Am. Med. Assoc.*, *188*, 711 (1964).

(18) J. Adriani and H. Dalili, *Curr. Res. Anesth. Analg.*, *50*, 834 (1971).

(19) H. Wilson, *Practitioner*, *197*, 673 (1966).

(20) *Medical Letter*, *11*, 70 (1969).

(21) "The Pharmacological Basis of Therapeutics," 5th ed., L. S. Goodman and A. Gilman, Eds., Macmillan, New York, N.Y., 1975, p. 391.

(22) "Tentative Findings of the FDA OTC Panel on Hemorrhoidal Drug Products," Information Copy, 1977.

(23) "The United States Dispensatory and Physician's Pharmacology," 26th ed., A. Osol, R. Pratt, and M. Altschule, Eds., Lippincott, Philadelphia, Pa., 1967, p. 428.

(24) O. Thulesius and J. E. Gjores, *Acta Chir. Scand.*, *139*, 476 (1973).

(25) F. M. Melton and W. B. Shelley, *J. Invest. Dermatol.*, *15*, 325 (1950).

(26) D. M. Aviado, "Sympathomimetic Drugs," Charles C Thomas, Springfield, Ill., 1970, pp. 95–494.

(27) "The Pharmacological Basis of Therapeutics," 5th ed., L. S. Goodman and A. Gilman, Eds., Macmillan, New York, N.Y., 1975, p. 501.

(28) E. Granet, "Manual of Proctology," Yearbook, Chicago, Ill., 1954, p. 59.

(29) "Summary Minutes of the FDA OTC Panel on Hemorrhoidal Drug Products, Rockville, Md., Nov. 21–23, 1976.

(30) G. K. Steigleder and W. P. Raab, *J. Invest. Dermatol.*, *38*, 129 (1962).

(31) "The Pharmacological Basis of Therapeutics," L. S. Goodman and A. Gilman, Eds., 2nd ed., Macmillan, 1955, pp. 730–743.

(32) J. Adriani, R. Zepernick, J. Arens, and E. Authemont, *Clin. Pharmacol. Ther.*, *5*, 49 (1963).

(33) W. C. Carey and T. G. Randolph, *J. Am. Med. Assoc.*, *175*, 539 (1961).

(34) *Journal of the American Medical Association*, *234*, 145 (1975).

(35) K. Genest and D. W. Hughes, *Can. J. Pharm. Sci.*, *4*, 4145 (1969).

(36) W. B. Deichman and H. W. Gerarde, "Toxicology of Drugs and Chemicals," Academic, New York, N.Y., 1969, p. 448.

(37) E. M. Boyd, in "Pharmacology in Medicine," 4th ed., V. A. Drill, Ed., McGraw-Hill, New York, N.Y., 1971, p. 1034.

(38) B. Korpassy and K. Kovacs, *Br. J. Exp. Pathol.*, *30*, 266 (1949).

(39) W. Goodson, D. Hohn, T. K. Hunt, and D. Y. K. Leung, *J. Surg. Res.*, *21*, 125 (1976).

(40) M. A. Valdes-Dapena and J. B. Arey, *J. Pediatr.*, *61*, 531 (1962).

(41) "AMA Drug Evaluations—1973," 2nd ed., American Medical Association, Chicago, Ill., 1973, p. 893.

(42) "AMA Drug Evaluations—1971," 1st ed., American Medical Association, Chicago, Ill., 1971, p. 586.

(43) L. Augsberger and R. T. Shangraw, *J. Pharm. Sci.*, *57*, 624 (1968).

(44) "Evaluations of Drug Interactions," 2nd ed., APhA, Washington, D.C., 1976.

(45) W. A. Ritschel, "Biopharmaceutical Development and Evaluation of Rectal Dosage Forms, Applied Biopharmaceutics II," College of Pharmacy, University of Cincinnati, Cincinnati, Ohio, 1973, p. 1160.

(46) N. A. Allawalla and S. Riegelman, *J. Am. Pharm. Assoc. Sci. Ed.*, *42*, 267 (1953).

(47) J. Anschel and H. A. Lieberman, in "The Theory and Practice of Industrial Pharmacy," 2nd ed., L. Lachman, H. A. Lieberman, and J. L. Kanig, Eds., Lea and Febiger, Philadelphia, Pa., 1976, pp. 247–269.

(48) S. Riegelman and W. J. Crowell, *J. Am. Pharm. Assoc. Sci. Ed.*, *47*, 115 (1958).

Product (Manufacturer)	Dosage Form	Anesthetic	Antiseptic	Astringent	Protectant	Other
A-Caine (A.V.P.)	ointment	benzocaine, 2% diperodon hydrochloride, 0.25%	—	zinc oxide, 5% bismuth subcarbonate, 0.2%	cod liver oil base	phenylephrine, 0.255% pyrilamine maleate, 0.1%
Americaine (Arnar-Stone)	suppository ointment	benzocaine, 280 mg (suppository) 20% (ointment)	benzethonium chloride, 0.1%	—	polyethylene glycol base	—
Anusol (Warner-Chilcott)	suppository ointment	pramoxine hydrochloride, 10 mg (ointment)	—	zinc oxide, 11% bismuth subgallate, 2.5% bismuth–resorcinol compound, 1.75% peruvian balsam, 1.8%	vegetable oil base	benzyl benzoate, 1.2%
Aphco (Amer. Pharm.)	suppository ointment	benzocaine	boric acid	bismuth salts peruvian balsam zinc oxide	—	—
BiCozene (Creighton)	cream	benzocaine, 6%	—	—	cream base	resorcinol, 1.67%
Blue-Gray (Columbia Medical)	suppository	benzocaine	boric acid	bismuth subgallate bismuth–resorcinol compound zinc oxide peruvian balsam	—	—
Calmol 4 (Leeming)	suppository	—	—	bismuth subgallate zinc oxide peruvian balsam	Norwegian cod liver oil cocoa butter base	—
Diothane (Merrell-National)	ointment	diperodon, 1%	8-quinolinol benzoate (salt), 0.1%	—	propylene glycol	sorbitan sequioleate
Epinephricaine Ointment (Upjohn)	ointment	benzocaine, 2.5%	secondary amyltricresols, 1%	zinc oxide, 2%	bland base	epinephrine, 0.2% vitamins A and D
Eudicane (Rexall)	suppository	benzocaine, 130 mg	8-hydroxyquinoline sulfate, 16.2 mg	zinc oxide, 260 mg bismuth subgallate, 64.8 mg peruvian balsam, 64.8 mg	cocoa butter	ephedrine sulfate, 4.05 mg
Gentz Wipes (Philips Roxane)	medical pad	pramoxine hydrochloride, 1%	cetylpyridinium chloride, 0.5%	hamamelis water, 50% aluminum chlorhydroxy allantoinate, 0.2%	propylene glycol, 0.10%	fragrance
Hazel-Balm (Arnar-Stone)	aerosol	—	benzethonium chloride, 0.1%	hamamelis water, 79.9%	water-soluble lanolin derivative, 20%	—
Hemor-Rid (Columbia Medical)	ointment	diperodon hydrochloride, 0.25%	—	zinc oxide, 5% bismuth subcarbonate, 0.2%	cod liver oil petrolatum	phenylephrine hydrochloride, 0.25% pyrilamine maleate, 0.1%
Lanacane (Combe)	cream	benzocaine	chlorothymol	—	water-washable base	resorcinol
Manzan Ointment (DeWitt)	ointment	benzocaine, 1%	phenol, 0.5% menthol, 0.2%	tannic acid, 1.5%	—	allantoin, 0.5% ephedrine hydrochloride, 0.2%
Manzan Stainless (DeWitt)	ointment	benzocaine, 1%	phenol, 0.5%	zinc oxide, 10%	—	allantoin, 0.5% ephedrine hydrochloride, 0.2%
Manzan Suppositories (DeWitt)	suppository	benzocaine, 1%	phenol, 0.5% menthol, 0.2%	zinc oxide, 96%	—	allantoin, 0.2% phenylpropanolamine hydrochloride, 0.2%

Product (Manufacturer)	Dosage Form	Anesthetic	Antiseptic	Astringent	Protectant	Other
Mediconet (Medicone)	medical pad	—	benzalkonium chloride, 0.02%	hamamelis water, 50%	ethoxylated lanolin, 0.5% glycerin, 10%	methylparaben, 0.15% perfume
Non-Steroid Proctofoam (Reed & Carnrick)	foam	pramoxine hydrochloride, 1%	—	—	petroleum mineral oil, 40%	—
Nupercainal Ointment (Ciba)	ointment	dibucaine, 1%	—	—	—	acetone sodium bisulfite, 0.5%
Nupercainal Suppositories (Ciba)	suppository	dibucaine, 2.5 mg	—	zinc oxide bismuth subgallate	cocoa butter	acetone sodium bisulfite, 0.05%
Pazo (Bristol-Myers)	ointment suppository	benzocaine, 0.8%	camphor, 2.18% eucalyptus oil, 0.25%	zinc oxide, 4%	petrolatum, 87.57% (ointment) lanolin, 5% (ointment) hydrogenated vegetable oil (suppository)	ephedrine sulfate, 0.2%
Perifoam (Rowell)	foam	pramoxine hydrochloride, 1.0%	benzalkonium chloride, 0.1%	hamamelis water, 35%	lanolin	allantoin, 0.3% methylparaben, 0.15% propylparaben, 0.05% alcohol, 5%
PNS (Winthrop)	suppository	tetracaine hydrochloride, 10 mg	—	bismuth subcarbonate, 100 mg	—	tyloxapol, 25 mg phenylephrine hydrochloride, 5 mg
Pontocaine (Winthrop)	cream ointment	tetracaine hydrochloride (equivalent to 1% base) (cream) base, 0.5% (ointment)	menthol, 0.5% (ointment)	—	white petrolatum (ointment) white wax (ointment)	methylparaben (cream) sodium bisulfite (cream)
Preparation H (Whitehall)	ointment suppository	—	—	—	shark liver oil, 3%	live yeast cell derivative (supplying 2000 units of skin respiratory factor) phenylmercuric nitrate, 0.01%
Preparation H Cleansing Pads (Whitehall)	pads	—	—	hamamelis water	glycerin	—
Proctodon (Rowell)	cream	diperodon hydrochloride, 1%	—	—	—	—
Rantex (Holland-Rantos)	medical pad	—	benzalkonium chloride	hamamelis water, 50%	lanolin	methylparaben alcohol, 7%
Rectal Medicone Suppositories (Medicone)	suppository	benzocaine, 50.4 mg/g	8-hydroxyquinoline sulfate, 5.55 mg/g menthol, 3.75 mg/g	zinc oxide, 75 mg/g peruvian balsam, 24 mg/g	cocoa butter vegetable and petroleum oils	—
Rectal Medicone Unguent (Medicone)	ointment	benzocaine, 20 mg	8-hydroxyquinoline sulfate, 5 mg menthol, 4 mg	zinc oxide, 100 mg peruvian balsam, 12.5 mg	petrolatum, 625 mg lanolin, 210 mg	—
Tanicaine Ointment (Upjohn)	ointment	phenacaine hydrochloride, 10.8 mg/ml	camphor, 15.1 mg/ml phenol, 13 mg/ml menthol, 4.3 mg/ml	zinc oxide, 0.17 g/ml tannic acid, 0.053 g/ml	—	atropine, 0.54 mg/ml
Tanicaine Suppositories (Upjohn)	suppository	phenacaine hydrochloride, 22 mg	phenol, 13 mg	zinc oxide, 390 mg tannic acid, 110 mg	—	atropine, 1 mg

Product (Manufacturer)	Dosage Form	Anesthetic	Antiseptic	Astringent	Protectant	Other
Tucks Cream and Ointment (Parke-Davis)	cream ointment	—	—	hamamelis water, 50%	lanolin petrolatum	—
Tucks Pads (Parke-Davis)	medical pad	—	—	hamamelis water, 50%	glycerin, 10%	methylparaben, 0.1% benzalkonium chloride, 0.003%
Vaseline Pure Petroleum Jelly (Chesebrough-Ponds)	ointment	—	—	—	white petrolatum, 100%	—
Wyanoid Ointment (Wyeth)	ointment	benzocaine, 2%	boric acid, 18%	zinc oxide, 5% peruvian balsam, 1%	castor oil petrolatum	ephedrine sulfate, 0.1%
Wyanoid Suppositories (Wyeth)	suppository	—	boric acid, 543 mg	zinc oxide, 176 mg bismuth subcarbonate, 146 mg bismuth oxyiodide, 30 mg peruvian balsam, 30 mg	cocoa butter	belladonna extract, 15 mg ephedrine sulfate, 3 mg

Index

A

D

F

G

H

I

O

P

Q

R

U